PHARMACOLOGICAL, CONVULSIVE AND OTHER SOMATIC TREATMENTS IN PSYCHIATRY

PHARMACOLOGICAL, CONVULSIVE AND OTHER SOMATIC TREATMENTS IN PSYCHIATRY

LOTHAR B. KALINOWSKY, M.D.

Clinical Professor of Psychiatry
New York Medical College
New York, N.Y.

HANNS HIPPIUS, M.D.

Professor of Psychiatry
Free University
Berlin, Germany

GRUNE & STRATTON NEW YORK AND LONDON

ACKNOWLEDGEMENTS

We gratefully acknowledge the contribution to this book made by the late Paul Hoch as co-author of the original volume published in 1946, and of subsequent editions. We also express our thanks and appreciation to Dr. Brenda Grant of London, England, for her extensive collaboration in the edition of 1961.

The bequest of a grateful patient, the late Franklin Wormser, who specified the use of this bequest for scientific endeavors by one of us (LBK), helped greatly to defray most of the expenses for manuscript preparation of this book.

As in all previous editions, the untiring support of Mrs. Hilda Kalinowsky in the technical preparation of the manuscript is greatfully acknowledged. Dr. Richard Abrams was extremely helpful in proofreading and making valuable corrections.

Dr. Henry M. Stratton, our publisher, who actually originated this whole undertaking by suggesting the first book exactly 25 years ago, again gave encouragement and assistance, and was particularly generous in his willingness to print the voluminous bibliography.

The Authors

Parts of this volume are revised from the 1961 volume listed below, which in turn was revised and updated from previous versions as follows:

Shock Treatments and Other Somatic Procedures in Psychiatry (Kalinowsky and Hoch), © 1946

Shock Treatments, Psychosurgery and Other Somatic Treatments in Psychiatry (Kalinowsky and Hoch), © 1952

Somatic Treatments in Psychiatry—Pharmacotherapy; Convulsive, Insulin, Surgical, Other Methods (Kalinowsky and Hoch with Grant), © 1961

all published and copyrighted by Grune & Stratton, Inc.

Library of Congress Catalog Card No. 72-75148
Printed in U.S.A.
(GL-B)

Contents

Preface

This monograph, which deals with all somatic treatments in psychiatry, grew out of an original book on Shock Treatments published in 1946. Even at that time, it had become evident that psychiatry was heading for great advances through the introduction of several new treatments developed almost simultaneously in the 1930's. Since patients suffering from the previously untreatable major psychoses benefited the most from these methods, their appearance had an enormous impact on all areas of psychiatry. Significant changes in the management of mental hospitals were made possible, and custodial care was replaced by a positive therapeutic approach with the goal of social rehabilitation.

Regrettably, it soon became noticeable that introduction of a new treatment was often regarded as competition with or replacement of previous therapeutic methods. To avoid this competitive situation, the original 1946 book was designed to offer a balanced view of the then available treatments. It has been with this in mind that the senior author, more closely connected with convulsive therapy, had invited the late Paul Hoch to contribute to the chapter on insulin coma therapy, in which he had more extensive experience. Later, pharmacotherapy became more and more important, and this again suggested a co-author primarily engaged in this type of work, who would guarantee a balanced view of pharmacotherapy and the previous somatic treatments. The choice of the new co-author in the present edition, a European psychiatrist experienced in psychopharmacology, was also meant to continue the international character of the book which had already been emphasized in its first writing, and which had been continued in the edition of 1961 by the collaboration of the English psychiatrist, Dr. Brenda Grant.

It has been tried to avoid the shortcomings sometimes seen in books written by many contributors with entirely different views. On the other hand, the present authors have made no effort to adhere strictly to identical views on all matters; and it is hoped that occasional differences of opinion between them, as reflected in the book, will not be confusing to the reader or interfere with a relatively uniform representation of the subject matter.

It was often difficult to decide whether, in this new volume, to eliminate previous discussions of certain treatments which presently seemed to have little or no practical value. This problem solved itself during the writing through some interesting incidents. As one example, the use of dilantin in non-epileptic psychoses, although originated by one of us, was now to have been omitted since it had long been replaced by the much more effective neuroleptic drugs. However, in the course of our writing, a new wave of interest arose when considerable publicity was given to attempts to use dilantin in treating a variety of psychiatric symptoms, and, rather than eliminating the section on this drug, it thus became necessary to update it. Another drug to have been omitted was malononitrile, which had been practically forgotten, but new and most interesting attempts at treating senile psychoses which turned out to have important theoretical links to malononitrile made revision of this discussion necessary.

The most difficult decision was how to deal with the once all-important insulin coma treatment. This historically first successful treatment of schizophrenia is still used in some hospitals here and abroad; and since the reasons for its discontinuation in others do not seem to be entirely valid, the chapter has been maintained, though in an abbreviated form. Aside from the wealth of physiologic and psychopathologic observations, the methodology of treatment evaluation in psychiatry, worked out for the first time in insulin coma treatment, has continued importance. Comparison of those data with statistics on later therapeutic methods demonstrates clearly that often different things are measured in evaluating different treatments, a point which is frequently overlooked by those who work with only one kind of treatment. Also, theoretical considerations relating to older treatments remain significant because evaluation of any theory on newer treatments is meaningful only if it takes into account similar therapeutic effects of other methods. It is our belief that all the information accumulated must remain available to the researcher engaged in subsequent therapeutic attempts, and that, even more than in the past, the entire group of somatic treatments must be regarded as one field of endeavor.

The chapter on pharmacotherapy was brought up to date by adding many new drugs and by reorganizing the material. Drugs available in some countries but not (or not yet) in others have been included. The index listing generic and trade names should make it easy for readers from different countries to orient themselves. In the text we tried to correlate chemical and pharmacologic data with clinical facts wherever present knowledge permits such correlation. Certain characteristics—such as pharmacologic properties and side-effects, so far as they are common to an entire group of drugs—have been discussed together rather than with each individual drug in order to avoid repetition. Although biochemical and pharmacologic research was included, clinical investigations were given primary importance. The same applies to the bibliography, where clinical papers have received preference.

The bibliography, although extensive and presenting a relatively large part of the volume, cannot claim to be complete. It is hoped, however, that index and bibliography together will help research workers engaged in a special problem find sufficient points of reference to gather further information, and that the clinician can easily obtain information on questions of special interest to him.

Although this book is limited to a discussion of the somatic treatments in psychiatry, the authors are fully aware that the psychodynamic approach remains the basis for the treatment of many psychiatric disorders. It is equally obvious, furthermore, that the somatic treatments have many psychological and particularly social implications which are frequently mentioned throughout the book, but which in themselves are not within the scope of a monograph on somatic methods.

Psychiatry is still—exactly as at the time of the first writing of this book in 1946—limited to purely empirical treatments of diseases whose origin remains shrouded in mystery. This state of affairs makes it all the more gratifying that active application of so many different therapeutic methods can restore the functioning of an increasing number of psychiatric patients. The awareness of constant progress, and the realization of the need for better integration of available treatments, encouraged us to rewrite this book.

The Authors

PHARMACOLOGICAL, CONVULSIVE AND OTHER SOMATIC TREATMENTS IN PSYCHIATRY

CHAPTER I

Historical Development

The history of somatic treatment procedures in psychiatry has not been a logical development. This is understandable in a field where the etiological and pathophysiological factors underlying the diseases are essentially unknown.

In the past, recommendations of organic treatment principally followed the trends of general medicine which inspired therapeutically-minded psychiatrists to apply new medical knowledge to their field. However, the really successful methods have been quite unrelated to developments in medicine and even in psychiatry. There is also no connection between the development of the various individual treatments. The one point which all organic methods have in common is that they are based on the belief that psychiatric conditions can be influenced therapeutically by nonpsychological methods.

The great strides made during the last few decades in active treatment of mental illness must be credited to psychiatrists who used clinical observations for their therapeutic attempts. Every new method originated in a psychiatric hospital rather than in research laboratories. This historical fact must be clearly recognized although it certainly should not discourage basic research. It is gratifying that the discoveries of the various treatment procedures, although empirical, subsequently gave great impetus to experimental investigations in psychiatry; and the hope for better understood and more effective treatments in the future lies in such investigations of ever expanding research facilities. However, the historical development of presently available treatments is a vivid demonstration of the need for clinical psychiatric research, which too often is downgraded by those engaged in basic research.

Therapeutic procedures applied in former centuries, which emphasized fright and intimidation, are often erroneously called the predecessors of the present day shock methods. Actually, they were strictly psychological procedures and have no place in a survey of organic treatment in psychiatry. They deliberately produced anxiety in conscious patients, whereas the patient under shock treatment is unconscious and, therefore, unaware of the treatment. This misnomer, "shock therapy," is partly to blame for the unwarranted comparison with medieval tortures.

Treatment procedures in psychiatry which should be included as organic methods of historical interest are the use of bloodletting, emetics, and purgatives. In the nineteenth century, surgical operations on various organs were recommended; castration as well as removal of the clitoris were based on theories regarding the effect of the genital organs on hysteria. In the beginning of this century the concept of focal infections as the cause of many illnesses led Cotton et al. to advise operations on tonsils, teeth, and other infectious foci, but Kopeloff and Kirby disproved the value of such procedures. Developments in the field of bacteriology inspired unsuccessful attempts to treat schizophrenia with various antitoxic and anti-infectious vaccines, autovaccines, and sera of recovered schizophrenics. An aseptic meningitis was produced by means of horse serum introduced into the subarachnoid space, and a "shock" with incompatible blood was also tried.

Progress in endocrinology suggested attempts with various glandular products, the thyroid gland being of particular interest. Efforts toward a better understanding of the role of hormones in psychiatric disorders have been recently revived in spite of therapeutic disappointments in the past. Increasing knowledge of the autonomic sympathetic and parasympathetic system has also been therapeutically utilized with no success.

The greatest effort has long been directed toward effective pharmacotherapy of mental illness. Older attempts had been limited to the symptomatic removal of the most disturbing manifestations of the psychosis. Later, efforts toward a pharmacological treatment of the illness itself became more and more the goal. Many of these attempts were based on some theoretical concepts which fully justified the therapeutic effort to prove their validity. Any historical sketch on pharmacotherapeutic attempts in psychiatry cannot leave unmentioned Kraepelin's systematic efforts in this direction at the end of the last century. It took more than fifty years until true progress was made in this area of psychiatric endeavor.

The first successful step in somatic therapy of mental illness was based on observations of clinical improvement in psychotic patients during intercurrent infections. In 1917 Wagner-Jauregg introduced malaria treatment in general paresis, the first successful treatment of a mental illness on a purely organic basis. However, the use of malaria and typhoid fever and later of heat-producing agents of a physical nature failed in other psychoses, indicating that the former were directed against the infectious agent of general paresis but not against the psychotic symptoms. This became even more obvious when penicillin began to replace the fever-producing methods in treating general paresis.

A promising approach to the treatment of the so-called endogenous psychoses developed out of the use of sedatives. In some countries, treatment with opium had long been routine for depressions, and large amounts of barbiturates had been recommended not only to sedate but to cure mental patients. An important step forward was made when Klaesi in 1922 used barbiturates for prolonged narcosis treatment. This therapy was first intended for schizophrenia but was later used even more for depressions. Continuous sleep treatment can be considered as the most important predecessor of shock treatments.

The new era of the so-called shock treatments started with the almost simultaneous and independent discovery of hypoglycemic coma treatment and of pharmacological convulsive therapy. The hypoglycemic coma technique developed from the symptomatic treatment of various types of psychiatric patients with insulin. Introduced in psychiatry by Steck, insulin was given with the double purpose of increasing the patient's weight and influencing excitement. It found particularly wide application in the treatment of morphine addiction. The decisive step from a purely symptomatic to a curative treatment was taken by Sakel when he made the important observation that deeper hypoglycemic states, occurring unintentionally during the symptomatic treatment of psychotics, actually had a beneficial effect on the psychosis itself. The hypoglycemic coma which Sakel's predecessors had tried to avoid became the focus of the new treatment of schizophrenia. Sakel presented the first report of his work in 1933 from the University Clinic of Vienna. The value of the technique, which was skilfully worked out in every detail, is apparent from the speed with which it was disseminated and adopted.

Less than two years later, in 1935, von Meduna reported attempts to treat schizophrenia with artificially induced convulsions. By a curious coincidence, the first two successful methods of treating schizophrenia were developed almost at the same time but starting from entirely different premises. Von Meduna worked from two facts: that epilepsy and schizophrenia are usually antagonistic to each other, and that schizophrenic symptoms may disappear, at least temporarily, after spontaneous convulsions. The same observation had previously led Nyiro to unsuccessful attempts at treating schizophrenics with transfusions of blood from epileptics. Von Meduna's systematic work was preceded by several similar attempts found in historical surveys by Diethelm and A. Kennedy. The first successful camphor treatment of a case of "mania" was reported as early as 1785 by Oliver in the *London Medical Journal.* The beneficial effect of hypoglycemic convulsions in insulin treatment was a factor in the later recommendation of combined insulin-convulsive treatment (Georgi), but it was not instrumental in the discovery of convulsive therapy. Sakel in his 1935 monograph on insulin treatment warned against the danger of epileptic seizures, but later fully recognized and stressed their therapeutic value, stating that the hypoglycemic shock may consist of either a coma or an epileptic seizure.

The great extension of insulin and convulsive therapy was demonstrated at the First International Meeting on Modern Treatment of Schizophrenia held in Münsingen (Switzerland) in 1937, over which M. Müller presided. It was here that Cerletti's assistant, Bini, first mentioned the possible use of the electric current as a convulsive stimulus in the treatment of schizophrenia. The new "electroshock" therapy was first demonstrated by Cerletti and Bini in 1938. Its development followed extensive experimental work in electrically induced seizures. It largely replaced pharmacological convulsive treatment, of which it is actually a technical modification and improvement. Following recognition of the value of convulsive therapy in the affective disorders as well, electric shock treatment became the most widely used organic therapy in psychiatry, prior to the introduction of new drugs in the nineteen-fifties. Historical attempts by Harms and some others to see the origin of electric shock therapy in the use of electricity in mental patients during the 18th and 19th century, or the treatment of certain psychomatic complaints in the 5th century A.D. with electricity-discharging fish (according to B. A. Finkelstein) are interesting but unrelated to present electric convulsive therapy because Cerletti and Bini rightly denied any effect of the electric current on mental illness. They used electricity only for the induction of the therapeutically effective convulsions. Efforts to apply various electric currents without convulsions failed to yield convincing therapeutic results. A newer procedure to induce convulsions by means of an inhalant, Indoklon, owes its promising introduction into psychiatric therapy to the purely incidental discovery of convulsive properties of a substance tested by the American pharmacologist Krantz for its anesthetic properties.

The history of the discovery of the shock methods has lately been under some dispute. Although the originators have given later accounts of their discoveries which differ considerably from previously known data, the first publications on these methods have to remain the source of orientation for the historical data. They are the original publication by Sakel on insulin coma treatment in 1933, the entirely independent introduction of pharmacological convulsive therapy by von Meduna in 1935, and the joint publication on electroshock therapy by Cerletti and Bini in 1938, after Bini had reported on the possibility of such treatment at the Münsingen meeting in 1937.

Almost simultaneously with the discoveries of the shock methods, Moniz in cooperation with Lima, in 1936, reported on another organic—this time surgical—approach to the treatment of mental illness. This was preceded by the work of Burckardt, a Swiss psychiatrist who in 1890 had treated psychotics by excision of parts of the cerebral cortex. Basing his work on various clinical considerations and on increased knowledge of the function of the frontal lobes, Moniz developed the surgical procedure of prefrontal leukotomy. This operation became more widely accepted as a result of the work of Freeman and Watts in the United States, and of a number of British workers. Undesirable side-effects in the sense of personality changes hindered the general acceptance of frontal lobe surgery. When the great value of the method, despite its side-effects, came to become more and more recognized, efforts were made to modify the original procedure. More restricted operations, and a more critical selection of patients led to more gratifying results. The advent of the neuroleptic drugs replaced psychosurgery in the majority of chronic schizophrenics. More recently however, it was recognized that, in properly selected cases, the more limited psychosurgical procedures continue to be an important therapeutic tool.

During the last decade, somatic treatment in psychiatry entered an entirely new era with the introduction of modern pharmacotherapy. In former times, the use of drugs in psychiatry had been mostly limited to what has been called "chemical restraint" by means of various sedatives. The use of some barbiturates for narcosuggestive and narcocathartic procedures represented a method of psychotherapy rather than a somatic treatment. When stimulants of the amphetamine group became known, they permitted only a temporary mood change in some depressed patients. In none of these instances, a basic change of symptomatology for any length of time could be achieved.

The first successful attempts to eliminate certain psychotic symptoms were made in 1952, when psychiatrists became acquainted with two entirely different drugs with almost identical effect. In France, Delay and Deniker reported on the usefulness of chlorpromazine. In July, 1952, Hamon et al. described the effect of this phenothiazine in a single case of manic excitement. The French discovery was based on the observation of anesthesiologists in "artificial hibernation" (Laborit) that patients under this drug became entirely indifferent toward surgical procedures, although they remained aware of their surroundings. Almost at the same time a similar effect was claimed for an alkaloid of the Rauwolfia root which had been used in India for a long time. Indian physicians had reported on this psychiatric drug in scientific journals even before the introduction of shock treatments. Swiss scientists deserve credit for the analysis and synthesis of this substance. A new wave of interest in pharmacotherapy swept through psychiatric centers in all parts of the world. Hope for a cure of all mental illness and for abandonment of previous treatments was expressed, but proved to be premature. Yet, the effect on the practice of psychiatry was undeniable; the interest of researchers of many disciplines in this new somatic approach was great, even in countries with predominantly psychodynamically oriented psychiatry.

Shortly after the advent of the neuroleptic drugs or "tranquilizers" other observers noticed the euphorizing effect of some drugs used in tuberculosis. This led to attempts to try these drugs in depressions which so far had been the almost exclusive domain of convulsive therapy. Again it was not a new biochemical discovery that led to the introduction of the first anti-depressant drug, iproniazid. Only subsequently the monoamine oxidase inhibiting action of iproniazid and several similar drugs was made responsible for the antidepressant effect. This theory neither led to the discovery of this group of drugs nor is it supported by the advent of newer tricyclic antidepressants like imipramine, amitryptiline and related drugs which are not monoamine oxidase inhibitors. The discovery of the important antidepressant imipramine highlights the continued importance of keen clinical observation in psychiatry. Imipramine, closely related to the phenothiazines, has been tried by Kuhn for its possible neuroleptic properties—which he failed to find; but he did observe a definite antidepressant effect which was confirmed by many subsequent observers.

The introduction of the major tranquilizers gave impetus to an ever increasing activity in pharmacotherapeutic research. While the Rauwolfia drugs lost importance in psychiatry, the number of phenothiazines increased, and other groups of drugs like the butyrophenones were added. Aside from the "major tranquilizers" more and more "minor tranquilizers" such as meprobamate, chlordiazepoxide and so on, were introduced. They are preferred to the older sedatives because of their lesser hypnotic effect and, today, probably belong to the most widely prescribed drugs in medicine including psychiatry, although they are not able to actually remove psychotic symptoms as the neuroleptics do.

Such "antipsychotic" effect can be claimed for an entirely different chemical substance, lithium salts, which have been long known in general medicine, and were later found to have an almost specific effect on manic excitement. Their particular interest lies in their recently recognized prophylactic value for both manic and depressive phases of the manic-depressive psychoses. If confirmed, this might make lithium an important clue to the biochemical understanding of this psychosis.

During the last few years, basic research in psychiatry has been strongly intensified and represents our main hope to arrive at a better understanding of the disorders we are treating, and to find treatments that are based on a better rationale than those we are using at present. For the time being, however, clinical observation and clinical research are still indispensable as is clearly illustrated by the historical development of our present treatments.

CLASSIFICATION OF PSYCHOTROPIC DRUGS (SEE P. 10)

Category	Representative members
Neuroleptics	(*a*) Phenothiazines (*b*) Butyrophenones (*c*) Thioxanthenes (*d*) Reserpine derivatives, benzoquinolizines
Anxiolytic sedatives	(*a*) Meprobamate and derivatives (*b*) Diazepoxides (*c*) Barbiturates
Antidepressants	(*a*) Monoamine oxidase (MAO) inhibitors (*b*) Imipramine and other tricyclic compounds
Psychostimulants	(*a*) Amphetamine, methylphenidate, pipradrol (*b*) Caffeine
Psychodysleptics (hallucinogens)	(*a*) Lysergic acid diethylamide (LSD) (*b*) Mescaline (*c*) Psilocybin (*d*) Dimethyltryptophan (DMT) (*e*) Cannabis (marihuana, hashish, etc.)

CHAPTER II

Pharmacotherapy

Introductory Remarks

The revolution which has been brought about in psychiatry by the development of the new drugs, the so-called neuroleptics, and later followed by the anti-depressants, has its most important effect in a more hopeful attitude toward therapy and prognosis in mental illness, especially in the psychoses. The fact that many chronic psychotics, previously regarded as unamenable to treatment, were shown to respond to drugs such as the phenothiazines led to a greater interest in other forms of therapy for them and to an attitude of therapeutic optimism. Their great value in states of acute excitement—without the hypnotic action of the drugs previously used—led to an entirely different atmosphere in the wards of many hospitals, and enabled a larger proportion of such patients to participate in social events and to benefit from the other hospital facilities.

The early claims by some workers for the new drugs have not been fulfilled, and it is realized that they improve symptoms only, rarely producing a deep-seated effect on the fundamental aspects of the illness. The main value of the neuroleptic drugs appears to be threefold: the benefiting of acutely disturbed patients, otherwise uncontrollable, particularly those suffering from schizophrenia, manic excitement, or toxic psychoses; a symptomatic improvement in chronic patients, enabling them to have more freedom and to participate in activities; and, finally, a greater stimulus for new fields of research.

Many observers, such as Brill and Patton, have noted the reduction of hospital population since the introduction of the tranquilizing drugs, as well as the decrease in the need for restraint and seclusion. However, comment has been made by some workers on what they regard as the more positive results obtained with the drugs in the United States as distinct from Europe. A. Lewis pointed out that in England an increased discharge rate preceded the introduction of the new drugs. The same was found by Shephard et al., while Waters and Northover demonstrated that also in Great Britain the introduction of psychopharmaca reduced the population in mental hospitals. In Europe it was particularly Ødegaard who expressed the opinion that psychopharmaca did not affect the number of hospitalized patients. He agrees with A. Lewis that reduced hospitalization rates started before the introduction of the new drugs. The same was found by Freyhan in an American hospital, where the separation rate had risen from 35 per cent in 1915 to 80 per cent in 1953. Statistical data by J.-E. Meyer et al. from a university hospital and a mental institution showed that the trend towards higher discharge rates coincided with the introduction of insulin and electric convulsive therapies, but that it was accentuated by the new drugs. All these statistics suggest that the era of pharmacotherapy had a lesser impact on mental hospital statistics in those countries like Great Britain and Scandinavia, where at that time extramural psychiatric care was already emphasized. A more conservative discharge policy may be explained by the lack of psychiatric facilities in the community, and thus nullifies the actual results of pharmacotherapy. The full potential of modern somatic treatments will only become evident with a greater expansion of social therapeutic measures. It has been postulated that the results are more remarkable in the American hospitals because of the understaffed and overcrowded conditions in some of them, so that part of the improvement, as measured by factors such as the discharge rates, could be attributed to the fact that patients who were never able to receive individual therapy responded to the drugs sufficiently to become accessible to work therapy and other methods. There is no doubt that, associated with this improvement in the mental condition of patients, there has been a complete change in hospital policy resulting in a greater degree of freedom for the patients, active attempts at resocialization, a decrease in the number of compulsory as distinct from voluntary admissions, as well as the establishment of research centers in mental hospitals. The relative part played by the drugs and by more intensive rehabilitation programs in the improvement of many patients is difficult to assess. What is important, however, is that in the new drugs an important new therapy has been added to a field which still has far too few effective treatments.

Nomenclature

The number of terms applied to the new group of drugs is confusing, since many of them do not adequately describe either the characteristic effects of the drugs or the factors which differentiate them from each other, from the earlier sedatives such as the barbiturates, or from stimulants such as the amphetamines. It is impossible to formulate a classification based upon their mode of action since this is still virtually unknown, and the most satisfactory method seems to be that which groups together those drugs with a similar chemical structure, and, at the same time, differentiates between substances with a predominantly sedative action and those which are mainly mood elevators.

The term "tranquilizer" was first applied to the action of chlorpromazine in calming disturbed behavior without the hypnotic effect induced by earlier drugs such as the barbiturates. A similar term "ataraxic," meaning the production of emotional equilibrium, has also been used to describe the characteristic effects of the large group of varied drugs which have since been developed. However, as many observers have pointed out, these terms do not define precisely any of the characteristics of these drugs, since other substances, such as bromides, have a similar action in producing sedation without sleep, and since the "tranquilizers" may also have a somnolent effect at the commencement of treatment and in large doses. The term "ataraxic" can be objected to on several scores: Drugs such as opium are also "ataraxics" and some patients, particularly neurotics, do not become "ataraxic" but alarmed by certain psychological side-effects, such as depersonalization, brought about by the drugs.

Neither do these terms distinguish between, on the one hand, the phenothiazines, which have a pronounced effect upon the psychoses, and, on the other hand, the milder sedatives, such as the meprobamate group, whose action is mainly on anxiety and tension and whose danger of addiction and withdrawal symptoms place them much closer to the barbiturates than to the phenothiazines. The term "neuroplegic," which has been used to cover the broad group of drugs described originally under "the tranquilizers," implies a paralyzing effect. Delay's suggestion that the phenothiazines and reserpine be placed in the category of "neuroleptic" drugs appears to be preferable to other designations.

At the International Colloquium on "Chlorpromazine and the Neuroleptic Drugs in Psychiatric Therapy" in Paris in 1954, Delay elaborated on the term "neuroleptic" as applied to the new drugs. The name was taken from Pierre Janet's term "psycholepsy," used to describe a fall in psychological tension. The neuroleptic drugs, by producing a fall in nervous or neurovegetative tension, caused a diminution in psychological tension accompanied by clinical relaxation. Delay contrasted this with the concept of "shock" in which there is a mobilization of defences in response to the production of an alarm reaction, and he likened the action of the neuroleptics to that of a *demobilization* of defences.

Delay has proposed the following classification of the new drugs based upon their predominant action:

(A) *Psycholeptics or Sedatives:* These drugs essentially depress mental tonus, leading to a slowing down of mental activity, a diminution of alertness, and, sometimes, somnolence, while the corresponding decrease in emotional tonus may lead to affective indifference. This group may be subdivided into:

1. *The hypnotics,* such as the barbiturates, whose principal action is on sleep.
2. *The neuroleptics,* such as the phenothiazines and reserpine. The characteristic picture induced by these two groups of drugs has been called by Delay the "neurologic syndrome," and is composed of psychomotor inhibition, modifying changes in the neurovegetative system, disturbance of tonus, and sometimes extrapyramidal effects, with a reduction of psychotic manifestations.
3. *The tranquilizers,* or as some call them *minor tranquilizers,* which have a sedative action on anxiety and, to some extent on agitation: They do not produce the neurologic syndrome, and they influence psychotic processes only mildly, if at all. Into this group fall drugs such as meprobamate.

(B) *Psychoanaleptics:* These drugs elevate mental tonus, increasing intellectual activity or alertness, as well as elevating emotional tonus. A distinction must be made between drugs such as the amphetamines which have merely a stimulant effect on mood, and that group of drugs which has been called "antidepressants" to emphasize their ability to alleviate psychotic depression, and which includes Tofranil and the amino-oxidase inhibitors. Both groups may be useful in depressions, but only the second one has a true antidepressive effect beyond mere stimulation and euphorization.

(C) *Psychodysleptics or psychotomimetics:* This refers to a group of drugs which can produce the so-called "model psychoses" and which have characteristically hallucinogenic and usually mild stimulant properties. Some of these, for example, lysergic acid, ditran and sernyl, have been used with some success in therapy as well.

We have, for the sake of convenience, classified the drugs to be discussed in a way similar to that proposed by Delay, since this affords a readily understandable means of differentiating drugs with fundamentally different properties from each other. Among these drugs are some, such as benactyzine and meratran, for which both stimulant and sedative actions have been claimed; these have been classified in the psycholeptic group, since here there are other drugs which are similar chemically. We prefer the term "anti-depressants" to such terms as "psychic energizers" or "thymoleptics," the latter term expressing their mood-elevating properties.

In this book, the newer drugs will be discussed first and more extensively. The hypnotics are omitted. Also the psychotomimetics are not discussed as far as their main significance for experimental psychiatry is concerned. Their occasional use in therapy will be mentioned here. Some other drugs, which were more or less successfully tried out prior to the present era of pharmacotherapy of psychiatric disorders, will be listed in a separate part of the book together with various physical treatments (Chapter VI).

Aside from Delay, many other authors proposed new classifications. He refers specifically to Cattell and Malitz, Kline, and S. B. Wortis. In view of the danger that too many different classifications might lead to confusion, a scientific group of the World Health Organization, in 1967, suggested a classification which tries to combine the principles of various previous attempts (see chart on page 6, WHO Techn. Rep. Ser. No. 371).

Neuroleptics, also known as "antipsychotics" and formerly "major tranquillizers" or "ataractics": drugs with therapeutic effects on psychoses and other types of psychiatric disorders. These drugs also have certain neurological effects, such as the production of extrapyramidal symptoms.

Anxiolytic sedatives, formerly called "minor tranquillizers": substances that reduce pathological anxiety, tension, and agitation without therapeutic effects on disturbed cognitive or perceptual processes. These drugs usually increase the convulsive threshold, do not produce autonomic or extrapyramidal effects, and often have potential for producing dependence.

Antidepressants: drugs effective in the treatment of pathological depressive states. Drugs in this category have sometimes been called "psychic energizers" and "thymoleptics."

Psychostimulants: drugs that increase the level of alertness and/or motivation. These effects are usually manifest in normal animals and humans.

Psychodysleptics: drugs producing abnormal mental phenomena, particularly in the cognitive and perceptual spheres. These drugs are also called hallucinogens, psychotomimetics, and in some cases psychedelics.

Methods Used in Drug Evaluation in Patients

The stages in the discovery and development of a new drug are, first, the recognition of a potentially useful biological effect in a chemical compound, second, the determination of the relative safety factors in animals and, finally, the establishment of activity, therapeutic efficacy, and safety in humans.

The problems of therapeutic evaluation of drugs in human studies are many and constitute a major difficulty in assessing the relative efficacy and toxicity of any new compound. In a number of cases the mere fact of being given a new drug by the doctor, who indicates his expectation of improvement, has a psychological effect upon the subject which can lead to inaccuracy in interpretation of the actual effect of the drug. The observers themselves may also allow their hopes to lead them to an over-optimistic view of the patient's improvement, and some drug studies are interesting not so much for their results as for the side-light which they throw upon the attitude of the doctor reporting, ranging from the cheerful optimist with wholesale improvements to the cautious and rather pessimistic obsessional with a questionable and moderate response in only a minority of cases. At the same time, the increased attention being paid to the patient group given the drug, as well as the question of spontaneous change in the illness pattern, which is particularly common in the neuroses, may produce misleading results. It has been shown, for example, many times that a percentage of neurotic patients will improve for a time on almost any new therapy, sometimes merely by regular hospital attendance to receive a placebo. Eisen et al. demonstrated that whether the investigator's attitude toward pharmacotherapy was favorable or unfavorable affected the frequency with which they attributed improvement to a drug.

The various techniques which have been used in drug assessment can be divided into two groups:

1. *The uncontrolled trial in which a group of patients is treated with a drug for a certain period of time, at the end of which the results are assessed:* This method is open to the objections previously stated and is of only limited value past the stage of preliminary evaluation. Where the patients being treated are chronic schizophrenics in a stationary state for many years and who can act to some extent as their own controls, this method of evaluation may be more acceptable than in acute psychotics or neurotics, where spontaneous remission is a far more likely occurrence. It may also be of assistance in making a rough assessment of the target symptoms of the drug and its toxic effects, so that more precise criteria for a controlled trial can be laid down.

2. *The controlled trial in which the drug under evaluation is compared with an inert substance called a placebo:* Since this alone, while obviating the psychological effects produced upon the patient by receiving a drug, does not eliminate the expectations of the observers, a "double blind" technique is

usually used. Here none of the medical or nursing staff participating in the trials knows which patients are receiving the drug and which the placebo, these being allocated at random by a neutral person who plays no part in assessing the therapeutic response. In double blind studies the new drug is compared either with a placebo, or with a drug with known therapeutic effect, or simultaneously with a placebo as well as a substance with known therapeutic effect. Aside from such comparative studies with groups, patients can also be studied individually with the double blind techniques, whereby the patient serves as his own control. Patients selected for such studies should be those with chronic and possibly stable psychopathological syndromes. The patients then receive the test drug, a placebo, and a known effective comparative drug in a varying, predetermined sequence, each of them for a few weeks or months. As an example, the first patient receives the test drug for the first month, a placebo for the second month, and the drug for comparison for the third month; the second patient receives the placebo for the first month, the substance for comparison afterwards, and the test drug at the end. The comparison of effects in the different treatment phases permits a good determination of the efficacy of the tested drug.

A usual selection system for the "double blind" trials is to match the patients into the number of groups required on the basis of such features as the duration and type of illness, and personality, thus enabling as many extraneous factors as possible to be eliminated. However, while the observers may not know which patients are on the drug, it is possible for them to guess in a number of cases because of the characteristic side-effects. This, moreover, is only one of the factors which may lead to misleading results in even the most carefully controlled trial.

The placebo effect has been discussed by Hankoff et al. and many other workers. It was summarized in some reviews by Shapiro, who gave a comprehensive history of the placebo effect. Although reports that placebos do equally well or even better than drugs are in the minority, this phenomenon needs explanation. The complexity of the issue is illustrated by Tanck et al. who, studying reserpine in chronic schizophrenics, found that the drug was more effective than a placebo, but that those patients who received reserpine first, followed by the placebo, showed greater improvement than those who received reserpine after the placebo. In a number of trials, it has been found that a supposedly inert substance was as effective in its therapeutic results as the trial drug, and in many trials some improvement is noted with the placebo. There may be several reasons for this—the encouraging effect of taking a drug at all, the increased attention received by the patient, and the influence of a milieu in which other patients may be improving on active drugs. In many instances, almost simultaneously with the larger use of drugs, an improvement took place in many chronic hospital wards through active social programs and increased freedom, and it may well be that, in such cases, neither the placebo nor the drug should be given credit but that it is the environmental change which has resulted in the alleviation of symptoms. This is an effective demonstration of the superiority of controlled trials, and perhaps explains claims made even for drugs which have relatively little value.

It is difficult to compare many of the studies on the same drug because of the variety of methods which have been used. There is no agreed scale of rating pre-trial behavior or improvement so that two different workers may mean very different things when they state that a certain drug has produced an improvement in 80 per cent of patients. Very few papers are at all detailed about those symptoms which specifically respond to a particular drug, called by Freyhan the "target symptoms," although this, as he rightly stressed, is the most important requirement for an appraisal of chemotherapy. It is well known by now that the phenothiazines are not a specific cure for schizophrenia or any other psychiatric disorder, and what is required is an evaluation of which clinical features are likely to respond to the drugs and which would be better treated by one of the older somatic methods.

There is often an inadequate period of trial of a drug, and there may also be an inadequate dosage. For example, some authors claimed no improvement after giving chlorpromazine and reserpine for a one week period to a group of patients reported as being tense, anxious, and emotionally disturbed, but for whom no more precise diagnoses were given. There is often an inadequate assessment of patients before and after the drug has been given: Concurrent treatments such as ECT are added; one drug is commenced too soon after cessation of previous therapy; and, all too often, the only diagnosis given for the patients is that of "chronic psychosis," by which one presumes that they are schizophrenics.

The effects of many of the drugs continue for some time after cessation of administration and may then still increase. Therefore, it cannot always be assumed in an investigation that improvement on a second drug after failure to respond to the first is evidence that the second drug is necessarily superior. Mendel, for example, has reported that patients first treated with prochlorperazine not only improved when perphenazine was substituted, but continued to improve when prochlorperazine was subsequently re-instituted.

Moreover, other environmental factors are not always taken into consideration—changes in the discharge policy of a hospital, in the ward personnel, or other changes important to the patient. The discharge policy of most American hospitals has been tremendously liberalized compared to five or ten years ago, and this has not been sufficiently realized in discussing the difference in the impact of the drugs here and abroad.

The role of the differing sedation thresholds in producing discrepancy of results has been emphasized, and Nash has advocated the administration of drugs on the basis of body weight or surface area to correct for differences in the volume of body fluids.

A wrong appraisal of results is often made because it is based upon variables (such as, employment figures, discharge rates, ability to participate in social functions) which fluctuate with other circumstances as well as with improve-

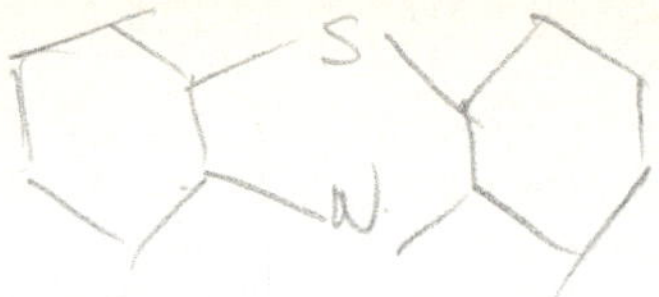

ment in the patient. It would be more worth while to attempt an assessment based, as far as possible, upon objective criteria which can be measured physiologically and psychologically, and which would provide a more impartial basis for results. There is something seriously amiss with methodology when wide discrepancies varying from "no improvement" to "complete remission in a large proportion of patients" are reported by different observers using the same drug in similar dosages in patients put into the same diagnostic category. It should not prove unduly difficult to design experiments controlled and described in detail so that their results can be validated by other observers, and there is still an obvious need for such carefully designed studies, despite the enormous volume of literature which has already been published on pharmacotherapy. The most important features of such studies should be a thorough pre-trial assessment using a number of different physiological and psychological techniques, elimination of as many extraneous factors as possible during the trial, and a post-trial assessment based upon the same techniques used previously.

THE NEUROLEPTICS

This group includes all those psychopharmaca whose pharmacological action resembles that of chlorpromazine, and which clinically influence such target symptoms as psychomotor excitement, tension, hallucinatory experiences, delusional thoughts, catatonic behavior, and schizophrenic depersonalization. All neuroleptics are furthermore characterized by more or less pronounced extrapyramidal motor side-effects.

To the neuroleptics being first the phenothiazines and the thioxanthenes which, together with some newer drugs can be classified as the group of "tricyclic neuroleptics." At present, the group of butyrophenones has—perhaps more so in Europe than in the U.S.—assumed an almost equal significance. By contrast, reserpine whose neuroleptic effect had been discovered almost as early as that of chlorpromazine, now plays only a minor clinical role. The other rauwolfia alkaloids and the benzoquinolizines which are structurally somewhat related to the rauwolfia drugs are therapeutically insignificant.

Phenothiazines and Other Tricyclic Neuroleptics

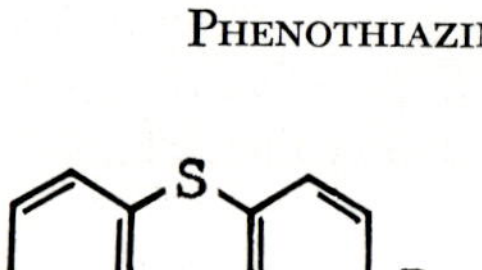

The largest group of tricyclic neuroleptics are the phenothiazines. They were first synthesized in 1883 by Bernthsen while investigating alternative procedures for synthesizing methylene blue. The phenothiazine nucleus consists of two benzene rings joined by a sulphur and nitrogen atom.

Phenothiazine itself was used for some time as a urinary antiseptic and antihelminthic, but ceased to be used because of its toxicity. In 1945, both French and German workers began an investigation of phenothiazine derivatives, and in 1950 chlorpromazine was synthesized by Charpentier.

New derivatives are formed by substitution at R_1 and R_2, as shown in the formula.

At R_1 the following substitutions can be made:

1. Dimethylaminopropyl side chain, as in chlorpromazine, promazine, triflupromazine, methopromazine, acepromazine and—finally too—methotrimeprazine.
2. Piperidine side chain, as in thioridazine, mepazine and propericiazine.
3. Piperazine side chain, as in perazine, prochlorperazine, butaperazine, thioproperazine, perphenazine, thiopropazate, fluphenazine and chlorimiphenine.

Compounds with a piperazine side chain at R_1 are more potent than those with dimethylaminopropyl or piperidine side chains, but have a greater tendency to produce extrapyramidal manifestations.

The substitutions at R_2 include halogens, methoxy, thiomethyl, acetyl and other organic radicals.

The phenothiazines as a group play a prominent role not solely because of their by now considerable number. Their particular importance lies in the fact that the discovery of the clinical effectiveness of chlorpromazine has been the point of origin for the entire field of modern psychopharmacotherapy. After the great significance of the phenothiazines for psychiatric therapy had been recognized, chemists all over the world tried to find new possibly still more effective drugs by systematically changing the chlorpromazine molecule. These efforts were successful up to a certain point. They led, for instance, to the discovery of substances like the tricyclic antidepressants which by now are almost as important as the neuroleptics. Also some other groups of neuroleptics have been discovered in this way. Today already three groups of tricyclic neuroleptics are known. They are the

Phenothiazines	(No. 1 to 6 and 9 to 20 of the list on the following page)
Azaphenothiazines	(No. 8 of list)
Thioxanthenes	(No. 7 and 21 to 23 of list)

The *phenothiazines* have become so numerous that it is hardly possible to present a complete list. Therefore, this survey is limited to 18 phenothiazine derivatives which are well proven products with brand names in the U.S. or in Europe. The innumerable experimental drugs are not mentioned. However, not included are those phenothiazines that are not psychopharmaca in a narrower sense as, e.g., antihistamines of the promethazine type, the antiparkinsonian drugs of the diethazine type, the antipruritic agents of the trimeprazine type, and the spasmolytics of the aminopromazine type. Finally, no detailed discussion will be given of some phenothiazine products which are psychopharmaca but whose effect is either very similar to that of other neuroleptics (as, e.g., acetophenazine—Tindal and carphenezine—Proketazine), or which are not used as neuroleptics but only as "minor tranquilizers" (e.g., piperacetazine—Quide).

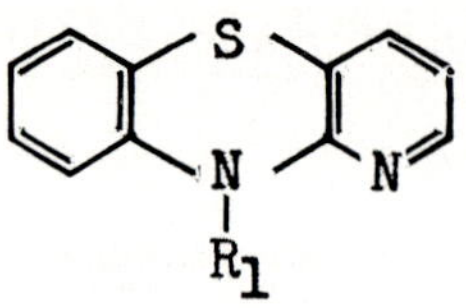

The *azaphenothiazines* remained a very small group and by now play hardly any role in psychiatric therapy. The group derives from the azaphenothiazine ring.

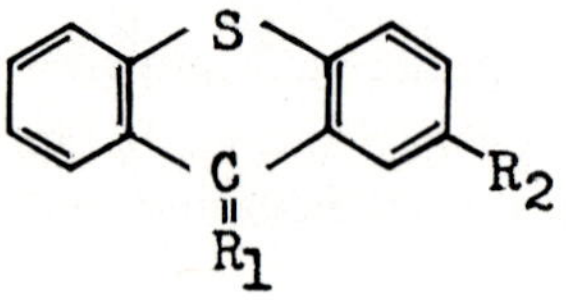

The *thioxanthenes* are a more important group. As diphenylmethane derivatives their chemical structure is analogous to the phenothiazine derivatives which can be conceived as diphenylamine derivatives. The products of this group derive from the thioxanthene ring.

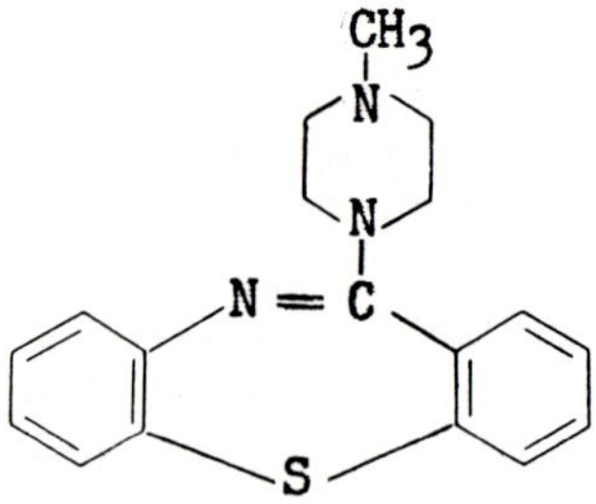

A fourth group of tricyclic neuroleptics described recently, differs from the hitherto known neuroleptics by having a seven-member central ring rather than a six-member central ring like the previously known neuroleptics. Thus, their chemical structure brings them nearer to the antidepressants (Bente et al.) which affords them a special theoretical interest. However, they will not be described in detail because so far the only commercially available product is the chlothiapine (see next formula) which is on the market in France as Etumine.

The following drugs belong to the group of *Tricyclic Neuroleptics*

1. Chlorpromazine (Thorazine, Largactil, Megaphen, Aminazin)
2. Promazine (Sparine, Prazine, Litranol, Verophen)
3. Triflupromazine (Vesprin, Vespral, Psyquil)
4. Methopromazine (Tentone, Mopazine)
5. Acepromazine (Plegecil, Notensil)
6. Methotrimeprazine, or Levomepromazine (Veractil, Nozinan, Neurocil)
7. Chlorprothixene (Taractan, Truxal, Solatran)
8. Prothipendyl (Tolnate, Dominal)
9. Thioridazine (Mellaril, Melleril)
10. Mepazine, or Pecazine (Pacatal, Lacumin)
11. Propericiazine (Neulactil, Neuleptil, Aolept)
12. Perazine (Taxilan)
13. Prochlorperazine (Compazine, Stemetil, Nipodal)
14. Trifluoperazine (Stelazine, Jatroneural)
15. Butaperazine (Repoise)
    Butyrylperazine (Randolectil)
16. Thioproperazine (Vontil, Majeptil)
17. Perphenazine (Trilafon, Fentazin, Decentan)
18. Thiopropazate (Dartal, Dartlan)
19. Fluphenazine (Prolixin, Permitil, Moditen, Antensol, Omca, Lyogen)
    Slow release drugs for intramuscular depots:
    Fluphenazine
    Enanthate (Prolixin enanthate, Moditen enanthate, Dapotum)

Fluphenazine
Decanoate (Lyogen Depot)
20. Chlorimpiphenine (Ponsital)
21. Clopenthixol, Chlorperphenthixene (Sordinol, Ciatyl)
22. Flupentixol (Fluanxol)
23. Thiothixene (Navane, Orbinamon)

Pharmacological Properties: Chlorpromazine is the most thoroughly investigated phenothiazine. Pharmacologically it is a many-sided broad-spectrum neuroleptic which serves as a yardstick for all newer neuroleptics. Chlorpromazine continues to be regarded as the prototype of the tricyclic neuroleptics. Therefore, the easiest way to describe the pharmacology of the tricyclic neuroleptics is to take chlorpromazine as the starting point.

Over the years opinions have varied as to the question which of the different pharmacological effects of chlorpromazine are most closely tied to its clinical action. Even now there is no general agreement on the pharmacological experimental designs which should be included in the screening of new potential neuroleptics. The least disputed assumption is that results of animal experiments are most promising for a neuroleptic effect, when extrapyramidal motor phenomena are seen. The extrapyramidal motor (cataleptic) effect had already been recognized as particularly characteristic for neuroleptics during pharmacological studies on chlorpromazine. Initially, however, it was assumed that perhaps other pharmacological effects are more closely related to the therapeutic action. Courvoiser and her co-workers, who reported on chlorpromazine in 1953, found that it had marked anti-adrenergic and local anesthetic properties, although there was no inhibition of the hyperglycemic response of adrenaline. It possessed mild anticholinergic and anti-histaminic actions, as well as a sedative, anti-emetic and hypothermic central action.

It potentiates the effects of certain drugs, especially morphine and the barbiturate derivatives. Chlorpromazine antagonizes the psychomotor stimulant actions of caffeine and amphetamine and some of the central actions of nikethamide and nicotine but not those of strychnine. However, it does not abolish seizures produced by either electrical means or by drugs. In addition to antagonizing apomorphine vomiting, its anti-emetic effect covers other types of nausea such as that induced by motion and radiation.

Courvoisier found a suppression of conditioned reflex response in animals, and it is of some interest that Archer, who in his experiments used thirst as the stimulus, found a lesser effect than did Courvoisier, whose stimulus was of an electrical and auditory type. Hostility in animals is reduced when the drug is given to them, and there is a reduction in spontaneous motor activity with, eventually, the development of sleep from which the animal, as distinct from one which is anesthetized, can be aroused by the usual stimuli. In Archer's experiments there was a reduction in motor speed in the maze performance but also some increase in the number of errors. Courvoisier noted that chlorpromazine depressed the oxygen consumption of guinea pig cerebral cortex slices in vitro and this has been confirmed by later workers.

Much attention has been devoted to the cerebral site of action of chlorpromazine and there is considerable evidence that one of the principal areas affected by the drug is the reticular formation. Wirth has noted that chlorpromazine depresses the excitability of the reticular formation, as well as all agents which stimulate it. It especially suppresses the activating action of adrenaline on the reticular zone. Wase et al. have demonstrated the specificity of chlorpromazine for the reticular formation radiochemically. As well as on the reticular formation, chlorpromazine acts on other sub-cortical structures in the midbrain, hypothalamus and rhinencephalon. This is in contrast to the barbiturates which act more strongly on the cerebral cortex and on the respiratory center in the medulla. Himwich, reviewing evidence concerning the effects of tranquilizing drugs, concludes that it is in the site of action that the reason for their difference from the barbiturates lies. Dell and his group showed experimentally that, after blockage of adrenergic intra-reticular mechanisms by the anti-adrenaline effect of chorpromazine, the spontaneous activity of these formations is diminished and they respond less to electrical and sensory stimuli. They no longer react to adrenaline liberated through nociceptive stimulation, and they become more sensitive to inhibiting influences. Therefore, the animal receiving chlorpromazine has a reduced spontaneous activity, falls asleep, and, if it is awakened, the waking state is not maintained. Olds, experimenting on animals with self-stimulating electrodes implanted in certain parts of the brain, found that those rats given chlorpromazine no longer administered stimulation to their brains when the electrodes were in the posterior hypothalamus, but continued self stimulation when the electrodes were in the anterior hypothalamus. He therefore concluded that chlorpromazine produces important changes in the posterior hypothalamus.

It seems according to Himwich that, while chlorpromazine in small doses inhibits the reticular system, large doses have an opposite excitatory effect. Stimulation of the mesodiencephalic alerting system produces characteristic low amplitude rapid waves in the electroencephalogram, and in small doses chlorpromazine blocks this pattern, but in large doses its action is reversed and the alerting system is stimulated.

The action of chlorpromazine in the brain stem was thoroughly investigated by many authors. The numerous findings led to different theories on the effects which are relevant for the therapeutic action (Bradley; Killam). Bradley holds that the action of chlorpromazine on the reticular formation of the brain stem is caused by suppression of those afferent stimuli which the reticular formation receives through collaterals from the ascending sensory pathways. Support for this hypothesis comes from results of micro-electrode recordings from neurons in the mesencephalic reticular formation. Chlorpromazine diminished fixing in response to sensory stimulation. Another hypothesis was developed by Killam who believes that chlorpromazine increases reticular activity. It then produces an enhancement of the filtering mechanisms in the reticular formation. The result is a reduced "flow-through" of inessential sensory information.

One of the most important pharmacological properties is an effect on the brain stem known as "catalepsy." Animals when placed in artificial unnatural positions, maintain such postures. Other remarkable effects on animal behavior have been described. Chlorpromazine decreases the aggressive behavior of many species (cats, fishes like betta splendens etc.) and increases their sociability. Many investigations have been made to define the effects of chlorpromazine on learning processes, for instance continued avoidance responses (Herz). In average amounts chlorpromazine abolishes conditioned responses, for example in rats, while nonconditioned responses are not diminished.

Aside from its blocking action on adrenergic mechanisms, chlorpromazine has been shown to have similar effect on the neurohormone, serotonin. Costa and Rinaldi found that animals receiving injections of 5-hydroxy tryptophan revealed larger concentrations of serotonin in the brain if they had been premedicated with chlorpromazine, indicating that, it least under certain conditions, chlorpromazine can block the breakdown of serotonin.

Of the other tricyclic neuroleptics *promazine* is pharmacologically very similar to chlorpromazine, but it is less potent when given in equivalent amounts. Also *methopromazine* and *acepromazine* have similar pharmacological properties as the other tricyclic neuroleptics with an aliphatic side chain. Finally, *triflupromazine* is similar to chlorpromazine. Animal experimentations with this drug have shown that it has both vagolytic and adrenergic blocking effects. It has powerful anti-emetic properties as well as antihistamine actions. It reduces amphetamine-induced overactivity in mice. There was no reduction in the incidence of metrazol or electrically induced convulsions. The action of morphine is potentiated.

Methotrimeprazine is a very powerful antihistamine and sedative drug with activities comparable to promethazine. It is similar to chlorpromazine in its autonomic activities, having both an anti-adrenaline action and a weak vagal depressant effect. It gives no protection against leptazol convulsions. It enhances the effects of barbiturates and ether anesthesia to about three times the degree that chlorpromazine does. It has less anti-emetic activity than chlorpromazine, but its action in depressing psychomotor performance in rats is about twice that of the latter. It is also about three times more effective in its hypothermic properties and about equal in its power to potentiate the analgesia of morphine.

Chlorprothixene was the first drug of the group of thioxanthenes, initiated by Petersen and Møller Nielsen. All the drugs of this group resemble in their pharmacological properties their structural analogues in the phenothiazine group. Thus, chlorprothixene is next to chlorpromazine, *clopenthixol* to perphenazine, *flupentixol* to fluphenazine, and *thiothixene* to thioproperazine. In general, the thioxanthene derivatives, in comparison to their structural analogues in the phenothiazine group have more anticholinergic and less "cataleptic" effects.

Prothipendyl as an azaphenothiazine derivative is a weak neuroleptic drug in pharmacological tests.

A new step in the development of phenothiazine derivatives was the investigation of the pharmacology of *thioridazine*. There are no pronounced antihistaminic, anti-emetic or anticholinergic actions, but there are moderate adrenalytic effects. It does not reduce body temperature as much as other phenothiazines do and it has a very weak cataleptic-inducing action in animals. Catalepsy production in animals has been correlated by Courvoisier with the occurrence of parkinsonism clinically. Thioridazine has not been reported to produce any gross extrapyramidal reactions, although muscular hypotonia has been reported on high dosage by May.

Haley et al. have noted that thioridazine has an adrenergic blocking effect, while Swinyard and his co-workers, in a comparison with chlorpromazine, found that it abolishes the conditioned escape response in animals as well as decreasing spontaneous motor activity, reducing the low frequency electroshock seizure threshold and prolonging hexobarbital sleeping time. They also found that the drug is only half as toxic as chlorpromazine in mice.

Taeschler and Cerletti found, when they estimated the effect of several phenothiazines on motor and emotional reactions in rats, that there was a close correlation between the inhibition of the conditioned avoidance response and the cataleptic effect. Mellaril was approximately 100 times less effective than perphenazine and 9 times less effective than chlorpromazine both in producing catalepsy and in the inhibition of the avoidance response. In the rat, there is a parallel between the cataleptic effect of a drug and the intensity of the side effects. Similarly, there is some degree of correlation between the anti-emotional effectiveness of a drug (i.e., its power to inhibit emotional defecation in rats) and the therapeutic efficacy. No correlation was found between the inhibition of the conditioned avoidance reaction and emotional defecation. The dose of mellaril required to prevent the emotional response was approximately three times lower than the "anti-escape" dose (i.e., that required to inhibit the conditioned avoidance reaction), while the opposite was true of perphenazine. Chlorpromazine inhibited both responses to about the same degree. Thus, mellaril, in contrast to the other phenothiazines tested, inhibits the emotional response more than the motor performance. Taeschler and Cerletti suggest that the suppression of psychovegetative reactions such as emotional defecation is a better predictor of the therapeutic efficacy of a drug than the inhibition of motor functions.

Mepazine which, like thioridazine, has a piperidyl ring in the side chain, was investigated by Nieschulz et al. in 1954. There is a similar, though not so pronounced, effect on the nervous system as occurs with chlorpromazine, but, unlike the latter, it has a marked depressant action on the parasympathetic nervous system. This accounts for both the often encountered atropine-like side-effects and its relatively week hypotensive action. Himwich et al. could demonstrate no blocking effect on the reticular formation. Mepazine possesses mild anti-pyretic and anti-histaminic properties.

Propericiazine which during the last few years has become very popular in France, also has a piperidyl ring in the side chain. However pharmacologically it is already close to the piperazine group of phenothiazine derivatives.

Perazine belongs with prochlorperazine, trifluoperazine, butaperazine, thioproperazine, perphenazine, thiopropazate, fluphenazine and chlorimpiphenine to the group of the strongly neuroleptic phenothiazine derivatives. Compared to chlorpromazine these phenothiazenes have a much stronger effect in many pharmacological tests. The broader action of the perazine derivatives becomes particularly noticeable in the catalepsy test. In various other pharmacological tests, however, the perazine derivatives are less effective than the corresponding promazine derivatives. From this one can infer that those pharmacological tests in which the perazine derivatives come off worse than the promazine derivatives, have little importance for the pharmacological screening of new neuroleptics. For it is undisputed that the perazine derivatives are clinically more potent than the promazine derivatives.

Prochlorperazine is, according to investigations by Courvoisier et al. four times more active than chlorpromazine both as an anti-emetic and in producing catalepsy in animals. When the drug is given to rats in a dosage of 10 mg. per g. of body weight, Ducrot and Koetschet showed that a state resembling flexibilitas cerea could be obtained, in which the animal can be moulded into abnormal postures which are sustained for a considerable period of time. The drug was 5 to 10 times less active than chlorpromazine in impairing the performance of mice attempting to regain their balance after being suspended from a horizontal wire.

Prochlorperazine is weaker than chlorpromazine in its adrenaline-antagonizing action, its anti-histaminic activity and its hypothermic effects. It has little, if any, vagolytic action, and only about one third of the power of chlorpromazine to potentiate the sedative actions of morphine, the barbiturates, and ether anesthesia. It is approximately as potent in reducing locomotor activity in mice, and its action on conditioned reflexes is rather different from that of chlorpromazine—the animals given prochlorperazine show a similar indifference to the conditioned stimulus as the animals given chlorpromazine, but, while those on the latter drug still respond to the unconditioned stimulus, the prochlorperazine-treated animals show, after about 5 or 6 hours, a state of catalepsy in which they often remain indifferent to the unconditioned stimulus.

Trifluoperazine possesses a marked antiemetic effect and approximately the same degree of adrenolytic and hypotensive activity as chlorpromazine but no parasympatholytic action. There is very little anti-histaminic effect and insignificant antispasmodic properties. It failed to show any anticonvulsant activity when tested in mice given maximal electroshock fits (Tedeschi et al.).

It is about six times as potent as chlorpromazine in depressing spontaneous motor activity in rats and approximately ten times more potent in its production of blockage of the conditioned avoidance response. Equivalent doses of trifluoperazine produced a more sustained catalepsy in rats than that found when chlorpromazine was given. All these properties have been shown by Taeschler and Cerletti to correlate with the intensity of the clinical side-effects of a drug, including parkinsonism and other extrapyramidal manifestations in animals. Clinically, trifluoperazine produces marked extrapyramidal side-effects in human subjects more frequently and more rapidly than chlorpromazine.

Butaperazine is exceptional in the group of all studied acidified perazine derivatives because of its pronounced pharmacological properties (Wirth et al.). It has strong cataleptic and antiapomorphine actions. In mice its barbiturate-potentiating effect is very distinct. In pharmacological tests studying the dampening effect of animal aggression, for instance in the Siamese fighting fish, betta splendens, the drug is very effective. The adrenolytic action corresponds to that of chlorpromazine from which it differs—like the other perazine derivatives—in its minimal effect on the arousal threshold of wakeful rabbits.

Thioproperazine was one of the first of those phenothiazine derivatives that are characterized pharmacologically by a combination of strong antiemetic and cataleptic action. Other central effects are minimal. Vegetative functions are hardly influenced by thioproperazine (Courvoisier et al.).

Perphenazine was shown in animal experiments to be at least five times more potent than chlorpromazine. It does not potentiate the barbiturates, is not a powerful hypnotic, and rarely produces drowsiness or lethargy unless given in very high dosage.

Thiopropazate has a pharmacological spectrum which resembles that of perphenazine. This is not surprising because, probably, the thiopropazate is hydrolized in the organism by unspecific esterases so that in vivo perphenazine develops.

Fluphenazine has very powerful anti-emetic properties, being 200 times as effective in this respect experimentally as chlorpromazine. It is also more powerful in blocking the conditioned avoidance response in rats: it has similar sympatholytic effects, and produces equivalent hypotension and reflex tachycardia. It has little sedative action in clinical doses, and there is no prolongation of the barbiturate or anesthetic sleeping time.

Fluphenazine enanthate and *fluphenazine decanoate* are two esters of fluphenazine which acquired special importance for practical therapy. Esterization of the OH-group in the end position of the side chain of fluphenazine with heptanoic acid results in fluphenazine enanthate; esterization with capric acid produces fluphenazine decanoate. Inhibition of avoidance tests, protection against d-amphetamine toxicity on the group behavior of mice, and the anti-apomorphine effect are prolonged for 15 days or more, while ordinary fluphenazine under the same conditions does not act longer than three days (Burke et al.; Boissier et al.). One injection of fluphenazine decanoate in doses of 10 to 30 mg. per kg. sedates male white mice for five weeks. These results of animal experiments suggested that these fluphenazine esters would be neuroleptics with slow-release action if used as intramuscular depots. This assumption was borne out by clinical results (Kinross-Wright et al.; and many others).

Chlorimpiphenine is similar to perphenazine, but its central action is more powerful and prolonged. It has sedative, cataleptic and hypothermal effects. In animal experiments testing the inhibition of conditioned avoidance responses, chlorimpiphenine is more active than perphenazine. The antiemetic activity tested on apomorphine induced vomiting in dogs is 21 times greater than that of perphenazine. Peripherally it exerts definite antiserotonin, antihistaminic and adrenolytic effects (Lenk et al.).

Chlorprothixene, discussed earlier, played the same role for subsequent thioxanthene derivatives with neuroleptic effect, as chlorpromazine did for the many later phenothiazine derivatives.

Clopenthixol, the perphenazine analogue in the thioxanthene series, is distinguished from chlorprothixene by a stronger inhibition of conditioned responses in rats, and by a weaker antiadrenaline and antiserotonin effect (Petersen and Møller Nielsen).

Flupenthixol has a stronger cataleptic action than clopenthixol. It has no hypnotic effect, and even large doses do not induce sleep in animals. Antiadrenaline, antiserotonin, and atropine-like anticholinergic effects are 10 to 15 times weaker than with clopenthixol.

Thiothixene, the latest thioxanthene derivative with neuroleptic action, is pharmacologically similar to thioproperazene and a very potent neuroleptic (Weissman).

1. Chlorpromazine (Thorazine, Largactil, Megaphen, Aminazin)

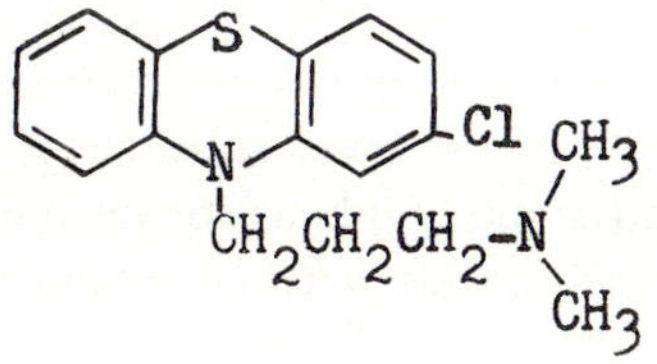

Chlorpromazine, 2-chloro-10 3-(dimethylamino)propylphenothiazine hydrochloride, was synthesized by French workers in the Rhone-Poulenc laboratories who were attempting to find a substance with more potent effects than the antihistaminic promethazine. Under the experimental number 456ORP, its clinical effects were reported by Laborit in 1951, who used the term "artificial hibernation" to describe the state which the drug produced in patients. When used in operative procedures, its effects were such that the patient, although fully conscious and aware of all the procedures, was indifferent to them and could sometimes be operated on without anesthesia. Laborit used in anesthesia the "Cocktail lytique," which was a combination of chlorpromazine with phenergan, atropine, hydergin and other drugs that act on the autonomic nervous system. The first psychiatric reports appeared in 1952 when Hamon, Paraire and Velluz reported on a case of manic excitement which subsided after 20 days treatment with chlorpromazine and pethidine, and Delay, Deniker and Harl wrote on the "Utilisation en Thérapeutique Psychiatrique d'une Phénothiazine d'action Centrale Elective (4560RP)." They described the typical response in the patient given chlorpromazine as being one of apparent indifference to external stimuli with emotional neutrality and decrease in initiative but without impairment of intellectual faculties or consciousness. They obtained spectacular results in most of the violent excitement states but inconclusive results in depressions, and noted that leucopenia and an activating effect on infections could occur. Later in the same year, Delay and Deniker reported on 38 cases of various psychotic disorders in which they had used chlorpromazine, in a paper entitled "The treatment of psychoses with a neurolytic method deriving from hibernation therapy," which was presented at the Congress of French Psychiatrists and Neurologists in Luxemburg in July, 1952. They were immediately aware of the therapeutic potentialities of the drug, and are rightly credited with the introduction of this drug into psychiatry.

Since then, there have been innumerable reports on its use in every type of psychiatric illness, and many new phenothiazines have been developed. Since many of the problems connected with chlorpromazine are valid for the other phenothiazines as well as for the Rauwolfia compounds, chlorpromazine which was the first of the neuroleptic drugs to be investigated in detail, will be taken to some extent as the model for the others, and problems pertaining to all of them will be discussed here. Subsequently, the specific features of the later drugs will be dealt with individually.

CLINICAL EFFECTS: On administration of the drug to patients, Lehmann and Hanrahan noted a fall in blood pressure which varied from 20 to 40 mm. systolic pressure and 10 to 30 mm. diastolic pressure, according to dosage and individual response. The hypotension may be greater in hypertensives and elderly arteriosclerotics than in normotensives, and is sometimes manifested by complaints of giddiness or, exceptionally, by fainting from which there is spontaneous and uneventful recovery. There was a compensatory tachycardia with an increase in pulse rate of 10 to 40 beats per minute. Distinct pallor and miosis were often found, and in single cases there was a mild hyperthermia of 99 to 101°F. for the first few days of treatment, but the fever subsided spontaneously, the temperature returning to normal (Anton-Stephens) or becoming subnormal (Lehmann and Hanrahan). The respiratory rate was not influenced. Dryness of the mouth and nasal congestion are frequent at the commencement of treatment.

Appetite is improved and there is usually a gain in weight, although some of the cases of Lehmann and Hanrahan complained of nausea and anorexia. They also noted that there was a tendency to constipation. Occasionally, there are complaints of a bitter or bad taste in the mouth (Winkelman). Experiments have shown that chlorpromazine both decreases gastric motility (Fournier) and inhibits gastric secretion (Dobkin et al.).

Delay and Deniker found an initial polyuria of up to 3 litres in 24 hours with some short term rises in blood urea. Dobkin et al., however, found a fall in blood urea levels, while Lehmann and Hanrahan noted no change, although there was urinary frequency without any other abnormality. Moyer and his co-workers found renal function to be unimpaired.

With large doses there is listlessness and a reduction of voluntary muscle power which may eventually be followed by the development of extrapyramidal manifestations to be described later.

No significant changes have been found in red cell or hemoglobin concentrations, except for a case of hemolytic anemia described by Cooperberg. The sedimentation rate tends to rise during treatment. There may be a fall in the white cells during the initial treatment stages, especially in the polymorphs, with sometimes an associated eosinophilia. In most cases, this has no clinical effects, and, in a case described by Anton-Stephens, a leucopenia was followed by a normal leucocyte response to infection. Sometimes, however, agranulocytosis develops (this will be discussed in the section on complications).

Since jaundice is another complication in patients receiving chlorpromazine, there have been many studies on liver metabolism. Bartholomew et al. performed liver biopsies and liver function tests in 25 psychotic patients before they received medication. Sixteen were normal and 9 showed minor subclinical disturbances. They were then given chlorpromazine, 100 mg. twice daily for three months. Clinical jaundice developed in two patients and subclinical hyperbilirubinemia in one. Definite histological changes were evident in the liver biopsy series from 5 out of 16 patients with normal livers prior to treatment and, in 8 out of the 9 with minor liver disturbances, there was increased pathology. Keup did a battery of liver function tests on schizophrenics receiving 100 to 375 mg. of chlorpromazine daily. He found exudative inflammatory changes in over half the patients even though only one developed jaundice and he attributed at least part of the changes to the drug. Hippius et al. found that in a group of schizophrenic patients the serum proteins showed definite abnormal levels electrophoretically before the onset of treatment, with a drop in the albumin and a rise to above normal in the globulin. During treatment with chlorpromazine and reserpine, the albumins decreased significantly further during the first week of treatment, and then, up to the 7th week, they increased up to normal levels. The globulins decreased to normal. In many of their patients, and in those of Cares, the serum alkaline phosphatase was increased without jaundice. The question of a true hepatotoxic effect of chlorpromazine must, therefore, remain in doubt. Hubble in 1941 showed that phenothiazine itself was hepatotoxic, but there has been no conclusive evidence from animal experiments that this is true for chlorpromazine. Lehmann and Hanrahan have also noted minor changes in serum proteins and in cephalin-cholesterol flocculation, the latter occurring in fifty per cent of cases. Keup believes that there are two types of liver reaction associated with chlorpromazine medication: a "cholestatic, mostly benign reaction of undefined origin, not related to the dosage given," which is equivalent to the obstructive type of jaundice; and, infrequently, "damage to the liver parenchyma, preponderantly of a mild nature and related to the dosage employed."

Sainz has noted that there is an increase in the excretion of riboflavin which is not correlated with clinical improvement. However, the phenothiazines also increase the blood levels of ascorbic acid, and it was found that the higher the increase, the greater the clinical improvement. He noted two distinct types of action on the central nervous system. There is, first, a general peripheral vagolytic effect with dilation of the pupils, dryness of the mouth, decreased gastric secretion and decreased peristalsis. This stage does not correlate with clinical improvement. The second autonomic action was called by Sainz central or insular vagolytic activity. Its effect is much more selective and, while dilation of the pupils and/or dryness of the mouth may persist, the intestinal manifestations are absent. Only this central effect correlated with the degree of improvement, the dryness of the mouth having the highest correlate.

The *psychological effects* of chlorpromazine are those used therapeutically, and will be mostly described in the section on results. Here only some general observations will be listed. There may be a short period of drowsiness, but this is usually mild in degree. Anton-Stephens called this the stage of "somnolence," and distinguished between this and both physiological sleep and barbiturate sedation. He considered that the intensity of the reaction might be related to the mental state, acutely disturbed patients being much more rapidly sedated than less disturbed ones. Winkelman limits medication in outpatients to bedtime until it can be tolerated in the day without drowsiness. He advises dexedrine to combat the somnolence which Blair and Brady oppose because dexedrine may lead to an exacerbation of the psychosis. As the drowsiness disappears, a state of calm and indifference develops, described by Anton-Stephens as "psychic indifference," both to surroundings and to symptoms, but with no diminution of intellectual faculties or alteration of awareness. There is a decrease in the distress caused by hallucinations, delusions, or tension, but no loss of contact with the environment. An opposite action of the drug will be described in the section on psychiatric complications.

An indifference to rather than unawareness of pain has been seen. A patient of Baker with painful inflammation of injection sites on one leg which resulted in flexion of both hips due to reflex spasm on walking, made no spontaneous complaint while on the drug, although later, when taken off largactil, she admitted that her leg had been very painful. This author also stresses the fact that, beneath drug-induced apathy, the underlying mood disturbance can still be elicited, and quotes a quieted manic who would briefly show flight of ideas and then relapse into silence.

As von Baeyer, in the German literature on shock treatments, distinguishes between the effect of the therapeutic agent itself on the psyche and the effect of the treatment on an illness, so do Sutter and Pascalis similarly differentiate between primary psychological effects of chlorpromazine and the secondary reaction on the part of the patient to the drug effect, which can differ considerably in various patients according to their personality structure.

PSYCHIATRIC INDICATIONS:

Schizophrenia: It is in the treatment of this disorder that chlorpromazine and other neuroleptic drugs have found their widest applications. The favorable response of many schizophrenics was recognized by Delay et al. in their early papers. They found that the best results both in quality and quantity were in the paranoid form, even in cases resistant to insulin and ECT. A third of their patients were able to leave the hospital and half showed considerable improvement even though remaining in the hospital. These results in paranoids were obtained no matter what the length of the illness was, unlike the catatonic and hebephrenic forms where the prognosis worsened with the duration of the psychosis. Acute catatonia responded favorably to chlorpromazine, but in the chronic case the drug had only a symptomatic effect on the aggressive and impulsive behavior. The hebephrenic group had the worst results, particularly in the quality of their remission. In this group, Delay and his fellow workers found that, in those cases with a history of less than three years, there were twice as many discharges as mere improvements in hospital adjustment or failures. Where the illness had lasted from 3 to 5 years, the discharges plus improvement in the hospital equaled the failures, while after 5 years the failures were double all the improvements.

Labhardt also emphasized the good results obtained in those chronic schizophrenics who no longer responded to insulin or ECT, and who constitute the "incurable" section of most psychiatric hospitals. He confirmed the better results in paranoid and catatonic cases and noted a better response in females. The symptoms which were most improved were aggression, as well as mannerisms and stereotypies, which are usually regarded as indicators of a poor outlook for recovery. In dull patients without initiative, there was often a worsening of symptoms and the appearance of an apathetic type of depression, a fact noted by many later workers. Contrary to the complete disappearance of delusions and hallucinations in the acute schizophrenic, chronic ones showed only a change in their emotional response to these symptoms. The most important feature was that chronic schizophrenics, of whom 205 were studied, could respond to the drug and return to the community. There is not room to list the numerous reports that have appeared since on the drug in chronic schizophrenia. It may suffice to say that the majority of them have concurred with these early findings.

Hyvert obtained optimal results with a treatment regime consisting of three weeks of intramuscular injections of 150 to 200 mg. of chlorpromazine three or more times daily, which was usually given in combination with hyaluronidase in doses up to 600 mg. because of the slowness of absorption and the painfulness of the injection. This was followed by oral amounts which were 50 per cent or more higher than the injections. Often if was necessary to resume the injections if the tablets did not maintain the improvement. With this elaborate regime 93 per cent of chronic schizophrenics improved, and of these, 35 per cent were discharged from the hospital. He also noted a much greater improvement in female patients, and on the assumption that this might be due to lack of estrogen, he gave estrogens in large doses to his male patients and was able to improve his results almost to the point obtained in women.

Many reports did not differentiate adequately between the effect of the drug in acute and chronic schizophrenics. There is agreement about the beneficial effect of chlorpromazine and other neuroleptics in acute catatonic excitement, where the older sedatives were often both ineffectual and dangerous because of the large amounts required. Also in acute paranoid schizophrenics the immediate results can be satisfactory. They are poor in catatonic stupor with some exceptions. In these hypokinetic syndromes, other drugs, such as stelazine, which will be mentioned later, are preferable to chlorpromazine.

In chronic schizophrenia, most authorities agree that many patients can be helped to some extent. Some claim excellent results with intensive treatment, while others (Baker, Elkes and Elkes, Anton-Stephens) found that most patients are merely improved by the drug. Actually its main benefit is to render the chronic patient more amenable to occupational and recreational therapy (Blair and Brady). One of the negative reports on the drug by Loftus et al. failed to note any improvement with either chlorpromazine in doses of 450 mg. daily or benactyzine in a double blind trial with 120 chronic psychotic patients treated over a twelve-week period. They believe that many reports contain unsuspected errors such as failure to evaluate the role of preferential treatment in the study groups, faulty criteria of improvement, especially reliance on the discharge rate, and neglect of other environmental causes of improvement. Many workers like Lehmann and Hanrahan, have rightly emphasized that the psychosis often persists beneath the quieted exterior and that the improvement is symptomatic only, with no effect on delusions and hallucinations. This is in contrast to the effect in acute cases, where the psychosis may be completely relieved. Even though chronic patients show only some amelioration, this is of great importance in such a serious and malignant illness, and it is obvious that the drug is worthy of trial in all chronic schizophrenics who have failed to improve with other therapies. The enormous effect of this therapeutic approach on mental hospitals has been stressed particularly in the American literature (Denber and Bird, Brill and Patton, and many others). Results with maintenance drug therapy in discharged hospital patients were reported in follow-up studies by Kris and Carmichael, who found a single daily dose of 50 to 150 mg. at bedtime sufficient for maintenance in the majority of cases: This also prevents drowsiness and helps to keep the patients at work. Pollack estimates that chlorpromazine reduces the relapse rate of released hospital patients to one fourth to one third of the usual rate.

The important question of how treatments with chlorpromazine and other drugs compare with the shock treatments, what the different indications are, whether and how the older treatments and pharmacotherapy can be combined, and many other problems which arise in connection with the new drug therapy of schizophrenia will be discussed elsewhere.

Depression: Favorable results in depression were reported in the beginning of chlorpromazine therapy, but have not been confirmed since, and there is no doubt that the anti-depressant drugs are much more effective. While agitation as a symptom in depression may be relieved by chlorpromazine, the underlying depression is often sharpened (Goldman). Baker found that even in favorable cases the depression recurred as soon as the drug was discontinued. Better results can be obtained in the reactive depressions where the drug decreases the tension associated with the adverse circumstances. Labhardt found that the periodically occurring depressions were not prevented by prophylactic chlorpromazine medication.

Manic Syndromes: All neuroleptic drugs have a calming effect on manic excitement, and render the patient less toxic, drowsy or inaccessible than would drugs such as the barbiturates. In an illness so prone to eventual spontaneous remission, it is difficult to assess how far the drug is curative and how far it serves only to lessen the symptoms which will return when the drug is stopped. Baker and others found that manics usually show a return of their symptoms, when the drug is withdrawn.

Labhardt has emphasized that the action of chlorpromazine is fundamentally different in schizophrenia, manic-depressive psychosis and neuroses. In his experience, it is possible to remove the basic symptoms in schizophrenia and to have a curative effect on the disease process. However, in the manic-depressive psychoses the drug effect is much more superficial with a temporary alleviation of symptoms only. The neuroses are never fundamentally influenced by chlorpromazine and at best certain associated autonomic symptoms disappear. Even this minor improvement could not always be maintained with maintenance therapy, especially when external factors proved disabling. On the other hand, schizophrenics who had improved or remitted with chlorpromazine exhibited excellent resistance to external stress. This is, incidentally, regarded by Labhardt as an argument against the view that neuroses are the precursors of schizophrenia.

When chlorpromazine is given in the early stages of a manic attack, it can prevent the development of the acute manic picture, but its use in high doses has to be carefully supervised, since we have seen manics who, treated with thorazine became acutely depressed within 24 hours, necessitating a course of ECT; and there have been a number of similar reports in the literature.

Symptomatic Psychoses: Symptomatic psychoses due to various causes were first observed by H. H. Meyer as being highly responsive to the effect of chlorpromazine. The etiology of the psychosis must be treated primarily wherever possible, but, whatever the cause, the symptomatology of these acute psychotic reactions responds extremely well to the drug. Meyer reported good results in acute post-traumatic psychoses, epileptic clouded states, eclamptic psychoses, delirium tremens, withdrawal psychosis in barbiturate addicts, psychoses consequent upon thyrotoxicosis and cardiovascular disturbances, as well as in other toxic and infectious conditions producing mental manifestations. Organic confusional states such as arteriosclerotic brain disease and senile dementia where there is agitation and disturbed behavior are also helped symptomatically, although of course the underlying disease process is not reversed. Bonello and Pollack reported good results in the relief of the mental and physical symptoms of Huntington's chorea, although again this was purely symptomatic. Thorazine was found to facilitate the management of disturbed epileptics when given by Bonafede in addition to their usual anti-convulsant medication. Miles describes a case of phantom limb pain with psychosis, both of which responded to the drug.

Alcoholism. Withdrawal from drugs: Delay et al. reported favorable results in delirium tremens in 1952, and Letailleur has used a technique which is based on the slow intravenous injection of chlorpromazine in a warm saline solution in combination with barbiturates such as nembutal. These injections are given during the acute phase and are followed by oral medication. Kammerer and Ebtinger, who also had good results, regard acute intoxication where there has been recent alcohol intake (chlorpromazine potentiates alcohol), serious infections and grave cardiovascular insufficiency as contra-indications for the drug. Friedhoff and Zitrin, in a comparative study of the actions of chlorpromazine and paraldehyde in delirium tremens, found that they were both non-specific therapies. Chlorpromazine had a slower onset of action, patients treated with it recovering in 8 days, while those on paraldehyde were better in 6. However, it had advantages in that the chlorpromazine patients could be more readily aroused for feeding and care than the others.

Today, the introduction of chlormethiazol (distraneurin) which is described in Chapter VI of this book, has largely eliminated the use of chlorpromazine and other neuroleptics in delirium tremens in those countries, where this new drug is available. It will probably soon find a still wider use in all countries, all the more as the danger of chlorpromazine for the circulatory system in patients with delirium tremens is increasingly recognized.

Kielholz was the first to recommend a combination of insulin and chlorpromazine for morphine and barbiturate withdrawal in addicts, emphasizing the improvement of sleep by means of this treatment. Friedgold and Ripstein, who had favorable results from a regime of initial injections of chlorpromazine (50 mg. i.v. followed by 100 mg. i.m., four hourly for 2 to 3 days), with subsequent oral medication, believe that two of the reasons for its success are the powerful anti-emetic action and the central and autonomic nervous system depression. Fraser and Isbell, however, did not consider that the drug helped to alleviate withdrawal symptoms, although, in their series of cases, they gave it orally or intramuscularly in smaller doses than the previous observers, which might account for their negative findings.

Cummins and Friend advise a combination of chlorpromazine with disulfiram (Antabuse) in treating alcohol withdrawal symptoms. Their regime consisted of an initial dose of 100 mg. of chlorpromazine with 500 mg disulfiram orally, followed by 50 mg. chlorpromazine in 6 and 24 hours' time. After a further 24 hours, disulfiram 50 mg. is given with 25 mg. chlorpromazine and then the disulfiram is continued in the same dosage daily for a week. The chlorpromazine suppresses the nausea and vomiting of the disulfiram-alcohol reaction and can be given intramuscularly if necessary. They found that the results were better with the combination than with chlorpromazine alone. Oral chlorpromazine may help to prevent the onset of delirium in cases where there are prodromal signs or where a sudden cessation of alcohol intake is necessary.

Psychoneuroses: Chlorpromazine and other neuroleptics are used extensively in neurotic patients, but here we know less what they accomplish than in the psychoses. One of the complicating factors is that most neurotic patients receive some form of psychotherapy in addition to the drug, and it is difficult to discern to what extent the drug or the psychotherapy should be credited for improvements. One of the first double blind studies of the value of chlorpromazine in the treatment of anxiety and tension states was that of Rees and Lambert. Their results showed 66 per cent improvement with the drug as compared to 10 per cent with the placebo. Continued treatment increased the favorable results in some cases, but in others the benefit was only temporary. In view of the relationship of chlorpromazine to phenergan and its vagolytic effect, Rees tried it in patients with asthma, hoping for a reduction in emotional tension. Although there was alleviation of anxiety, the incidence of asthma attacks remained the same, possibly one of the factors being that chlorpromazine is more anti-adrenergic than vagolytic. Garmany et al. and Silverman found that tension and anxiety were the symptoms most benefited, and that the results were not good if there were predominant depressive or hysterical features. Silverman noted that some obsessional states were improved, and stated that no obsessional patient should undergo leucotomy before chlorpromazine has been tried. However, long-term results in obsessional neurosis have been disappointing (Hoch), with frequent relapse and inability to maintain any improvement (Trethowan and Scott). Moyer who obtained remissions varying from complete recovery to relief of symptoms in 94.9 per cent of patients diagnosed as tension states and 90 per cent with anxiety neuroses, failed to obtain improvement in conversion hysteria.

In general, it is agreed that the action of chlorpromazine in the neuroses is much less spectacular than in psychoses, and that its main role is one of symptomatic relief of tension with little, if any, effect on the underlying neurotic mechanism. Because of its calming abilities it has been used in a number of psychosomatic disorders, such as certain skin lesions and migraine, where anxiety is considered to play an important etiological part. As emphasized by Winkelman, personality disorders and chronic hypochondriasis are not improved, the latter group of patients often making much of the drug's side-effects. Hoch concluded that if a psychoneurosis does not have anxiety or tension as the main symptoms, or if vegetative-nervous-system manifestations are not in the foreground, these drugs are ineffective. In the subsequent chapter, the role of drugs in psychotherapy will be discussed.

Disturbed Children: Heuyer in 1955 reported very favorable results in children with schizophrenia, post-encephalitic personality changes, and epileptic psychoses, although with sometimes increased convulsions in the latter group. There were apparently fewer neurological or vascular side effects than in adults. Its greatest value is in the hyperkinetic schizophrenic child (Freedman et al.). The action is similar to that in adults with mainly symptomatic improvement. Drugs in child psychiatry were extensively studied by B. Fish.

Good results have also been obtained in disturbed mental defectives, and Bair and Herold demonstrated an average increase in IQ of 10.4 points in a group of hyperactive defectives after they had received chlorpromazine for 60 days. Adamson in a controlled study found that, in a group of mentally retarded children, the placebo group showed improvements such as a reduction in tension and self mutilative behavior during the first 6 weeks of the trial in 80 per cent, but then gradually regressed until only 40 per cent showed improvement by the eighth week of treatment. In contrast, 90 per cent of the chlorpromazine group showed improvement maintained over the entire 8 week period on a dosage of 100 to 400 mg. The familial and post-encephalitic forms of mental deficiency responded less well than mongols, those with congenital malformations, or defect as a result of cerebral trauma or degenerative disease. It is of interest to speculate on the environmental causes of the improvement in the placebo group; such factors as increased attention, as well as more subtle alterations in staff attitudes, probably played a part. Although Ison found no significant increase in IQ scores in defectives treated with thorazine for 30 days, there was some evidence that a greater degree of motor relaxation had been produced in those patients as distinct from the controls.

Effect on Induced Psychosis: Schwarz and his co-workers have reported that, when given intramuscularly in small doses, chlorpromazine has a blocking effect on LSD and mescaline psychosis. Denber and Merlis have utilized its action on mescaline psychosis in a treatment procedure for acute and chronic schizophrenics. They gave 0.5 g. of mescaline intravenously at the rate of 2 cc. per minute and then talked to the patient, but without attempting interpretation. Mescaline produced a free flow of conflictual material in a setting of anxiety and tension, which was later successfully relieved by the administration of chlorpromazine 50 mg. intramuscularly. The relief of tension brought about by chlorpromazine enabled the patient to look at the psychotherapeutic material obtained during the interview in a state of tranquility.

MODES OF ADMINISTRATION: Chlorpromazine can be given orally, intramuscularly, or intravenously, diluted as an injection or more usually by drip. It can cause subcutaneous necrosis and should always be given by deep injection into the large muscle masses, preferably the glutei. Oral administration can be in the form of sugar coated pills, a syrup, or sustained release capsules, which were found by Kris to be especially valuable in the maintenance treatment of discharged and working hospital patients.

The French workers have made extensive use of the intravenous drip method. Denber has described the method used by Requet, who gives agitated patients 50-100 mg. of chlorpromazine in 350 cc. of sterile saline intravenously over a period of 3 to 4 hours. This treatment can be continued twice daily for up to 15 days, the average length being 10 days. The only danger is the occasional production of a periphlebitis. McNair used a similar technique in patients with acute anxiety, giving up to 25 treatments. Both Baruk in France and Neri in Italy used a 4 per cent solution of largactil which corresponded to 1 mg. per drop, but both found frequent reactivation of latent infections of various kinds. Lecomte who also uses a continuous drip technique for disturbed patients, commences with intravenous sodium amytal which is followed by chlorpromazine.

It has sometimes been observed that patients may show little response to oral doses as high as 1200 mg., but will respond to small intramuscular injections of 25 mg. three times daily. Tuteur has raised the question of a "gastrointestinal blood barrier," preventing adequate absorption of oral chlorpromazine, to explain this. Many authors started routinely with intramuscular administration followed, after alleviation of the most disturbing symptoms, by oral administration. The vast majority of patients are probably treated orally only.

Combinations with Other Drugs: In the beginning of psychiatric drug therapy many authors preferred to administer chlorpromazine together with other drugs, especially with sedatives. Today, these methods have only very little importance.

"Artificial Hibernation" was first used in 1952 by Deschamps producing narcosis of two weeks by using chlorpromazine to potentiate the effects of relatively small quantities of barbiturates. In addition, phenergan and diparcol were used; diparcol has a vagal blocking action which complements the antiadrenergic action of chlorpromazine. Charatan found that 150 mg. of chlorpromazine, 0.6 g. of barbiturate, 150 mg. diparcol and 50 mg. phenergan were required to produce 12 to 14 hours sleep per day. Particularly in the French literature there are numerous reports on the combination of barbiturates with chlorpromazine as safer than barbiturates alone. Such sleep treatment, also given in the Soviet Union, can be used in many psychiatric conditions, including neuroses and addiction. Usually, small amounts of chlorpromazine are used to avoid the dangers of circulatory collapse. While there are no comparative studies on sleep treatment with the barbiturates alone and in combination with chlorpromazine, it appears that the former is, because of its dangers, applicable only for short periods up to three weeks, whereas combination with neuroleptic drugs is considered a more innocuous treatment which can be used whenever prolonged action is required, e.g., as maintenance treatment when the acute illness is over.

Dosage: There is no general agreement as to whether the course of treatment should be short and intensive or more prolonged with a lower dosage. Neither is there any concurrence as to the optimum dose level which will produce the maximum benefit. In schizophrenia, doses of 75 to 150 mg. daily were advocated by Alsen and Johansson, and from 800 up to 3600 mg. by Kinross Wright. The exact amount required will depend on the individual reaction to the drug and has to be determined by clinical assessment. It has been claimed that dosages are lower in Europe than in the United States. Some authorities have considered that the maximum therapeutic efficacy is obtained on quite low doses. Delay, and Ayd felt that results could not be improved by giving more than 300 mg. or 500 mg. daily, respectively. Pollack thought that the dose which gave the greatest degree of benefit in his cases was 800 mg. Denber and Bird found that, on the average, females required a higher dose than males.

Treatment should commence with small doses, 25 to 50 mg., three times daily, particularly in those patients most liable to hypotensive effects such as elderly arteriosclerotics and hypertensives. In those patients who are extremely disturbed, higher initial doses, possibly given intramuscularly, may be necessary. With this type of patient, where there is often a high tolerance to sedatives, there should be great care if chlorpromazine is combined with barbiturates, especially if given by intravenous administration, since the two drugs potentiate each other. We have seen a case of severe vasomotor collapse in a hypertensive patient with an agitated organic reaction who was given large doses of intravenous sodium amytal and thorazine within a short space of time.

For children, manufacturers recommend that those under 5 should be given 1 mg. per kg. body weight two or three times daily, while those over the age of 5 should receive one third to one half of the adult dose.

Tolerance develops, according to Sainz, between the second and third month of medication, necessitating an increase of dose to maintain the clinical improvement. Also, Rees and Lambert found that relapses occurred under constant dosage in 78 out of 117 cases of anxiety states. On the other hand, Feldman obtained no evidence of tolerance formation. Of his patients, 85.4 per cent on annual review were receiving dosages identical to or smaller than those they were receiving a year ago. Part of the explanation for this discrepancy of findings may be that, during the early stages of treatment, to keep the improvement or to increase it, more of the drug must be given; but, once the maximum benefit is obtained, the maintenance dose can be kept constant.

Neurotics, however, are notoriously prone to fluctuate in their condition no matter what medication is given, and so the amount of a drug required to maintain an improvement in them would not necessarily remain constant.

DURATION OF TREATMENT: Much controversy has raged over the question of how long a patient, particularly a schizophrenic, should remain on the drug if it is helping him. Kinross-Wright has divided these patients into those with an acute illness, where the drug can be withdrawn within a month; chronic patients without many paranoid or obsessive features, where a daily maintenance dose is required which can be progressively reduced; and those with fixed paranoid or obsessive features who require a maintenance dose for an indefinite time. In chronic patients, where the illness is ameliorated by the drug but where the basic symptomatology is unchanged, most observers have noted relapse when the drug was stopped. Pollack reported that the continued use of a small maintenance dose of chlorpromazine caused a marked reduction in the relapse rate. Winkelman found that the relapse rate after the drug was discontinued was 80 per cent in six months. Good et al. noted that chlorpromazine could be withdrawn from chronic schizophrenics for ten to twelve weeks without any noticeable change, but after this period there was a marked deterioration. This is in contrast to the observation by Brooks, Ayd, and many others that patients relapse almost immediately after the medication is discontinued. Good saw no relationship between the duration of previous chlorpromazine treatment and relapse after its withdrawal; but a resumption of the treatment after three months without it has the same beneficial effect as if treatment had been continuous. Ayd was able to observe the effects of prolonged administration of chlorpromazine over a period of two to four years without untoward side-effects on the blood, kidneys or liver, but Feldman still saw skin rashes and parkinsonian syndromes as well as low white blood counts in a small minority of cases after two years of medication.

Acute schizophrenics with short duration of illness, if treated with the drugs, should be tentatively withdrawn after two or three months to see whether the symptoms have actually disappeared or whether they have only been covered up by the drug. The quite different problem in acute and chronic schizophrenics will be discussed extensively later. In chronic schizophrenics, medication can and should be administered indefinitely without untoward effects.

2. *Promazine (Sparine, Prazine, Liranol, Verophene)*

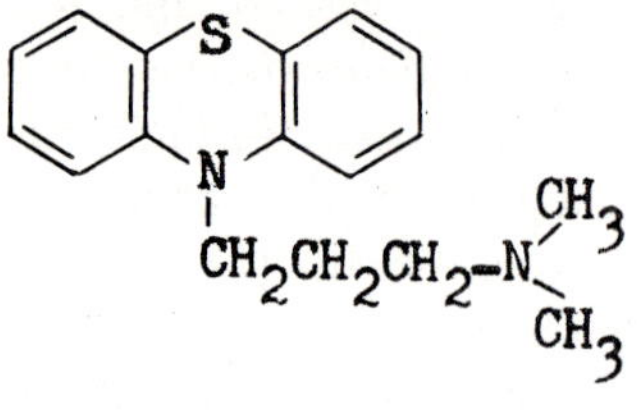

Promazine is 10-[3-(dimethylamino)propyl]-phenothiazine.

RESULTS OF CLINICAL INVESTIGATIONS: It has been used for the treatment of the same psychiatric conditions as chlorpromazine, but a number of studies have demonstrated that it is less effective.

In a study of its action in schizophrenia, the Veterans Administration obtained results on 800 patients treated for 12 weeks in four groups, which received either 400 mg. of chlorpromazine, 400 mg. of promazine, 180 mg. of phenobarbital, or a placebo daily. It was shown that promazine, while being more effective than either the placebo or barbiturate, was not as potent as chlorpromazine, and the superiority of the latter has been established by other studies such as those of Fleming et al. and Gilmore and Shatin. Rudy et al. found it superior to mepazine.

Fazekas et al. claimed good results in delirium tremens and the withdrawal symptoms of heroin addiction. He used intravenous injection of 200 to 300 mg. of sparine within 5 to 10 minutes and then maintained the patient on oral medication for a few days. If sparine alone failed to control symptoms, he advised its combination with 100 to 200 mg. of pentobarbital sodium intravenously. It has also been extensively recommended for use in geriatrics since it was claimed that it had less hypotensive effect than chlorpromazine. As with most neuroleptic drugs, patients tend to relapse when medication is stopped as shown in an otherwise favorable report by Fink and Vlavianos.

Being a less potent neuroleptic than chlorpromazine, promazine is widely used outside of psychiatry (Fazekas et al.). In obstetrics it serves to prepare women for childbirth, and it is recommended for such post-partum conditions as eclampsia (Matthews; Bielefeld). It should not be overlooked, however, that promazine is transmitted through the placenta to the fetus in whom high blood concentrations are found, when promazine is administered intravenously to the mother.

Promazine is still widely used in alcoholism, although recent reports are more critical. Thus, Schwarz et al., in a double-blind study, did not find promazine more effective than placebo in prophylaxis or treatment of withdrawal symptoms in alcoholics.

Mode of Administration and Dosage: It may be given orally either in tablet form, or as a suspension in the form of promazine embonate, or by injection. It does not produce as much muscle tenderness, pain, or local tissue reaction after intramuscular injection as does chlorpromazine. Opinsky et al. report a case of arterial thrombosis with gangrene after the inadvertent arterial injection of sparine, and it is advised that, when the drug is administered intravenously, it should be diluted with equal amounts of saline.

The usual oral dose is up to 1000 mg. daily in divided doses, although some workers have given larger amounts. Intramuscularly, it can be administered in amounts up to 200 mg. every 4 to 6 hours. For intravenous use, 50 to 150 mg. should be given slowly and can be repeated in 15 minutes if the desired calming effect is not obtained, provided that the total given does not exceed 300 mg.

3. *Triflupromazine (Vesprin, Vespral, Psyquil)*

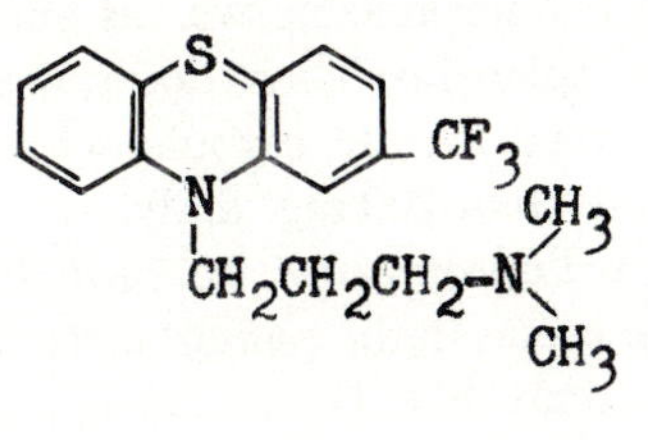

Triflupromazine is 10- [3-(dimethylamino)-propyl] -2-(trifluoromethyl)-phenothiazine.

Results of Clinical Investigations: There has been a number of favorable reports on the value of vesprin. Hegarty reported enthusiastically on the drug used in chronic disturbed schizophrenics. The paranoid group had the best results. Ilem and Sainz considered results superior to chlorpromazine in acute schizophrenics as measured by both the greater number of remissions and the better quality of the improvement. In the chronic group, the paranoid and catatonic patients obtained the greatest benefit. Among the neuroses, only the obsessive-compulsive group was improved, while in the other groups there was a high incidence of akathisia which was very disadvantageous. They did not consider it superior to chlorpromazine in the therapy of manics, where there was a slowing of the psychomotor excitement but no change in affect and thinking. It was of no value in depressions, but the agitation and insomnia in cases of senile dementia was relieved, although the patients still remained confused. Another favorable report was published by Pennington.

There have been a number of papers on the effects of trifluopromazine in the treatment of alcoholic psychoses. Fox used it to cover the withdrawal symptoms because advantages are that the drug is less hypotensive and has less potentiating effect on alcohol or sedatives. Because of the dangers of sudden collapse in these patients with a high blood alcohol, the author commenced with small doses, usually 20 mg. intramuscularly which was repeated if the patient did not go to sleep. One side-effect noted was the development of hyperventilation in a few patients which occasionally necessitated the drug being withdrawn.

The frequently mentioned lack of adequately controlled studies applies as well as to the other phenothiazines. One of the relatively few controlled trials which attempted to measure the degree of improvement in terms of objective criteria was that of Hegarty and Dabbs who compared a group of schizophrenics treated with vesprin to a similar group given a placebo. While there was a marked improvement in the vesprin-treated group as compared to the control group, the main response was in the sphere of social behavior and in the diminution of the florid schizophrenic symptoms such as delusions and hallucinations. There was a much smaller improvement in fundamental thought disorder assessed objectively by psychological tests. Walsh et al., in a similar controlled trial, compared vesprin with both chlorpromazine and a placebo. They also found that no therapeutic differences could be demonstrated by tests in favor of either of the two drugs as compared to the placebo. However, it is of interest that the nursing staff, when asked to assess the patients' progress, regarded a larger proportion of the chlorpromazine- and vesprin-treated patients as "much improved" than those on the placebo. It may be that there are some elements of response to the drugs which the tests are inadequate to measure, or that any improvement is superficial and not associated with any change in the deeper psychotic mechanisms. Contrary to the findings of Walsh et al., Roebuck and his co-workers reported that triflupromazine was as effective as chlorpromazine and more effective than a placebo. Their doses were rather lower since none of the patients, who were mainly chronic schizophrenics with a very poor prognosis, received more than 200 mg. daily.

The contradictory conclusions of reports on triflupromazine are probably due to a relatively larger number of acute schizophrenics in the patient material of favorable studies. In chronic schizophrenics some, like Hanlon et al., reported favorably, while most authors came to negative conclusions (Smith et al.). Altogether, triflupromazine seems to be equal but certainly not superior to chlorpromazine. Today, it is, therefore, used in some countries less as a neuroleptic than an antiemetic (Goethe).

MODE OF ADMINISTRATION AND DOSAGE: It may be given orally, as tablets, capsules, or as an emulsion, or intramuscularly or intravenously. The use of the easily swallowed emulsion is particularly appropriate in the management of the geriatric patient. The emulsion is non-irritating, which is a further advantage since it has been noted that phenothiazines in tablet form can produce sloughing of the mucous membrane of the mouth in some patients, particularly senile or catatonic schizophrenics who hold the tablets in the mouth for a prolonged period.

The dosage used by various investigators has been variable; and some, such as Roebuck et al. and Azima et al., have claimed that a daily oral dose of under 200 mg. is sufficient in chronic schizophrenic cases, while Ilem and Sainz gave up to 1200 mg. daily. For acute cases, their dosage was even higher, the maximum being 6000 mg. daily in a paranoid schizophrenic who, despite this massive dose, displayed only a moderate degree of extrapyramidal signs, readily controlled by parsidol. Psychoneurotics were given an average of 100 mg. daily, the maximum level being 400 mg. daily.

4. *Methopromazine (Tentone, Mopazine)*

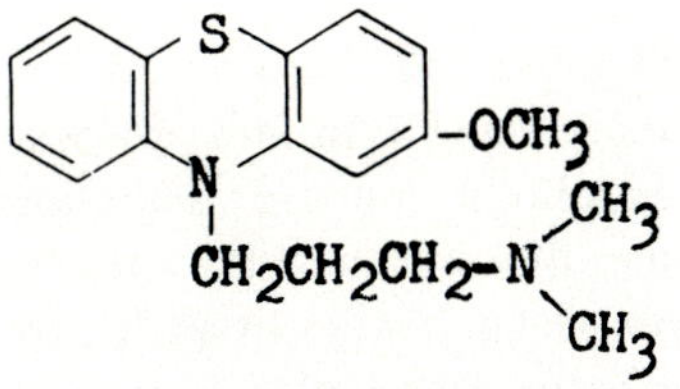

Methopromazine which is 10- [3-(dimethylamino)propyl] -2-methoxyphenothiazine, was first reported on by Delay et al. Gosline et al. found that it was not very potent but had fewer side-effects than many of the other phenothiazines. Today, it is hardly used as a neuroleptic in schizophrenics, but as a tranquilizer in anxiety and tension states. In these conditions it is sufficient to give 30 to 100 mg. daily, while in hyperactive patients 100 to 500 mg. are needed.

5. *Acepromazine (Plegicil, Notensil)*

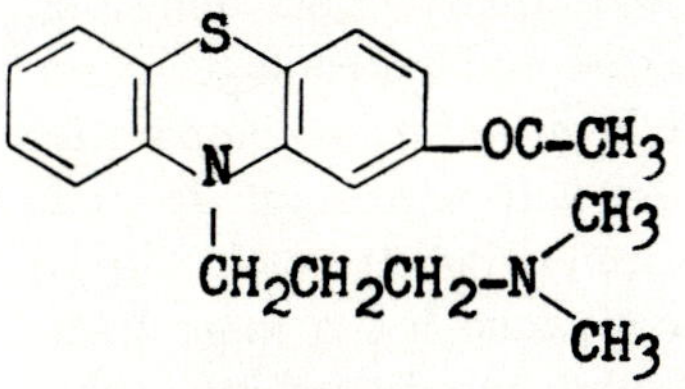

Acepromazine is 10- [3-(dimethylamino)-propyl] -2-acetylphenothiazine. Like methopromazine this drug has never been widely used. While the first clinical investigations (Delay et al.) seemed to show that acepromazine acts as a neuroleptic in schizophrenics and manics, its potency, compared to the newer neuroleptics, is so weak that this drug today has hardly any place in the pharmacotherapy of the psychoses.

A favorable report in the American literature is by Tolan et al. who also reviewed the literature of the drug. They gave 40 to 120 mg. and found significant improvements in behavior. There was a low incidence of parkinsonism but some incidents of confusion and excitement. Simpson found the drug to be of no value in chronic psychotics and noted that it could increase aggression and overactivity, while at the same time it did not activate withdrawn patients. Urquhart and Forrest used it in doses of 75 mg. three times daily and concluded that neither this drug nor promazine was effective enough to replace chlorpromazine and reserpine. Given intravenously in a dose of 100 mg. by Ferguson it had some action in suppressing overactivity. In chronic schizophrenics O'Reilly et al. found it largely ineffective. Attempts to obtain better results with larger doses led to hypertension and occasional convulsions (Collard and Maggs).

6. *Methotrimeprazine or Levomepromazine (Veractil, Nozinan, Neurocil)*

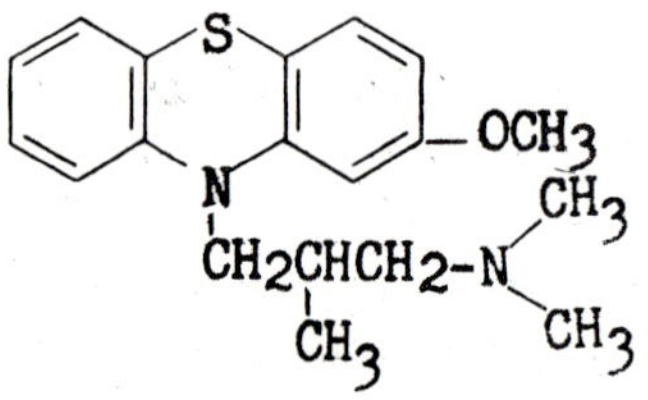

Methotrimeprazine or levomepromazine is 10- [3-(dimethylamino)-2-methylpropyl] -2-methoxyphenothiazine.

Results of Clinical Investigations: Methotrimeprazine has been used in all the conditions in which chlorpromazine has been found to be indicated, but its main difference from other phenothiazines is that claims have been made for the efficacy of methotrimeprazine in depressions, particularly where there is agitation and anxiety; that methotrimeprazine has more sedative effect than chlorpromazine (Tölle); and that methotrimeprazine has remarkable analgesic properties (Lasagna and De Kornfeld).

The first clinical reports on the drug were by Sigwald et al., who found improvement in a varied patient group, including manics, schizophrenics, depressions of neurotic and psychotic type, and anxiety and phobic states. Deschamps and Madre similarly found good results in depressive illnesses, and they noted a better response in psychotic than in neurotic depressions. Trelles et al. found improvement in a small group of elderly melancholics some of whom had failed to respond to ECT. In general, the neurotic depressions, apart from those where there is considerable anxiety, do not respond well, but good results have been reported in other types of depression, including that associated with marked hypochondria. Sigwald et al. regard the main indication as the endogenous depressions, especially with associated anxiety and delusions. Again, various studies have differed as to the degree and percentage of improvement in each diagnostic category. There have been so far no comparative studies between methotrimeprazine and any of the anti-depressant drugs to ascertain the relative efficacy, speed and degree of remission. It would appear from the studies performed so far that methotrimeprazine has a more beneficial effect on the anxiety and agitation associated with the depression, rather than on the depressive mood itself, and, while it may be a useful adjuvant to the treatment of these illnesses, the primary therapy is still either ECT or one of the antidepressants. When these treatments remove the depression but fail to remove the concomitant anxiety and restlessness, methotrimeprazine is indicated, although this drug has always been used more in Europe than in the United States.

The marked sedative hypnotic effect of methotrimeprazine lends itself very well to the removal of acute psychotic excitement states, where intramuscular application is well tolerated because, contrary to chlorpromazine, methotrimeprazine has no tissue-damaging effect (Bucci and Saunders). Its parenteral use in agitated geriatric patients was recommended but may lead to hypotension and intensify confusion (Sarwer-Foner et al.).

There have been favorable reports of the use of the drug in chronic schizophrenia by observers such as Baker and Thorpe, who found in a controlled trial that the drug was as effective as chlorpromazine. Quinn et al. have compared the action of methotrimeprazine with both chlorpromazine and a placebo in chronic schizophrenia, and also found that the results with methotrimeprazine were at least as good as with chlorpromazine, but that, in general, the beneficial effects of both drugs, although undoubtedly present, were of a moderate nature only, involving improvement in active psychotic symptoms such as delusions and hallucinations and in social and work activities. They discuss the discrepancy that they found between the medical and nursing staff's assessment of the patients, the nursing staff giving a higher improvement rate to the placebo group, and at the same time putting a higher percentage of medicated patients into the "worse" category.

The drug has similar actions to chlorpromazine in manic and other excitement. In the neuroses, the results are variable as with the other phenothiazines. Baruk et al. found that there was considerable improvement in obsessional neuroses, some of whom showed a return to more normal behavior patterns and a decrease in obsessional thinking. Faure et al. found that in mentally defective children the drug produced a decrease in anxiety and a lessening of disturbed behavior.

Methotrimeprazine proved to be very effective in self-destructive children (Mizes et al.). Svennebye et al. noticed that in children daily doses of 100 mg. may lead to "false" positive reactions in tests for phenylketonuria which is rarely seen in related phenothiazines like chlorpromazine or promethazine.

Sigwald and his co-workers have used methotrimeprazine in a group of neurological disorders including upper motor lesions and parkinsonism, and obtained temporary symptomatic improvement with intravenous injections in doses of 25 to 50 mg. Their most interesting finding was the relief of post-herpetic neuralgia as well as in the pain of acute herpes zoster and of trigeminal neuralgia with doses up to 400 mg. This analgesic effect was later taken up by several others. Lasagna and De Kornfeld evaluated this effect in postoperative pain. Given orally, the drug did not relieve pain more than a placebo, and larger oral doses caused dizziness and drowsiness. However, if given by injection methotrimeprazine provided pain relief comparable to that achieved with similar doses of morphine. Montilla et al. found that the dosis ratio of morphine to methotrimeprazine is 10 to 15 mg. for subcutaneous injections. The same dosis ratio between morphine and methotrimeprazine (2 to 3) was found by Bloomfield et al. for intramuscular injections. The strong analgesic effect is important because it was demonstrated that methotrimeprazine does not cause addiction (Fraser and Rosenberg).

Mode of Administration and Dosage: The drug may be administered orally, intramuscularly, and also intravenously, but there is a danger of postural hypotension. Lambert et al. gave the drug by slow intravenous infusion of 50 to 100 mg. to psychotic patients.

The dose required is approximately two thirds that of chlorpromazine in comparable cases. The usual intramuscular dose is 25 mg., and this should be given with the patient recumbent. In cases of severe excitement, a systemic dose of 50 mg. can be given provided that precautions are taken to check the pulse and the blood pressure carefully. The commencing oral dosage should be between 25 and 50 mg. daily for ambulatory patients and 100 to 200 mg. in severely psychotic cases. This may be gradually increased to a total of 1000 mg. if necessary, provided that the side-effects do not become severe. Since children are particularly prone to the side-effects of hypotension and drowsiness, they should receive a total daily dose of not more than 40 mg.

7. *Chlorprothixene (Taractan, Truxal, Solatran)*

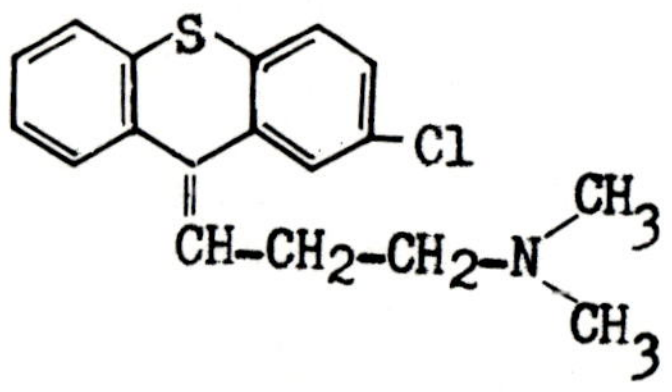

Chlorprothixene, the oldest known member of the thioxanthene group of tricyclic neuroleptics, is 2-chloro-9-(3-methylaminopropylidene)thioxanthene. It differs from chlorpromazine by having a carbon atom instead of a nitrogen atom in the central ring of the tricyclic ring system, where the basic side chain is inserted. Of the two possible isomeres of the compound the one with neuroleptic effect is the trans-isomere.

Results of Clinical Investigations: Chemical synthesis and pharmacological studies suggested that chlorprothixene in its clinical aspects would be closely related to its corresponding phenothiazine analogue, chlorpromazine. Therefore, Ravn in Denmark carried out extensive uncontrolled trials in schizophrenics, and stressed the relief of tension and agitation, and the "antipsychotic" effect in paranoid syndromes. Like Ravn, Arnold in Austria found it useful not only in schizophrenics and manics but also in depressions. He, therefore, called it a "broad spectrum neuroleptic." This surprising antidepressive effect of a neuroleptic drug was seen by Feer et al. and Pöldinger in Switzerland, as the greatest advantage of chlorprothixene, and Chantraine and Pairoux concurred. In the United States Kruse stressed already in 1960 the antidepressive properties of the drug which, according to Geller are more marked in low doses of 50 mg. and less, while the neuroleptic effect is more pronounced in daily doses of 100 mg. and more. Gross and Kaltenbäck denied a true antidepressive effect but found the neuroleptic action particularly suitable for the agitation of depressed patients without intensifying depressed mood. Many other investigators like Barsa and Saunders in the United States questioned the antidepressive effect which may be partly explained by attempts to force antidepressive action with high doses (Haydu et al.; Denber et al.).

Hoffet and Cornu and most others found fewer side-effects than with chlorpromazine. Even high doses of chlorprothixene give minimal extrapyramidal symptom as also seen in a double blind study by Remvig and Sonne who compared chlorpromazine and chlorprothixene in schizophrenics and manics with a dose ratio of 15 mg. chlorprothixene to 25 mg. chlorpromazine. In a cooperative double blind study of the Veterans Administration (Lasky et al.) chlorprothixene given for 24 weeks, was slightly superior to chlorpromazine, thioridazine and fluphenazine, equal to triflupromazine, and better than reserpine. Today the well tolerated chlorprothixene, though also used in hospitalized schizophrenics, probably has its main application in the after-care of discharged psychotics (Flegel et al.) as well as in neurotics.

In disturbed geriatric patients Smith and Barron recommend chlorprothixene because of the relative absence of side-effects including hypotension. Initial mild drowsiness tends to disappear after a few days. In disturbed children Harman and Winn found that the calming effect leads less often to regression than when chlorpromazine is given. In brain damaged children Kohlmann and Rett noted that the calming effect of chlorprothixene improves functioning only in erratic children but lowers performance in less disturbed brain damaged children due to diminished concentration and impaired visual motor coordination. In non-brain damaged problem children Grünewald et al. showed in a double-blind study that cognitive learning was not influenced by doses up to 45 mg. daily. Here, contrary to brain damaged children, special performances requiring a careful survey of alternatives like learning of differentiation in the experimental situation, was significantly improved. Although visual motor coordination became slower, the children made fewer errors in the test.

The tranquilizing effect of larger intramuscular doses of chlorprothixene has also been used in the treatment of psychoses due to alcohol (Alsen and Frey; Neumann and Peters).

Mode of Administration and Dosage: The dosage of chlorprothixene, like that of chlorpromazine, varies widely. In depressed patients oral doses of 15 to 50 mg. daily are sufficient. In schizophrenics 100 to 500 mg. are necessary, and maintenance doses of up to 150 mg. are adequate. Acute excitement states are controlled by intramuscular injection of 30 to 100 mg. which can be repeated without danger, and Hagopian and Crossfield used initial doses of up to 900 mg., whereby hypotension is best prevented by bedrest. Parenteral use of chlorprothixene has the advantage of small amounts of fluid (50 mg. in 1 ml.) and a good local tolerability. Fincle and Johnson demonstrated in a double-blind study that the tolerance to high doses can be improved by gradual increase. In ambulatory patients injections are inadvisable because even 25 mg. may have too much of a dulling effect (Simpson). Barsa and Saunders who recommend combination of chlorprothixene with other drugs such as more potent neuroleptics, also showed the usefulness of a new liquid preparation (20 mg. in 1 ml. of juice) for long term treatment. This syrup with a sweet, pleasant tasting, fruit flavored base is also suitable in child psychiatry.

8. *Prothipendyl (Tolnate, Dominal)*

Prothipendyl is 10-(3-dimethylaminopropyl)-l-azaphenothiazine. Chemically it is closely related, among the phenothiazines, to promazine from which it

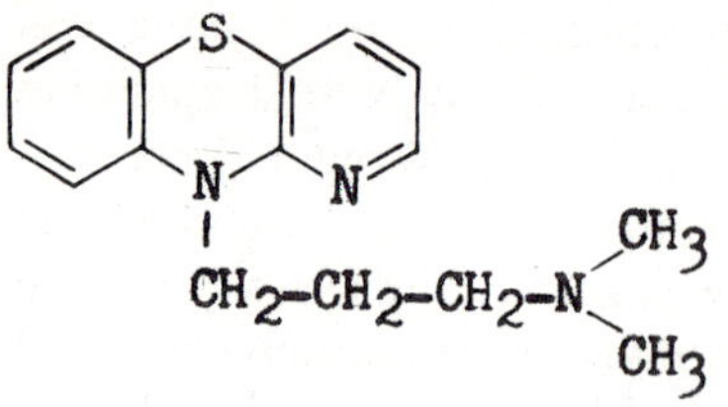

differs in the substitution of one of the two benzol rings of the phenothiazine ring system by a pyridine ring.

Clinical Results: When prothipendyl was introduced, Quandt as well as Hift and Kryspin-Exner pointed out that the drug is much better tolerated than chlorpromazine. Even in large doses no extrapyramidal motor symptoms were seen; and Richter and Müller showed that prothipendyl even controls Parkinson tremor, oculogyric crises and torticollis if given intravenously up to 0.65 mg./kg. In spite of this advantage it is not widely used because as a neuroleptic it is weaker than chlorpromazine and much weaker than the piperazinyl-phenothiazine and the butyrophenones. It is more popular for agitated patients in general medicine.

McKenzie and Rosewell-Harris as well as Jude et al. showed its usefulness for behavior disturbances of mentally subnormal patients. It is also indicated, whenever phenothiazines are ruled out because of allergies, jaundice, severe extrapyramidal symptoms or agranulocytosis (Edelstein and Assael). Since it does not have the hypotensive effect of chlorpromazine (Koranyi et al.), it still has a place in geriatric patients (Jessel; Messmer).

Mode of Administration and Dosage: In psychoses results comparable to other neuroleptics can only be obtained with high doses up to 1200 mg. In acute excitement states intravenous or intramuscular injection of 80 to 240 mg. are effective. Oral doses of 240 to 480 mg. daily can be given over a long period.

9. *Thioridazine (Mellaril, Melleril)*

Thioridazine, 2-methylmercapto-10 [2-(N-methyl-2-piperidyl)-ethyl] -phenothiazine, is the most widely used phenothiazine derivative with a piperidyl ring in the side chain.

Thioridazine was preceded by an earlier piperidine derivative known as NP 207 which was the chlorine analogue of thioridazine. This drug with a chlorine atom as substituent in the phenothiazine ring instead of the methylmercapto-group of thioridazine, never got beyond the experimental stage, because it was found to produce retinal degeneration. This retinopathy due to piperidylchlorophenothiazine (NP 207) should not be confused with the pigment deposits in lens and cornea, and in the skin, noticed since 1964 in many phenothiazine derivatives. The retina changes due to NP 207 come closest to the hereditary retinitis pigmentosa (Meier-Ruge) and were first reported in 1956 (Verrey; Kinross-Wright; Malitz and Hoch; Goar and Fletcher). They appear in spots and sometimes over a wider area (Burian and Fletcher), usually after eight weeks. Impaired vision in the sense of nightblindness disappears, when the drug is discontinued, although the pigmentation could still be seen after years.

Thioridazine, although chemically closely related to NP 207, fortunately fails to cause retinopathies except in very rare instances, when the drug was given in high doses for a long time. May et al. reported four such cases in treatment-resistant chronic psychotics who received up to more than 100,000 mg. given over an average of 43 days, i.e. daily doses of up to 4000 mg. Other cases after large doses were described by Weekley et al.; Connell et al.; Leinefelder and Burian; Hogopian et al. Visual disturbances usually preceded ophthalmoscopic findings, the latter probably representing already morphologic changes. In the usual daily dose of up to less than 600 mg. Applebaum showed that thioridazine is not damaging to the eyes as proven by the millions of patients treated over the years with this drug.

Clinical Results: Thioridazine has found such a wide application because of the relative absence of such side-effects as drowsiness which gives it a great advantage over chlorpromazine. Equally significant is that even patients on large doses show few extrapyramidal motor symptoms. Since it has been demonstrated again and again that good clinical results can be obtained with thioridazine without extrapyramidal side-effects, the often made assumption became doubtful that therapeutic action of a neuroleptic is related to its extrapyramidal motor effect. Most workers found thioridazine as effective as the majority of the other phenothiazines but very free from the serious toxic effects which are found with these other drugs. Kinross-Wright, who reported good results in a group of psychotic and neurotic patients, considered it to be as potent as chlorpromazine, milligram for milligram. Hollister et al. observed improvement in a large proportion of chronic schizophrenics previously refractory to other treatments. Neither of these trials was controlled; nor was that of Cohen, who reported results comparable to chlorpromazine in a group of hyperactive psychotics, while Barsa and Saunders found it less effective.

Reeves, in a controlled trial, found that thioridazine relieved the symptoms of anxiety, apprehension, functional fatigue and insomnia, tension headache and anxiety associated with duodenal ulcer and hypertension. In the latter group, there was a reduction in blood pressure of 30 to 40 mm. systolic and 5 to 10 mm. diastolic, but in the remaining patients the pressure was not significantly changed. Haug compared the results with thioridazine (mellaril) to those obtained with a placebo and with previous chlorpromazine treatment in a group of chronic schizophrenics. Chlorpromazine and thioridazine were equally effective, but chlorpromazine acted more rapidly and caused more apathy than mellaril, which was slower in action but did not interfere with the patient's functioning. Haug, therefore, concluded that the latter drug is indicated in the chronic case, while chlorpromazine should be used in acute syndromes. Rémy has found that, in a comparison of chlorpromazine and mellaril, the percentage helped was practically the same. However, when the relief of individual symptoms was compared, it was found that mellaril was more effective in states of agitation, excitement, delirium, and in depressive states with negativism. Delay also reported that mellaril was as effective as chlorpromazine and that the patients tolerated it better. There was less drowsiness and slowing of thought than with chlorpromazine, but he found it less effective in chronic psychotics and in cases with great agitation. He noted recovery and marked improvement particularly in manics and acute delirium. Aivazian agreed with Delay that acute schizophrenics are benefitted much more than chronic cases. He found that those symptoms favorably influenced were anxiety, tension, insomnia, anorexia and hallucinations, while the drug had much less effect on delusions, somatic complaints, withdrawal, negativism and depressive manifestations.

Over the years thioridazine has been included in various extensive, methodologically sound double-blind studies comparing mostly thioridazine and chlorpromazine, all coming to the conclusion that the therapeutic effect of the two drugs in acute and chronic schizophrenics is very similar (Borup Svendsen et al.; Waldrop et al.; Herman and Pleasure). Side-effects were also similar, but thioridazine showed fewer extrapyramidal signs. The NIMH Psychopharmacology Service Center Collaborative Study Group has compared the results in acute schizophrenics treated with thioridazine, fluphenazine, chlorpromazine and placebo. There was a highly significant difference in therapeutic efficacy between the drugs as a group and placebo (Goldberg et al.), but no significant difference between any of the three drugs. Side-effects differed with chlorpromazine and thioridazine showing a high incidence of drowsiness, dizziness, faintness and weakness. Thioridazine had no more extrapyramidal effect than placebo, but the highest incidence of anticholinergic side-effects like dryness of the mouth. A double-blind study by Hanlon et al. comparing thioridazine with chlorpromazine, triflupromazine, prochlorperazine, perphenazine, thiopropazate, triflouperazine and fluphenazine revealed no differences between these eight neuroleptics after 30 days. However, analysis of the more severely ill patients showed that thioridazine is a weaker neuroleptic than prochlorperazine, perphenazine and fluphenazine. In spite of some contradictory findings, thioridazine proved to be the best tolerated phenothiazine derivative.

The relative absence of extrapyramidal signs is of theoretical interest because in the opinion of Leger it contradicts the view that neuroleptic and extrapyramidal action are interdependent. In clinical practice the well tolerated thioridazine is increasingly used in long term treatment. It can be given for years without losing its effect (Leonhardt; Leger and many others). The lack of side-effects enables patients to participate in work therapy (Denys). This was also seen in hyperactive and aggressive mentally retarded children and adolescents (Abbott et al.; Rinsley). Thioridazine was equally valuable in the prevention of relapses and the rehabilitation of discharged patients.

The good tolerability of thioridazine extended its indications to the treatment of withdrawal symptoms of addicts (Mulvaney), psychopathological manifestations of epileptics without increasing the incidence of seizures (Kami and Mandel) and, geriatric patients (Judah et al.; Felger; Fleischl). In child psychiatry Wallinga recommends thioridazine in combination with psychotherapy for emotionally disturbed children, while Mises and Borenstein were able to keep children with anxiety in school with the help of this drug. The control of tension and anxiety in neurotic and psychosomatic disorders is facilitated by the absence of habituation which is a danger with many other drugs used in these conditions (Smith). Therefore, thioridazine is widely used in private psychiatric practice (Reeves; Bercel). Belin and Griffiths reported relief of anginal pain resistant to trinitroglycerine with 30 mg. daily of thioridazine.

Thioridazine is one of the few phenothiazines that have some antidepressive effect as first shown by Flügel et al. Later Bauer confirmed this "thymoleptic" effect and found that retarded depressions respond less well than those with hypochondriacal symptoms and delusions. Of other target symptoms in depressions agitation responded only if not very severe, and obsessive-compulsive symptoms not at all. In a double-blind study Overall et al. found the antidepressive effect of thioridazine equal to that of imipramine. In France, Schnetzler and Lamand confirmed this antidepressive effect, which Soulairac et al. saw only in affective psychoses but not in depressed schizophrenics or alcoholics. According to Nayrac et al., the anxiolytic effect of the drug makes it more useful in neurotics than in endogenous depressions.

Therapeutic use was made of a special side-effect of thioridazine. In 1961 Singh reported one and Freyhan three patients who, under thioridazine treatment, noticed loss of ejaculation with maintained erection. Further cases were reported by Green; Heller; Taubel. On this basis Singh as well as Nistri and De Luca suggested the use of thioridazine in the treatment of ejaculatio praecox, which Doepfmer did successfully with small doses of 25 to 75 mg., and which Haider used to control excessive masturbation. The unintentional loss of ejaculation may lead to severe anxiety (Greenberg and Carillo), and it appears that thioridazine has more endocrine effect than generally assumed.

Mode of Administration and Dosage: Hollister began treatment with 50 mg. orally three times daily increasing gradually over 25 days to 1600 mg. which was maintained for about three weeks, and then reduced to a maintenance level of 400 to 600 mg. daily. Kinross-Wright went to a maximum of 2400 mg. in chronic psychotics with a maintenance dose of 300 mg. No eye changes were noticed, but in view of the previously mentioned retinal changes patients on more than 100 mg. daily should be controlled ophthalmologically. Also Delay and co-workers recommend relatively high doses of 600 to 900 mg. in acute psychosis, and delusional syndromes may respond only after three months of large doses. Maintenance treatment of chronic patients requires an average of 300 mg. daily, and lower doses are sufficient for the prevention of relapses in ambulatory patients. In neurotic and psychosomatic conditions, a daily dose of 20 to 60 mg. may be sufficient. Anxiety states often require doses as high as those used in psychoses. The amount given in children is 10 to 40 mg. daily.

Intramuscular administration is purely tolerated according to Delay et al. Brill had good results with injectable thioridazine in acute alcoholic psychoses giving five or six deep intragluteal injections of 25 mg. a day. Slow release (Spacetabs) are available only in some countries.

10. *Mepazine (Pacatal, Lacumin)*

Mepazine or Pecazine is 10-[3-methyl-3-piperidylmethyl]-phenothiazine. It was introduced a few years after chlorpromazine by Hiob and Hippius. Like

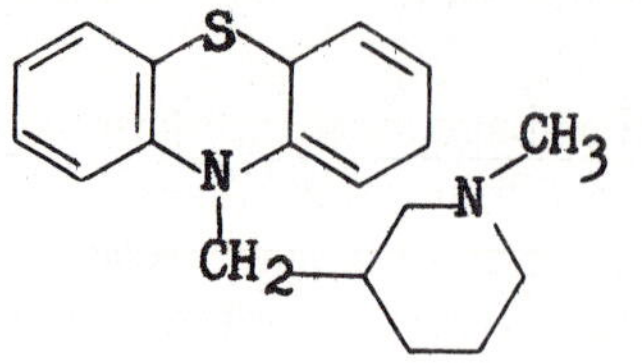

promazine it is a chloride-free tricyclic neuroleptic, and it was hoped that these chloride-free phenothiazine derivatives would have the therapeutic effect of chlorpromazine with fewer side-effects. This hope was not fulfilled and today mepazine plays an unimportant role in psychiatric therapy.

Results of Clinical Investigations: Reports on the efficacy of mepazine are varied. The first investigators found it effective as a neuroleptic but certainly not superior to chlorpromazine (Hiob and Hippius; Bowes). While Denber and also Kline and Jacobs found it ineffective, Feldman as well as Werenberg reported favorably. Lomas compared chlorpromazine with mepazine in chronic schizophrenics and found mepazine less toxic but also much less effective. In acute schizophrenia Bowes advised a combination of the two drugs as being very effective and reducing the incidence of side-effects. This he attributed to their mutually antagonistic autonomic effects. Even without controlled studies it was evident that mepazine is inferior to chlorpromazine and the piperazinyl-phenothiazines. Since such chlorpromazine side-effects as jaundice, allergies and agranulocytosis were also observed in mepazine, this drug represents hardly a progress.

Like thioridazine, mepazine has some antidepressive effect which is theoretically interesting because both these drugs have no extrapyramidal symptoms, and also their vegetative side-effects like dry mouth, impaired accomodation, and urinary disturbances show their relationship to the tricyclic antidepressants (Nieschulz). The strong anticholinergic action, characteristic for the antidepressants, but also present with mepazine, explains that the deliria described in treatment with tricyclic antidepressants, were first observed after mepazine by Hiob and Hippius.

Mode of Administration and Dosage: Mepazine may be administered orally or intramuscularly. The average dosis in schizophrenics lies between 250 and 400 mg. daily, and maintenance doses below 250 mg.

11. *Propericiazine (Neulactil, Neuleptil, Aolept)*

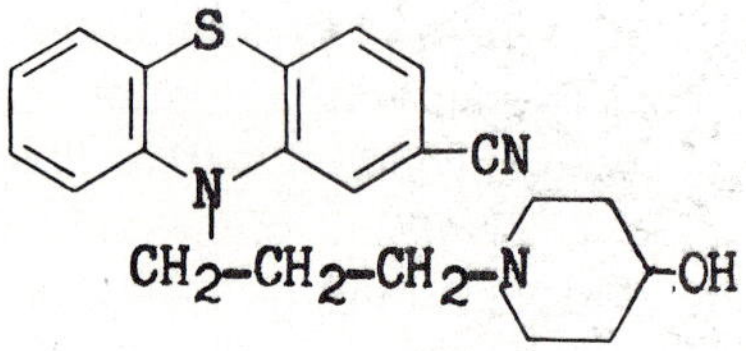

Propericiazine is 2 - cyano - 3 - [(4 - hydroxy - 1 - piperidino) - 3 - propyl] - 10-phenothiazine. This drug is little known in the United States but widely used in Europe, especially in France. It differs from other piperidyl-derivatives such as thorazine in that the piperidyl ring does not include a part of the typical 3-carbon-atoms of the side-chain but is at the end of the side-chain. Therefore, propericiazine is a link between the piperidyl group and the piperazinyl group of phenothiazines which is true not only for the chemical structure but also for its clinical effects.

Result of Clinical Investigations: In France, where Deshaies; Chanoit et al. and Volmat et al. gave the first reports, propericiazine was recommended for the very broad field of behavior and character disorders. In schizophrenics it is suitable for maintenance treatment because it is a stronger neuroleptic than the phenothiazines of the promazine group and the other piperidyl derivatives, and, therefore, comes close to the effectiveness of the piperazinyl derivatives. Yet, it has neither the inhibiting effect on drive nor the extrapyramidal action of piperazine-phenothiazine (Harrer), and the initial damping effect is short. Also in the United States Turns et al. preferred it in chronic schizophrenics. St. Jean et al., in Canada, found it similar to chlorpromazine as did Rajotte et al. in a controlled study. Remarkable was the effect of propericiazine on otherwise treatment-resistant somatic delusions and dysesthesias of pseudoneurotic schizophrenics (Hippius). This might be explained by its distinct central analgetic effect which has also been used in pain (Harrer). A large cooperative study of hospitals in Luxemburg and Belgium found the drug at least as effective as other phenothiazines in reducing aggressiveness and impulsiveness in character disorders (Bobon et al.).

Mode of Administration and Dosage: Propericiazine can be used orally as tablets and as drops. In psychoses the dose is 75 to 150 mg. daily, and should be increased gradually because of circulatory disturbances. In maintenance therapy 30 to 80 mg. are adequate, and in behavior disturbances 10 to 30 mg.

12. *Perazine (Taxilan)*

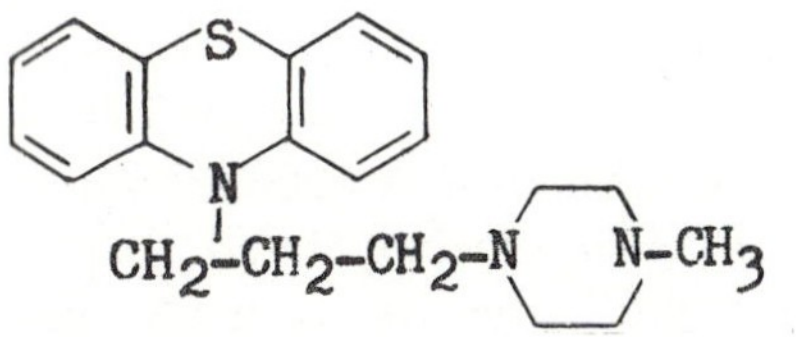

Perazine, 10-[3-(4-methyl-1-piperazinyl)propyl]-phenothiazine, is a representative of the piperazine group of phenothiazines with such other neuroleptics as prochlorperazine, trifluperazine, butaperazine, thioproperazine, perphenazine and fluphenazine. Perazine is a neuroleptic thus far only introduced in Germany (Enss et al.). Like all piperazinyl-derivatives, it acts faster and is more potent than the promazine-derivatives but has fewer side-effects. Therefore, it is especially useful for long term treatment and can be given for years in chronic schizophrenics. In episodic cases of schizophrenia it also reduces recurrences (Hippius and Selbach). Maintenance therapy with perazine delays schizophrenic defect states. The advantage of perazine over other piperazinyl derivatives used in long term therapy, became even more important since persistent dyskinesias were reported after long use of highly potent neuroleptics (Uhrbrand and Faurbye). This occurs in about 20 per cent of cases treated with high potency neuroleptics over a period of five years but only in about 5 per cent in perazine treated patients. Contrary to other drugs of the piperazine group, perazine has also been used successfully in depressions (Tölle), and is particularly useful in depressive syndromes of schizophrenia.

Mode of Administration and Dosage: Perazine has a great therapeutic latitude. It has a strong initial sedative effect useful for the treatment of acute psychosis. In paranoid and hallucinatory psychoses initial doses of 150 to 300 mg. daily can be quickly raised to 400 and 800 mg., and in excitement states up to 1500 mg. The initial effect can be increased by intramuscular injections (50 mg. in 2 ml. ampules). The dosage for perazine corresponds more with that of chlorpromazine than with other piperazine derivatives. The usual maintenance dose is 75 to 400 mg. daily in women, and 150 to 600 mg. in men (Enss et al.).

13. *Prochlorperazine (Compazine, Stemetil, Nipodal)*

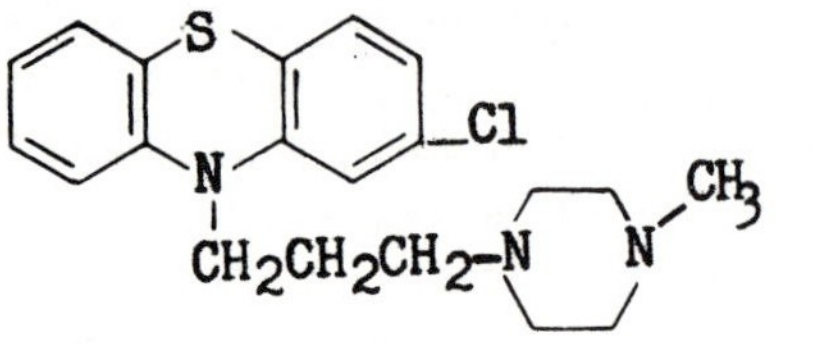

Prochlorperazine is 2-chloro-10-[3-(4-methyl-1-piperazinyl)propyl]-phenothiazine. In the United States prochlorperazine was the first drug of the so-called piperazine group of phenothiazine derivatives. It is widely used in Canada and France but practically unknown as a neuroleptic in Germany, where perazine, its chemical analog without chlorine, takes it place.

Results of Clinical Investigations: Like the other phenothiazines, prochlorperazine has been used extensively in schizophrenics, particularly the chronic group. Broussolle et al. reported that in this type of illness it was the paranoid patients who responded best while Milne and Berliner found that in their trials the simple and hebephrenic patients, a group in which the results are usually very poor, were most benefitted. The drug is active in smaller doses than chlorpromazine, and it also produces its therapeutic action more rapidly than chlorpromazine with less drowsiness. These features and its effectiveness were confirmed in four simultaneously presented American reports by Kline et al., Denber, Goldman, and Freyhan. A patient whom Goldman changed from chlorpromazine to prochlorperazine, stated that he felt much less depressed and less sleepy, therefore better able to work and drive a car. Galbraith et al. considered the drug as effective as chlorpromazine as judged by its ability to maintain improvement in chronic schizophrenics previously treated with chlorpromazine. They could distinguish, however, no precise criteria for its use as distinct from the other phenothiazines. Dransfield, in a trial with 50 aggressive and disturbed male psychotics, did not feel that the results justified the substitution of compazine for chlorpromazine, especially since there would seem to be a much greater expectation of parkinsonism. Denham, however, thought that the drug was more effective than chlorpromazine in the control of persistent delusions and hallucinations. Those schizophrenics who had only thought disorder without abnormal psychomotor behavior did less well or failed to benefit at all. He made no direct comparison with chlorpromazine, the patients who had been previously treated with chlorpromazine, acting as their own controls. A study by Pennington in chronic psychotics showed 10 per cent recovery and 57 per cent improvement. The drug often has an enlivening effect upon apathetic, withdrawn and regressed schizophrenics. Prochlorperazine has also been found of benefit in the acutely disturbed psychotic, and Goldman has commented that combination with ECT, which was advocated by Vallade et al., is free from danger. Broussolle was particularly impressed by the value of the drug in acute manics. Its immediate action seems to recommend it for psychiatric emergencies.

Pilkington treated a group of 88 mental defectives with prochlorperazine for two months and found it particularly valuable in the hyperactive group as well in those with affective disturbances. These defectives with a concomitant schizophrenic illness did poorly, while among epileptics the low grade adults obtained the most benefit.

The results with the drug in the psychoneuroses are not spectacular, and there is a paucity of adequately controlled studies. Winkelman observed that it relieved anxiety in neurotic patients, and that there were few complaints by hypochondriacs about the side-effects. McFoos noted a relief of tension when the drug was administered, but there is a tendency for many neurotics to improve for a time with any medication, and no placebo group was used.

Prochlorperazine has also been tried in the treatment of alcoholic psychoses, withdrawal symptoms in drug addicts, and in the control of hyperactivity in psychotic geriatric patients, a group in which Rothstein and Lacerva obtained good results. Its powerful anti-emetic action makes it particularly useful in the control of the nausea and vomiting associated with drug or alcohol withdrawal. In fact, prochlorperazine was initially used as an anti-emetic in general medicine for the treatment of Ménière's syndrome, migraine, and other conditions in which nausea and vomiting are common.

Since the extrapyramidal motor symptoms can be well controlled with antiparkinsonian drugs, prochlorperazine proved to be quite successful in maintenance therapy (St. Laurent et al.). However, they are more frequent than with chlorpromazine. Delay et al. compared them with postencephalitic symptoms and took them as a point of origin for their study of the theoretical significance of the extrapyramidal action of neuroleptics.

As with the other phenothiazines, it is difficult to lay down any criteria for the use of prochlorperazine as compared to other neuroleptic drugs. There is still a lack of sufficient critical assessment of the precise value of each of the phenothiazines in mental illness, and while this is so it will inevitably prevent the most adequate use being made of any of them.

Mode of Administration and Dosage: The drug may be given orally as tablets in the maleate form or as a solution in the methanesulphonate form. The methanesulphonate may be administered as a syrup containing 5 mg. in 5 cc. The drug can also be given rectally in suppositories or by deep intramuscular injection.

The usual starting dose for the treatment of psychotic disturbances is from 25 to 75 mg. daily orally, this being gradually increased to the level at which the maximum benefit is obtained. This may require a daily dose of 250 mg. or over. Where there is acute excitement, 25 mg. by injection may be given up to three times daily. The rectal route has the disadvantage of uncertain absorption and lack of complete control over the actual dose which the patient is receiving.

14. *Trifluoperazine (Stelazine, Jatroneural)*

Trifluoperazine is 10-[3-(4-methyl-l-piperazinyl)propyl]-2-(trifluoromethyl)-phenothiazine.

RESULTS OF CLINICAL INVESTIGATIONS: There have been numerous very positive reports on trifluoperazine and there seems to be no doubt that it is an extremely effective phenothiazine. One of its main benefits, as noted by Barsa et al., is that it activates the chronic withdrawn and apathetic or depressed schizophrenic. It is often more successful in this type of patient than chlorpromazine which tends to increase the withdrawal and depression. Because of its activating effect, prolonged use can sometimes lead to hyperactivity, irritability and sleeplessness.

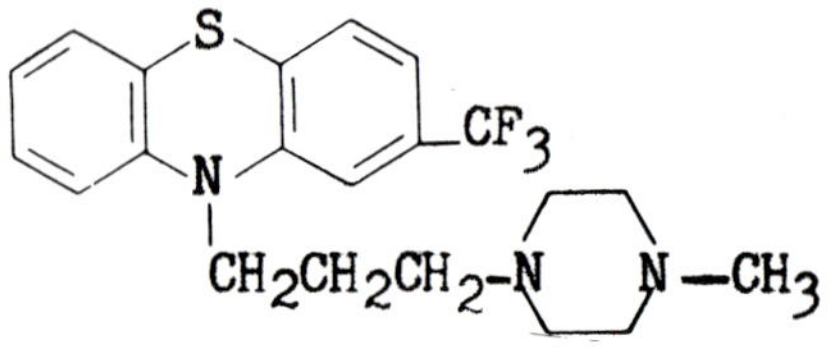

Improvement in a percentage of chronic schizophrenics treated has been reported by many observers, including Kruse, Barsa et al., and Tolan and Peppel. These were not controlled studies but dealt with patients who had been refractory to other forms of treatment and so could, to a certain extent, act as their own controls. The best response was found in withdrawn and regressed patients who became more alert and responsive. Allen, in a study of schizophrenics resistant to other neuroleptics found it to be of benefit also in deluded and hallucinating chronic schizophrenia. The value of trifluoperazine in the treatment of chronic "anergic" schizophrenics was confirmed by Reznikoff. Later, the activating effect was confirmed in several controlled studies, e.g., by Hollister et al. in a cross-over study on chronic schizophrenics and by Weckowicz and Ward on matched groups. This effect on apathetic schizophrenics became so important because the neuroleptics known until 1960, influenced "productive" symptoms, but the "defect" symptomatology remain uninfluenced.

The stimulating effect of trifluoperazine is less noticeable in nonschizophrenics but exists even in normals. These psychological effects were studied by Lehmann and Knight. They found that trifluoperazine tends to reduce the response to perceptual stimuli, so dampening the sensory input, and at the same time it tends to reduce psychomotor speed and to improve concentration, attention and abstractive ability. In other words, it also increases the patient's ability to handle the sensory input. They compared these results to those obtained with chlorpromazine and found that, while the latter drug had a similar dampening effect on sensory input, it was not so effective as trifluoperazine in those tests involving ability to handle this input.

Good tolerability and minimal circulatory effects make trifluoperazine suitable for involutional psychoses (Hader et al.). The absence of tiredness is an advantage for ambulatory treatment (Gearren). In child psychiatry Fish noted that it stimulated withdrawn hypoactive children to more competent locomotion and dexterity. There are also reports on resocialization of hyperactive children with behavior problems. Altschuler describes impressive results in obsessive-compulsive syndromes treated with relatively high doses of 60 to 90 mg. daily. When he made a placebo control after six months, patients relapsed but improved again, when trifluoperazine was reinstituted.

Gunn, who studied the drug in a group of chronic psychotics with long-standing illness, found for stelazine what has been noted by other observers that, while there is often a gain in weight, when patients receive phenothiazines, because of the increased appetite and probably also the relief of psychotic symptoms, when such cases develop extrapyramidal symptoms, there is weight loss. He did not find that the drug produced any untoward effects when combined with ECT, and also commented that, in two patients given anesthesia during the course of their therapy with trifluoperazine, no abnormal fall in blood pressure or tachycardia has been noted by the anesthetists. Freed found that there were no side-effects even when the drug was used in combination with intravenous barbiturates given as premedication for ECT. He observed that trifluoperazine relieved both pre-treatment anxiety and post-shock excitement.

Goldman has reported that small doses of trifluoperazine are rapidly effective in relieving the hallucinations of delirium tremens. In one acutely disturbed patient the hallucinations disappeared within six hours of his being given 5 mg. of the drug intramuscularly. Feldman similarly found that trifluoperazine had a better effect than chlorpromazine on delusions and hallucinations, but that the latter had a more beneficial action on factors such as aggression, sociability, tension, self-mutilation and appetite. Madgick et al. noticed that many of their patients became markedly euphoric. MacDonald and Watts considered the drug as effective as insulin in a group of paranoid schizophrenics.

Some beneficial results have also been claimed in neurotics of certain types. Goddard found that it was helpful in both chronic and acute anxiety but had little effect on obsessive-compulsives. The same author noted poor results in agitated depression, despite the reported euphorizing action in some schizophrenics. May et al. in a double blind trial saw that phobic symptoms, particularly those associated with considerable tension, were especially helped. Those cases with a predominantly depressive element did not respond.

While the number of controlled trials which have been carried out with trifluoperazine is small compared to the number of papers published on its use, it seems to have a definite place in the treatment of certain types of mental illness, most especially in chronic schizophrenics who are either withdrawn and apathetic or deluded and hallucinated.

Mode of Administration and Dosage: It may be given either orally or intramuscularly. The same precautions regarding site and depth of injection as for the other phenothiazines apply to stelazine also. Injections should not be given at intervals of less than four hours, because there is the possibility of a cumulative effect. Dosage should not exceed 10 mg. in 24 hours by injection. For patients who hide or refuse tablets, stelazine concentrate, which can be mixed with liquid or a semi-solid food, may be used.

Severely agitated patients may be given initial intramuscular injections in doses of 2 mg. three times daily. When the patient will take oral medication, an initial dose of 5 mg. three times daily can be given for psychotics, gradually increasing by 5 mg. increments until the maximum response is obtained. Barsa et al. gave a maximum of 30 mg. four times daily in some of their cases over a period of 5 to 7 months, and the majority received 60 to 80 mg. Hollister et al. consider 60 mg. the maximal dose, but usually 30 mg. are adequate.

For neurotics smaller doses can be administered, commencing with 1 to 2 mg. two or three times daily and increasing to a maximum of 10 mg. daily. Care should be taken that complaints indicative of early extrapyramidal stimulation, such as restlessness and inability to keep still, are not mistaken for anxiety symptoms and the dosage increased with a resultant aggravation of motor disturbance. Feldman has pointed out the importance of gradually raising the dosage scale, because the narrow dose range means that patients are more susceptible to dosage variations.

15. *Butaperazine (Repoise, Randolectil)*

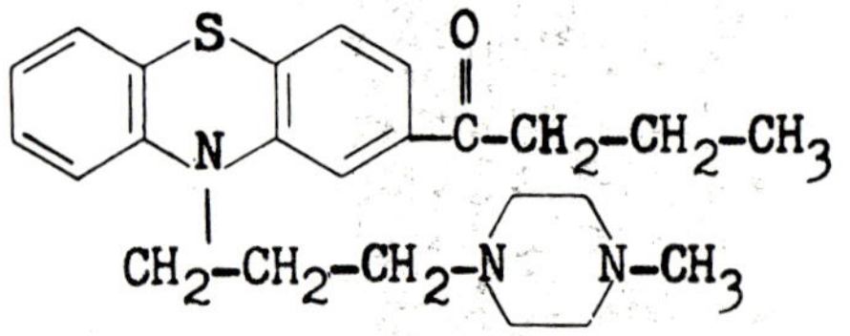

Butaperazine or butyrylperazine is 10-[3-(4-methyl-1-piperazinyl)-propyl] -phenothiazine-2-yl-1-propanone. Like all other piperazine derivatives butaperazine is a very potent neuroleptic. In clinical investigations of several piperazine phenothiazines Flügel et al. found the butyryl derivative to be most effective. Delusions and hallucinations respond best (Bente et al.). In the United States Denber et al. could not confirm these results even with ten times higher doses, and also failed to see any dyskinesias which the European workers found in 45 per cent of their patients. Equally surprising discrepancies between American and European patient material were seen by Bente et al. in EEG studies. Some American reports on butaperazine were more favorable. Mandel and Philip compared it with trifluperazine in a controlled study with a double-blind cross-over design, and found no significant difference between the two drugs in effectiveness and in incidence of side-effects. The great similarity with trifluperazine shows that butaperazine belongs to the strongest phenothiazine neuroleptics. Comparing it with chlorpromazine and perphenazine Gerz found butaperazine faster acting and more tranquilizing without causing undesired sedation. Sharply et al. comparing butaperazine and perphenazine in a double blind study found the two piperazinyl derivatives of similar therapeutic effectiveness in chronic patients, but butaperazine had more extrapyramidal side-effects.

MODE OF ADMINISTRATION AND DOSAGE: Butaperazine removes acute excitement states with intravenous injections of 10 mg. which can be repeated if necessary. It also can be injected intramuscularly. In general, even acute psychosis respond to oral medication with 10 to 30 mg. Larger doses up to 300 mg. did not improve the effect (Denber et al.). Maintenance doses are 5 to 10 mg. daily.

16. *Thioproperazine (Vontil, Majeptil)*

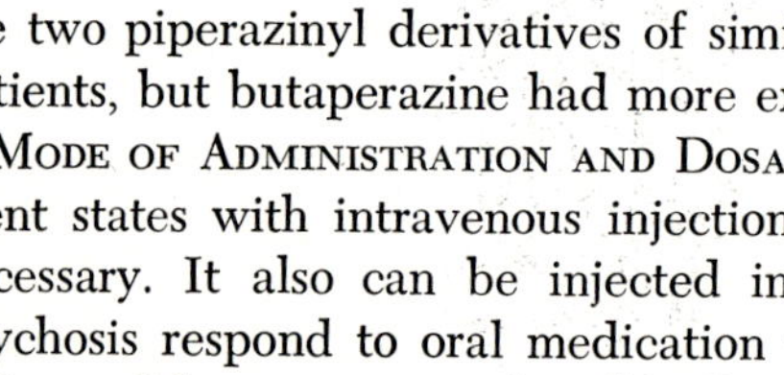

Thioproperazine, N-dimethyl-10-[3-(methyl - 1 - piperazinyl)propyl] - phenothiazine-2-sulfonamide, is considered to be the strongest phenothiazine neuroleptic available.

RESULTS OF CLINICAL INVESTIGA-

TIONS: Thioproperazine was developed in France. Delay et al. reported enthusiastically about the drug, but since it is highly potent, they feel that it should be given on and off, possibly in a hospital. It has the most frequent and varying extrapyramidal motor side-effects of all phenothiazines which makes it most interesting for the study of these phenomena. These symptoms are, according to Delay, so pronounced that the therapeutic effect can be judged only after discontinuation of the drug, all the more as it also causes indifference and despondency as well as sleep disturbances. In treatment resistant patients these side-effects must be accepted. Denber et al. find the drug highly potent, while Kurland and Vasconcellos had poor results possibly due to a rather low dosage. Denham and Carrick who treated a group of 40 male schizophrenics with a length of illness from 2 to 40 years, found that 21 of them showed a complete remission of their symptoms and that these were the group who had the most marked extrapyramidal side-effects. Others with lesser degrees of this neurological phenomenon showed improvement, but less than the other group, while the one patient who did not improve had no extrapyramidal manifestations. They noted that, with discontinuous treatment, the improvement began when the drug was withdrawn and the extrapyramidal symptoms began to resolve. Often symptoms such as hallucinations disappeared about 48 hours after the end of the first course of treatment, but severely deteriorated patients might require several courses. Hordern et al. question the usefulness of thioproperazine. Although in a controlled study it turned out to be superior to fluphenazine and a placebo, they found that the many dystonic crises caused so much anxiety in the patients and among the nursing staff that they want the drug limited to few selected cases. Moffat and McLeod also doubt the value of such a risky drug.

MODE OF ADMINISTRATION AND DOSAGE: The drug may be given by the "continuous" or the "discontinuous" method. In the former, the initial few days' doses are given intramuscularly, followed by oral administration in a range from 10 to 35 mg. daily. A "discontinuous" method to avoid the distressing side-effects of the drug has also been used. Delay et al. recommend commencing with a dosage of 10 mg. daily and increasing every two days by 10 mg. until the patient is receiving 50 mg. daily. The drug is then withdrawn and recommenced later at a higher dose. Coirault et al. applied the same technique but with a higher dosage so that what they described as "chemical shock" is produced. Deshaies et al. have given the drug intravenously as a slow infusion of 10 mg. or a slow injection of 1-3 mg. as well as orally increasing slowly for several weeks. Denham and Carrick also used the discontinuous method, giving 30 to 50 mg. three times daily in gradually increasing doses for five days, until a state of maximum muscular hypotonicity ensued. Then the drug was stopped and, if there was a total complete remission, the patient was kept on a maintenance dose of 2.5 to 10 mg. daily; whereas, if there was a continuation of symptoms, further courses of treatment with higher doses were given.

17. *Perphenazine (Trilafon, Fentazin, Decentan)*

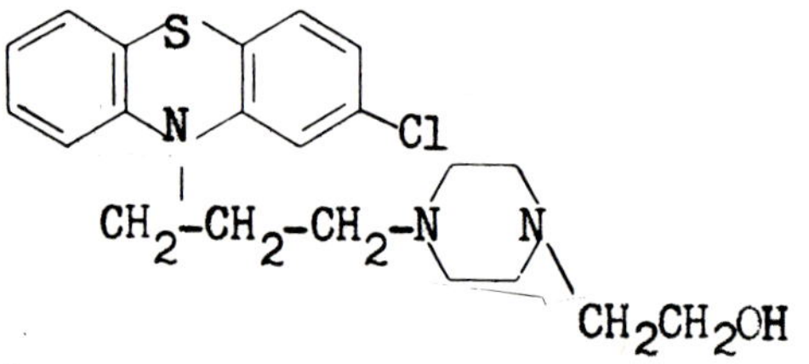

Perphenazine is 4-[3-(2-chlorophenothiazine-10-yl)propyl] -1-piperazine-ethanol. The drug, one of the oldest neuroleptics of the piperazine group, has been administered, according to Ayd, to millions of patients, but is now more popular in combination with antidepressants, in such drugs as Etrafon and Triavil. It seems that in Europe the often massive side-effects prevented a wider use (Cornu).

Results of Clinical Investigations: Cahn and Lehmann found the drug of benefit in manics and in all types of schizophrenia, as well as in one patient with an acute epileptic psychosis. They found no benefit in depression; this opinion has been shared by Ayd, who found, however, that perphenazine relieved the associated anxiety and agitation in the same way as does chlorpromazine. Frühman and Gross noted an increase in depression in patients with endogenous depressions. Ayd observed that the greatest improvement was in the acute cases and that chronic psychotics and neurotics benefitted little from the drug. He found a combination with ECT to be both safe and effective. In chronic schizophrenia some improvement in accessibility and response to the environment was reported by O'Riely and by Cohen and Freireich. Lingjaerde and Schiøth considered the indications for perphenazine in this condition to be the same as those for chlorpromazine, except that the former appeared to have a more stimulating effect on sluggish and apathetic patients.

This stimulating effect which perphenazine has in common with some other piperazine phenothiazines has been stressed by many workers. It might be partly explained by the findings of Shelkunov that in animals prolonged administration of perphenazine leads to an activation of central adrenergic processes. The dual ability of the drug to act as an ataractic, calming aggressive patients, and a stimulant activating sluggish and rigid patients (Illberg) makes perphenazine useful as maintenance drug in the rehabilitation of schizophrenics. Thus, Jaquith et al. were able to reduce in schizophrenics rehospitalization rates to lower the duration of hospitalization and to improve adjustment at home. Barbour used perphenazine in many chronic patients on an ambulatory basis. According to Gerz, the patients feel subjectively better with perphenazine than with the stronger vigilance-damping other phenothiazines, are less somnolent, and complain less of drowsiness and "dragged-out" feeling. The extrapyramidal symptoms are a drawback but Hanlon et al. showed in a double-blind study that prophylactic anti-parkinsonian drugs like benztropine mesylate do not interfere with the therapeutic results. Casey et al., in a comparative study, found that perphenazine 50 mg., chlorpromazine 635 mg., triflupromazine 175 mg., and prochlorperazine 90 mg. daily were equally effective; but the greatest number of side reactions, particularly extrapyramidal features, were produced by perphenazine and prochlorperazine. One interesting feature of this investigation was that patients who received phenobarbital also showed some of the side effects associated with the phenothiazines, such as restlessness, autonomic reactions as shown by dryness of the mouth or blurred vision, and even abnormal hepatic tests and blood changes, as well as depression or agitation. When Freyhan compared perphenazine with prochlorperazine and trifluoperazine, he found that it occupied, both as regards its power of psychomotor inhibition and the production of extrapyramidal reactions, an intermediate position between the other two drugs. It reduced psychomotor activity in smaller doses than prochlorperazine and had a high incidence of extrapyramidal side effects.

Tension and anxiety symptoms, but not depressive manifestations were reported by Maragoni to respond well to the drug. Hinton differed from this in finding that the beneficial action in neurotics was greater on the depressive mood than on the anxiety symptoms. Larson et al. studying the effect of high doses of perphenazine up to 768 mg. in chronic, semi-regressed patients, found that the drug has a wide margin of saftey, but that its maximal clinical effect can be achieved by the lower doses usually employed.

Several investigators studied the effect of perphenazine on thyroid function. In 1962 Cranswick et al. found increased protein-bound iodine in the serum in 11 out of 32 perphenazine-treated patients. This was confirmed by Oltman and Friedman but denied by Ayd, and Hollister et al. The patients with increased protein-bound iodine had no clinical symptoms of a hyperthyreosis. Later Cranswick and Simpson reported that crystallized perphenazine contains traces of iodine which in the organism becomes electively bound to certain serum proteins and thus increases the concentration of protein bound iodine in the serum. Recently, these views were supported by Mølholm-Hansen and Stersboek-Nielsen.

Modes of Administration and Dosage: Perphenazine is usually given either orally or by intramuscular injection. In the latter case, the injection should be given with the patient either sitting or lying down in order to avoid any hypotensive effects. The drug can also be administered intravenously, but the injection should be well diluted with glucose saline or normal saline and injected slowly not exceeding 5 mg.

For acute psychotic cases, the drug may be given initially by intramuscular injection, usually 5 mg.; but 10 mg. may be given where there is gross excitement. This dose can be repeated in six hours, and a total of 30 mg. may be injected over a 24-hour period. Orally, the dosage for disturbed patients is 8 mg. three or four times daily, but a total of up to 64 mg. has been given in some cases. For less severely disturbed patients, 2 to 4 mg. three or four times may be sufficient.

18. *Thiopropazate (Dartal, Dartalan)*

Thiopropazate, 4-[3-(2-chlorophenothiazine-10-yl)-propyl]-piperazine-ethyl-acetate, is the acetic acid ester of perphenazine. Since the thiopropazate molecule is split by unspecific esterases into the perphenazine molecule and acetic acid, it is most probable that perphenazine and not thiopropazate becomes active in the organism.

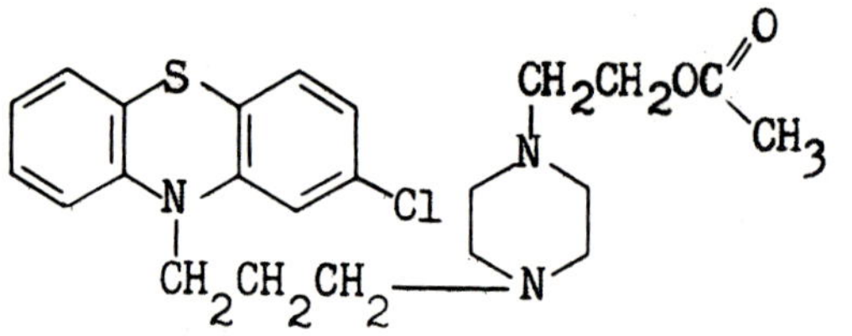

Results of Clinical Investigations: There have been relatively few trials on the use of dartalan. Edisen and Samuels have reported the results of a double blind trial in which a group of mostly schizophrenic patients were treated with the drug. They found that a number of these patients were improved, the symptoms helped most markedly being depersonalization, withdrawal, flattened affect, anorexia, anxiety and delusions. Patients with mood depression gave better results with the placebo. Hamilton et al. also conducted a trial in which the drug, given in a dosage of 30 mg. daily, was compared with chlorpromazine 300 mg. daily and a placebo, while at the same time the interaction of all three substances with occupational therapy was assessed. They attribute an absence of any significant difference over the eight-week treatment period between the placebo and chlorpromazine as possibly due to the low dosage or to the short period of treatment. Both drugs, but especially chlorpromazine, exerted a significant inhibitory action on any improvement produced by occupational therapy. At an assessment two weeks after the commencement of the trial the thiopropazate-treated patients showed a significant improvement, confirming earlier suggestions that the drug exerts its therapeutic action speedily. At the end of eight weeks the results with thiopropazate were still superior to those obtained with chlorpromazine, the placebo or occupational therapy.

Thiopropazate has been used successfully by some authors in the treatment of Huntington's chorea.

Mode of Administration and Dosage: It is normally given orally. The usual initial dose is from 10 to 30 mg. daily, depending on the severity of the illness, and gradually increasing to between 40 and 160 mg. per day (Matthews).

19. *Fluphenazine (Prolixin, Permitil, Moditen, Antensol, Omca, Lyogen)*

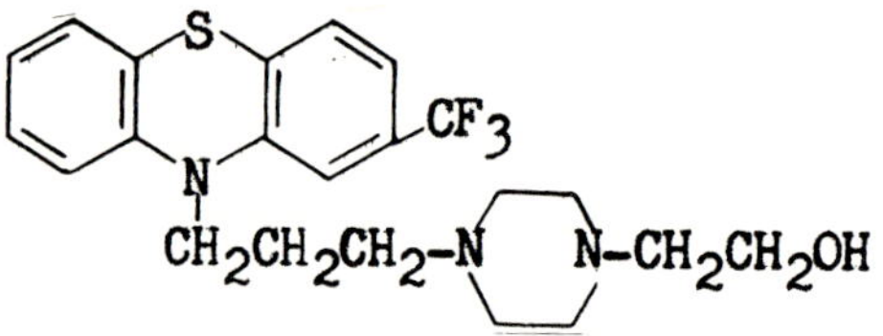

Fluphenazine is 4-[3-(2-trifluoromethyl)phenothiazine - 10 - yl] - propyl-1-piperazine-ethanol.

Since fluphenazine like perphenazine has a hydroxyl group in para-position of the sidechain, it can form an ester as alcohol with organic acids. Perphenazine, when in form of an ester with acetic acid, becomes thiopropazate (see 18) whose action is identical with the original compound. The ester of fluphenazine with organic acids having a longer carbonchain, forms compounds with a much longer duration of action than the non-ester fluphenazine. The fluphenazine esters are the first depot neuroleptics. Best known are fluphenazine enanthate and fluphenazine decoanate. Fluphenazine enanthate (trade names: Prolixin enanthate, Moditen enanthate, Dapotum) is a compound of the original drug with heptanoic acid (CH_3-$(CH_2)_5$-COOH), dissolved in sesame oil. Fluphenazine decanoate (trade name: Lyogen Depot) is a compound of the original drug with caprinic acid. During the last few years these two depot preparations have been widely used.

Results of Clinical Investigations: This very potent neuroleptic has all the advantages and disadvantages of this group, the latter characterized by marked extrapyramidal symptoms. The advantages of quick onset of neuroleptic effect and strong so-called anti-psychotic action were still enhanced by the depot preparations.

In the first clinical investigations fluphenazine was used as neuroleptic for the psychoses, and as tranquilizer for the neuroses. Darling has reported good results in a group of mixed psychotic and neurotic patients, and Niswander and Karacan found that improvement in their patients could be sustained on 1 mg. of the drug daily following the initial response. They obtained over-all improvement in 63 per cent of recent, mainly psychotic, admissions. Their results were good in schizophrenics, manic-depressives, psychoneurotic reactions and involutional psychoses. Personality disorders and sufferers from chronic brain syndrome were not improved. Taylor was impressed by the anti-delusional and anti-hallucinatory activity of fluophenazine, and its action in diminishing tension and anxiety in psychoneurotics. Holt and Wright similarly found that the drug exerted a controlling action on delusions and hallucinations, and emphasized the extremely rapid onset and prolonged duration of action. Moore stressed the adaptability for outpatient maintenance treatment as a definite advantage of fluphenazine. In a double-blind study with cross-over design Millar found fluphenazine clearly superior to chlorpromazine. In the large NIMH study on fluphenazine, chlorpromazine and thioridazine, fluphenazine did not do better than chlorpromazine. Remarkable results in Huntington's chorea were obtained by Korenyi and Whittier.

Mode of Administration and Dosage: The drug has a sustained action and can therefore be given as a single daily dose, although, if necessary, doses at 12-hour intervals may be given. For neurotics, 0.5 to 3 mg. orally daily is the usual dose; while for psychotic disturbances the initial dose should be 0.5 mg. increasing to a level high enough to control the symptoms; 180 mg. daily orally has been given in some cases (Darling), although the more usual level is up to 10 mg. daily. In doses below 1 mg. daily fluphenazine is used as tranquilizer, and Morrow gives it as adjuvant to psychotherapy in doses of 1 to 3 mg. In recent years French authors (e.g., Gayrat and Lambert) recommended extremely high doses of 300 to 1000 mg. in otherwise treatment-resistant schizophrenics. Surprisingly, extrapyramidal side-effects are less in doses over 100 mg. than in small doses of 10 to 25 mg. A patient of Kruse, treated for a month with 20 to 45 mg., developed extrapyramidal symptoms only, when the dosis was reduced to less than 2 to 5 mg., and they disappeared only, when the dosis was still further reduced. Denzel gave 1500 mg. to a schizophrenic whose tolerance to the drug was also tested with intravenous injection of 345 mg. within 90 minutes. In these large doses fluphenazine has a calming effect, whereas low dosage after longer application has rather a stimulating effect. In children with behavior problems Waites and Keele recommended 0.5 to 50 mg. daily.

Results of Clinical Investigations: Systematic studies on maintenance treatment of schizophrenics have proven that maintenance doses of a neuroleptic lower the relapse rate and delay, at least temporarily, the development of schizophrenic defect states (Selbach and Hippius). The concept of neuroleptic medication as a symptom removing compensatory treatment led to the search for depot preparations. After successful treatment in the hospital discharged patients often neglect to take their medication, relapse, and have to be readmitted. In these instances depot preparations help to prevent what has been called "revolving door psychiatry."

Kinross-Wright et al. were the first to recommend this new method of drug therapy. The need for such depot preparations was soon demonstrated by many other favorable reports on fluphenazine enanthate. Winthrop stresses their importance particularly in uncooperative patients like acute manics, but also in difficult treatment situations as they exist in developing countries. Comparing fluphenazine enanthate injections with oral unesterized fluphenazine Ravaris et al. and Haider saw no difference in clinical effect. After discontinuation of depot therapy Ravaris et al. saw 90 per cent relapses. The unpleasant extrapyramidal side-effects led Kline and Simpson to the routine use of anti-parkinsonian drugs. Whittier et al. noticed these side-effects with particular frequency in older patients.

Fluphenazine decanoate, introduced by Simpson et al., gives fewer extrapyramidal side-effects. This was confirmed by Kurland and Richardson who believe that the decanoate requires even fewer injections than the enanthate.

Mode of Administration and Dosage: In these long-acting fluphenazines intramuscular injections of 12.5 to 25 mg. are usually sufficient for a period of two weeks (Hsu et al.; Kingstone). Compared to two weeks' oral medication, this represents a saving of two-thirds of the dose. The intervals between injections can be reduced to one week in case of relapse, and prolonged to a month, when the patient remains symptom-free. The depot preparations are well tolerated and do not give local infiltrations at the site of injection.

20. *Chlorimpiphenine (Ponsital)*

Chlorimpiphenine is 1-methyl-2-oxo-3-(4-[3-(2-chloro-phenothiazine-10-yl)-propyl]-1-piperazine-ethyl)-imidazole.

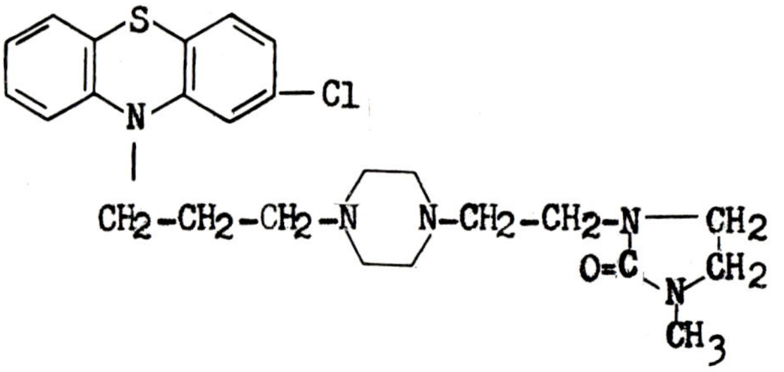

Structurally chlorimpiphenine is closely related to perphenazine and thiopropazate. In contrast to the latter, this compound is not hydrolyzed by unspecific esterases in the end-group of the side chain because there is no ester linkage.

RESULTS OF CLINICAL INVESTIGATIONS: So far only uncontrolled clinical studies are available. They show that chlorimpiphenine is a strong neuroleptic both in therapeutic efficacy and in side-effects, and is comparable to perphenazine. Its pronounced anti-psychotic effects set in rapidly which makes it useful in excitement states of paranoid and catatonic schizophrenia and in manic excitement. Like other piperazine phenothiazines, chlorimpiphenine has an activating effect on disturbances of affectivity and drive, and, therefore, is useful in hebephrenics, simple schizophrenics and schizophrenic defect states (Berzewski and Hippius; Schäpperle and Schwarz).

MODE OF ADMINISTRATION AND DOSAGE: The dosage ranges between 5 and 30 mg. daily. In excitement states the drug should be given by intramuscular injection.

21. *Clopenthixol (Sordinol, Ciatyl)*

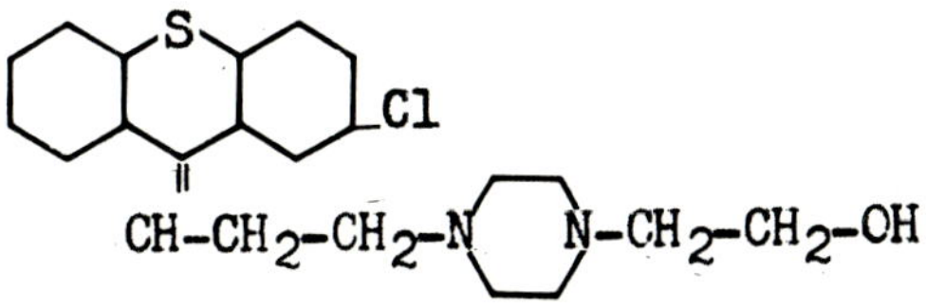

Clopenthixol or chlorperphenthixene, 4-[2-chloro-9-thioxanthenylidene)propyl] - 1 - piperazine - ethanol, is the thioxanthene analogue to the phenothiazene derivative perphenazine.

RESULTS OF CLINICAL INVESTIGATIONS: The first report by Ravn and Rud in Denmark on the favorable effect on schizophrenics was soon confirmed by other European authors. Clopenthixol resembles in its effects the potent neuroleptics of the piperazine group of phenothiazenes. It is fast acting, but in the beginning patients are often drowsy and sleep a good deal. The therapeutic action is similar to that of perphenazine, but Gross and Kaltenbäck find clopenthixol superior to perphenazine. Korda et al., in a controlled study, found no difference to chlorpromazine. In chronic psychoses Ban et al. found it very effective. Even otherwise totally treatment-resistant cases may still respond to clopenthixol (Wolpert et al.). It is useful in acute psychoses with productive symptomatology and, in small doses, for continuous medication in easily relapsing psychoses and those with residual symptoms (Marx). Extrapyramidal and dulling side-effects suggest its use in the hospital (Bjorn and Rasmussen). Reduced libido under clopenthixol, an unpleasant side-effect, was considered by Cahn as possibly useful for therapeutically desirable reduction of sexual activity.

MODE OF ADMINISTRATION AND DOSAGE: The dosage range is between 10 and 180 mg. daily. Arnold and Deisenhammer give up to 400 mg. daily. As maintenance dose 5 mg. once a day may be sufficient (Marx).

22. *Flupentixol (Fluanxol)*

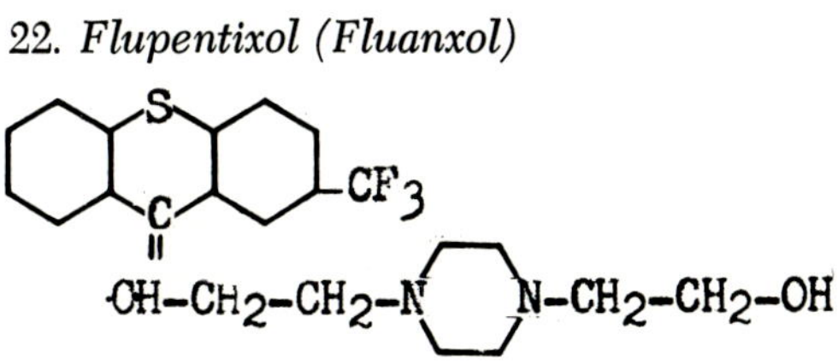

Flupentixol, 2-trifluoromethyl-9-{3 - [4 - (2 - hydroxylethyl) - 1 - piperazinyl] - propylidine} - thioxanthene, is the most potent neuroleptic among the thioxanthene derivatives.

RESULTS OF CLINICAL INVESTIGA-

TIONS: Contrary to clopenthixol, flupentixol has no marked sedative and fewer motor inhibitory effects than other thioxanthenes (Pöldinger). This profile of action makes the drug well suited for long-time treatment of chronic paranoid schizophrenics (Gross and Kaltenbäck). Like all highly potent neuroleptics flupentixol has a stimulating effect which makes it useful also in schizophrenic defect states. It also has an anxiolytic effect (Pöldinger).

MODE OF ADMINISTRATION AND DOSAGE: Flupentixol as a highly potent neuroleptic is effective in doses of 1 mg. three times daily, and in maintenance treatment even 0.5 mg. three times daily. It is only available for oral medication.

23. *Thiothixene (Navane, Orbinamon)*

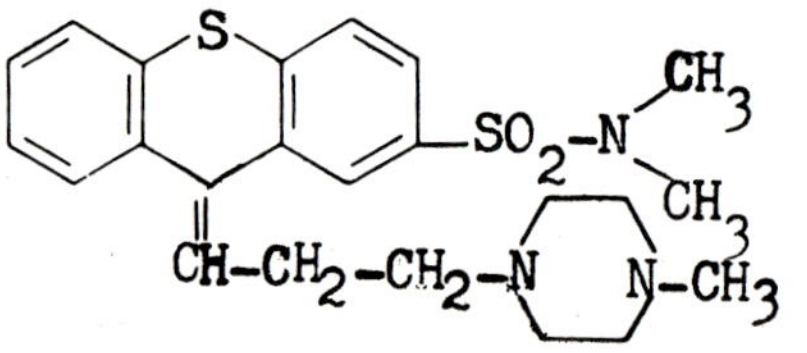

Thiothixene, 1 - methyl - 4 - [3 - (2-sulfamylthioxanthen-9-ylidene) - propyl]-piperazine, is the analogue of thioproperazine. On a milligram-per-milligram basis, thiothixene is the most potent thioxanthene which makes its position comparable to that of thioproperazine in the phenothiazine group.

RESULTS OF CLINICAL INVESTIGATIONS: Since 1965 numerous investigations demonstrated the efficacy of thiothixene in acute as well as chronic schizophrenics. Sugerman et al. showed that thiothixene, next to floropipamide, was the most effective of more than 20 neuroleptics investigated by them. Others are less enthusiastic. Hekimian et al. noted some antipsychotic action but little effect in chronic schizophrenics. According to Delay, inert chronics respond fairly well, but the drug is inadequate in severe psychomotor excitement states and in manics. This was confirmed by Simeon et al., although these and other authors were occasionally impressed by spectacular individual cases. Thus, Davison et al. mentioned a schizophrenic of 22 years of illness, who after 12 weeks' treatment with thiothixene could be discharged from the hospital. In a double-blind study Gallant et al. gave schizophrenics who were known to be non-reactors to placebo, either 20 mg. thiothixine or 800 mg. of thioridazine. Therapeutic results were identical; but side-effects differed, thiothixine giving extrapyramidal symptoms, while lethargy, seen with thioridazine, was absent. This profile makes thiothixine similar to the potent neuroleptics of the piperazine phenothiazines. Therefore, Kurland et al. consider thiothixine equally useful in acute and chronic schizophrenics. In the latter group an important target symptom for thiothixine is apathy which does poorly in neuroleptics with sedative action. This lack of sedative action makes it also useful, when psychotherapy or occupational therapy are given simultaneously (Haase et al.).

MODE OF ADMINISTRATION AND DOSAGE: Initial dosis of 2 to 10 mg. daily should be increased slowly to 15 or 30 mg. In some cases up to 60 mg. are given. The drug is available only in capsules for oral therapy.

Side-Effects and Complications of Phenothiazines and Other Tricyclic Neuroleptics

Chlorpromazine, as the first drug to be studied extensively, exemplifies many of the side-effects common to all neuroleptic drugs. Other drugs have only some of the side-effects, and again in others certain complications do not seem to occur. For the sake of brevity, most side-effects and complications will be discussed for chlorpromazine as an example, only adding some remarks on other drugs. Some distinction should be made between those side-effects which are part of the normal action of the drug, among which most authors include the extrapyramidal syndromes, and toxic reaction such as agranulocytosis or jaundice. In this section, side-effects and complications will be discussed together under the particular system of the body which they primarily affect. At the same time, the mode of their production and their significance, if any, in treatment will be clarified as far as possible.

From a theoretical point of view there might be no sharp distinction between side-effects linked to the therapeutic action, and complications. Thus, persistent dyskinesias after long-term neuroleptic treatment are a complication, but the extrapyramidal effect of neuroleptics is generally considered an integral part of their therapeutic action. Also, vegetative symptoms are part of the drugs' action. Highly potent neuroleptics have strong extrapyramidal, and only minimal vegetative side-effects. Theoretically interesting is that the vegetative side-effects known from chlorpromazine are similar to those characteristic for the tricyclic antidepressants. Systematic investigations of the side-effects of tricyclic antidepressants and tricyclic neuroleptics have shown that these two groups have much closer relations than could be expected from their therapeutic action profile. Thus, several neuroleptics also have an antidepressant effect in low doses, and it happened to be these neuroleptics that have fewer extrapyramidal and more vegetative side-effects.

Two main groups of either unpleasant or actually dangerous side-effects can be distinguished, namely somatic and psychiatric manifestations. They may occur after an overdose, for instance in suicidal attempts, or in the course of therapeutic administration. In this section only the latter will be described distinguishing between those after short-term use of weeks, and long-term use over several years. Finally, symptoms due to discontinuation of neuroleptics must be mentioned.

Disturbances of Somatic Functions

1. Neurological Side-Effects: It appears that extrapyramidal symptoms, as the most frequent side-effects of neuroleptic drugs, were not immediately recognized. Early observations were reported by Steck; Haase; Giacobini; and Osterman. These symptoms are more frequent with the piperazine derivatives than with chlorpromazine. Freyhan distinguishes three main types:

a. *Parkinsonism,* which varies in degree from diminished drive and lassitude to the fully developed syndrome with rigidity, tremors, salivation, cog wheel rigidity, slowness of walking, mask-like facies and other typical features.

b. *Dyskinetic Syndromes* in the form of speech and swallowing difficulties due to hypertonicity of regional muscle groups, perioral spasms with, frequently, an involuntary protrusion of the tongue, torticollis, mandibular tics, oculogyric spasms, hyperextension of the neck and trunk, with the spine being curved backward from the hip, myoclonic muscle twitching and torsion spasms. Characteristically, these manifestations wax and wane, and there is often sweating, pallor and sometimes fever. Consciousness is never impaired. Other names for this syndrome are hyperkinetic-dystonic crises or excitomotoric syndrome (Delay et al.).

c. *Akathisia:* This term was first used in 1902 by Haskovic, and Kinnier Wilson described it as one of the features of parkinsonism. It is characterized by restlessness, localized by patients in their muscles, and inability to sit still. They describe it as "quivering," and Haase, in a self-observation, experienced a sensation in his legs which forced him to move them around.

Freyhan found a sex difference in that parkinsonism was twice as frequent in women, and akathisia and dyskinesia were more often seen in males. The dyskinetic reactions occurred very early in the treatment, 85 per cent in the first three days; parkinsonism later. Neither of the two syndromes depend on high dosage, although Haase thinks that dyskinesia may have some relation to a too rapid dose increase. Dyskinesia, contrary to parkinsonism, is a transitory phenomenon. Mild cases may be managed by dose reduction. Severe dyskinesias of sudden onset can be treated by intravenous injection of anti-parkinsonian drugs. In addition, oral medication of kemadrin, 10 to 20 mg., is recommended as initial dose followed by smaller doses of anti-parkinsonian drugs with each dose of the phenothiazines. In parkinsonism Freyhan does not recommend the routine use of anti-parkinsonian agents, since some of them such as disipal, are mild stimulants and may complicate therapy. The treatment of akathisia is more difficult, and in some cases the neuroleptic must be discontinued. Akathisia is often mistaken for an agitated depression. Hodge rightly points out that it is not accompanied by mood changes.

Milder hypokinetic extrapyramidal syndromes have been called "parkinsonoid" by Staehelin. It is usually noticed after ten days. Symptoms are a slowing down of psychomotor activity with a fixed posture, absence of associated movements of the arms on walking, a degree of mask-like facies, occasional trembling of the tongue and facial seborrhoea. Haase has pointed out that the most common evidence of this syndrome is a change in the handwriting in the form of micrographia, which he found in 86 per cent of his cases, while the more severe symptoms of parkinsonism were present in only 5 per cent. The gradual decrease in the size of the handwriting was found by him to be closely correlated with the lessening of impulse on the part of the patient, resulting in a diminution of both physical and mental activity.

Both Haase and Gratton have compared the extrapyramidal effects of high doses of the neuroleptic drugs with the sequelae to encephalitis lethargica. Gratton describes "phenothiazination" as a "chemical reversible encephalitis" and distinguishes a somnolent, an akinetic-abulic, and a turbulent phase. The somnolent phase lasts from 2 to 7 days with chlorpromazine and 15 or more with reserpine. It is more prominent with chlorpromazine than with the piperazine derivatives. The akinetic-abulic phase was first described by Flügel and Bente. In this state there is no rigidity or tremor, but relaxed musculature with trembling, salivation and seborrhoea with expressionless facies. Mentally, it is characterized by diminished emotional irritability and drive, with relaxation and a more complacent attitude to previously disturbing factors. They found the EEG in this state to show, in about a third of the cases, a continuous, often monorhythmical, bilateral synchronous theta activity in the anterior brain with marked decrease of psychosensory reactions. This tracing was similar to that found in akinetic epilepsy and certain forms of stupor. They could rarely obtain this state, which they regarded as a desired therapeutic effect, with chlorpromazine alone, and they found that, in 77 per cent of cases, a pronounced degree of the syndrome could be produced by giving 250 mg. of chlorpromazine and 7 mg. of reserpine. In the akinetic-abulic state, the normal sleep rhythm is no longer apparent, and the patients sometimes sleep during the day and lie, relaxed but awake, at night. A turbulent phase with anxiety and affective disturbance also occurs.

Like other observers, Gratton found a 2:1 incidence of extrapyramidal signs in favor of women. He also showed that synthetic estrogenic hormones will facilitate the appearance of these reactions in both men and women. Another endocrinological factor, hypoparathyroidism, favoring dyskinetic syndromes was recognized by Schaaf and Payne.

The most interesting question is whether these extrapyramidal syndromes play a part in the therapeutic mechanism, and a number of workers have advised their production by means of high doses of drugs in order to obtain the maximum improvement in patients. Staehelin concluded that there was a therapeutically beneficial correlation between chlorpromazine therapy and the "parkinsonoid" reaction, and Haase has suggested that one of the reasons for the successful action of the drug in states of hypermotility might be that, as indicated experimentally, one of the chief areas affected is the reticulo-corticostriate circuit of the brain, "the spot where impulses are first translated into motion." Such correlation of improvement with the production of extrapyramidal signs would suggest that those areas of the brain which form the reticular formation and the basal ganglia are being acted upon by the drug. A definite relationship, in each individual case between extrapyramidal side-effects and clinical improvement does not exist. Simpson and Kunz-Bartholini even noticed the most pronounced extrapyramidal symptoms in patients with unsatisfactory results.

At the International Colloquium in Paris in 1955, Freyhan developed his concept that the effectiveness of chlorpromazine is singularly dependent on hypermotility and abnormally increased initiative, no matter whether such states originate from anxiety or are the manifestations of organic, affective or schizophrenic psychoses. He believes, and the clinical evidence is in favor of this, that all psychopathological states manifesting themselves in a final common pathway of hypermotility, impulsiveness and emotional tension can be effectively modified by the drug. He explains clinical response in relation to the patient's awareness of reduced motility and impulse. Manics, hyperactive schizophrenics, and other agitated and impulsive patients, can be slowed down beneficially, while those who are retarded and depressed are made worse. In the case of neurotics, there is a considerable variation. Those who need intensified activity to neutralize their anxiety, such as many obsessionals, may react unfavorably to the loss of initiative and drive and experience mounting anxiety. Others with much tormenting anxiety and self concern may experience a loss of drive as a desirable passiveness. This may account for the often contradictory results in neurotics and for the poorer benefits in this group in general, since their overactivity is often merely a symptom of an underlying conflict, unlike that of the psychotic which may well be dependent on more straightforward physiological mechanisms.

It seems that akathisia and dyskinesia, as distinct from the hypomotility of parkinsonism, are not beneficial therapeutically. The question has arisen, in view of the rather distressing nature of the fully developed extrapyramidal syndrome, whether the same results can be obtained by giving anti-parkinsonian drugs in association with the tranquilizer, in order to obtain the benefits minus parkinsonism. Most authors feel that this combination does not interfere with the theraputic results. The extrapyramidal symptoms usually rapidly disappear after the drug is stopped, although caution is advised in Parkinson's disease which Fernandes and Leitao regard as a contraindication. Dangerous, sometimes fatal incidents, with board-like rigidity and difficulty in swallowing were seen. Genetic factors may contribute to the degree of drug-induced parkinsonism as suggested by the report of patients with an advanced degree of the syndrome whose mothers had died from Parkinson's disease. Myrianthopoulos et al. found that blood relatives of patients with extrapyramidal side-effects due to neuroleptics have a higher incidence of non-drug related pyramidal syndromes than the relatives of patients without extrapyramidal side-effects. Kruse who observed three cases, where extrapyramidal symptoms (restlessness) persisted for up to 18 months after cessation of the phenothiazine, suggests, in view of the fact that these patients were aged 50 or over, that a predisposing factor might be vascular changes in the extrapyramidal system.

Where there is difficulty between the restlessness due to the physiological effect of the drug itself and the enhanced anxiety that sometimes occurs, particularly in neurotics, an anti-parkinsonian agent may be given which will relieve the physiological symptoms due to extrapyramidal stimulation but not those of psychological origin. When pregnant women are treated with phenothiazines, the newborn may develop extrapyramidal symptoms (Hill et al.).

The frequency of extrapyramidal signs differs with the various neuroleptics. At the one end are drugs like levomepromazine, thioridazine and mepazine which have little or no extrapyramidal action or may even have an anti-parkinsonian effect. At the other end are thioproperazine, thiothixene and several piperazine derivatives which almost regularly cause more or less pronounced extrapyramidal manifestations, and always more than the corresponding promazine derivatives. Akathisia, too, is mostly limited to piperazine derivatives. Always the intensity of these side-effects depends on the dosage, as do the hypokinetic phenomena. Contrary to this, the dyskinetic symptoms in the beginning of therapy depend primarily on the rapidity of the increase in dosage.

Noteworthy in this connection are the recent observations that extremely large doses of highly potent neuroleptics, even if rapidly increased, cause surprisingly few extrapyramidal symptoms (Gayral and Lambert).

Since 1959 attention has been drawn to persistent hyperkinesias which may occur after long-term neuroleptic therapy. French authors were the first to mention these motor phenomena which occur at the earliest after three months of treatment, and sometimes even after years (Broussolle and Rosier; Sigwald et al.). They occur primarily in the region of the head and consist of rolling movements and protrusion of the tongue, chewing and smacking, or grimacing of the lower face. In the extremities choreiform, athetoid, torsion-dystonic or ballistic hyperkinesias occur. They may be limited to more hyperextension of the big toes and may be easily overlooked. Sometimes strange swaying movements of the trunk are observed. Occasionally torticollis is seen (Harenko). Some patients have periodic respiratory disturbances which may persist during sleep, while most other symptoms mostly disappear during sleep (Hunter et al.). Uhrbrand and Faurbye saw these late hyperkinesias in 15 of 155 patients treated with perphenazine. Predisposing factors are advanced age and brain damage like trauma, vascular conditions, brain surgery such as lobotomy (Hunter et al.). Studies on larger groups of unselected hospital material did not confirm these predisposing factors (Heinrich et al.). There is only a slight sex difference predisposing to these symptoms (20 per cent females to 10 per cent males). It is still debated whether highly potent neuroleptics lead to persistent hyperkinesias more often than weaker neuroleptics. There is evidence that even drugs with little extrapyramidal effect such as thioridazine may cause late hyperkinesias. Their frequency does depend on the total amount given. Several investigations comparing dosage and intensity of extrapyramidal action revealed that late hyperkinesias are the more frequent the larger the intensity of extrapyramidal action had been during the total treatment time (Heinrich et al.). Contrary to the sudden hyperkinetic-dystonic symptoms after short medication, late hyperkinesias set in slowly, and are often not noticed by the patient himself. Sometimes they appear only after discontinuation of the drug which had been well tolerated for months. Often they disappear, when treatment is reinstated. The late hyperkinesias do not respond to antiparkinsonian drugs. They may, however, still cease after months, although it must be assumed that they are irreversible hyperkinesias (Degkwitz and Wenzel). Therefore, the concept that severe extrapyramidal symptoms are necessary for maximal therapeutic effect needs careful reexamination (Schmidt and Jarcho).

Other neurological side-effects are rare. Robie presented a case who showed a typical picture of tabes on chlorpromazine, 25 mg. t.i.d. for five weeks. There were Argyll Robertson pupils, a positive Romberg sign, extreme ataxia, loss of vibration sense up to the knees, speech garbling, memory defects, absent knee reflexes, and muscle weakness in the neck. The entire picture resolved spontaneously with no residual effects after ten days off the drug. A similar syndrome due to overdosage of trifluoperazine was seen by Rudy et al. Such neurological syndromes as "pseudotabes," spastic paresis, and others are rare, and were interpreted as "decompensation phenomena" based on individual disposition by Helmchen and Hippius.

Convulsions may occur with all neuroleptics but are rare and seem to occur preferably with chlorpromazine and promazine (Logothetis). They also depend on the dosage and occur relatively often in acute poisoning due to suicidal attempts. Also a fast increase of dosage may lead to convulsions. Graff et al. reported convulsions after three 8 mg. tablets of perphenazine taken over 26 hours by a woman, eight weeks pregnant, with no history of epilepsy. Blair and Brady saw convulsions at any stage of the treatment, Logothetis mostly either within the first few days of medication or after sudden increase in dosage. Schlichter et al. observed that 11 out of 12 patients on 4000 mg. of chlorpromazine daily, developed seizures. Most convulsions occur in patients who never had had them before. They are typically grand mal in character and Szatmari reported two cases of status epilepticus. Doussinet found frequent temporal localization in the EEG. Fabisch demonstrated that chlorpromazine, in doses of 0.3 to 0.5 mg./kg. body weight intravenously, can increase abnormal phenomena in the EEG of epileptic patients, in a way similar to overbreathing or photic stimulation. Focal EEG changes without convulsions were seen by Helmchen and Künkel.

Chlorpromazine has repeatedly increased the incidence of convulsions in post-lobotomy patients. Paganini and Zlotow did not see convulsions in lobotomized patients who never had convulsions after the operation; but they did see recurrence of convulsions and occasional status epilepticus in those who had had previous convulsions.

Shaw et al. have drawn attention to central nervous system manifestations in children, such as seizures, muscle spasms, nystagmus, vomiting and respiratory difficulty which gave rise to diagnoses of neurological and infectious disease in a number of cases. All recovered completely when the drug was withdrawn.

2. Vegetative Side-Effects: Pharmacological evidence already suggested that the clinical use of neuroleptics would lead to numerous vegetative side-effects, both peripheral and central ones. They are most frequent in the beginning of treatment. Later on the organism adjusts to them by restoring the vegetative equilibrium. The clinical characteristics of these vegetative syndromes depend on the interplay of the manifold central and peripheral vegetative effects of the drugs. The result is a combination of sympathetic and parasympathetic symptoms. Phenomena of parasympathetic irritation due to adrenolytic effect are predominant. The addition of sympathetic symptoms is understandable because many neuroleptics, similar to the tricyclic antidepressants, have, aside from an adrenolytic action, also a definite anticholinergic effect. The outcome is a manifold, often apparently contradictory picture; and it often remains an open question what is peripheral, and what central effect. Since regulatory mechanisms are involved, it can be assumed that there is always some central effect.

Vegetative phenomena are hypotension or, occasionally, hypertension, bradycardia or tachycardia, palpitations, stenocardiac complaints, hypersalivation or dryness of the mouth, diarrhea or constipation, fever or hypothermia, perspiration or anhidrosis, flushes or chills, pallor or reddening of the skin, tiredness and sleepiness or sleep disturbances, polyuria or disturbances of micturition, loss of appetite or bulimia, nausea, vomiting, hyperperistalsis or intestinal atonia (paralytic ileus), miosis or mydriasis, impaired accommodation.

These symptoms are less apparent with the piperazine derivatives than with the drugs of the promazine group and those neuroleptics which are related to the tricyclic antidepressants.

3. Cardio-vascular Symptoms: Facial pallor is often noticeable in spite of warm and dry skin and good peripheral circulation, particularly after parenteral application or high oral dosage. Delay and Deniker noted redness and flushing of the cheeks soon after the drug had been given.

Hypotensive effects are frequent. Blood pressure readings after intramuscular administration usually drop within 30 to 40 minutes an average of 30 to 50 mm. systolic and 20 to 30 mm. diastolic (Cohen). A compensatory tachycardia of 20 to 40 per minute may lead to the complaint of palpitations. The blood pressure drop is maximal in three to four hours, with usually a return to pre-injection levels within four to six hours. There may be dizziness on assuming the erect posture, with concomitant clouding of vision and feeling of imbalance. Syncopal attacks may occur, more often in those over 60. In some cases of cerebral arteriosclerosis, cerebral vascular hypotension may result in memory defect, difficulty in retention and possibly clouding of consciousness. Foster et al. recommend the use of noradrenaline rather than adrenaline to restore the blood pressure because of phenothiazine reversal of adrenaline action.

Goldman has quoted instances where a lowered blood pressure, produced by chlorpromazine, has led to vascular accidents such as coronary occlusion in elderly patients. Pauly reports two coronary thromboses during the course of chlorpromazine therapy, one of whom died. Nayrac and Graux observed three cases of sudden death in patients on chlorpromazine, which they attributed to the fall in blood pressure with consequent irreversible collapse or vascular occlusion in the heart or cerebrum. In the first German paper on chlorpromazine, H. H. Meyer reported on a fatality in a 50 year old woman with hypertension who, under moderate doses of megaphen, collapsed and died a few days later. Tschudin has recorded a cardiac death in a catatonic excitement and this has been mentioned repeatedly since. It is a warning that, in the severe excitement states where cardiovascular collapse is always a danger, the neuroleptic drugs should be administered with caution. Their use is invaluable in many cases and the advantages outweigh the dangers, provided that as small a dose as possible is used and the patients are carefully observed. The greatest care is required in the agitated psychoses of old age with hypertension and coronary atheromatosis.

The intensity of blood pressure changes differs with the various neuroleptics. Those of the piperazine group with strong extrapyramidal action have comparatively little effect on blood pressure. It can be considerable with the promazine derivatives and the phenothiazines with the piperidyl ring. Especially larger doses and intravenous injections cause a fall in systolic and diastolic pressure with subsequent tachycardia. This is due to peripheral vasodilatation in skin and muscles which leads to orthostatic hypotension, experienced by the patient as weakness, darkness before the eyes, and dizziness. In severe cases it may lead to collapse, particularly in patients with preexisting circulatory lability (Kaplan). Severe collapses were seen in patients with pheochromocytoma (Brody; Lund-Johansen). In these patients reversal of the adrenaline action by the phenothiazines may lead to severe circulatory collapse. Dramatic fall in blood pressure under phenothiazines suggests the possibility of a pheochromocytoma (Lund-Johansen).

4. FATALITIES: Sudden death with tricyclic drugs drew much recent attention to the circulatory effects of neuroleptics and all other psychopharmaca. Hollister and Kosek reported six such fatalities in patients with a normal heart during treatment with phenothiazines, presumably due to ventricular fibrillation followed by irreversible cardiac arrest. Other sudden fatalities may be due to suffocation after aspiration of food or vomitus (von Brauchitsch and May). Such deaths can be credited to neuroleptics only indirectly. A direct effect of the psychotropic drugs must be assumed, when sudden unexpected death occurs under an Adams-Stokes syndrome with sudden pallor, clouded sensorium, unconsciousness, pulselessness, and inaudible heart sounds. Autopsy in such cases offers no explanation for the cause of death. Leestma and Koening studied the medical world literature by means of a computerized search system. Reviewing their own two cases and 73 cases from the literature, they came to the conclusion that there are three types of death from phenothiazines, namely aspiration with asphyxia, irreversible cardiac arrest, and catastrophic hypotension. The most important effect of phenothiazines on the cardiovascular system is the ability to exert alpha-adrenergic blockage and to produce epinephrine reverses, the production of repolarization defects in the EKG, depressive effects on ATP-ase action in the heart, quinidine-like action on the heart, and the ability, alone or in combination with pressor amines, to produce cardiac arrhythmias.

EKG studies in patients with normal heart were initiated by these reports on sudden deaths. Findings of usually reversible polarization disturbances were prolonged PQ- and QT-intervals, flattening, inversion, broadening and deformation (splitting, notching) of the T-wave, lowering of the ST-interval. The frequency of such EKG changes depends on type and dosage of the neuroleptic. They were seen with thioridazine by Kelly et al. in some cases already after 200 mg. daily, while Wendkos saw the first T-wave changes only after daily doses of 600 mg. and more. Huston and Bell found that thioridazine up to 300 mg. leads to EKG changes in 50 per cent, doses of up to 900 mg. daily in 70 per cent of all patients. At a symposium in Montreal there was consensus of opinion that all phenothiazines may give, more or less frequently, such EKG changes.

Gastro-intestinal symptoms consist mostly of spastic colitis with diarrhea and constipation. More significant intestinal atonies (Kline and Jacobs), occasionally lead to paralytic ileus (Warnes et al.). Such incidents occur in neuroleptics with strong anticholinergic action like mepazine and chlorprothixine.

5. Bladder Disturbances: Bladder disturbances are also explained by anticholinergic action. Paralysis of the detrusor muscle leads to disturbances of micturition and sometimes to complete occlusion of the bladder making catheterization necessary (Kline and Jacobs). On the other hand, chlorpromazine and other phenothiazines have some antidiuretic effect. Edemas on face and legs may occur (Barsa and Kline).

Other anticholinergic effects are visible complants due to impaired accommodation and dryness of the mouth. These harmless but subjectively highly unpleasant vegetative side-effects are worse in the beginning of the treatment, probably depend on the dosage, and diminish spontaneously in the course of treatment.

Nasal congestion, often persistent, may interfere with breathing through the nose. Large oral doses of neuroleptics occasionally lead to nausea and vomiting which is surprising since neuroleptics in general have an antiemetic effect. They seem to be central phenomena because simultaneous disturbances of equilibrium are often present.

Central disturbances of temperature regulations express themselves in elevation of temperature without evidence of an infection early in treatment. Blair and Brady found that there was often an exacerbation of the psychosis in association with this; and that it was a prognostically favorable sign. Ayd has described a fatal case of hyperpyrexia with chlorpromazine. Shapiro gave a survey on hyperthermia in connection with a case due to trifluoperazine.

6. Endocrinological Side-Effects: Endocrinological disturbances due to neuroleptic therapy are relatively frequent but often so slight that they may go unnoticed. In view of certain theories on the site of action of phenothiazines, the frequency of endocrinological changes is not surprising (von Brauchitsch). Khazan et al. found them in 5 per cent of all patients. Swelling of the mammae and galactorrhea are seen with chlorpromazine and other phenothiazines (Mendels). The lactation is similar in composition to that seen in post-partum, but there is no lactosuria. Phenothiazines probably do not effect the endocrine glands themselves but the anterior hypophysis and the hypothalamus. In patients with galactorrhea overproduction of lactotropic hormone with deficiency of luteinizing hormone was found by Kulcsar et al. Hilbert saw false positive reactions in pregnancy tests. The occasional menstrual disturbances with amenorrhea or oligomenorrhea are probably also hypothalamic (Kulcsar et al.; Destounis). However, it must be remembered that menstrual disturbances also occur in untreated psychotics. In males gynecomastia was seen with occasional frontal adiposity and striae suggesting Cushing's disease. Disturbances of ejaculation were discussed in the section on thioridazine, although this side-effect is not limited to thioridazine, and was seen by Ditman with chlorprothixine.

Weight gain is comparatively frequent in long-term neuroleptic treatment.

Still unexplained is the effect of neuroleptics on the endocrine function of the pancreas. Cooperberg describes the appearance of diabetes together with jaundice about two weeks after cessation of therapy. He points out that Charatan and Bartlett showed there could be impaired glucose tolerance after a single injection of chlorpromazine. He suggests that the sudden appearance of the diabetes might be due to the stress reaction of the drug on the liver in a potential diabetic, but considers it possible that chlorpromazine might have a more direct effect in precipitating diabetes. Glycosuria alone has been noted. In Saint Elizabeths Hospital in Washington, Thonnard-Neumann found an increase of diabetes in female patients from 4.2 per cent before the introduction of phenothiazines to 17.2 per cent in 1966. Withdrawal of the drug led to a remission of this "phenothiazine diabetes" in 25 per cent of the patients. Opitz and Loeser found that neuroleptics counteract substances which decrease the blood sugar level. However, there are also observations of hypoglycemic effects (Hippius et al.).

7. Biochemical Side-Effects: Biochemical side-effects of tricyclic neuroleptics are usually only revealed, when special chemical studies of the serum are undertaken. They should be known, however, because otherwise there is danger that if biochemical changes are found, they are wrongly interpreted. In systematic electrophoretic investigations of serum-protein-fractions under neuroleptic treatment, Hippius et al. found an almost constant increase of α_2 globulins which later in treatment again disappear. It may be accompanied by increased sedimentation rate. Bengzon et al. investigated the effect of neuroleptics on the activity of various serum enzymes. Such enzyme activity findings have practical importance in connection with jaundice due to tricyclic neuroleptics (see later). Increased enzyme activity prior to treatment might become normal during medication.

8. Hematopoietic System: Harmless changes in the blood picture under neuroleptic treatment are frequent. Transitory eosinophilia has its maximum in the second to fourth week. In the beginning of treatment short-lasting leucopenia and eosinopenia occur which do not require discontinuation of the drugs. Long-term therapy may lead to relative lymphocytosis and monocytosis. The most frequent complication is agranulocytosis. Several deaths have been reported (Hippius and Kanig). The agranulocytosis may be related to dosage because the most frequent reports refer to neuroleptics which must be given in doses higher than 100 mg. daily, for instance, chlorpromazine, promazine, thioridazine, mepazine, perazine. Actually, agranulocytosis is possible in all tricyclic psychopharmaca, although it is rare in those given in lower doses. If one combines all tricyclic psychopharmaca, the frequency of agranulocytosis in 0.001 to 0.002 per cent, as assumed by the AMA Council on Pharmacology and Chemistry in 1956, is considered too low by Hippius and Kanig because many cases are not diagnosed. Agranulocytosis before the fifth week of treatment, affects mostly middle-aged and older patients, and has a mortality rate of 30 to 40 per cent. Regular blood controls during the first ten weeks of treatment are advisable in order to recognize this complication early. Since agranulocytosis due to phenothiazines develops slowly, immediate discontinuation may prevent further aggravation. After chlorpromazine recurrent agranulocytosis was seen by Pollack, and patients who developed this complication before the sixth week of treatment usually had been treated with chlorpromazine before.

The onset may be acute with high fever and oral inflammations to the point of necrosis with regional lymphadenitis. Intestinal inflammations may be complicated by a jaundice which is unrelated to the usual chlorpromazine jaundice starting between the second and fourth week of treatment with the drug. The blood picture shows disappearance of neutrophiles. There is not always correlation between clinical symptoms and blood picture. Agranulocytosis may appear in general sepsis or pulmonary complications (Tuteur).

Treatment should be preventive by means of regular blood counts and discontinuation of the drug if the white count falls below 4,000. If the count rises again and the drug is continued in small doses, the patient and his family must be warned to report any sore throat immediately. Once the condition has developed, antibiotics, and cortisone or ACTH should be given. Blood transfusions are of doubtful value, and Tuteur believes that one of his fatalities was due to the transfusion.

The specificity of the noxious drug may be considerable. Thus Bashkaran et al. saw a complete myelophthisic anemia with fatal outcome during the tenth week of prochlorpromazine therapy in a patient who previously had tolerated chlorpromazine well. This patient had a completely aplastic bone marrow, and also the formation of red blood corpuscles and thromocytes was involved. Such cases are rare, but still rarer is the involvement of red cells and thrombocytes alone. After prochlorpremazine Fischer and Gottreich have described a case of severe anemia without evidence of granulocytic impairment, which recovered; the patient subsequently received courses of triflupromazine and trifluoperazine without any complications. The already mentioned case by Cooperberg of hemolytic anemia which developed together with diabetes, cleared up completely after three months. A recurrent thrombocytopenia after thioridazine was seen by Aivazian. In such cases blood coagulation can be impaired. On the other hand, thromboses were also seen and may become a dangerous complication of neuroleptic therapy. Häfner and Brehm assume an incidence of thrombosis in 3 per cent of all patients treated with neuroleptics. They may lead to thrombophlebitis or—even fatal embolism (Suchenwirth). Thrombophlebitis may also be a complication of intravenous infusion of phenothiazines. Maurice described the development of phlebitis, mostly of the large veins of the legs in 5 out of 180 patients, three of whom died.

9. Disturbances of Liver Function: One complication of phenothiazine therapy is the development of jaundice of an intrahepatic obstructive type. The estimated incidence of this varies slightly. Ayd gives it for chlorpromazine as 1.4 per cent, Rees as 1.5 to 2 per cent, Doughty as 0.8 to 1.4 per cent, and Blair and Brady as 0.1 to 4 per cent. The general consensus of opinion is that it is an allergic reaction to the drug (Cook and Sherlock), but no criteria for its prediction have been established except for a significantly high incidence of previous allergic reactions in those who develop it. It usually occurs in the first month of treatment, but is not dependent on high dosage since Ayd found it in patients on 75 to 200 mg. daily. In a few instances, the jaundice appeared one to two weeks after the phenothiazine drug was stopped. Its occurrence is not related to sex or to diagnosis, nor to the route of adminis-

tration of the drug, but it occurs most often in those over 40. It may lead to unnecessary surgery if the jaundice is not recognized as drug-induced.

The onset of the jaundice may be preceded by a transient eosinophilia, chills, fever, abdominal pain, persistent or intermittent nausea with occasionally vomiting and pruritus. Bartholomew et al. cite a case in which acute abdominal pain simulated an acute abdominal emergency. These prodromal symptoms last for about a week and they disappear when the jaundice develops, apart from the pruritus which persists. The jaundice is of the obstructive type with dark urine and pale stools, a raised serum alkaline phosphatase, bilirubinemia and usually unimpaired parenchymal function of the liver as shown by the usual tests. In general, it subsides within 4 weeks, but cases have been reported in which it lasted for as long as 197 days.

Some clinicians withdraw the drug; others do not, claiming that the jaundice clears up anyway. Most agree that it is safe to recommence the phenothiazine when the jaundice subsides. The patients with jaundice should be on a low fat diet with parenteral fat soluble vitamins and intravenous glucose if necessary.

The typical liver histology is biliary stasis with infiltration of the portal tracts by polymorphs, among which eosinophils are numerous during the first week but are replaced later by lymphocytes. In the typical case, portal-zone fibrosis and hepatic cellular damage are either slight or absent. Suggestions as to the mode of causation include the idea that increased permeability of the cholangioles may result from hypersensitivity to the drug (Editorial British Med. J.), that there is inspissation of bile and interference with its flow due to a change in its composition brought about by the action of the phenothiazine on the liver (Stein and Wright), or that there is a disturbance of the motility of the bile ducts (Besson). Menguy et al. observed increased tonus of the sphincter Oddi.

Aidin recommends the estimation of serum glutamic-oxalacetic transaminase to avoid confusion with other types of obstructive jaundice since it is greatly increased in jaundice due to phenothiazines. The most sensitive tests during treatment appear to be the serum alkaline phosphatase and the bromsulfalein retention. The alkaline phosphatase often rises, but Cares et al. did not find it a very accurate predictor of impending icterus, and prefers serum bilirubin estimations over the first four months.

Although the usual phenothiazine jaundice is harmless, liver deaths have been reported. Boardman in 1954 had a fatal case, a 45 year old woman with mitral stenosis, in whom liver microscopy showed a toxic hepatitis. Elliot et al. report the death of a patient from aseptic liver necrosis within eight days after the dose of chlorpromazine being increased to 1600 mg. daily. Kalk has observed a case of acute yellow atrophy.

There is evidence that, in a minute number of cases, the jaundice may be followed by more permanent damage. Melrose and Roy studied two patients who had had chlorpromazine jaundice six months and one year previously, respectively. In both cases, there were persistent histological changes but no biliary cirrhosis. In one case, the liver function tests remained abnormal.

Myers and his fellow workers observed a case in which, one year after the onset of chlorpromazine jaundice, biliary cirrhosis, confirmed by biopsy, and portal hypertension were present. Kalk followed with biopsy studies in one case the transition from liver changes with cell degeneration and periportal fibrosis into a biliary cirrhosis. Kelsey et al. also reported cirrhotic changes in 2 apparently recovered patients out of 20, but he could not with certainty attribute this to chlorpromazine, since they had received other drugs and had previously suffered from diseases which could have involved the liver. Liver damage has not been reported in patients who have taken large amounts of phenothiazines in suicide attempts. It appears that the restoration of normal liver histology and function may be delayed in a small number of cases, and patients who have had this complication should be watched carefully afterward with regard to recovery of liver function and the possible development of biliary cirrhosis.

Lambo has suggested, in view of his finding that allergic manifestations to chlorpromazine, including jaundice, are very rare in Africans and Chinese but common in the Europeans in the same area, that there may also be some racial susceptibility involved.

Lomas and Winkelman both regard previous liver damage as contraindication. This opinion is not shared by Moyer et al. and Kinross-Wright; but both found that patients with hypoproteinemic states or chronic alcoholism and pregnant women seem predisposed to phenothiazine jaundice. Isaacs et al. suggests that chlorpromazine should not be given when infectious hepatitis is endemic, the patient is malnourished or has liver disease, and where other potentially hepatotoxic agents are being used or estrogens have been given.

Significant is the statement by Hollister that the incidence of phenothiazine jaundice gradually decreases, although more and more patients are treated with phenothiazines. This is maybe due to the fact that today chlorpromazine is used less, and the highly potent neuroleptics more. Chlorpromazine is the phenothiazine which most often causes jaundice. The few, mostly single, observations of jaundice due to other phenothiazines suggest that it is a relatively rare occurrence in such drugs as promazine, levopromazine, mepazine, prochlorperazine and thioridazine (Kähler).

10. Dermatological Side-Effects and Ocular Opacities: All phenothiazines are potentially allergenic. Like jaundice, the severe allergic skin manifestations due to phenothiazines also became less frequent. Chlorpromazine caused allergic reactions on skin and mucous membranes in approximately 10 per cent of patients mostly between the second and fourth week of treatment. Aside from the intake of the drugs, contact of a phenothiazine derivative with the skin may also lead to allergies. In the beginning of psychopharmacology more than half of the nursing personnel developed contact dermatitis before the tablets were coated. This does not exist with the newer neuroleptics.

All types of generalized drug eruptions of the skin may occur. Cohn, in an early paper, described different types of dermatitis. Less frequent are allergic symptoms like facial edemas, asthma, allergic arthritis. Antiallergic medication during these manifestations (second to fourth week of treatment) usually makes it unnecessary to stop the neuroleptic.

Different from the allergic side-effects is the photosensitivity of patients under phenothiazine medication. It is partly dosage-dependent and persists during the whole period of treatment. Patients under phenothiazines have a lower skin erythema threshold (Degkwitz) and must be warned against sun bathing which may lead to severe skin eruptions.

Recently observed skin pigmentations are also related to sunlight. The parts of the skin involved are those that are exposed, like head, neck, hands and so on. Other pigmentary deposits were found in the eyes, particularly in the lens, cornea and sclera, occasionally also in the conjunctiva. The skin changes appear as reddish, bluish, bluish-greyish and slate grey pigmentations.

The first extensive report on these skin pigmentations and ocular opacities was published by Greiner and Berry in 1964. They saw skin pigmentations in 70 females all of whom had been on large doses of 500 to 1500 mg. of chlorpromazine for at least three years. Most such observations were made on chlorpromazine-treated patients. Probably other phenothiazines, or perhaps even all tricyclic psychopharmaca can lead to such pigmentations in skin and eyes (Margolis and Goble).

Statements regarding the frequency of lenticular opacities must take into consideration that approximately 11 per cent of the general population over 40 years of age have such pigmentary deposits anyway (Delong). Rubin and Slonicki studied the biochemical origin of these skin and eye pigmentations due to the phenothiazines. It is possible that the understanding of their development would help to explain the chemical quality of those receptors in the central nervous system which are responsible for the action of neuroleptics.

Psychiatric Side-Effects

Psychopathological symptoms which were not present before and appear only during neuroleptic medication, can be either activated symptoms of the disease for which the patient is treated, or undesired side-effects of the neuroleptic drug administered. Hippius pointed out that the second possibility is frequently overlooked but must be properly recognized in order to decide on the continuation of treatment.

Apathy, lassitude and lack of initiative are frequent side-effects. Neuroleptics with a dampening effect like chlorpromazine may cause somnolence and even sopor and comatose states, particularly, when these neuroleptics are used in combination with barbiturates and similar drugs. Even without such combinations drugs like chlorpromazine produce drowsiness in the initial stage. This is less noticeable with the phenothiazines of the piperazine group. The patients are easily awakened by the usual stimuli and rapidly become alert again. There is no interference with nocturnal sleep, even when the patient sleeps most of the day. The hypersomnia which occurs in 85 per cent of patients (Cohen) disappears within about seven to ten days. In contrast, a small number (0.5 per cent) develop insomnia. There are often vivid dreams.

Disturbances of wakefulness are often seen with the piperazine derivatives in the sense of sleep disturbances. Sometimes it comes to a complete dissociation or inversion of the sleep rhythm. The strongest effects were seen by

Delay and Deshaies with thioproperazine. The patients were active in the morning, but at about noontime, 3 to 4 hours after ingestion of the drug, they lay down and complained of fatigue, restlessness combined with inability to walk, and heaviness of the limbs. At the same time, there was a difficulty with speaking and echolalia might occur. The symptoms reached their zenith by about the seventh to ninth hours. There might be insomnia with inversion of the sleep rhythm, and motor restlessness developed after 24 hours. Patients showed, at first, depression or anxiety, which was followed after about 48 hours by relaxation and euphoria.

The most striking psychiatric complications are delirious and confusional states. Neuroleptics precipitate such dramatic syndromes less often than antidepressants, but they do occur in neuroleptics with dulling effect, and in those which also have anticholinergic action. Confusional states were seen by Blair and Brady in about 2 per cent of chlorpromazine-treated patients, mostly with high doses, and a patient of Kinross-Wright died in a toxic, confusional state due to chlorpromazine. Acute delirious states are most frequently seen in the beginning of treatment, and set in suddenly, often at night. Older patients go into a delirium more often than younger ones, in whom they occur only with larger doses, particularly, when the amount is quickly increased. The manifestation rate in all drugs depends not only on the amount but also on the speed with which the dosage is either increased or, also, decreased (Helmchen and Hippius). The acute delirious states with their multitude of symptoms must be distinguished from more gradually developing amnestic syndromes in which confusion rather than productive and motor phenomena predominate. The syndromes vary from slight confusional states to fully developed Korsakoff syndromes, and are observed almost exclusively in older patients.

After long-time maintenance treatment with neuroleptics in schizophrenics, depressive states and disturbances of initiative may occur. They usually resemble endogenous depressions, but sometimes are more similar to schizophrenic defect states with lack of initiative. If these depressive syndromes improve after discontinuation of neuroleptic therapy, the conclusion is justified that they were side-effects of the drug. The differential diagnosis is often difficult because depressive episodes may also occur in untreated schizophrenics. Their pharmacogenic etiology may be assumed, when the depression is accompanied by physical side-effects of the drugs like hypotension, Parkinson symptoms, akathisia (Simonson; Helmchen and Hippius). Comparison of groups of schizophrenics with and without drug therapy showed that depressive symptoms were considerably higher in the drug-treated group. The more a neuroleptic drug affects the extrapyramidal motor system, the more frequently it leads to depressive symptoms (Gerle). In such patients it has been recommended to combine neuroleptic medication with an antidepressant. Depressive symptoms under neuroleptic therapy may also be, at least partly, due to reactive neurotic factors inherent in the patient's personality. This is particularly so, when depressive mood becomes apparent in the first days of treatment. Hegarty described depressive symptoms in hallucinating and inaccessible patients, when they first begin to benefit from medication. This may be a direct drug effect but may also be due to secondary reactive factors. Individual psychodynamic constellations can often be clearly seen as the root of abnormal reactions to the experience of unpleasant physical side-effects such as dyskinetic syndromes (Helmchen and Hippius). Another possibility is that depressive symptoms become more evident after the removal of the schizophrenic symptomatology. It can also be assumed that sometimes after a good therapeutic effect of neuroleptic treatment, the patient's awareness of his illness leads to a depressive reaction (Cohen et al.).

Withdrawal Symptoms

There is no evidence that chlorpromazine or other phenothiazines have any of the addictive properties of drugs such as the barbiturates; so, on these grounds, there is no fear of giving it for long periods of time. However, withdrawal symptoms occur. Brooks has described them as tension, fear, restlessness, and, on the physical side, vomiting, often severe, insomnia, and increased perspiration. They develop on the second day after abrupt cessation of chlorpromazine and gradually subside by the tenth day. Patients under other drugs, particularly reserpine, show fewer withdrawal symptoms. In chlorpromazine withdrawal, symptoms are suggestive of excessive adrenaline liberation as a reaction to the withdrawal of the anti-adrenergic effects of chlorpromazine and might be helped by drugs such as hyoscine and atropine.

Battegay examined 81 patients who for years had been on neuroleptics, or on neuroleptics combined with anti-parkinsonian drugs, and whose medication was then abruptly stopped. Such sudden withdrawal may lead to the above mentioned withdrawal symptoms that can be interpreted as symptoms of vegetative irritation. Furthermore, sudden discontinuation of neuroleptics can elicit or increase an extrapyramidal tremor. Sometimes a hyperkinetic-dystonic syndrome of the mouth and throat region may appear only, when the medication is stopped. Finally the persistent hyperkinesias may also follow sudden withdrawal. Older people are especially prone to these withdrawal symptoms. Although all these various manifestations after sudden discontinuation of neuroleptics are undoubtedly withdrawal symptoms, they certainly are no evidence of an addiction or habituation because no such patient presents a psychological dependence (Battegay).

Overdosage

Overdosage usually occurs in connection with suicidal attempts. The signs and symptoms of phenothiazine overdosage are similar to those found in overdosage with anti-histamines. There is coma, sometimes accompanied by convulsions with severe hypotension, the blood pressure in some cases being unrecordable, tachycardia, tachypnea, hypothermia, absent tendon reflexes and severe stomatitis. In a case described by Vallet and Lepetit, the ingestion of 52 tablets of 25 mg. of chlorpromazine resulted in a coma followed by transitory excitement. There were no sequelae and the depression, which had produced the suicide attempt, was successfully treated with ECT. Aubertin et al. had a similar case where 40 tablets of 25 mg. had been taken. They used gastric lavage, heart stimulants and strychnine, and again the patient made a complete recovery. Samuels, who had a patient who took over 5000 mg., advises against the use of stimulants because of the danger of convulsions. He advises noradrenaline to raise the blood pressure, broad spectrum antibiotics, artificial respiration if necessary and intravenous fluids to maintain fluid balance. Like the other observers, he found no sequelae in his patient. Angst saw two patients in whom 6.3 gr. of chlorpromazine and 3.75 gr. of thioridazine respectively, had only led to somnolence. Overdosage of neuroleptics is actually only dangerous, when barbiturates or other hypnotics are taken simultaneously. In Europe, Pöldinger gave a survey on acute intoxications with neuroleptics, and recently, in the United States, Davis et al. published a careful and extensive compilation of cases of acute overdosage of tricyclic neuroleptics.

Contraindications

There are few contraindications against the use of neuroleptic drugs. Infections are considered a contraindication by some because they may be aggravated. On the other hand, tuberculosis is not a contraindication as demonstrated by Pleasure and also by Maccagnani. Cheng, however, found increased weakness and loss of weight, and in schizophrenics with tuberculosis he had better results with lobotomy.

Some authors have regarded liver damage as a contraindication, as well as extrapyramidal diseases and circulatory debility (Fernandes and Leitao). It should not be given in coma due to alcohol or the barbiturates, nor in cases where there has been a previous agranulocytosis. Great care is necessary in administering the drug to patients with severe cardio-vascular disease, particularly marked hypotension or cardiac failure.

Sigwald warns against the use of chlorpromazine in ambulatory patients with vascular conditions such as coronary disease, severe generalized arteriosclerosis, and arterial hypertension. If the doses are slowly increased, chlorpromazine is somewhat better tolerated. Circulatory disturbances, though not solely depending on age, can have much more serious consequences in older patients. Sudden fall in blood pressure and its impact on an already impaired heart can lead not only to cardiac but also to cerebral vascular complications.

Pregnancy is a possible contraindication during the first three months. This question arose because many neuroleptic drugs are used in non-psychiatric patients because of their antiemetic action. One of these indications is hyperemesis gravidarum. Although Favre-Tissot et al. assume that phenothiazines have no teratogenic action, it appears safer to limit neuroleptic treatment in the beginning of pregnancy to patients in whom they are strongly indicated. There is no contraindication later in pregnancy, and patients with previous post-partum psychoses may be given prophylactic medication with neuroleptics towards the end of a new pregnancy. The question has also been asked whether patients on maintenance therapy should use contraceptives to avoid possible untoward effects on the fetus in case they become pregnant.

Determination in Body Fluids

Qualitative and quantitative determination of phenothiazines and their metabolites in tissues and body fluids has not only theoretical and scientific interest. In long-term treatment it is important to find out with relatively easy laboratory test whether an ambulatory patient actually takes the drugs. Such tests are available for blood and urine. Dubost and Pascal found that chlorpromazine gives a red color reaction with sulphuric acid, which can be estimated colorimetrically and used to ascertain the amount of both free and conjugated chlorpromazine in blood and urine. The concentration in the blood after various levels and routes of administration does not exceed 4 to 6 mg. per litre. Only a small percentage appears in the urine, oxidized to the sulphoxide which has a mild tranquilizing effect. The fate of chlorpromazine in the body is not fully known, although the evidence suggests that there is considerable destruction in the organism, the most likely site for this being the liver.

Forrest and Forrest have described a simple test for approximately estimating the daily intake of the drug from urine examination. One ml. of urine is added to 1 ml. of a solution containing 4 parts of 10 per cent H_2SO_4 and 1 part of 5 per cent ferric chloride (this establishes a *p*H of 1 or less, an acidity at which no interference by aspirin-containing drugs is possible). The mixture is shaken in the test tube, and the amount of chlorpromazine is estimated according to color reaction from pale violet for doses under 200 mg. to definite violet for up to 600 mg., dark violet for up to 1000 mg., and nontransparent deep inky violet with dosage of more than 1000 mg. The presence of chlorpromazine in the urine may interfere with the results of some other biochemical tests; those based on color changes after the addition of oxidizing agents if bile pigments are present, and the urinary pregnancy tests.

Forrest et al. have developed rapidly applicable urine tests for most phenothiazines and related drugs. These tests proved to be very helpful for many purposes in this field. Similar urine tests are now available for the thioxanthines (Mellinger et al.).

Electroencephalographic Findings

Extensive EEG studies have been done with all neuroleptics (Brazier). They mostly served the purpose to clarify the mode of action of these psychotropic drugs. The EEG records also have practical importance because they seem to have certain prognostic significance and, furthermore, help to establish whether an ambulatory patient actually takes the prescribed neuroleptics. EEG studies with chlorpromazine were made by Lehmann and Hanrahan, who found that chlorpromazine did not appear to alter the basic character of the EEG with the patient awake. When the drug is given intravenously in the proper dosage, EEG somnolence is induced (Bente and Itil). The most important difference from the EEG of spontaneous sleep is that there is a special tendency for rhythmical protracted waves to be found with a simultaneous abatement of the rapid activity such as sleep spindles. Therefore, during chlorpromazine sleep there is a greater predominance of those mechanisms which check excitation than is found in normal sleep. Fink has described the typical EEG picture during chlorpromazine administration as showing delta activity, desynchronization of the record, and a decrease in the amount of fast activity. The drug also induces spontaneous seizure activity in patients who have not had fits prior to its administration and whose pretreatment records were normal. Fink states that chlorpromazine acts by altering brain function and that the delta shift is most effective in changing behavior, with desynchronization of the record being least effective.

Bente and Itil attempted to classify the neuroleptics on the basis of different EEG patterns. Another goal of some EEG studies was to recognize which patients may be stimulated by large doses of neuroleptics to have convulsions.

Reinert has made a study of the EEG changes when ten schizophrenics were treated with doses of promazine rising to 2000 to 4000 mg. per day. There was a high incidence of EEG abnormalities which were correlated to some extent with the dosage. The results also indicated that convulsions were more likely to occur when the dosage was suddenly increased by a substantial amount than with large but continued dosage. All the EEG records returned to the pre-treatment state when the drug was stopped.

EEG studies which were undertaken in attempts to determine the prognosis of neuroleptic therapy are discussed in the next section on prognostic tests.

Prognostic Factors and Tests

Soon after the introduction of chlorpromazine many authors tried to establish prognostic criteria for neuroleptic therapy. As far as clinical assessment is concerned, prognostic criteria are the same as in all other treatments. Thus, schizophrenics with short duration of illness and florid symptomatology have a favorable prognosis, while hebephrenics have the poorest prognosis. In addition, various tests were used to refine prognostication.

Rathod and Rees made a study to determine whether any definite criteria could be established in terms of the autonomic response to mecholyl and adrenaline for the use of chlorpromazine in disturbed psychotics. A group of disturbed female patients showing psychomotor overactivity or marked tension or agitation was chosen, and half were given the active preparation and the other half the inert placebo. This was followed by a changeover of the two groups, the first receiving the placebo, and the other group chlorpromazine. 48.1 per cent showed improvement with the placebo, 74.1 per cent with chlorpromazine. Changes in blood pressure response to mecholyl and reduction in the amechol score were correlated positively with clinical improvement, whether this occurred with chlorpromazine or with placebo.

Alexander and Moore found that schizophrenics showing an adrenaline-mecholyl test pattern similar to those of depression (adequate response to adrenaline, enhanced muscarinic hypotensive response to mecholyl), respond well to ECT; those with epinephrine precipitable anxiety do better with insulin and the new drugs. The response to all types of treatment declined with duration of illness, most markedly for ECT and insulin, somewhat less for drug therapies and psychotherapy, and least for frontal lobotomy.

A study of EEG correlates with improvement was made by Andermann. Patients responding to the drug with increase in the amount and stability of the alpha rhythm improved better than those with no increase in the alpha rhythm. Furthermore, the appearance of alpha activity in the temporal zone seems to correlate with improvement. He concludes that patients having little or no alpha activity are likely to benefit from chlorpromazine administration, while those having habitually stable high voltage alpha activity are not. Patients on drugs who still show deficient alpha activity in their EEG tracings may require a higher dosage of the drug. He explains this with the alteration of a ruminative personality with little alpha activity to a passive dependent personality with abundant alpha activity.

A somewhat different approach was taken by Helmchen and Künkel who made extensive studies on EEG changes produced by the neuroleptics themselves. The fast appearance of paroxysmal dysrhythmias makes for a fast clinical improvement. On the other hand, focal changes in the EEG impair the clinical prognosis.

Several authors question correlations between EEG changes and clinical effect. Hollister et al. failed to see such correlations in EEG studies with thioridazine; but Borenstein, also studying thioridazine, did find certain correlations between clinical symptomatology before treatment and during treatment on the one hand, and EEG tracings before and during neuroleptic therapy on the other hand.

Combination with Other Treatments

1. Combination with Psychotherapy: The neuroleptic drugs are helpful in psychotherapy by alleviating acute anxiety and tension and so enable the patient to face problems calmly and discuss them. In hypochondriacal patients, it can, like most other drugs, be harmful in that it tends to focus their attention upon the side-effects, and this becomes an obstacle to any real psychotherapy.

Some psychoanalysts have criticized the use of chlorpromazine on the grounds that partial relief of the anxiety will greatly decrease the motivation for psychotherapy and that drug administration implies that psychotherapy is unnecessary or at best is secondary to the drug. Winkelman has adequately replied to these criticisms and has endeavored to demonstrate the important role that chlorpromazine, given in conjunction with psychotherapy, can play in suitable cases. He found that chlorpromazine reduces acting out, so producing both a change in the patient's environment and an increased degree of ego control. The strength and severity of superego prohibitions and commands appear to be diminished, and possibly the instinctual demands of the id are also reduced. At the same time, the ego is strengthened, both by a reduction in anxiety and a reduction of inhibition, which enables the patient to bring the unconscious and preconscious levels of functioning into everyday life. Regression is facilitated because there is a diminution of the psychic intolerance toward painful stimuli occurring in the regressed state. The only negative aspect is that drowsiness, lethargy and apathy reduce to some extent the effectiveness of ego function, because they deprive it of the use of much energy and drive towards action.

Azima and Wittkower have employed chlorpromazine with psychoanalysis to induce prolonged sleepiness with partial disorganization and regression. Ostow has spoken of long-term phenothiazine administration as doing essentially the same thing to intrapsychic structure in the release of energy as does catharsis and working-out psychoanalytically. A book by Sarwer-Foner deals with the dynamic aspects of the drug.

2. Combination with ECT: The combination of a neuroleptic drug with electric convulsive therapy was first discussed by Foster and Gayle, and since then there has been much controversy about both its efficacy and, most important, its safety. There have been reports of fatalities due to its use by Weiss, Freeman; and others. We [L.B.K.] know of several unpublished fatalities, where the causal relationship could hardly be doubted. The main danger lies in its hypotensive effect. Weiss, who reports a patient who sustained a disturbing vasomotor collapse after ECT while receiving 450 mg. of chlorpromazine daily, found that a marked fall in blood pressure occurred immediately following the treatment, but that this was not present after subsequent treatments when chlorpromazine was omitted. He postulates that the hypotensive action of chlorpromazine is intensified by ECT. Other very experienced clinicians like Sargant, do not hesitate to combine ECT and chlorpromazine. The introduction of piperazine-phenothiazines and of the butyrophenones with their relatively slight hypotensive effect made the combination of ECT and neuroleptic therapy safer. We still prefer to delay ECT, when a patient is under neuroleptics if such delay is not harmful to the patient. ECT during or shortly after reserpine therapy is contraindicated.

Goldman sees the danger in the muscle relaxant. Since this and thiopentone may be potentiated by phenothiazines Barker and Baker prefer unpremedicated ECT in combined treatment. However, we know of a fatality in an unpremedicated ECT after chlorpromazine had been instituted. Ollendorf saw no danger even if ECT is given with a muscle relaxant, although he works with very large doses of chlorpromazine—2100 mg. as the optimum—in acute and chronic schizophrenia. He begins with three shock treatments, and, at the same time, commences a course of chlorpromazine, rapidly rising in dosage to the maximum level. Before the end of the treatment, which usually lasts for one month, three more shock treatments are applied. Blair and Brady found no untoward effects with the combination, but took the precaution of omitting the chlorpromazine on the morning of the treatment. This omission of the morning dose is highly advisable and is now routine procedure with many psychiatrists combining ECT and pharmacotherapy. Keeping the patient lying flat for a period after treatment should help to minimize the risks from hypotension.

The question of the efficacy of the combination of ECT and chlorpromazine has also been much discussed. Various authors have considered whether the drug shortens the course of treatment required in depression or in schizophrenia, whether it diminishes the period of post-ECT confusion, and whether it relieves some of the pre-ECT apprehension. Lesse found that chlorpromazine in combination with ECT did not influence any of these things and that its main value was in the control of acutely disturbed patients so that they could receive shock treatment more easily and in the control of post-ECT restlessness. He did not consider the combined treatment dangerous, but did not recommend it except in the cases specified, since there was no evidence that the results were better. Furtado was able to reduce the number of ECT required to treat involutional melancholia to three or four, but he considered the therapy of those cases with hypertension to be safer with ECT alone.

Today, when ECT is given alone, it will often be followed by neuroleptic medication in order to stabilize or to maintain the therapeutic result obtained with ECT.

3. Combination with Insulin Therapy:

a. Insulin Coma: There are a number of objections to the use of chlorpromazine in conjunction with insulin coma treatment. First, chlorpromazine is liable to produce drowsiness if given before the treatment, making it impossible to assess accurately the depth of coma in some cases. We regard it as wise to discontinue this drug when the patient commences insulin because it may also give rise to confusion with hypoglycemic reactions later in the day. According to Engelmeier, the drug also favors unusually early and abrupt coma, even in previously insulin resistant patients. Barbiturates are safer for the control of hypoglycemic excitement; and, although Webb used chlorpromazine in doses of 100 mg. about an hour after the injection of insulin for this purpose without untoward effect, we have heard of a death when the drug was given parenterally in a hypoglycemic excitement.

b. Modified Insulin: This combination has been used in the treatment of the alcoholic psychoses, particularly delirium tremens. Recently, Dally and Sargant have described its utilization in the management of anorexia nervosa. They gave chlorpromazine orally, increasing from an initial dose of 150 mg. daily to a maximum of 1000 mg. daily if necessary. Modified insulin therapy was given concurrently, commencing with 5 units and increasing gradually each day until there was drowsiness and sweating. This regime was continued, with reassuring psychotherapy, until the weight was near to normal again. Insulin and chlorpromazine were then reduced and the patient discharged if eating was satisfactory. There was follow-up psychotherapy, and a maintenance dose of chlorpromazine was thought to be beneficial in preventing relapse in some cases. The group of patients treated in this way was compared to those treated by other methods over the previous 20 years. It was found that the chlorpromazine-insulin treated group showed a greater weekly weight gain and a shorter period of hospitalization. The authors regard the combination of the two drugs as essential to the success of the treatment, because if either of them was stopped before the weight was back to normal, there was a likelihood of relapse. They warn against the hypotensive effects of chlorpromazine in these emaciated patients, and, to guard against any untoward reactions, kept the patients in bed until weight was almost back to normal.

4. Combination with Other Drugs: Lately, combinations of drugs are more and more used with two different objectives. One is to improve the therapeutic result by combining two or more drugs ("therapeutic combination"); the other is to counteract undesirable side-effects ("corrective combination").

The pharmaceutical industry has begun to offer standard formulae of combinations of drugs acting on different target symptoms. We feel strongly that the treating psychiatrist himself should be best equipped to select drugs for simultaneous use against different target symptoms. The potentiating effect of such drugs as the phenothiazines and other drugs has to be taken into consideration; also the possible cumulative action of identical side effects of drugs from different groups must be carefully weighed. If this is done, the psychiatrist, acquainted with the complex psychopathology of an individual patient will be able to combine drugs in a more individualized manner and in this way improve considerably his often discouraging results with pharmacotherapy.

The first drugs to be combined were chlorpromazine and reserpine. Barsa and Kline thought that this combination has a potentiating effect and reduces the turbulent phase of reserpine therapy. They considered this combination to be indicated for long-term maintenance in chronic, deteriorated schizophrenics with apathy and withdrawal. Feldman noticed that this combination produces the highest incidence of parkinsonism. Flügel and Bente used the two drugs together for the induction of an "akinetic-abulic" syndrome because of the belief that optimal therapeutic results were correlated to strong extrapyramidal symptoms. This therapy was abandoned, when it was seen that extrapyramidal symptoms are not necessary for therapeutic results. It was then tried to prevent these side-effects with combinations of phenothiazines and anti-parkinsonian drugs. Dally lists for this corrective medication anti-parkinsonian drugs like benzhexol hydrochloride (Artane), 6 to 15 mg. daily; benztropine hydrochloride (Cogentin) 1 to 2 mg. daily; procyclidine hydrochloride (Kemadrin) 15 to 30 mg. daily; orphenadrine hydrochloride (Disipal), 150 to 300 mg. daily; biperidine hydrochloride (Akineton), 2 to 6 mg. daily. The treating physician himself must add these drugs to the neuroleptics. Only in Germany a product Phasein, combining the neuroleptic reserpine with orphenadrine found wider application.

Another type of combined drug therapy is based on the experience that more potent neuroleptics like fluphenazine, perphenazine and so on, have only little initial calming effect. Therefore, such patients as disturbed paranoids may, for a time, require a second neuroleptic like chlorpromazine not so much for its "anti-psychotic" as for its initial dampening effect.

Combinations of phenothiazines with tranquilizers which have a more immediate calming effect, are used in syndromes accompanied by anxiety. Combinations of phenothiazines with hypnotics are helpful in insomnia, particularly in depressions (Dally). Finally, combinations of phenothiazines and antidepressants are used in schizophrenics who under neuroleptic therapy become depressed and have no drive. However, the main indication of this combination are agitated depressions.

THE RAUWOLFIA ALKALOIDS

The effects of the phenothiazine derivative chlorpromazine in psychoses had not yet been generally recognized, when the rauwolfia alkaloid *reserpine* became known as another neuroleptic drug. Chemically chlorpromazine and reserpine belong to entirely different groups; pharmacologically, though, they are quite similar.

In the beginning of the psychopharmaco-therapeutical era it looked as though reserpine and chlorpromazine were neuroleptics of equal value. In the meantime, however, the phenothiazines and related drugs are entirely in the foreground, while reserpine plays only a minor role as a neuroleptic. Chlorpromazine became the point of departure for the development of a large number of similar neuroleptics. Already minimal changes of the relatively simple structure of its molecule led to new, easily synthesized effective neuroleptics. In contrast, the group of rauwolfia alkaloids which all have a rather complicated chemical structure, remained small. While in the phenothiazine group newer neuroleptics have become more potent, the rauwolfia alkaloids introduced after reserpine, were without exception less potent than the mother substance. In the course of time, it also became apparent that reserpine compared to chlorpromazine is less effective and its action slower. Reserpine scored even less well in comparisons with the more potent phenothiazines. After a while, reserpine maintained its place as a neuroleptic in patients in whom the phenothiazines had to be discontinued because of side-effects like agranulocytosis or jaundice; but this indication also ceased, when the butyrophenones were discovered. It also became apparent that reserpine causes just as frequent, though different side-effects as chlorpromazine (Cieslak).

Today reserpine is rarely used in the treatment of acute psychoses, although still as a neuroleptic for the maintenance therapy of chronic psychotics. Even here it is mostly used in combination with drugs like orphenadrine (Phasein). Nevertheless, the rauwolfia alkaloids must be discussed extensively because the study of their biochemical action led to important conclusions regarding the effects of neuroleptic drugs in general.

The main alkaloid of the root of rauwolfia serpentina is *reserpine* (3,4,5-Trimethoxybenzoyl-methyl-reserpate).

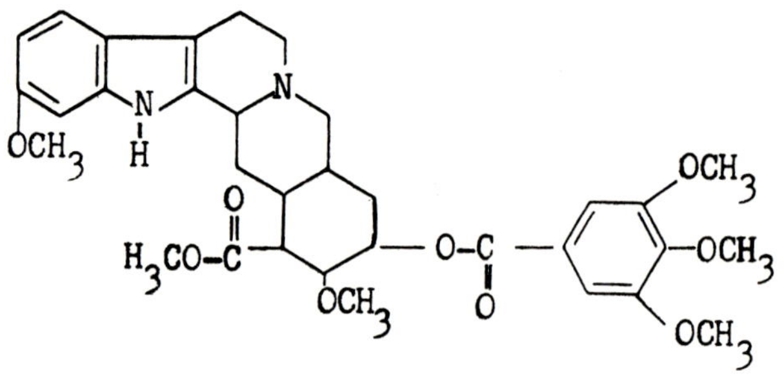

Another rauwolfia alkaloid with neuroleptic effect is *deserpidine* (11-Desmethoxyreserpine; trade name: harmonyl) which has been isolated from the root of rauwolfia canescens.

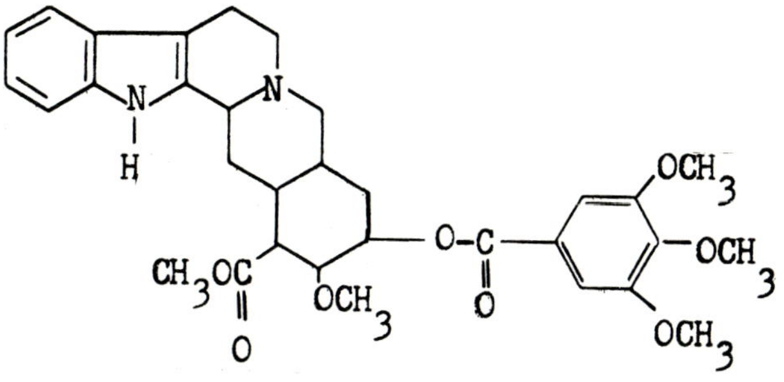

Deserpidine possesses all the uses and actions of reserpine but is less potent, although it seems to have a more rapid action. It is claimed that lethargy and mental depression are not so marked with this drug.

Rescinnamine (3.4.5-Trimethoxy-cinnamoyl-methylreserpate; trade name: Moderil) is an example for rauwolfia alkaloid which is being used mostly as a minor tranquilizer. It has less sedative action than reserpine.

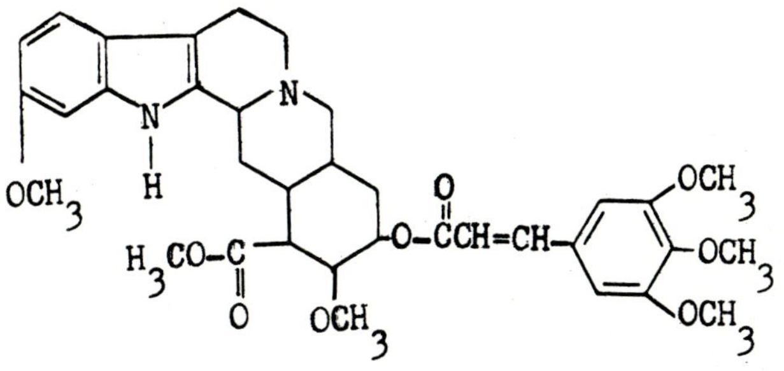

Furthermore there are extracts from the rauwolfia root, i.e., raudixin, raupina, and also alkaloid admixtures like rauwiloid, raupentina.

Malamud et al. compared reserpine, rescinnamine and deserpidine with a placebo, and found all three rauwolfia derivatives to be significantly more effective. At the termination of treatment, when the results with the three drugs were compared, the results from reserpine therapy were best, while at the six-months follow-up the results from rescinnamine were best. Deserpidine was rated first in allover effectiveness.

Biochemical Effects: Although reserpine plays a minor role in therapy, numerous biochemical investigations continue to be published regarding distribution in various tissues, metabolism, site and mechanism of action of this drug. Even though it is still not yet clearly established on what biochemical qualities the clinical therapeutic effect is based, it is the generally accepted view that reserpine exerts its effect through its action on the biogenic monoamines in the central nervous system. Reserpine leads to a depletion of granular depots of 5-hydroxytryptamine (serotonin), noradrenaline and dopamine in the cells of the central nervous system. These biogenic monoamines are obviously transmitter substances and, therefore, important for the functioning of the nervous system. After liberation from these depots the biogenic amines can be metabolized and are no longer fulfilling their physiological functions as transmitter substances in the central nervous system (Himwich and Himwich). According to these theories reserpine acts through diminished concentrations of transmitter substances in the central synapses.

Pharmacological Properties: The fact that reserpine does not act directly but through its effect on physiological distribution models and through changes in concentration of monoamines in the central nervous system, probably explains the delayed onset and the long duration of its action. In animal experiments it leads to hypotension, some hypothermia, bradycardia, slow respiration, miosis, increased gastric secretion and a number of endocrine effects such as stimulation of ACTH and prolactin secretion from the anterior hypophysis, adrenal cortical hypertrophy, decreased secretion of gonadotropin from the anterior hypophysis, decreased production of thyreotropic hormone, decreased secretion of thyroxin, antidiuretic effect (von Brücke and Hornykiewicz). A particularly important pharmacological action is a cataleptic effect which can be demonstrated in animals, and which plays an important part in the screening of neuroleptic substances (Bein et al.).

Reserpine has a marked central sedative action, but animals treated with it are arousable for short periods by stimuli and there is no evidence of any analgesic effect. Weiskrantz and Wilson investigated the results of reserpine administration and amygdaloid nucleus lesions in rhesus monkeys, both of which produce a taming effect on the animals so that, instead of withdrawing and possibly attacking the observer, they become placid and allow themselves to be petted. They found that those monkeys given reserpine made far fewer avoidance responses to a painful stimulus (electric shock) than normal animals, while in those monkeys who had had amygdaloidectomy, greater intensities of the shock were required to elicit avoidance behavior and their responses were slower. Both normal and brain-operated animals responded eagerly to a food reward, but the reserpinized monkeys did not approach the food tray spontaneously and chewed their food for only a few minutes if it was held in front of their mouths for some time. The reserpine effect was unaltered by amygdaloidectomy, thus excluding the amygdaloid nucleus as the target area for the drug's action. However, complete removal of the associated brain areas including the prepyriform area, the anterior temporal lobe, anterior part of the insula and posterior orbital area as well as the amygdaloid nucleus had similar behavioral results to those found when reserpine was administered. On the basis of their findings, the authors suggest that the role of reserpine is to block the impulses arising in these areas so that they do not activate the hypothalamus.

Clinical Effects: Barsa and Kline have described three stages in the course of treatment with serpasil:

1. The *sedative* stage in which the patient is quieter and drowsy. Duration about 3 to 10 days.

2. The *turbulent* stage in which he becomes more disturbed and there is an exacerbation of delusions and hallucinations. They stress the importance of persevering with treatment through this stage. Duration up to 3 weeks.
3. The *integrative* stage in which the patient becomes more cooperative, friendly and interested in the outside environment.

During the sedative stage, the patients may complain of lassitude, fatigue and drowsiness, but they can usually be aroused. Their appetite is good and they are cooperative. During this stage, Mielke kept his patients in a darkened room to decrease external stimuli to a minimum. The drug produces a hypotensive action, less marked in normotensives than in those with hypertension and most pronounced after parenteral administration. There is often an associated bradycardia. Flushing of the skin may occur, which disappears after the first few doses. There is often an increase in appetite which may lead to great weight gain.

Similar to the results of animal experiments, in clinical use the drug produces in addition to its cardiovascular action, slowing and deepening of respiration, ptosis, miosis, increased salivation, vasodilatation of the conjunctiva, reduction in perspiration and swelling of the nasal mucous membrane resulting in nasal congestion. There may be an accompanying drop in body temperature, ankle or facial edema, and diarrhea. Increased volume and acidity of gastric secretions have been demonstrated.

Rinaldi and Himwich studied the effect of reserpine on the electrical activity of cortical and subcortical structures. At first they thought that reserpine did not produce any EEG changes, in contrast to the barbiturates which give rise to a typical sleep pattern in the electroncephalogram. Using increasingly large doses, however, the authors obtained definite changes from the reticular formation of the tegmentum and the thalamic diffuse projection system in the form of a persistent EEG pattern of alertness. Thus, it appears that reserpine is a stimulator of the mesodiencephalic alerting system in contrast to the depressant action of the barbiturates. In animal experiments (Killam and Killam) reserpine stimulates the limbic system which may exhibit spontaneous seizure activity (Himwich). Bente and Itil also found no electroencephalographic changes with low dosage, but, with prolonged use of 7 to 12 mg. of reserpine daily, there was a protraction of the basal rhythm, and dysrhythmical theta and delta activity appeared in the fronto-central and temporal regions. With an increase of dosage to 40 mg. daily, these changes became more prominent, and there were phases of both decreased tension and high tension wave complexes with fronto-central predominance.

Schneider used the Funkenstein test to measure sympathetic reactivity and concluded that, when patients had either normal or increased sympathetic reactivity, reserpine decreased this. But, where initially sympathetic reactivity was decreased, the usual action of reserpine was to increase it.

Bernstein, who used serial estimations of the same test, noted that the development of a parasympathetic predominance could be the herald of a depressive illness. He also observed that it took about two weeks after the discontinuation of reserpine for the parasympathetic predominance to disappear. On the basis of this, he advised that ECT should not be given during this period because of the dangers of hypotension.

Reserpine potentiates the action of alcohol and this may constitute a major problem in patients taking the drug (Kopman and Hughes).

MODES OF ADMINISTRATION AND DOSAGE: The drug may be given orally, intramuscularly or intravenously. The intravenous dose used by Noce et al. was 0.2 mg./kg. body weight; but, in general, this route of administration does not appear to have any advantages over the intramuscular one, and, while Noce et al. found no side-effects apart from vertigo, Rea and Fazekas report a death from shock six hours after an intravenous injection of the drug. Bein et al. noted that there was no great difference in the speed of action of reserpine when it is given either orally or intramuscularly, the main effects being observed after about 6 to 24 hours. This is in contrast to chlorpromazine, where intramuscular injection can produce effects within 10 to 60 minutes. The accumulation of reserpine in the body is also slow, so that the maximum effect may not be observed for several days. It has been observed that intramuscular injections of reserpine are not so painful and do not so often produce the local reactions found with chlorpromazine. At the same time, there seems to be little difference in efficacy between the oral and intramuscular routes.

For acutely disturbed patients, an initial dose of 2.5 mg. intramuscularly should be given in order to ascertain whether they are liable to any undue hypotensive effect. This dose may be repeated in about 30 minutes if necessary. At the same time, oral medication should be commenced. Barsa and Kline, who commenced their treatment of disturbed psychotics with an initial 5 mg. dose intramuscularly, continued to give this injection together with 3 mg. orally daily for 10 days. If the patient had responded at the end of this time, the oral dose was continued, but the injections were decreased in frequency and gradually discontinued. If there was no improvement, the intramuscular dose was increased; but, with continued failure to respond, it was finally eliminated while the oral medication was continued. They found that the optimal maintenance dose was 3 mg. orally daily, and this conclusion was also reached by Moore and Martin. The latter two authors used higher initial doses, giving 10 mg. intramuscularly (at night) with 3 mg. orally daily for up to seven weeks. Ferguson gave even higher doses up to 80 mg., Avenarius et al. up to 90 mg. Bleuler and Stoll found a dose of 10 mg. of reserpine daily to be equivalent to 200 mg. chlorpromazine.

The question of duration of treatment is important, and in general the same considerations apply as for chlorpromazine. Hollister et al. maintain that in chronic schizophrenics the period of treatment should be at least three months at a maintenance level of up to 8 mg. daily before therapy is abandoned as being ineffectual. Ayd has reported that treatment with reserpine can be continued over a period of up to three years without untoward effect. The dosages given were 5 to 15 mg. daily orally, and, while parkinsonism usually occurred when the daily dose exceeded 5 mg., this was controlled by the appropriate medication. Delay et al. have also stressed that, whereas improvement with chlorpromazine may become apparent within a few weeks, reserpine may have no pronounced effects for several months and then suddenly produce an unexpected response which disappears when the drug is discontinued and reappears when it is resumed.

Complications of Treatment: *Central nervous system: Extrapyramidal reactions* occur with great frequency and are of the same type as with the phenothiazines, namely, parkinsonism, dyskinesia and akathisia. Most patients during treatment display a generalized tremulousness which may be controlled by cogentin and is possibly a sign of commencing extrapyramidal reaction to the drug. Some of the German workers such as Habel have used a reserpine-orphenadrine combination called Phasein in order to avoid the extrapyramidal symptoms. Scheurle was unable to demonstrate any difference in therapeutic results when patients were treated with reserpine alone and developed extrapyramidal manifestations or when a reserpine-orphenadrine combination was given to prevent these complications. He concluded that the extrapyramidal or the other side-effects of the drug, such as the turbulent phase and the autonomic-vasomotor manifestations, were not a necessary component of its beneficial results. Bleuler and Stoll have noted that, in contrast to chlorpromazine, the majority of patients who respond to reserpine show at least mild extrapyramidal reactions. Barucci found organic brain symptoms favoring extrapyramidal side-effects.

The remarks made in the section on extrapyramidal manifestations in chlorpromazine apply in general to reserpine also. However, Haase has attempted to make a distinction between some of the extrapyramidal symptoms found following chlorpromazine administration and those occurring with reserpine. With reserpine a greater degree of rigor and increased salivation are often found. The tremor with chlorpromazine is a fine-beat one, whereas reserpine in doses of 6 to 8 mg. daily may cause a rough-beat tremor resulting in a total inability to write. In a study of the handwriting of patients on these two drugs, he noted that there was a tendency for the writing to expand during the phase of stimulation produced by low doses of reserpine. He did not find that reserpine achieved the optimum therapeutic effect of chlorpromazine, since there was a considerable degree of disabling limitation of movement with it—in contrast to chlorpromazine, where the impulse reduction was linked to a minimum of motor immobility. Generalized chorea with athetosis, commencing within three days of the cessation of the drug therapy, was reported by Muir.

Other neurological side-effects to be considered are a rare *mid-brain syndrome* and *convulsions.*

The mid-brain syndrome, consisting of hyperpyrexia, ocular palsies and decerebrate rigidity was seen particularly in mental defectives, and it is suggested by Kline et al. that it probably only develops in damaged or defective brains. The only treatment is to withdraw the drug immediately.

Convulsions occur in about 1 per cent of patients receiving the drug, usually during the first six weeks of treatment. Deaths in status epilepticus have been observed.

Psychiatric Side-Effects and Complications: Lethargy, apathy and increasing withdrawal are frequent. Stimulants such as ritalin and drugs such as orphenadrine can be used. They are not so successful when the patient has become completely withdrawn, and in this state glutethimide (doriden) has relieved some patients.

The turbulent phase which may be preceded by restlessness and agitation is treated by Kline et al. with benztropine methane-sulfonate (Cogentin). This restlessness and agitation in the beginning occurs for a considerably long time, when further reserpine increase is avoided because of the turbulent phase. Actually the turbulence can be overcome by increase of the dosage (5 to 10 mg. daily). Contrary to this phenomenon, restlessness and agitation in connection with akathisia occur only after prolonged treatment with reserpine and will not be diminished by higher dosage which would rather intensify this syndrome. Often this akathisia also remains uninfluenced by anti-parkinsonian drugs like benztropine (cogentin) and biperiden (akineton), and requires discontinuation of reserpine.

Insomnia, particularly on low doses, dreams and nightmares are frequent. This results from the fact that REM-phases are increased by reserpine (Hartmann). Increased eroticism has been noted. Toxic confusional syndromes are probably due to overdosage.

Depression has been reported, often even in patients on small doses for hypertension. They might only complain of anhedonia or a lack of feeling, but can become depressed to the point of psychosis. Depressive symptoms will begin about four weeks after initiation of therapy but sometimes do not occur until the patient has been on the drug over a year. Occasionally, transient depression may follow an injection. The picture is typically that of an endogenous depression with feelings of guilt and hopelessness accompanied by early morning wakening, and suicide is a real danger. Withdrawal of the drug may be sufficient to produce a spontaneous recovery from the depression; but, in some cases, antidepressants may be required. The first symptom of depression should be a signal for immediately stopping the drug. It is not yet known how effective a combination of reserpine with one of the antidepressant drugs would be in preventing this complication.

Other Complications: As a result of the drug's influence upon the *gastro-intestinal tract,* appetite is often increased, although there may be anorexia. Weight gain may follow the increased food intake. Cramp-like abdominal pain and diarrhea may occur with nausea and vomiting. Sometimes these symptoms are relieved by cogentin or doriden; but if these drugs are not successful, the anti-cholinergics such as belladonna are invariably effective. Perforation of gastric and duodenal ulcers has been reported, some with fatal outcome. There were also hemorrhages from such ulcers (Freyhan) and melena. Hollister failed to show any evidence of a blood coagulation disorder in such patients, and the effect of the drug is most probably a direct one on the gastric mucosa, increasing the stomach movements and the secretion of acid and gastric juice. In Hollister's patients with hematemesis and melena, only one showed radiological evidence of an ulcer, and he believes the effect of the drug is to produce small gastric erosions or exacerbate old ulcers rather than to induce new areas of ulceration.

Cardio-vascular complications which may occur are bradycardia and hypotension manifesting as dizziness or syncope. Kline et al. found a combination of atropine and ephedrine useful, as well as stimulants such as dexedrine. They note a tendency for patients with a cardiovascular disease to decompensate more easily when on the drug. Liebaldt has reported a number of patients who died with signs of circulatory collapse—or suddenly without any premonitory signs—and there have been unexplained deaths recorded in the literature. This is especially a danger in elderly patients in whom large doses should be avoided. Liebaldt noted that, among his group of fatalities, a majority died either a few days after reserpine had been commenced or after the dosage had been increased. These fatalities are probably due to interference with permeability in the brain. Addition of orphenadrine at least partially compensates the disturbed permeability (Liebaldt).

A host of other side-effects has been listed in the literature, such as nasal congestion which can be treated with local anti-histamines, edema of face and extremities, frequency of micturition, and nocturnal incontinence, increased thirst, muscular cramps and twitchings, paresthesias, pupillary constriction. Dermatitis is rare, but a seborrheic dermatitis has been described and can be treated with anti-histamines and hydro-cortisone. Urticaria due to allergic sensitivity to the drug has been seen, and Cahn reported a severe angioneurotic edema. Endocrinological disturbances are impotence, loss of sexual desire, lactation, gynecomastia, and menstrual irregularities such as menorrhagia or amenorrhea.

Reduced resistance to intercurrent diseases was seen by Kline et al. in patients on both chlorpromazine and reserpine. They also require larger doses of antibiotics. Patients in bed developed trophic ulcerations more readily (Scheurle). Thrombophlebitis has been reported. Shortness of breath, a sensation of "smothering," and aggravation of bronchial asthma were seen.

Sure observations of blood dyscrasias are not known. Liver damage has also not been reported. The only exception is a fatal case of acute yellow atrophy reported by Maggs and Ellison in a patient receiving 12 mg. reserpine daily for three weeks.

A number of inadequately explained fatalities in patients under reserpine have already been mentioned elsewhere. In reserpine-treated patients, deaths due to possible lack of cough reflex were described by Wardell. The majority of fatalities during reserpine therapy reported by Liebaldt, are also unexplained, and so are some single fatalities mentioned in various reports on reserpine treatment.

Overdosage results in a marked longlasting hypotension with bradycardia. In some cases the patients became somnolent and even comatose. These comas are accompanied by intense skin flushes and swelling of the nasal mucosa, and the patients are endangered by collapse. The acute intoxication should be treated with noradrenaline or similar pressor drugs and by intravenous infusion of glucose in saline. Intravenous drip of 5 per cent glucose in saline with 4 mg. lacterenol per 1000 ml. can be used with the flow adjusted to maintain the pressure at normal level. There have been no reports of deaths from excessive ingestion of the drugs for suicidal purposes.

Chronic intoxication is marked by bradycardia, gastric hyperacidity and intestinal hypermotility.

CONTRAINDICATIONS: Because of the side-effects of reserpine the following conditions should be regarded as contraindications: peptic ulcer and other ulcerative conditions of the bowels, although it has been recommended in ulcerative colitis; asthma thromboses; tendency to edema; comatose conditions, such as those due to the barbiturates or alcohol; depression or a history of previous depressions. The drug should be withdrawn prior to surgery, since there may be a considerable hypotension and bradycardia in patients receiving reserpine who are anesthetized (Ziegler and Lovette). It should not be administered in association with ECT because fatalities have occurred.

Since the effect of reserpine persists for days and weeks (Freedman and Benton), medication must be stopped at least for a week prior to anesthesia for surgery or ECT. Even without anesthesia the combination of ECT and reserpine is strongly contraindicated. There have been a number of reports of alarming reactions when ECT is given to patients receiving reserpine. Hypotensive shock and apnea have been seen following the treatment, and fatalities have occurred. Foster and Gayle found in a number of their patients a typical picture of low blood pressure, absent or weak pulse, and difficulties with breathing in the post-ECT period, which was followed by confusion and lethargy during the rest of the day. One patient who died showed pulmonary and cerebral edema but no anatomic cause of death. Liebaldt, in his collection of patients who had died suddenly without any premonitory signs or with signs of circulatory collapse, also included one following ECT. Foster and Gayle state that a minimum of seven days should elapse between the cessation of reserpine therapy and the administration of ECT, and there is no doubt that a combination of the two treatments is contraindicated because of the dangers involved. It would appear that the hypotensive effect of reserpine combines with the hypotension which can occur following ECT to produce a state of severe shock.

The combination of reserpine and iproniazid, as recommended by Radinger et al. for regressed and apathetic patients, requires caution. The depletion of biogenic amines from intracellular depots together with the monoamine oxidase inhibition may produce severe confusion and possibly dangerous excitement.

CLINICAL INVESTIGATIONS: The present limited use of rauwolfia alkaloids has been mentioned in the beginning of this chapter. Here, only a few clinical studies will be listed.

Schizophrenia: The first American report on the drug was by Kline in 1954, who observed its effects in a group of chronic schizophrenics, and stressed the fact that reserpine did not fundamentally alter the schizophrenic process but had a symptomatic effect, particularly on violent and disturbed behavior. Using the incidence of assaults and restraint in the ward as a measure of the sedative action, Kline found that the number of both was considerably reduced in the reserpine-treated patients. Another early and very enthusiastic report in the same year was by Noce et al., who were so impressed by the sedative action of serpasil in violent and disturbed patients that they considered it would supplant ECT in a large proportion of cases. Delay et al., reporting in 1955, found the action of reserpine to be more variable and the results more inconsistent than with chlorpromazine.

Flach made a study of the symptoms which were most frequently improved by reserpine, and he found that the drug was most beneficial where there was tension or fear and anxiety in association with the psychotic manifestations, withdrawal, thinking disorder and delusions being relieved in association with alleviation of the affective disturbance. He found that depression in schizophrenia was often relieved—in contrast to the effect in endogenous depression where the gloomy mood may be deepened.

The studies of reserpine's action in schizophrenia indicate that the drug is, in general, capable of producing symptomatic improvement in this psychosis; in some cases complete remission of the illness can occur. Thus, in the beginning of pharmacotherapy, when chlorpromazine and reserpine were the only neuroleptics available for the treatment of schizophrenia, reserpine was used for a very short time in the acute, productive schizophrenic. Even then very few authors found it superior to ECT and insulin. For a considerable time reserpine maintained a place in chronic schizophrenics, and in such cases it can be more effective than ECT. Avenarius et al. obtained some results with high doses (30 to 90 mg. daily) in treatment-resistant, symptom-poor schizophrenics (hebephrenics, simple schizophrenia, pseudoneurotic schizophrenia). The activating effect with such high doses in defect states is quite surprising. J.-E. Meyer et al. combined such high doses from the beginning with orphenadrine (300 to 1200 mg.) which is not only anti-parkinsonian but also activating.

In chronic schizophrenics it is desirable to try all the available neuroleptic drugs, for a reasonable period of time, to find the one which is most effective. Reserpine, in particular, should be maintained for at least three months, since improvement is often slow. There are some entirely negative reports, such as, for instance, a double-blind study by Freedman evaluating reserpine and the rauwolfia derivate harmonyl and coming to the conclusion that neither drug is more effective than a placebo.

Depression: The general consensus of opinion is that reserpine is ineffective in depression and that it is contra-indicated in those retarded depressions without agitation or anxiety, since the condition may become worse. Reserpine can precipitate a psychotic depressive reaction, and it seems that its use should be avoided in endogenous and involutional depressions and in patients with a history of such depressions. There have been some reports of its beneficial effects in the schizophrenic depression, although possibly for these states phenothiazines such as stelazine might give more satisfactory results. It can help to restore sleep and relieve agitation and hypochondriasis in psychotic depression as noted by Delay. A trial which decisively demonstrated the lack of any fundamental response in depression with reserpine was that of Shepherd; all failures subsequently recovered with ECT.

More favorable results in depression were reported with a German preparation *Phasein,* which is a combination of reserpine and orphenadrine, the latter counteracting both depression of mood and parkinsonian side-effects (Habel). Van Andel has studied the effect of orphenadrine on reserpine-treated patients before and after extrapyramidal symptoms appear. He found that the psychiatric symptoms were sometimes exacerbated when orphenadrine was given prematurely. However, when the drug was administered after the appearance of the extrapyramidal symptoms, a depressive mood was replaced by euphoria together with control of the neurological reactions. If at all, it seems that reserpine is only effective in combination with other drugs such as orphenadrine but also with doriden (Glutethimide). After initial medication with reserpine an "inversion" of the doriden effect is achieved which makes the good therapeutic results of the doriden-reserpine combination understandable.

Mania: A good response has been observed in some patients with manic excitement. Here again, however, the drug should be given with some caution in view of its depression-producing potentialities, and the phenothiazines, the butyrophenones, and lithium should be used first.

Watt reported favorably, but Mielke was not so impressed by the response in his manic patients, who tended to change from gaiety to annoyance when the drug inhibited their exaltation and the rapidity of their stream of thought. However, Delay et al. found that some cases of manic excitement which did not respond to chlorpromazine were quieted by reserpine, although they often had to raise the dose of the drug progressively in order to combat a return of the excitement.

In view of the obviously uncertain effect of reserpine in manics, it was soon replaced by the more potent neuroleptics from the group of phenothiazines, thioxanthines and butyrophenones, the latter (e.g. haloperidol) having the advantage that in manic excitement states they can be easily used intravenously. In less severe manic states today lithium salts are the treatment of choice.

Psychoneuroses: In general, the results with reserpine in this group of patients are not encouraging. Many of them complain a great deal about the side-effects of the drug. Moore and Martin found that the patients most helped were those who were underweight, particularly cases of anorexia nervosa and chronic anxiety states. Ferguson, who made a comparative study using reserpine and a placebo in anxious neurotics, found that on the basis of objective tests there was no difference between the drug and the inert preparation. When assessed on a clinical basis, however, a number of the reserpine group were rated as improved. Tension headaches are a symptom reported as particularly benefitted by the drug. Hare et al., who compared reserpine 2 mg. t.d.s.; amylobarbitone sodium 2 gr. t.d.s.; and a placebo in anxiety neurotics over a period of a week, found the barbiturate successful in alleviating anxiety symptoms in most patients, but reserpine ineffective. It should be observed, however, that the evidence indicates that reserpine is much slower acting than the barbiturates, and that a week is possibly too short a period for its full effect to become manifest. However, the phenothiazines and the rauwolfia alkaloids are not as effective in the rapid alleviation of some psychoneurotic manifestations as the barbiturates and the minor tranquilizers.

Epilepsy: While reserpine used alone may induce or increase epileptic fits, there have been a number of reports about its efficacy when used in conjunction with anticonvulsant medication, in controlling the irritability and moodiness often found in the epileptic patient. Brooks reported that the addition of reserpine to the dilantin-phenobarbital regime in his patients not only improved behavior very markedly but decreased the incidence of seizures by a third. Lambos found that, once the fits were controlled by other medication, reserpine decreased irritable outbursts which had been unrelieved by the anticonvulsants.

Organic Psychoses: Previously reserpine had been recommended for a great number of organic psychoses. In the meantime it became evident that withdrawal symptoms respond much better to tranquilizers like diazepam or chlormethiazol. In delirium tremens reserpine is now considered contraindicated. Occasionally it is still used in acute and chronic brain syndromes of old age. In the latter group, particular care should be exercised and the dosage kept low, since such patients, often with hypertension and atherosclerosis, are most prone to hypertension and vasomotor collapse following administration of the drug. The symptoms most helped in these patients are irritability, agitation and querulousness. Reserpine remains useful in the treatment of Huntington's chorea. It has been found to relieve some of the disturbing involuntary movements of choreo-athetosis. It has been used to control the overactivity of mentally defective and psychotic children, and Lambos reported good results in nocturnal enuresis. Fisher and Teller found beneficial effects in tuberculous patients with a concomitant psychosis.

Other Neuroleptics

Benzoquinolizine Derivatives

For a while the benzoquinolizine derivatives were interesting because their action is similar to that of reserpine (Pletscher et al.) but, contrary to reserpine, they can be far more easily synthesized, while the alkaloid reserpine must be isolated from rauwolfia serpentina. Today the benzoquinolizine derivatives—like reserpine—have little importance in psychiatric therapy.

Like reserpine, several benzoquinolizine derivatives decrease 5-hydroxytryptamine (serotonin) and catecholamines (especially norepinephrine) in the brain, but release little or none of these biogenic amines in the periphery. Compared to reserpine, their action on the monoamines in the brain is shorter, lasting for only 24 to 30 hours; they are less potent and have a faster onset of action. The monoamine depletion is antagonized by pretreatment with monoamine oxidase inhibitors. In the brain benzoquinolizines prevent the reserpine induced decrease of 5-hydroxytryptamine but not that of norepinephrine. In animal experiments they have a tranquilizing but no hypnotic effect. Other actions are potentiation of narcosis, hypothermia, enhancement of pentylenetetrazol convulsions, decrease of conditioned reflexes, and prevalence of parasympathetic tone in the autonomic system (Pletscher et al.). Some benzoquinolizine derivatives cause moderate hypotension but do not have the gastrointestinal effects of reserpine (Quinn et al.). They are rapidly eliminated and do not have the cumulative effect of reserpine. In the EEG they cause slow waves with high voltage interrupted by bundles of spikes, similarly to the EEG pattern of chlorpromazine.

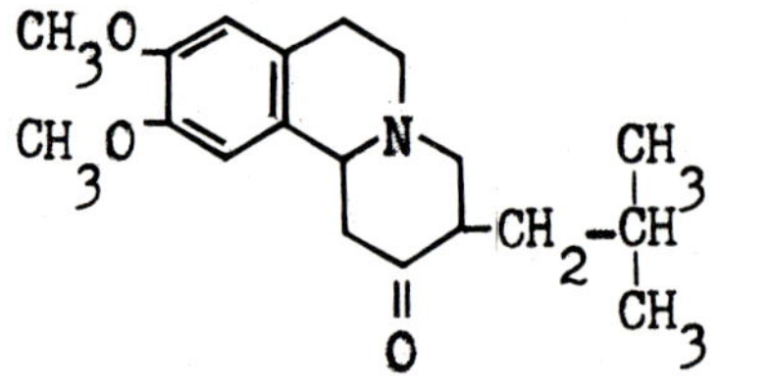

TETRABENAZINE (3-isobutyl-1,2,3,4,6,7-hexahydro - 9,10 - dimethoxy - 2 - oxo-benzo-(a)quinolizine (Nitoman) is the only benzoquinolizine used clinically.

It differs from reserpine in that it is less hypotensive, and patients do not appear to pass through a turbulent phase. The other side-effects are similar to those of reserpine and the phenothiazines but less pronounced. An average dosis of 75 to 150 mg. may cause a Parkinson syndrome which led Sattes to use tetrabenzaine in Huntington's chorea. Initial hyperkinetic-dystonic reactions occur in 1 to 2 per cent of the patients. Other side-effects are sweating, dry mouth, drowsiness, ataxia, metrorrhagia, lactation, moderate hypotension, bradycardia. Blood dyscrasias and liver damage have not been reported. Psychiatric side-effects are depression, anxiety, excitement and insomnia.

According to Voelkel and Dresler, it appears to have less effect on hyperactivity and tension and more on delusions, hallucinations, and thought disorders. Stockhausen reported that it had a marked anti-hallucinatory effect in schizophrenia, but that the hallucinations of general paresis remained unaffected. He also observed that females required a lower dosage than males and showed a better response to the drug, which has been described as reducing the disorganized thinking of schizophrenia as well as diminishing the intensity of delusions and anxiety.

Smith compared it with a placebo and reserpine in chronic schizophrenics and found that, although both drugs produced significantly better results than the placebo, reserpine was better than nitoman. However, there was a difference in the length of time that the patients took to respond, the reserpine-patients not showing improvement until the third month while the nitoman-patients responded during the first month. Lingjaerde has reported that those psychotic symptoms most helped by the drug were negativism, aggressiveness, agitation, hallucinations, and restlessness, but that there was little effect on autism, apathy, insomnia, or lack of insight. Voelkel and Dresler point out that, unlike reserpine, it does not prolong post-ECT apnea, and it has been combined uneventfully with this treatment. These authors also found a good response in depressions with hypochondria, agitation, and delusions of guilt, in contrast to the retarded group where the drug was ineffective.

Lingjaerde summarized his own and other studies up to 1962 in a monograph and, on the basis of 1300 cases, comes to a definitely positive opinion on tetrabenazine. However, Wright and Kyne compared tetrabenazine with thioridazine, trifluoperazine and reserpine in a controlled study on schizophrenics, and came to the conclusion that tetrabenazine is the least reliable drug.

Mode of Administration and Dosage: The drug can be administered orally, intramuscularly or intravenously. Orally 35 to 300 mg. have been given daily.

By the parenteral route the dose is 50 mg. Painful infiltrations have been observed occasionally after subcutaneous administration.

Several other benzoquinolizines studied by Voelkel, do not differ in their action from tetrabenazine.

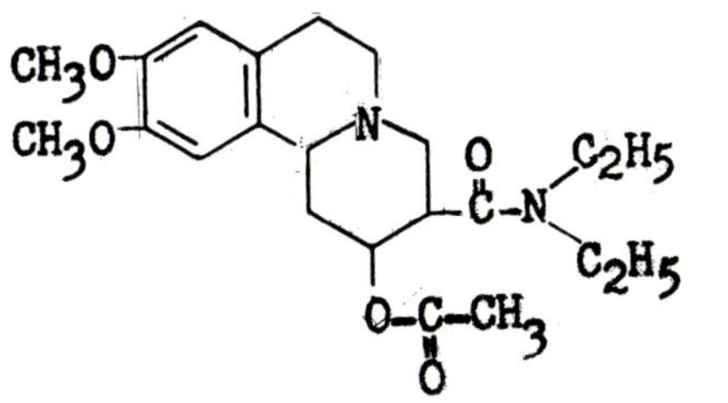

Benzquinamide (2-hydroxy-3-di-aethycarbamyl-9,10-dimethoxy-1,2,3,4,6,7-hexahydro-11bH-benzoquinolizine (Quantril) alone has a special place. It depresses the conditioned avoidance response in animals with dosages which have no effect on the monoamine content of the brain. Only in very high doses it makes for a weak amine depletion in the central nervous system (Weissman and Finger). Even in large doses benquinamide has no chlorpromazine-like effect in psychotics (Bishop and Gallant) but acts similarly to barbiturates and tranquilizers (Smith, Sainz). Bishop and Gallant warn against its use in psychotic patients with a depressive component, especially if they are suicidal.

Oxypertine (Forit)

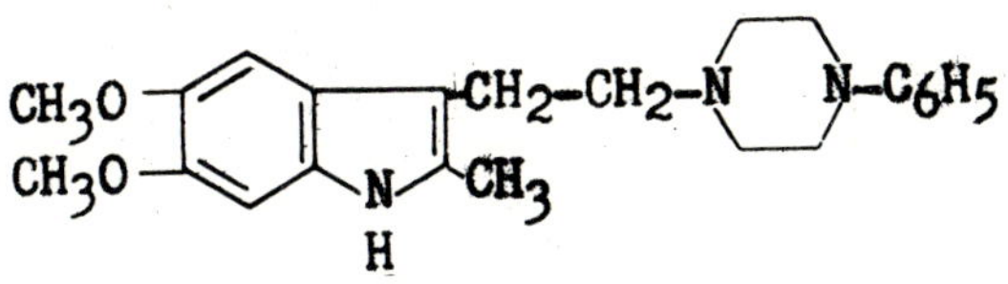

Oxypertine (5,6-dimethoxy-2-methyl-3-[2-(4-phenyl-piperazinyl)-aethyl]-indol) is the first representative of a new group of psychopharmaca which may or may not gain major importance in psychiatric pharmacotherapy. But merely the fact that oxypertine is an indole derivative roused interest in this drug because of its chemical relation to serotonin, dimethyltryptamine, LSD, reserpine, and etryptamine. Older and more recent theories regarding tryptophane metabolism and the biochemistry of schizophrenia have thereby found new impetus (Durell and Pollin).

In 1962, Archer et al. were the first to direct attention to the chemically new group of indolyl-ethyl-piperazine derivatives. Wylie and Archer as well as Abdul Hameed and Haley compared in pharmacological investigations oxypertine and similar substances with chlorpromazine. Already the pharmacological studies revealed that oxypertine has different effects. Aside from tranquilizing properties, it also has a stimulating effect. This strange two-fold action was confirmed by clinical investigations whose results were summarized by Skarbek and Jacobsen in 1965. These differences in clinical effect depend to a certain degree on dosage. The stimulating effect prevails with lower doses (20 to 40 mg. daily), the tranquilizing effect with larger amounts. Flament et al., however, found that in schizophrenic defect states also higher amounts have an activating effect. Their pilot study at the National Institute of Mental Health was the reason that most later investigations concentrated on autistic schizophrenics with diminished drive. This usefulness of oxypertine in schizophrenic defect states was confirmed in several controlled studies (Calwell et al.; Durell and Pollin). The patients become more responsive to their surroundings. Also after treatment-free intervals this contact improving, antiautistic effect on chronic schizophrenics can be reproduced on the same patient under double-blind conditions (Skabek and Hill). Hollister et al. demonstrated with rating scales (BPRS) that oxypertine at least equals the effectiveness of tricyclic neuroleptics. In double blind studies by Hunt comparing trifluoperazine and oxypertine, the latter drug proved to be equal—but not superior—to trifluoperazine.

Side-effects are few. Parkinsonian syndromes and, sometimes in the beginning of treatment, hyperkinetic-dystonic syndromes occur. Dizziness, tremor, nausea and vomiting have been seen.

Mode of Administration and Dosage: Initial intramuscular injections were recommended, but in general oral medication of 60 to 320 mg. daily is adequate. Some authors gave up to 560 mg. without improving the therapeutic result.

The Butyrophenones

The butyrophenones are a group of neuroleptics which chemically is related neither to the phenothiazines nor to reserpine. However, pharmacologically their action in animal experiments is very similar to that of the phenothiazines. It was this similarity that led to their discovery. Originally the butyrophenones were synthetized in connection with studies on structural modifications of morphine-like analgesics with central action. During pharmacological investigations of such substances which are chemically related to pethidine and meperidine, Janssen et al. encountered manifestations such as catalepsy which were otherwise seen only in phenothiazines and reserpine. This suggested clinical investigations of these pharmaca as neuroleptics with possible effect on schizophrenic and manic psychoses. Such studies were performed in 1958 in Liège by Divry et al. who confirmed clinically what has been anticipated on the basis of animal experimentation, namely that the butyrophenones are effective neuroleptics. Since 1958 Janssen et al. synthetized and studied pharmacologically a large number of butyrophenone derivatives (Janssen in 1967 more than 5000 tertiary amines structurally related to haloperidol). Several are now available commercially, and in some the generic and trade names are identical:

1. Haloperidol	(Haldol, Serenace, Haloperidol)
2. Triperidol	(Triperidol)
3. Methylperidol	(Luvatren, Luvatrena)
4. Floropipamide	(Dipiperon, Piperonyl)
5. Benperidol	(Frenactyl, Glianimon)

Aside from these there are other commercial products which either have no clinical significance, e.g. Fluanison (Soulairac et al.) or, although being neuroleptics, are used in other indications, e.g. the neuroleptanalgesic droperidol (Bobon et al.). Finally, numerous butyrophenones were found to be effective neuroleptics but have not yet been commercially introduced, e.g. spiroperidol (Bobon et al.) and fluspirilene (Haase et al.).

Pharmacological Properties: Neuroleptics of the butyrophenone group reduce the spontaneous motility of test animals already in low doses, while larger doses induce catalepsy. In monkeys higher dosage causes agitation. Reactions to sensory stimuli are diminished. The butyrophenones are amphetamine antagonists and inhibit several effects of apomorphine and tryptamine. The hypnotic barbiturate action is increased. Adrenaline effects like mydriasis and hypertension are more or less suppressed. Vegetative effects are primarily due to inhibition of the sympathetic system, while the parasympathetic system is hardly affected. Like neuroleptics, the butyrophenones cause hypothermia (Janssen).

Comparison of various butyrophenones show that triperidol and haloperidol have a strong and lasting cataleptic action, are distinct amphetamine and apomorphine antagonists, and have comparatively few vegetative effects. Floropipamide has a weak extrapyramidal motor effect but shows very distinctive anti-tryptamine activity. In experiments on monkeys floropipamide has a quieting effect, while haloperidol and triperidol may cause agitation.

1. *Haloperidol (Haldol, Haloperidol, Serenace)*

Haloperidol is 4′-fluoro-4(4″-chlorophenyl)-(4′-hydroxy)-piperidine-butyrophenone.

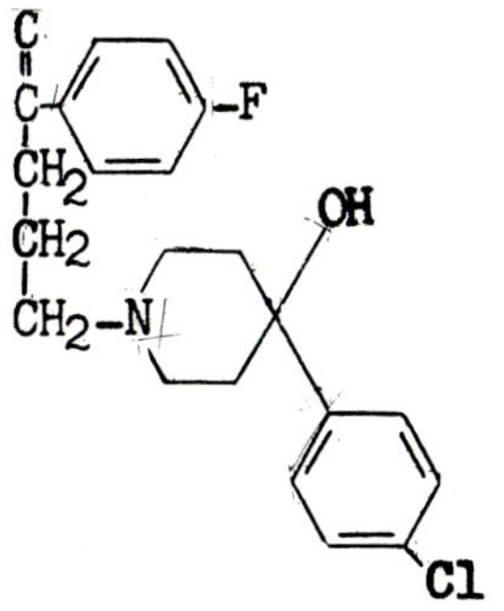

Haloperidol first investigated by Divry et al., is still the prototype of this neuroleptic group. Most clinical effects as well as side-effects of haloperidol are found in greater or lesser intensity with the other butyrophones. Triperidol is two or three times stronger, methylperidol definitely weaker than haloperidol. Floropipamide differs the most from it.

Favorable results with haloperidol in mania, schizophrenia, and acute delirium have been reported, especially in Europe. In the U.S. Denber et al., in 1959, were the first to investigate haloperidol in a clinical study on psychotic women but could not confirm the good results of European workers. In subsequent years Denber repeated these investigations with the same unsatisfactory results. Therefore, Denber and Collard expressed the opinion that the great divergencies in the response to haloperidol between American and European workers may be due to differences in environmental and genetic background. This could not be proven conclusively. It should be mentioned that Denber's patients received up to 200 mg. daily which is ten times the dosage given by European authors. However, later investigations in the U.S. with lower doses of 10 to 20 mg. daily, confirmed the Eurpean results (Holstein and Chen). In Great Britain Danik and Coverdam obtained similar positive findings. In paranoid schizophrenics and manic excitements haleperidol improvements aided the open-door policy and shortened hospitalization. Also, Paley et al. proved beyond doubt that haloperidol is an effective neuroleptic. Delay et al. found that hebephrenic patients were rarely helped, and that in depression, while the anxiety was relieved, the underlying mood did not change. Haloperidol might be regarded as a neuroleptic drug by the standard of Delay's classification because of its apparently powerful anti-psychotic effect and the fact that extrapyramidal symptoms, similar to those found with the phenothiazines and reserpine, readily occur.

Kristjansen used tofranil with haloperidol in depressed patients with good results. He noticed that side-effects, such as dizziness, loss of appetite and weight, and fatigue, were more common in patients over 65. However, Sugerman et al., in a controlled study, found haloperidol particularly valuble in disturbed geriatric patients because doses up to 4 mg. daily avoid the hypotension seen in other neuroleptics, and even one mg. daily appears to be adequate as maintenance dosis in most cases. By now, haloperidol is increasingly accepted in the treatment of schizophrenia also in the English speaking countries. Its use in manics, and particularly in delirium tremens and other deliria is still rare, while in Europe it is considered as singularly effective in these conditions. Oles also obtained the best results in manic states, and agrees with Delay et al. that agitated depressions and chronic hebephrenics did poorly. In child psychiatry haloperidol is not particularly well received in the U.S. and Britain. In controlled studies Burk and Menolascino reported on emotionally disturbed, retarded children, and Barker and Fraser in overactive and aggressive children. In a careful double-blind study in children with severe behavior disorders Cunningham et al. demonstrated a statistically significant calming effect. The children on haloperidol were rated as less overactive, less destructive, less restless, less resentful and less disobedient.

Of special interest are the surprising results with haloperidol in the Gilles de la Tourette syndrome, where still in 1959 Eisenberg et al. found pharmacotherapy including tranquilizers ineffective. Seignot was the first to report good results with haloperidol in this otherwise uncontrollable tic syndrome. Subsequently, this was confirmed by many others (Challas and Brauer; Lucas; Shapiro and Shapiro). Chapel et al. emphasized that haloperidol even influences the troublesome coprolalia which makes the social adjustment and rehabilitation of these otherwise socially rejected patients possible.

Side-effects of haloperidol are primarily extrapyramidal motor symptoms which Oles found in 80 per cent of all cases. In this respect haloperidol resembles the piperazine sub-group of phenothiazines. Himwich and Glisson demonstrated that these extrapyramidal effects are due to a significant selective reduction of dopamine in the caudate nucleus. Therefore, patients under haloperidol have an increased excretion of the principal dopamine metabolite, homovanillic acid (Bruno and Allegranza). Fast increase of dosage in the beginning of treatment may lead to hyperkinetic-dystonic syndromes of neck, mouth, throat and tongue muscles which, like the later developing parkinsonian symptoms, are relatively well controllable with such anti-parkinsonian drugs as cogentin or biperidin. Some authors recommend to combine haloperidol with anti-parkinsonian drugs routinely (Shorodin). Considerably less controllable is the akathisia which occurs with larger doses and often makes discontinuation of the drug necessary. In individual cases long-term haloperidol therapy may lead to persistent dyskinesia (Degkwitz and Luxemburger).

All other somatic side-effects play a minor role compared to the extrapyramidal symptoms. This is a great advantage of haloperidol and other butyrophenone derivatives over the phenothiazines. Oles found no evidence of blood dyscrasias or liver damage. Delay et al. saw in 5 patients a syndrome with perspiration, dehydration, hyperthermia, and a clouded state. By stopping the drug and giving fluids, a fatal outcome can be avoided but instances of death are known as a consequence of this so-called syndrome malin which is not dosage-dependent and occurs early in the treatment. Divry et al. saw hypotension and bradycardia, and reported one fatality due to cardio-vascular collapse. In general, vegetative side-effects due to haloperidol are rare. On the basis of a questionnaire and survey of the literature Gerle registered the side-effects in 12,500 patients treated with haloperidol. Hypotension and tachycardia are usually slight. Nausea, loss of appetite and diarrhea may occur. Allergic skin reactions are extremely rare. Endocrine symptoms and agranulocytosis were never seen. Jaundice occurred in 18 cases, 12 of which occurred in two relatively small groups in Italy, and only six in the remaining 12,000 patients. Gerle, therefore, concludes that haloperidol has no liver toxicity high enough to be of significance for its clinical use. In accordance with Delay et al., this survey also revealed sleep disturbances after long use of haloperidol, particularly in patients developing akathisia.

Already in 1963, Delay et al. showed that, aside from extrapyramidal motor symptoms, the psychiatric side-effects play a most important role. Haloperidol may cause depressive syndromes as also seen in other potent neuroleptics (Helmchen and Hippius). Therefore, depressed patients, particularly endogenous depressions, should not be given haloperidol. Waelkens considers depressions and neuroses, cerebral vascular disease, and coronary sclerosis as contraindications to the drug which should also be avoided in parkinsonian and other brain stem syndromes. The manufacturers finally point out that the safety of the drug in pregnancy has not yet been established.

EEG changes in patients were found to be similar to those occurring with the phenothiazines. In animal experiments with rabbits, Shimizu et al. showed similarities in terms of the acute effects on the arousal system and on hippocampal seizure discharges but differences regarding the chronic effects on the arousal system and regarding "activated" sleep. The sleep induced by haloperidol resembles more natural than chlorpromazine-induced sleep. The latter shows more slow waves than sleep induced by haloperidol or natural sleep.

Mode of Administration and Dosage: Haloperidol is orally and parenterally effective. Its success in Europe is perhaps explained by the fact that it was the first neuroleptic available in drops which are tasteless and easy to take (1 ml = 20 drops = 20 mg.). This facilitates gradation of dosage in long-term maintenance therapy (1 drop = 1.0 mg.), where in chronic schizophrenics 1.5 to 2 mg. daily are sufficient (Flegel). Low dosage is also recommended in children and geriatric patients.

In acute schizophrenics and manics 5 to 10 mg. daily are given. In severe excitements 5 mg. of haloperidol can be given intravenously. This was also recommended in cases of delirium before chlormethiazol was introduced. If an excitement state is not arrested within 20 minutes, further injections of 5 mg. intravenously or intramuscularly can be given in intervals of 20 to 30 minutes. This is possible because haloperidol, contrary to the phenothiazines, has little circulatory effect. Thus, side-effects due to phenothiazines are often an important indication for the use of haloperidol and other butyrophenone derivatives.

2. *Triperidol*

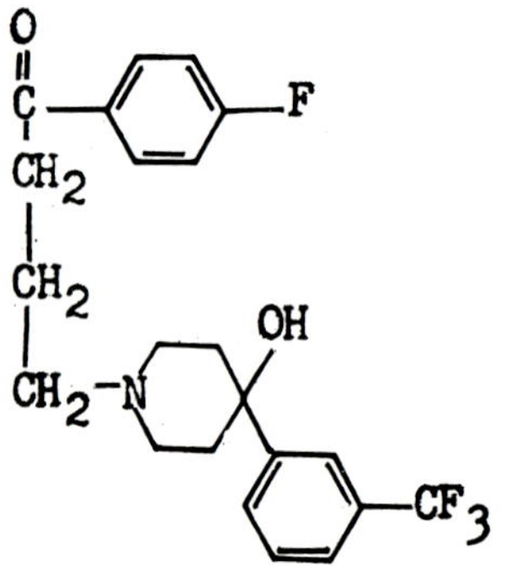

Triperidol is 1[3-(4-fluorbenzoyl)-propyl] - 4 - hydroxy - 4(3″trifluormethyl - phenyl)-piperidin-hydrochloride.

Pharmacological and clinical actions of triperidol closely resemble those of haloperidol. Its neuroleptic potency is estimated as three times stronger than that of haloperidol, and, therefore, can be given in lower doses. The close relationship to haloperidol is not surprising because chemically these two butyrophenone derivatives differ only in the phenyl group of the molecule, where triperidol has a $-CF_3$ group in the meta position and haloperidol a chlorine atom in the para position.

Already the first clinical investigations revealed the usefulness of triperidol in the treatment of schizophrenic defect states (Divry et al.). Dullness, lack of drive and initiative may be improved, and resocialization made possible. Other target symptoms are impaired affective contact and autism. This good effect on schizophrenic defect states and hebephrenics was not confirmed by Gross and Kaltenbäck who saw the best results in acute schizophrenics with psychomotor excitement and hallucinations. The same was seen by Hollister et al. in 57 newly admitted acute schizophrenics treated for six weeks with triperidol and studied with rating scales (brief psychiatric rating scales—BPRS—and inpatient multidimensional psychiatric scale—IMPS). Their comparison with other neuroleptics showed that triperidol is equal or even superior to the most potent tricyclic neuroleptics. Their computerized results showed a particular superiority in paranoid schizophrenics, where they consider it the drug of choice. This finding would further substantiate the idea of Hollister et al. and Klett and Caffey that certain drugs have different effects on different schizophrenic subtypes.

In double blind studies Gallant and his co-workers compared triperidol first with chlorpromazine, then with chlorpromazine and haloperidol (Pratt et al.) and finally with trifluoperazine and phenobarbital. They also concluded that trifluperidol acts faster and more intensively than other neuroleptics, not only in certain subtypes of schizophrenia but in all groups of acute schizophrenics and even in chronic schizophrenics which would make it the drug of choice in all schizophrenics. The same superiority was found in a double blind study by Fox et al.

These enthusiastic opinions should not obscure the often pronounced side-effects. While vegetative and vasomotor phenomena are minimal, extrapyramidal symptoms can be severe. The initial dyskinesias and Parkinsonian syndromes can be controlled with anti-Parkinsonian drugs. A greater problem are the not infrequent akathisias, often complicated by persistent insomnia. This should lead to discontinuation of the drug, all the more as triperidol as a very potent neuroleptic may occasionally lead to persistent dyskinesias.

MODE OF ADMINISTRATION AND DOSAGE: Slow increase of medication is recommended to limit side-effects. Gallant and co-workers suggest an initial daily dose of 0.5 mg. up to a maximum of 6 to 8 mg. Others gave up to 12 mg. The average dose is 0.5 to 2 mg. daily. Modifications of dosage is facilitated by liquid triperidol (20 drops = 1 mg.). In severe psychotic excitement 2.5 to 5 mg. of triperidol intravenously or intramuscularly can be administered.

3. *Methylperidol*

Methylperidol (Luvatren) is 1-[3-(4-fluorbenzoyl)-propyl]-4-hydroxy-4(p-tolyl)-piperidine-hydrochloride.

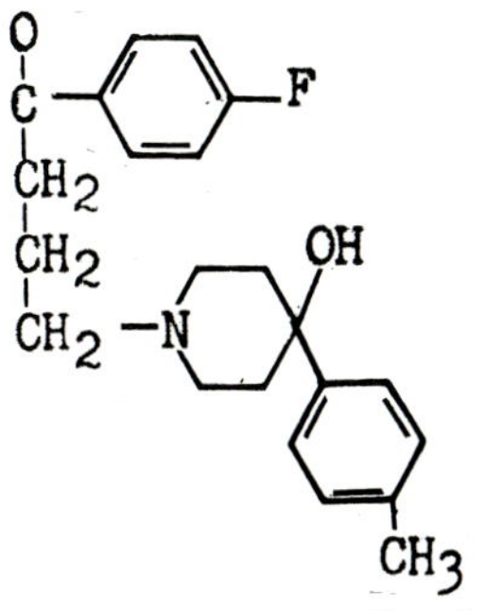

Methylperidol is chemically related to haloperidol and triperidol but pharmacologically and clinically weaker than the two other butyrophenon derivatives (Angst and Pöldinger; Gastager and Gruber). Even parenteral application has a minimal effect on psychomotor excitement and delusions. The best results were seen by Angst and Pöldinger in non-disturbed paranoid, hallucinatory schizophrenics. The drug may have a place in continuous treatment and rehabilitation because side-effects are few except for occasional initial dyskinesias (Uytterschaut and Jacobs).

MODE OF ADMINISTRATION AND DOSAGE: 15 to 60 mg. orally are sufficient. Doses up to 300 mg. are well tolerated but hardly improve the results. Methylperidol is available in 5 mg. tablets and in solution, but where parenteral application is necessary, more potent butyrophenone derivatives should be used.

4. *Floropipamide*

Floropipamide (Dipiperon) is 1-[3-(4-fluorbenzoyl)-propyl]-4-piperidino-piperidin-4 carbonic acid amin.

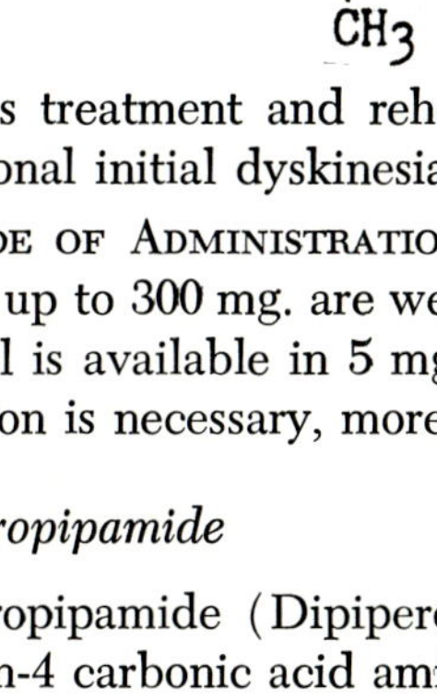

Floropipamide occupies a special place among the butyrophenone derivatives because it has the lowest extrapyramidal effect. As a relatively weak neuroleptic its usefulness is limited to rather bland psychotic syndromes; and the minimal side-effects make it suitable for long-term therapy of schizophrenics.

Like most butyrophenone derivatives this drug was first clinically investigated in Liège (Belgium) by Bobon, Collard and co-workers.

It soon became apparent that floropipamide not only influences productive symptomatology like hallucinations but also autism, contact difficulties, negativism and mutism which are often resistive to other neuroleptics. Bobon and co-workers also found that floropipamide effect on sleep disturbances in psychoses. Administered during the day, it has no immediate hypnotic effect, but it procures nocturnal sleep, thus regulating the wake-sleep rhythm. This "delayed hypnogenic effect" was confirmed by Sugerman. Bente et al. studied statistically the determinining factor of the floropipamide effect in 300 patients and found that it depends more on the course of the psychosis than on the target symptoms. All authors are particularly satisfied with the results in long-term therapy and with the absence of side-effects (Nuyts; Flegel and Neller; Gross and Langner). The only disadvantage, particularly in older patients, is a hypotensive effect (Nuyts).

Mode of Administration and Dosage: Floropipamide is given orally in tablets of 40 mg. The average dosis of 120 to 360 mg. daily can also be maintained in long-term therapy.

5. *Benperidol (Frenactyl, Glianimon)*

Benperidol is 1-3-(4-fluorbenzoyl)-propyl-4-2-oxybenzimidazolinyl-(1)-piperidin-tartrate.

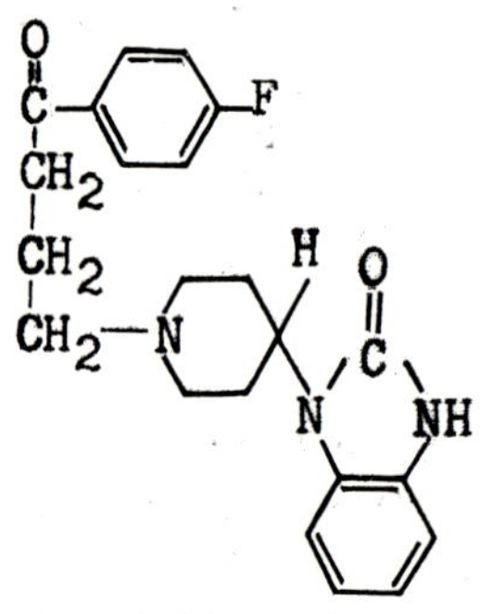

Benperidol is one of the most potent neuroleptics available. Bobon et al. who were also the first to investigate clinically this butyrophenone derivative, thought in the beginning that benperidol in small doses of approximately 3.5 mg. daily had a good effect on psychomotor excitements without showing marked extrapyramidal manifestations. Later it turned out that the drug causes very definite parkinsonian and, relatively often, hyperkinetic-dystonic syndromes. Measuring the degree of extrapyramidal action on handwriting, Haase et al. found that the extrapyramidal motor effect of benperidol is about 350 times stronger than that of chlorpromazine and eight times that of haloperidol.

Clinical studies, mostly done in France and Belgium, revealed a strongly inhibiting effect on motor excitement (Monroy et al.; Basset et al.). Furthermore, Flügel and Pfeiffer saw favorable results in hebephrenics. Coliard and Lecoq, in a double blind study with placebo in neuroses, found the tranquilizing effect of benperidol unsatisfactory. Hypersexuality in 30 patients treated by Sterkmans and Geerts, responded so well to relatively small doses of 0.7 to 2.5 mg. daily that the authors called the benperidol effect "a temporary, therefore reversible neuroleptic castration." With proper dosage results are practically always satisfactory. Schmidt and Daudet were able to lastingly influence behavior disorders of disturbed oligophrenics with 0.4 to 0.8 mg. of benperidol.

The drug is also useful for the restlessness and agitation of symptomatic psychoses, deliria and particularly agitated senile psychoses, where Miletto and Sacco emphasized its minimal vegetative side-effects.

Mode of Administration and Dosage: Benperidol is available orally as liquid for individualized gradated dosage. In severe excitement intravenous or intramuscular use of 0.5 to 2 mg. is effective. The dosis for acute psychosis lies between 1.5 and 5 mg. daily, for long-term treatment between 0.6 and 1.5 mg.; but penperidol is rarely used for maintenance treatment because of the extrapyramidal side-effects.

TRANQUILIZERS

The term "tranquilizers" is being used in different, often contradictory ways. Originally the neuroleptics were called "major tranquilizers," while other drugs which had a calming effect but were ineffective in the psychoses, were called "minor tranquilizers." The latter will now be surveyed. Sometimes the barbiturates are included in this group, but more often the tranquilizers are designated as "mild non-barbiturate sedatives" in contrast to the barbiturates. In order to overcome the confusion created by these different definitions of tranquilizers, more recently the term "anxiolytic drugs" was introduced. However, this term also leaves unclear whether older sedatives like the barbiturates belong to this group. We limit ourselves here to a description of the modern sedatives, although barbiturates in small doses may often have similar therapeutic effects. In spite of many objections the most commonly used name for these drugs is still "tranquilizers."

A. Substituted Diols

Meprobamate (Miltown, Equanil, Mepavlon, Aneural, Cirpon)

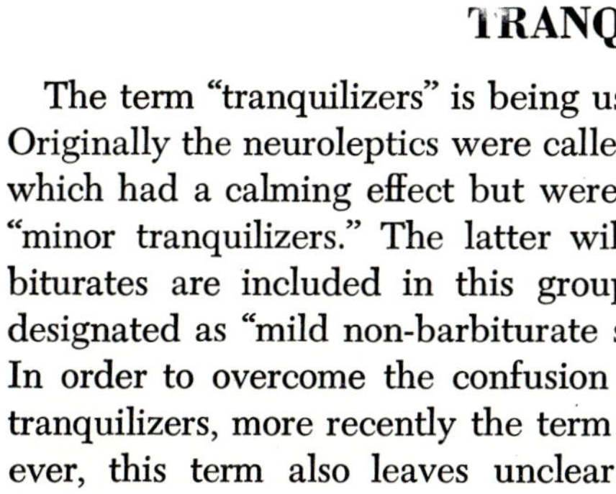

Meprobamate, 2-methyl-2-n-propyl-1, 3-propanediol dicarbamate, was developed from mephenesin (3-0-toloxy-1, 2-propanediol), which was introduced in 1946 as a muscle relaxant. Since the hydroxyl groups of mephenesin are rapidly oxidized, its action is of short duration, and a search was made for derivatives with more prolonged activity. A series of dicarbamates derived from 2- substituted 1, 3-propanediols were subsequently tested and found to have marked anticonvulsant effects of long duration. In 1951 Berger and Ludwig reported upon meprobamate, which they observed to have pronounced muscle relaxing powers and anticonvulsant activity as well as a taming effect upon monkeys.

Physiological and Pharmacological Properties: Berger observed that the drug was readily absorbed and was excreted in the urine conjugated with glucuronic acid. High doses in animals produced a flaccid muscle paralysis, affecting skeletal muscles only, and sedation. With lower doses, there is muscular relaxation. Its onset and duration of action are about eight times longer than that of mephenesin. It antagonizes the convulsive and lethal effects of leptazol and strychnine as well as electrically induced convulsions. Barbiturate anesthesia is prolonged. The drug acts upon the multineuronal reflexes of the central nervous system depressing them; it has little direct action on muscle, peripheral nerve, or monosynaptic reflexes. No change in cardiac, respiratory or autonomic function was noted. After the oral administration of 200 mg./kg. of body weight of meprobamate, monkeys became tamer while retaining their appetite and interest in the environment. In patients on high doses of 10 g. per day for four weeks Shagass et al. found that the EEG pattern was similar to that induced by the barbiturates. Fast activity was increased; the alpha rhythm was frequently slowed; and the theta activity augmented. This is compatible with the resemblance of the drug to the barbiturates, particularly its production of habituation and withdrawal symptoms on high dosages.

Mercier and Dessaigne reported that meprobamate reduced cortical excitability in animals and prevented EEG after-discharges from spreading to the opposite hemisphere by a blocking action at the diencephalon. The response of the reticular activating system to both direct and indirect stimulation was reduced, but cortical epileptic discharges were suppressed to an even greater degree, so that it appears that the cortical depressant effect of the drug is predominant. Meprobamate also reduced the hypertension provided by stimulation of the hypothalamus, the reticular formation, and the sciatic nerve. It has been found useful in the treatment of neurogenic hypertension and its action in this condition may be due to a depression of the hypothalamic-bulbar vasoconstrictor centers (Berger and Ludwig).

Results of Clinical Investigations: The main use of meprobamate is in the treatment of the neuroses, especially anxiety and tension states. There is much conflicting evidence as to its efficacy, some trials having apparently demonstrated its superiority over both a placebo and barbiturates, while other similarly controlled experiments have recorded opposite results. Uhlenhuth et al., in a comparison of meprobamate, phenobarbital, and a placebo, attempted to discover the degree of interaction between the attitude of the doctor prescribing the drug and the responses of the patients receiving it. They found that the reaction of the patients was very dependent upon the attitude of the doctor toward drug therapy. These patients were chronic neurotics who, after receiving treatment over long periods of time, had probably become acutely sensitive to the attitude of the doctor treating them and tended to respond in accordance with what they thought he expected. Rickels et al., on the other hand, found that meprobamate was preferred to amobarbital, prochlorperazine and a placebo by a group of acute neurotic out-patients as judged by the fact that fewer patients receiving it dropped out of therapy and that it particularly relieved insomnia, irritability, and mild depression. Two negative studies, those of Moriarty and Batterman et al., did not find meprobamate superior to a placebo or to butabarbital respectively. Hinton, in a controlled trial, found that, when compared with a placebo for 4 weeks, meprobamate failed to produce a significantly higher level of improvement than the placebo, although symptoms of anxiety, tension, and phobic ideas were relieved to some extent.

Insomnia, anorexia and somatic symptoms were not relieved. Observers such as Gardner and Selling have been impressed by the alleviation of anxiety; but, as shown by the number of negative reports, its beneficial effects are by no means unequivocal. Laties and Weiss, in a review of the studies on meprobamate up to 1958, observed that they provided no evidence of its superiority over barbiturates or a placebo in anxious neurotic out-patients, although there were indications of its efficacy in alcoholics and hospitalized patients with anxiety symptoms.

There is the disadvantage of producing a dependence on the drug as with the barbiturates; and treatment should be confined to a fairly short period of time during the acute stages of a neurosis. The drug should never be prescribed indefinitely because of the danger of habituation. Heller and his coworkers have noted that, in fact, the drug has most benefit in those patients who have an illness of recent onset and only moderate severity, accompanied by a fairly acute onset of symptoms. They found that anxiety states, reactive depressions, and obsessional neurotics were helped by the drug, but that hysterics did not respond. Lehmann and Sirnes observed that unless there was improvement with the drug in the first few days of treatment there was no point in continuing it. Psychosomatic conditions such as neurodermatitis and tension headaches have also been reported as being favorably influenced by the drug. Although it is not an analgesic, it may change the attitude toward pain.

Meprobamate has been given in the psychoses, and, while it may have some effect in relieving anxiety in pseudoneurotic schizophrenics and agitated depressions, it is less effective than the phenothiazines or reserpine for this purpose, and it has no effect on the underlying psychosis. It has been administered to control the withdrawal symptoms in alcoholism, but again there is no evidence that it has any advantages over the phenothiazines. Its use in the alleviation of pre-ECT apprehension and post-ECT confusion has also been recommended, but West and da Fonseca did not find that it made any significant difference in their patients, and the same authors noted very little change in the objective somatic concomitants of anxiety such as sweating, tachycardia, and tremors, although there was some subjective relief of tension. No side-effects have been reported from its use in conjunction with ECT.

Barsa and Kline, who found no improvement when meprobamate alone was given to chronic psychotic patients in doses up to 4 Gm. daily, reported that a combination with chlorpromazine in patients previously refractory to phenothiazine therapy, produced a sustained improvement in behavior and mental content in about one third of them. Hift et al. found that in mild endogenous depressions meprobamate in conjunction with psychotherapy is safe, and that depressions due to incipient arteriosclerotic dementia might also benefit.

Mode of Administration and Dosage: The drug is administered orally as tablets or a suspension; 400 to 800 mg. three times daily is usually sufficient for the control of neurotic symptoms. For children over three years of age, 100 to 200 mg. two or three times daily should be the initial dose, with a gradual increase to obtain the desired clinical effect. The drug should always be withdrawn slowly, particularly where high doses have been given, because of the risk of producing a withdrawal psychosis and convulsions.

HABIT FORMATION AND WITHDRAWAL SYMPTOMS: There seems to be no doubt that meprobamate can produce dependency and withdrawal symptoms which are similar to those with the barbiturates or alcohol. Ewing and Haizlip found, in patients who were withdrawn from the drug after receiving 3.2 to 6.4 Gm. for forty days in a double blind study, not only insomnia, vomiting, tremor, muscle twitching, overt anxiety, anorexia and ataxia, but some hallucinosis with anxiety and tremors similar to delirium tremens. In addition, three of the patients had grand mal seizures. In animal experiments, Swinyard et al. found that the withdrawal syndrome was quicker in onset and shorter in duration than the one which occurred with barbiturates in their studies; but one of us [L.B.K.] has shown that the time of onset also differs in barbiturates, and changes with their excretion time. Phillip et al. reports two cases, one of psychotic depression and the other of a paranoid reaction, when meprobamate was withdrawn. Lemere found that, in contrast to chlorpromazine and reserpine, increase of the medication by the patient was common, particularly in abstinent alcoholics.

It is obviously wise to avoid, as far as possible, long-term medication with meprobamate, particularly without adequate supervision and especially in those individuals whose personality or type of illness predisposes them to dependence upon drugs. Meprobamate should preferably be used for short periods of treatment in the acute cases to help patients over a crisis. It should be emphasized that the tense psychotic can also become dependent upon the drug, and we have seen a post-lobotomy schizophrenic undoubtedly dependent upon meprobamate, who began to require increasingly large doses to control her anxiety.

OVERDOSAGE: The usual picture of a large overdose of meprobamate is the development of coma accompanied by loss of the deep reflexes, marked muscle relaxation, hypotension which may reach shock levels, fixed dilated pupils, and respiratory collapse. In lesser degrees of intoxication, there may be drowsiness with incoordination of motor movements and of speech. Myoclonic seizures can occur during the coma.

Treatment of acute meprobamate poisoning should consist of gastric lavage, intravenous infusion if necessary, oxygen to prevent cerebral anoxia, and vasopressors such as norepinephrine to raise the blood pressure if there is gross hypotension, as well as prophylactic antibiotics if unconsciousness is prolonged. Heberden and Cooper advise the use of leptazol in a dose of 3 ml. intravenously for the termination of coma. They found that this produced an immediate restoration of consciousness in a comatose patient who had ingested 8 Gm. of meprobamate. Allen and Black applied bitemporal cerebral electrostimulation, which they had to maintain for two hours, together with intravenous levarterenol bitartrate to restore the blood pressure in a severely collapsed patient.

Powell has reported two fatal cases after the ingestion of 12 Gm. and 20 Gm. of the drug. Another fatal case, due to pulmonary edema, occurred several days after the suicide attempt; and Kamin and Shaskan reported on a fatal case after ingestion of 47.6 Gm. (119 tablets).

SIDE-EFFECTS AND COMPLICATIONS: It has been reported that meprobamate, in doses of 800 mg., produces no impairment of mental or physical efficiency. Marquis et al. found that the drug given alone did not interfere with the skills required for driving a car safely, and that the impairment produced by alcohol was not increased. Loomis and West, however, in a similar test of performance with a simulated car driving apparatus, found that meprobamate in a dose of 400 mg. produced some impairment of performance, which was less intense than that with chlorpromazine or secobarbital. Reitan could demonstrate no impairment of visal-motor co-ordination, motor speed, problem-solving, or attention with normal doses of the drug, although when meprobamate was given in a total dose of 1600 mg. before the test, performance was significantly better with the placebo.

Hift et al. have described experiments with self-administration of the drug in a single oral dose of 400 to 600 mg. Within 5 to 10 minutes, a sensation of pressure in the head or dizziness was experienced which lasted for about 15 minutes and was followed by a feeling of "gay indifference" lasting 2 to 3 hours. A dose of 1.2 Gm. produced greater degrees of this feeling, but was followed by tiredness and disturbances of concentration lasting for 4 to 6 hours. Drowsiness may occur, usually disappearing as treatment proceeds. This is particularly marked in patients who increase the dose themselves and in such cases may proceed to euphoria, dysarthria, and incoordination (Lemere).

Hypersensitivity reactions have been described. They occur during the first few days of therapy, and, in some instances, may commence shortly after the first dose of the drug is taken. Holoubeck et al. describe the case of a patient who developed a generalized erythematous rash just over an hour after taking one meprobamate tablet. This was followed by chills, fever, nausea, and vomiting, with leucocytosis and neutrophilia. This condition cleared up uneventfully; but, when the patient took a further one and one-half tablets some time later, a similar reaction occurred with the signs of shock. The fever and rash subsided following treatment with corticosteroids and antibiotics.

The rash may be urticarial or an erythematous maculopapular eruption, sometimes becoming purpuric. There may be intense itching, and Friedman and Marmelzat noted that it tended to appear in both sexes initially in the pelvic girdle area. No abnormality of the platelet count has been reported in those patients who develop a purpuric type of skin eruption. This may be accompanied by swelling of the small joints or by edema of the lower extremities, resembling the allergic reactions seen with many other drugs. Antihistamines may be tried, but they have not been found to be as efficacious as corticosteroids.

Other types of sensitivity reaction which have been described are intestinal hyperperistalsis with rice water diarrhea, temporary diplopia due to paralysis of the extra-ocular muscles, and a paradoxical reaction of severe excitement (Friedman and Marmelzat). All of them occurred after 1 to 2 tablets and were relieved by withdrawal of the drug. Angioneurotic edema has been reported (Selling), as well as bronchospasm. Van de Erve and Childs suggest that previous mephenesin administration may predispose to a cross-sensitization reaction. Stroud regards early recognition of the skin eruption as being of great importance, since he found that initial reactions were often milder than subsequent ones which developed when the prodromal signs were ignored.

Adlin et al. have observed a fatal reaction after the ingestion of 600 mg. of meprobamate. There was a sudden onset of purpura accompanied by dermatitis, pyrexia, and oliguria. Autopsy revealed renal tubular degeneration.

Erythema multiforme has been reported (Stroud) in patients taking the drug over a period of two months. In one case, collapse occurred and prolonged therapy was required with steroids. Hypotension may occur in old people given large doses (Scott et al.). Epigastric discomfort, anorexia, and nausea occur, and two patients with peptic ulcer, reported by Hift et al., had to be taken off the drug because of severe vomiting.

A single case of aplastic anemia with fatal outcome was reported by Meyer et al. in a woman taking only 200 mg. daily for a week.

Other Tranquilizers Related to Meprobamate

During the last few years numerous drugs have been introduced which are closely related chemically and pharmacologically to meprobamate, or to its mother-substance, mephenesin (Berger and Ludwig).

Drugs related to mephenesin are:
1. Phenaglycodol (Ultran)
2. Mephenoxalone (Trepidone)
3. Promoxolane (Dimethylane)

Drugs similar to meprobamate are:
1. Emylacmate (Striatran, Nuncital)
2. Hydroxyphenamate (Listica)
3. Phenylpropanol Carbamate (Gamaquil)
4. Carisoprodol (Soma, Sanoma)
5. Tybamate (Solacen, Tybatran)

Most of these drugs combine the clinical effect of a minor tranquilizer with that of a muscle relaxant. As numerous as these substances are, they do not play an important role in psychiatric therapy.

B. Carbinole and Amide

Methylpentinol (Oblivon C)

Methylpentinol is 3-methyl-1-pentyn-3-ol-carbamat.

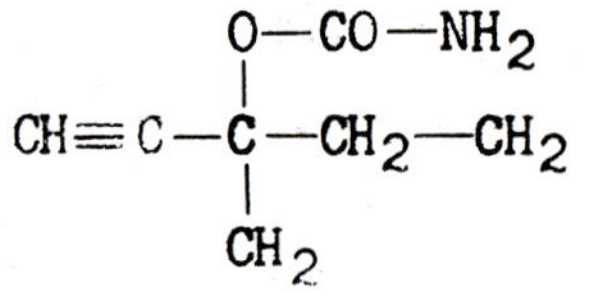

Oblivon has been used as a mild sedative in a dose of 600 mg. Bockner reported improvement of tension, anxiety and panic reactions with a daily dose of up to 2 g. Marley and Bartholomew, who gave patients 2 g. daily for five days, observed a large number of toxic central nervous system effects including nystagmus, ptosis, pupillary abnormalities, loss of facial muscle tone, ataxia, dysarthria, tremors, mood changes, impaired concentration and attention, body image and subjective time distortions, illusions and possibly hallucinations, as well as EEG abnormalities. In a chronic paranoid psychosis, Broussolle et al. reported improvement in behavior; but, after the drug had been stopped for eight days and was restarted, a state of shock followed by epileptic convulsions appeared.

Chemically closely related to methylpentinol is ethchloroynol which is also used as a tranquilizer and sedative.

Ectylurea (Levanil, Nostyn)

Ectylurea is cis-(2-thylcrotonoyl)-urea.

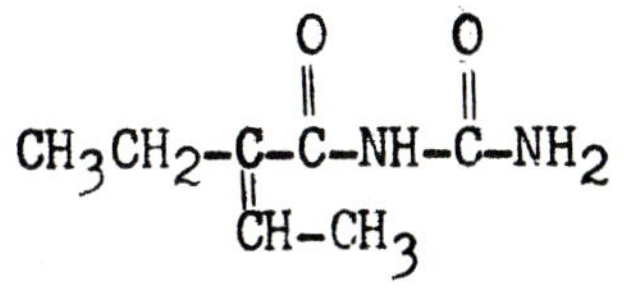

It has been used in the treatment of tension and anxiety. Beneficial results with minimum toxicity have been claimed by Bauer et al. with 300 mg. three or four times daily. There was no evidence of mental depression or of habit formation. The chief side-effect was drowsiness, although a few patients complained of nervousness. Nausea, rashes, and dizziness have been reported as occurring occasionally. The impression of these authors that the drug is ineffective in the psychoses, was confirmed by Baker who, in a controlled trial comparing this drug with chlorpromazine and a placebo, gave up to 1200 mg. daily. In another study, Campanella and Guida observed that ectylurea is most beneficial in anxiety states, while psychoses and obsessional neuroses fail to respond. Ferguson used the drug for the relief of anxiety in elderly patients.

C. Diphenylmethane Derivatives

1. *Orphenadrine (Disipal, Mephenamine, Norflex)*

Orphenadrine is β-dimethylamino-ethyl-2-methylbenzhydrylether.

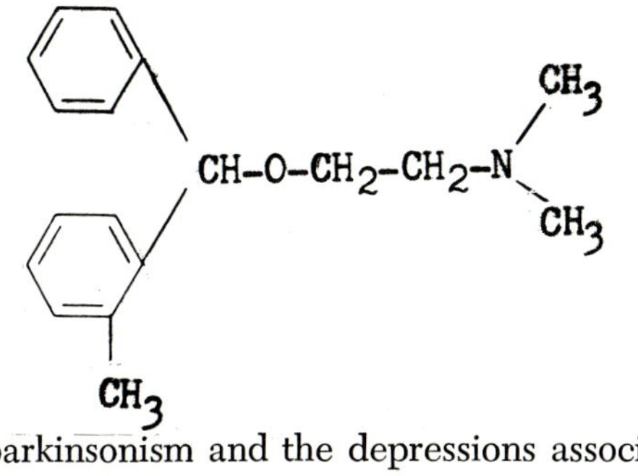

This drug was originally used in the treatment of Parkinsonism and as a muscle relaxant. It was noticed that it also exerted an euphorizing effect in such patients, and this led to its trial in depressive states by Robitscher and Pulver in doses of 50 mg. three or four times daily.

Its main value is in the treatment of depression associated with parkinsonism and the depressions associated with degenerative diseases in the senium (Meulenbeld). It has been used with the neuroleptic drugs, as mentioned earlier, to prevent the development of extrapyramidal symptoms. There is evidence that when it is given alone to schizophrenics the psychotic symptoms may be increased (Van Andel).

A combination of reserpine and orphenadrine, used in Germany under the trade name "Phasein," has already been mentioned. Here, orphenadrine is supposed to overcome the psychological and neurological side-effects of reserpine. Langley and Robin, however, who gave it in doses of 50 mg. three times daily, report that in a small series of only ten patients they could find no evidence that the combination of disipal with reserpine was of clinical value in mitigating the less severe extrapyramidal or other side-effects of reserpine.

2. *Phenyltoloxamine (PRN, Bristamine)*

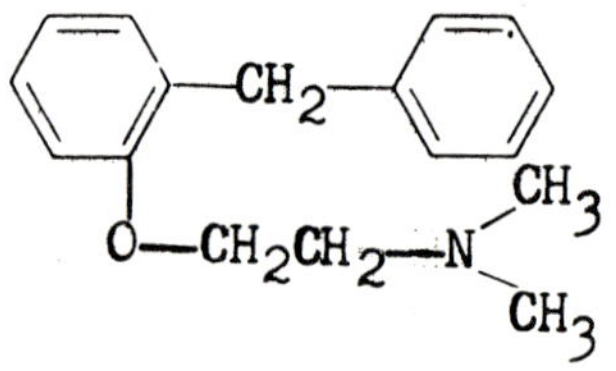

Phenyltoloxamine, N,N-dimethyl-2-(α-phenyl-0-toloxy)-ethylamine, has been used in an oral dosage of 100 to 200 mg. as a mild sedative in neurotics. It is said to have similarities in action to both meprobamate and secobarbital (Remmen et al.).

3. *Azacyclonol (Frenquel)*

Azacyclonol is α-diphenyl-4-piperidine-methanol.

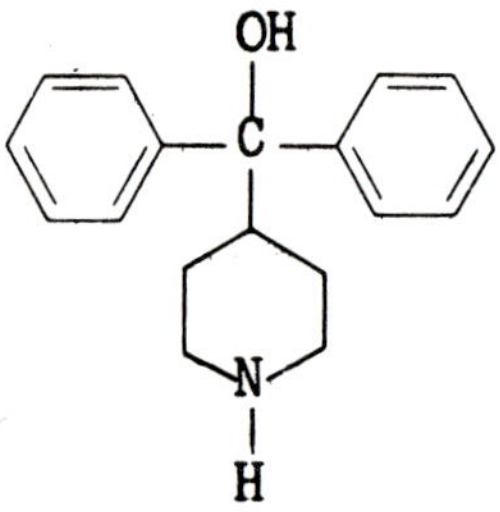

This drug was introduced by Fabing and Hawkins, who found that azacyclonol acted as a partial or complete blocking agent against the development of LSD 25 and mescaline experimental psychoses when given to healthy subjects prior to ingestion of these drugs. When injected intravenously during these experimental psychoses, it abruptly ends them. Because of this action, its use in acute schizophrenia was advocated, but clinical trials have largely produced disappointing results. Fabing and Hawkins themselves reported that 5 out of 14 acute schizophrenics remitted on the drug, but Sarwer-Foner and Korcanyi could find no anti-psychotic activity when they gave the drug orally. These authors point out the now well-recognized fact that the "model psychoses" differ from schizophrenia in a number of ways, and that, in the retention of some degree of insight and the prominence of distortions of apperception, they are more like the toxic psychoses.

Hargreaves examined the effect of the drug on hallucinations in chronic schizophrenics in a double blind trial, finding it to be of no value in these patients and to be without any anti-hallucinatory action. A similar trial by Lascelles et al. reached the same conclusion. Rosner et al., who in a double blind study compared the drug to pipradol, found that it produced no change in psychotic behavior. Rinaldi et al. were more enthusiastic, finding that a large proportion of chronic disturbed schizophrenics were helped. However, it should be noted that improvement also occurred with the placebo in his cases. While azacyclonol has little value in the treatment of schizophrenia, intravenous trial with the drug in the toxic psychoses might yield better results, as noted by Proctor and Odland.

No serious toxic effects have been reported from the use of the drug, which is usually administered orally in an initial daily dose of 100 mg. rising to 300 to 400 mg. per day in divided doses.

4. *Hydroxyzine (Atarax, Masmoran, Placidol, Vistaril)*

Hydroxyzine is 2-(2-4-(p-chloro-α-phenylbenzyl)-1-piperazinyl-ethoxy)-ethanol.

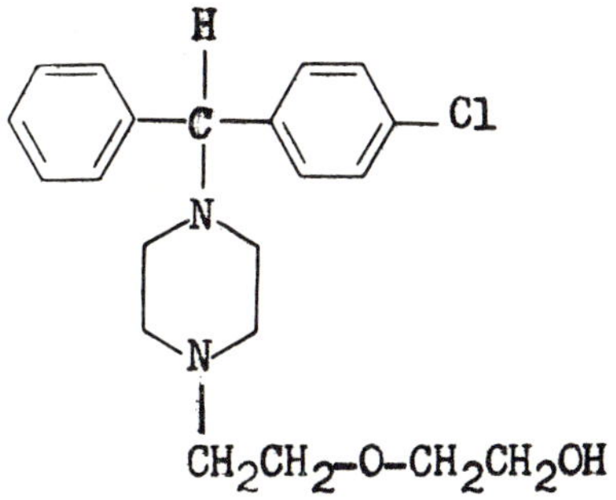

Hydroxyzine is a benzhydrol derivative with adrenolytic, anticholinergic, antiemetic, antihistaminic and antispasmodic properties. It has hypotensive and hypothermic actions. Like chlorpromazine, it has been found to produce a small rise in the threshold for arousal by direct electrical stimulation of the reticular formation.

It has been used as a sedative in the treatment of neurotic tension, anxiety, and over-activity in dosages of 10 to 300 mg. orally daily. Zubiani, starting with 75 mg. daily, orally or parenterally, and increasing to 400 mg. daily, administered the drug to schizophrenics with limited effect. Hallucinations did not disappear but the patients became emotionally indifferent to them. There has been no convincing evidence that hydroxyzine produces any significant change in psychotic states and even in the neuroses. Middlefell and Edwards found that the drug was no better than a placebo in the relief of tension in neurotics and in mild depressive states. Settel, in an uncontrolled trial, reported that the most outstanding feature of the drug was its ability to convert exaggerated responses to stress into normal ones. However, although tension and anxiety symptoms were relieved while the patients were on the drug, as soon as it was stopped they immediately experienced a recurrence of the symptoms and requested more of the drug. Seneca also had results in mild tension symptoms and psychosomatic complaints. Ayd states that the most successful use of hydroxyzine has been in the treatment of ambulatory anxious neurotic patients, either with acute symptoms or with an abrupt flare-up of chronic anxiety. Obsessive-compulsive neuroses, hysteria, hypochondriasis, and character disorders do not respond. Some workers, including Smigel et al., have reported that mild emotional upsets and hyperactivity in geriatric patients are helped by hydroxyzine. Hyperkinetic children as well, who may require up to 300 mg. daily, especially those with brain injuries, sometimes respond. Segal and Tansley saw favorable results with 20 mg. daily in maladjusted subnormal children.

The side-effects observed include hypotension, paradoxical excitement, drowsiness, dryness of the mouth, rhinorrhea, itching, headache, and increased peristalsis. Increase in frequency of epileptic attacks has been reported in a few cases (Muratorio).

Chemically related to hydroxyzine, is meclizine (Bonine, Bonamine, Peremesine) which is a widely used antiemetic drug.

5. *Benactyzine (Suavitil, Phobex)*

Benactyzine is 2-diethylaminoethyl-benzilate.

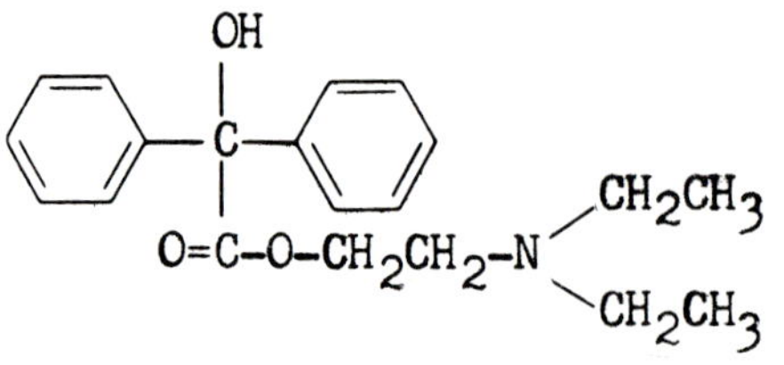

It produces sensations of giddiness and heaviness with difficulty in concentrating and a tendency to over-estimate the passage of time. Larger doses have an atropine-like effect, with dryness of the mouth and difficulty in accommodation. It protects animals against experimentally induced neuroses (Jacobsen).

It has been used in neurotic states, particularly in obsessional-compulsive and anxiety neuroses. It has also been found useful by some observers in mild cases of depression. In a rather sceptical study, Kinross-Wright and Moyer found its greatest value in the reduction of emotional reactivity to stress. The average dose was 3 to 16 mg. daily. Ayd, who administered the drug in doses up to 50 mg. daily to patients with predominant anxiety and obsessional thinking, found improvement in only a small number, while the medication often had to be stopped because of its unpleasant anticholinergic side-effects. Seager and Leitch found no difference between the drug and a placebo in a small number of neurotic patients when benactyzine was given in a dosage of 6 mg. daily over a two-week period. They observed no euphoriant effect and no evidence of withdrawal symptoms.

Jensen found it useful in neurotics with anxiety, obsessions, or sleeping disturbances; and Feinblatt et al. in phobic states. Both Plichet and Jacobsen observed favorable results in obsessive-compulsive patients. More recent negative reports, however, found the drug to be of no value in out-patients with anxiety states (Hargreaves et al.; Harrington and Mayer-Gross). Thus, benactyzine falls into the ever-widening group of drugs whose efficacy is still unproven.

The main side-effects reported are palpitations, dizziness, dryness of the mouth, difficulty in accommodation, feelings of depersonalization, clouding and slowing of thought, impairment of concentration, and manual clumsiness in performing complicated tasks with doses over 8 mg. daily. Kinross-Wright and Moyer found that there were subjective feelings of mental confusion, drowsiness, feelings of unreality, emotional lability, heaviness of the limbs, ataxia, and skin rashes with doses in excess of 12 mg. Cattell and Malitz find it contraindicated in "hostile" patients.

A combination of benactyzine with meprobamate was introduced by L. Alexander. The trade name of this combination is deprol which contains 1 mg. benactyzine hydrochloride and 400 mg. of meprobamate which has been used fairly widely to treat depression and anxiety in psychoneurotics. The side-effects of both benactyzine and meprobamate may occur, although it is claimed that the combination reduces them to a minimum. The initial dosage of deprol is 1 tablet four times daily, increasing to 3 tablets four times daily if required. L. Alexander obtained 57 per cent recoveries in depressions within eight weeks which was better than the spontaneous recovery rate within this period.

There have been a number of favorable reports upon the use of the drug in neurotic depression, including that of Ruchwarger, whose patients received concomitant psychotherapy; that of McClure et al. where a lesser degree of improvement was also observed in the placebo group; and that of Bell et al. Lathrop, who compared meprobamate with benactyzine and deprol in a controlled trial with ambulatory and pseudo-neurotic schizophrenics, found that meprobamate alone produced a greater over-all improvement than the other two drugs.

From what is already known about the effects of benactyzine and meprobamate in psychoses, it is not anticipated that deprol would have any dramatic effect upon psychotic depression. Pennington has reported improvement in depressions associated with chronic schizophrenia, involutional psychosis, senility or arteriosclerosis; but this was mainly in the sphere of improved behavior and social relations as distinct from the fundamental effect on the depressive process. It would appear that the best type of case for deprol therapy is the anxious and depressed neurotic.

6. *Captodiame (Suvren, Covatix, Covatin)*

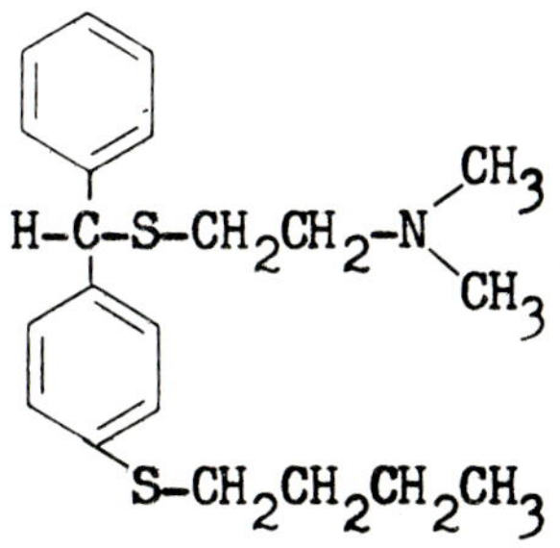

Captodiame, p-butylthiodiphenyl-methyl-2-dimethylaminoethyl-sulphide-hydrochloride, is a derivative of diphenyl-hydramine with two main actions: (1) psychotonic, similar to that of meratran and amphetamine, and (2) thymolytical, similar to reserpine and chlorpromazine. Sarro and de la Cruz, who were among the first to report on it, concluded that it was particularly effective in the irritability and anxiety of neuroses. Its main effect seems to be as a mild sedative. No complications from its use have been reported.

D. Benzodiazepine Derivatives

In 1960, chlordiazepoxide was introduced as the first benzodiazepine derivative. Since then some other structurally related drugs have been developed. This group of psychotropic drugs is unrelated to any other tranquilizer, or neuroleptic, or antidepressant drug. Today the benzodiazepine derivatives are the most widely used of all psychopharmaca.

1. *Chlordiazepoxide (Librium)*

Chlordiazepoxide, 7-chloro-2(methylamino)-5-phenyl-4-oxide, is the subject of innumerable publications.

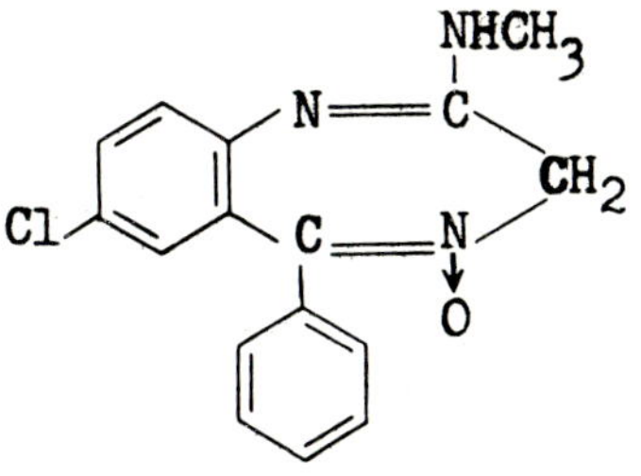

Physiological and Pharmacological Properties: Randall et al. has reported on its properties, which are a combination of some of those possessed by chlorpromazine, meprobamate, and phenobarbital. Librium possesses tranquilizing properties which are similar to those of reserpine and chlorpromazine, including a taming effect on vicious monkeys without depressing motor activity.

It exerts no autonomic blocking effects, however. The drug is anticonvulsant and has muscle relaxing properties considered to be greater than those of meprobamate. Spinal reflexes are depressed. It produces considerable stimulation of appetite. In very large doses, the blood pressure is lowered and the heart rate slowed. The EEG after chlordiazepoxide administration is similar to that found with the barbiturates and meprobamate, namely, a greater speed of activity accompanied by an increased synchronization (Sternbach et al.).

Results of Clinical Investigations: The dosage of the drug, which is usually administered orally, varies from 5 to 150 mg. daily. For elderly patients and children, 5 mg. should be the initial dose. It can be given intravenously in doses of 50 to 100 mg., particularly for sedating acute alcoholic psychoses (Ticktin and Schultz).

Since its introduction it has been claimed that chlordiazepoxide has achieved good results in practically every psychiatric disorder. Anxiety and phobic states, obsessional neurosis, schizophrenia, depression, alcoholism, and epilepsy are stated to have been treated successfully. Tension states, functional gastrointestinal disturbances, tension headache, spastic colon, and the anxiety associated with peptic ulcer in the psychosomatic sphere have also been alleviated. Tobin et al. advise that 25 to 50 mg. of the drug should be taken before neurotics face a stressful situation. Kinross-Wright et al. found the main benefits to be in the relief of anxiety, agitation, and aggression, and it would appear that the principal use of the drug will be in the treatment of neurosis. After many non-controlled investigations there are by now also a larger number of reports on controlled studies which show that chlordiazepoxide is clearly more effective in neurotic anxiety than placebo (Jenner et al.; McNair et al.).

Complications and Side-Effects: A number of side-effects have been reported. Drowsiness is common; a daily dose of 30 to 60 mg. may produce a reduction in spontaneous activity with difficulty to concentrate. Among the central nervous system side-effects are ataxia, motor hyperactivity, headache, and dysarthria.

A paradoxical reaction with hyperactivity, increased drive, and elated affect can occur. Increased irritability with acute rage reactions has been reported. Tobin et al. noted a "dissociative reaction" characterized by depersonalization and confusion and sometimes accompanied by anxiety or changes in spatial and temporal perception. Increased verbal productivity has been observed. Nausea and constipation—but also increased appetite with excessive gain of weight—have been seen. Menorrhagia, loss or increase of libido, urinary frequency, and some skin reactions were noted. Robinson has reported that syncope, without any prodromal warning signs, or vertigo, lasting for about five minutes, can occur on the second or third day of treatment.

Urinanalysis and liver function and blood tests have all been found to remain normal. A patient observed by Kinross Wright, took 625 mg. of the drug in a suicidal attempt and showed no ill-effects following gastric lavage, but another of his patients, a well-controlled epileptic, developed seizures.

Chlordiazepoxide, like barbiturates and meprobamate, causes withdrawal convulsions, and apparently also deliria if used for any length of time, and then suddenly discontinued. According to Hollister et al., withdrawal convulsions occur relatively late on the seventh or eighth day which is in accordance with the slow decrease of chlordiazepoxide in the blood.

2. *Diazepam (Valium)*

Diazepam is 7-chloro-1,3-dihydro-1-methyl-5-phenyl-2H-1-4-benzodiazepin-2-one.

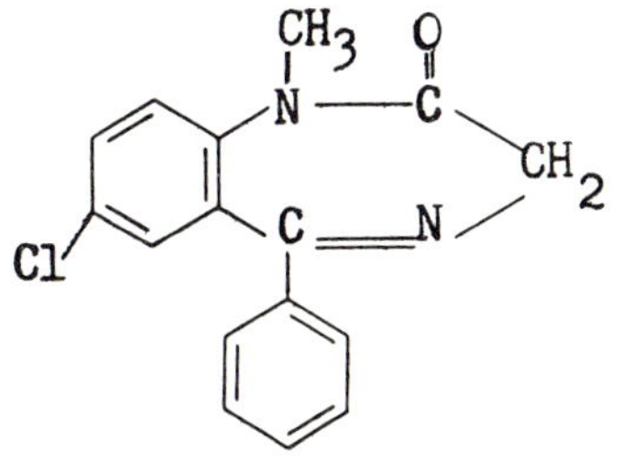

This tranquilizer was introduced a few years after chlordiazepoxide, and by now is used with the same frequency if not even more than chlordiazepoxide. In pharmacological experiments diazepam proved to be two to three times more potent than chlordiazepoxide (Sternbach et al.), and its therapeutic dosage is lower. The dosage range is between 2 and 80 mg. maximally. In general 2 to 30 mg. daily are quite sufficient.

In efforts to clarify the mode of action, neurophysiologic-pharmacological experiments have demonstrated that diazepam, like all other benzodiazepines, probably acts selectively on the limbic system, and particularly on the nucleus amygdalae, the hippocampus and the septal region. The limbic system consists of phylogenetically old brain structures which represent centers of cerebral integration and regulation for affectivity and vegetative organ functions. This site of action explains the indications of diazepam. Primarily symptoms like anxiety, tension, restlessness, excitement, and dysthymia are influenced as long as they are not symptoms of a psychosis. Therefore, diazepam is mainly used in neuroses. Also, neurotic symptoms superimposed on organic manifestations respond to it. Finally, it is widely used in physical complaints and symptoms which have no organic basis, so-called functional symptoms (Randall et al.). Diazepam was compared with chlordiazepoxide by Aivazian. It appeared that anxiety reactions with depressive manifestations responded more readily to diazepam, while chlordiazepoxide was more effective in anxiety without depression. Both drugs were ineffective in obsessive-compulsive symptoms. Diazepam seems to have a potentiating effect on acohol in the sense of delusions, restlessness and aggressiveness. Other indications are related to the muscle-relaxant properties of the drug (Hoff et al.). Thus, diazepam is recommended in spastic syndromes after strokes, and in multiple sclerosis, in parkinsonism, and it is also used in obstetrics. To be noted is the anticonvulsant action of diazepam that makes it possible to control a status epilepticus with intravenous doses of 10 to 20 mg. (Gastaut et al.; Prensky et al.). Relatively large doses are necessary to treat patients with otherwise treatment-resistant cardiac phobias; in such cases slowly increased oral doses of 30 to 50 mg. daily are recommended.

The side-effects are identical with those of chlordiazepoxide. Addiction does occur, but considering the wide use of the drug, this hardly seems to be a serious problem (Czerwenka-Wenkstetten et al.). When diazepam is suddenly discontinued, withdrawal symptoms like restlessness, perspiration, palpitations and, in some cases, delirium and convulsions have been reported (Hollister et al.; Barten).

3. *Oxazepam (Serax, Adumbran, Praxiten)*

Oxazepam is 7-chlor-1,3-dihydro-3-hydroxy-5-phenyl-2H-1,4-benzodiazepin-2-one.

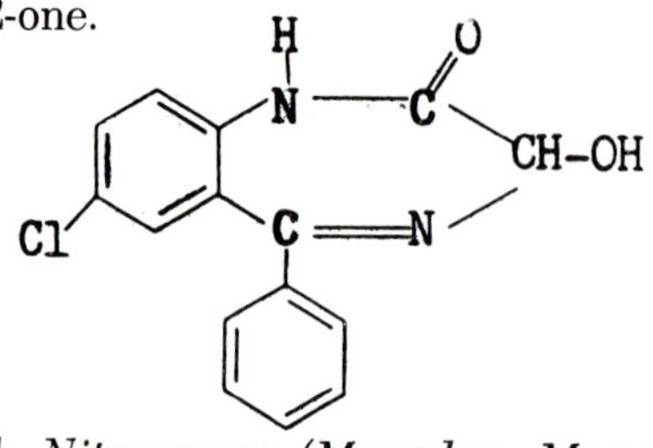

In pharmacological and clinical studies this benzodiazepine derivative proved to be weaker than chlordiazepoxide and diazepam (Sternbach et al.; Gerz; McPherson and Le Glassicke). Oral doses of 10 to 50 mg. are given.

4. *Nitrazepam (Mogadon, Mogadan)*

Nitrazepam is 1,3-dihydro-7-nitro-5-phenyl-2H-1,4-benzodiazepinone-10.

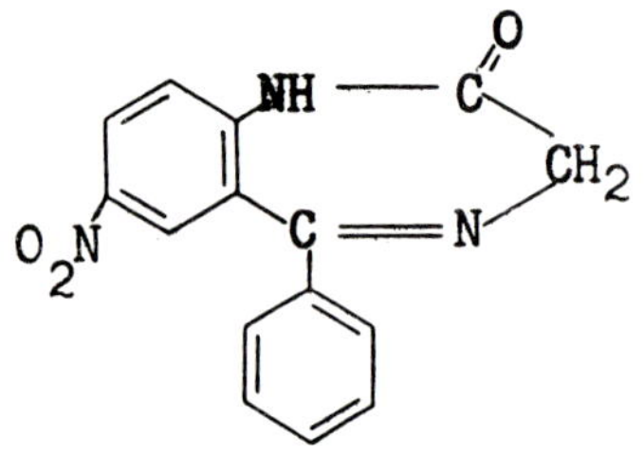

The sedative effect which had already been found to be stronger with diazepam in comparison to chlordiazepoxide, is still more pronounced with nitrazepam. Therefore, this benzodiazepine derivative is primarily used as a sleeping tablet. In a double-blind study on patients from a general practice in whom 5 to 10 mg. nitrazepam were compared with 50 to 100 mg. of butobarbiton and 250 to 500 mg. of glutethimide (Doriden) the patients preferred nitrazepam because of its faster and longer action. However, many complained of tiredness the next morning. Geriatric patients tolerate nitrazepam usually well in small doses of 2.5 to 5 mg. However, in patients with cerebral arteriosclerosis the drug may lead to nocturnal restlessness and slight confusion (Wyss and Mäder). Nitrazepam is effective in small children with Salaam seizures (Gibbs and Anderson).

THE ANTIDEPRESSANTS

This group includes all those drugs which have an elevating effect upon mood, and so ranges from the monoamine-oxidase inhibitors to the tricyclic antidepressants such as imipramine. A distinction should be made between the antidepressants and the psychostimulants. The psychostimulants, such as amphetamine, merely produce a temporary and superficial euphoric mood, often accompanied by the side-effects of overstimulation, such as feeling "jittery," without any lasting change in the underlying condition. It is true, the "psychostimulant" drugs may be of some value in the alleviation of mild depression due to reactive factors, but there is no evidence that any of them have a fundamental effect on psychotic depression. Contrary to this the "antidepressants" with the two subgroups of tricyclic antidepressants and MAO inhibitors are capable of influencing the depressive psychosis, and can in favorable cases completely relieve the depression. Their action is in this respect more similar to that of ECT, and, like it, they may produce a swing over into hypomania. The stimulants, far from being curative, may cause a deeper rebound depression, when their stimulant action wears off.

The synthesis and use of the antidepressants has not produced the same revolution in attitude as that which occurred with the major tranquilizers (neuroleptics), mainly because endogenous and involutional depression were, in the majority of cases, illnesses which could be relieved in a fairly short time with ECT. However, the development of drug therapy for depression is important for a number of reasons. ECT, although still the most reliable and widely used treatment for depressions, has certain disadvantages: the patients are often fearful of it; there are dangers inherent in the use of an anesthetic prior to its administration; the memory impairment which can occur may be a source of great distress, particularly to professional people; and, even when the treatment is received on an out-patient basis, it involves some absence from work. The administration of drugs instead of ECT, where successful, avoids these disadvantages. The relative indications for convulsive and drug therapy will be discussed later; but, although the drugs can be substituted in some cases where ECT would otherwise have been necessary, they have certainly not completely replaced it as a treatment for depression. They do, however, sometimes produce remission in the type of case which is resistant to ECT, particularly neurotic and certain chronic depressions, often the most difficult to treat. But, while one would welcome the day when all depressions could be treated chemotherapeutically, it has certainly not yet arrived, and one of the most important features of the new anti-depressants is the stimulus that they have given to further investigation into the etiology and psychopathology of depression and into more effective ways of relieving it.

In 1957, Kuhn reported in Switzerland on his first therapeutic attempts in depressive states with an iminodibenzyl derivative, imipramine, which had been developed a few years previously by Häflinger and Schindler. Because of its structural relationship to the phenothiazines, Kuhn had used it first in schizophrenia but with poor results. Then he observed that the compound had a definite effect on depressions. As in the case of chlorpromazine, it was again due to the clinical observations of a psychiatrist that imipramine was introduced, and thereby a new group of psychopharmaca discovered. After the findings of Kuhn had been confirmed by many investigators, chemists and pharmacologists directed and continue to direct their efforts towards the development of new antidepressants. Their point of departure is always the chemistry and pharmacology of imipramine. The iminodibenzyl nucleus in the molecule of imipramine differs from the phenothiazine molecule only in that the sulphur atom of the latter is replaced by a two-carbon chain in the central ring. Thus, imipramine has a seven-member central ring, and thereby differs from the neuroleptically effective phenothiazine derivatives which have a six-member central ring. Later it appeared that also many other tricyclic compounds with antidepressive effect have such seven-member central ring (Bente et al.). Contrary to this, almost all tricyclic neuroleptics have, like the phenothiazines, a six-member central ring.

Main indications for the tricyclic antidepressants are endogenous depressions including involutional melancholia. In the treatment of reactive and neurotic depressions antidepressants are usually only adjuvants. The choice of individual drugs among the increasingly large group of tricyclic antidepressants depends on the symptomatology of an individual patient, whereby the target symptoms of Freyhan play an important role. Kielholz developed an outline for the classification of depressions which is useful for the selection of tricyclic antidepressants according to such target symptoms as depressive mood, psychomotor retardation, and agitation. If psychomotor retardation predominates, those tricyclic antidepressants are indicated which, in their therapeutic action, are closest to the MAO inhibitors (desipramine, nortriptyline, protriptyline). If these drive-increasing antidepressants are given to retarded depressed patients, it should be remembered that the antidepressant effect may set in later than the effect on drive. This may activate suicidal impulses which were not active as long as the retardation persisted. Therefore, these drugs should be used for the initial treatment of severely retarded depressions only under careful clinical observation. The relation between drive and mood is better balanced in drugs like imipramine, monochlorimipramine, noxiptyline, dibenzepin, dimethacrine, melitracene. These tricylic antidepressants can, therefore, readily be used in ambulatory patients. Another important consideration in the use of an antidepressant in ambulatory treatment is how well a drug is subjectively tolerated, i.e. the intensity and frequency of vegetative side-effects.

Imipramine not only influences depressive mood and retardation but also the interference with the feeling of vitality (Vitalgefühle). This disturbance which is so characteristic for endogenous depressions responds well to imipramine and dibenzepin. If a depressive mood is combined with anxiety, restlessness and a feeling of being driven, tricyclic antidepressants like amitriptyline or trimepramine are indicated, as they also are in hypochondriacal depressions. Anxious and agitated depressions sometimes respond well to imipramine and related antidepressants, although these drugs may increase anxiety and intensify agitation. In such syndromes amitriptyline and similar drugs are more promising from the start. In psychotic depressions with a clear-cut depressive delusion treatment with tricyclic antidepressants is only successful when combined with a neuroleptic (see combination with other treatments).

One of the most important requirements for therapeutic success with tricyclic antidepressants is the continuation of a maintenance dose after clinical improvement has been obtained. Azima recommends continuation of maintenance therapy for three months after the improvement has become stabilized. In this way, he obtained excellent results in psychotic depressions, but only half as many improvements in neurotic depressions. There are negative reports, such as one by Lemere, who found that in office practice only 22 out of 137 patients with similar types of depression had benefitted from Tofranil, while H. Strauss reported 80 per cent favorable results in similar material. In general, there seems to be a greater tendency in the European rather than in the

American literature to consider ECT the more reliable method in depressions. However, this trend does not always reflect the actual situation. In our psychiatric wards of general hospitals which emphasize short hospitalizations, ECT is still much more frequently used, because of the time and money saving factor. The suicidal risk and the frequent reluctance of ambulatory patients to accept the numerous though usually harmless side-effects may explain why, in many instances, tricyclic antidepressants are not given a real chance. The favorable figures reflected in most publications on these drugs demonstrate their optimal results and potentialities, while in actual practice other considerations often arise.

Tricyclic Antidepressants

The following drugs belong to the group of tricyclic antidepressants:

1. Imipramine (Tofranil)
2. Desipramine (Pertofrane, Norpramin)
3. Monochlorimipramine (Anafranil)
4. Trimepramine (Surmontil, Stangyl)
5. Amitriptyline (Elavil, Tryptizol, Saroten, Laroxyl)
6. Nortriptyline (Aventyl, Nortrilen, Acetexa)
7. Noxiptyline (Agedal)
8. Protriptyline (Vivactil, Concordin, Maximed)
9. Dibenzepin (Nevoril, Noveril)
10. Opipramol (Ensidon, Insidon)
11. Dimethacrine (Istonil)
12. Melitracene (Trausabun, Dixeran)
13. Iprindole or Pramindole (Tertran, prondol)

Basically, the various tricyclic antidepressants do not differ pharmacologically or clinically from each other. Therefore, their biochemical and pharmacological properties can be discussed together.

Biochemical Effects: The tricyclic antidepressants are not monoamine-oxydase inhibitors. They have no direct effect on the metabolism of the biogenic amines in the CNS, but under their influence there is increased concentration of biogenic amines at the adrenergic receptors in the CNS. This occurs because the tricyclic antidepressants prevent the inactivation through re-uptake of the biogenic amines.

It is possible that in the organism not the tricyclic antidepressants themselves but their N-Desmethyl-compounds (Nor-compounds) are effective. This would explain that various pharmacological effects such as the reserpine antagonism are observed immediately after administration of desipramine, but only after a latency period in the case of imipramine and amitryptiline.

Pharmacological Properties: Some of the properties of the tricyclic antidepressants are similar to those of the phenothiazines. Imipramine was originally characterized as a weak chlorpromazine. Almost all tricyclic antidepressants—with the exception of desipramine—have a sedative effect in high doses, and often lower the body temperature. The centrally sedating effect shows in an inhibition of the spontaneous motility of experimental animals in a potentiation of barbiturate effect and in the antagonism to centrally stimulating substances. However, in low doses imipramine may intensify the effect of amphetamine. Learned behavior is impaired by the tricyclic antidepressants.

A basic difference between tricyclic antidepressants and phenothiazine derivatives is that only the antidepressants counteract the central inhibitory and extrapyramidal motor (cataleptic) effects of reserpine and tetrabenazine. Therefore, the "tetrabenazine reversal" or "reserpine reversal" plays a special role in the pharmacological screening of antidepressants. Furthermore, a characteristic of tricyclic antidepressants is their peripheral and central anticholinergic effect which is most pronounced with amitriptyline. Sigg has postulated that the basis of the action of antidepressants such as imipramine may be an activation of central adrenergic mechanisms by a sensitizing effect on central adrenergic synapses.

The electroencephalographic studies with tricyclic antidepressants are of special interest. Monnier and Krupp demonstrated in electroencephalographic studies that imipramine specifically depresses the reticular formation, evoking a sleep brain wave pattern and preventing EEG alerting; and they compared its action with that of chlorpromazine and reserpine. Chlorpromazine is synergistic with imipramine in preventing EEG alerting, while reserpine antagonizes the depression of the reticular formation produced by imipramine, causing EEG alerting. Van Meter et al. observed that in rabbits large doses of imipramine induce convulsant activity in the amygdala and hippocampus, eventually spreading to the rest of the brain. Fink found that intravenous administration of the drug to patients produced desynchronization and an increase of theta rhythms. This pattern is similar to that found with experimental anticholinergic compounds such as benactyzine, and coincided with behavioral alerting and euphoria.

Clinical Effects: Favorable results have been claimed for all tricyclic antidepressants within the range of 60 to 80 per cent. In one of the earliest investigations on results with imipramine Schneider and Crot in 60 per cent of all types of depression with 40 per cent failures. If a clear line is drawn between endogenous and neurotic or reactive depressions, it appears that the endogenous depressions, with a recovery rate of 74 per cent, show a much better response than the neurotic depressions, with a recovery rate of 52 per cent. The figures of this study, which we chose at random, reflect rather well the results obtained by the majority of workers. The generally better results in hospitalized patients might be explained by the fact that endogenous depressions are more frequently admitted to hospitals than neurotic depressions. It may also be added that unpleasant side effects are more likely to interfere with the willingness of out-patients to continue taking the drug, which could be another explanation for the more favorable results in hospital statistics. All psychiatrists agree that results are best in retarded depressions, while agitated depressions respond poorly or not at all. In many reports it is emphasized that mild or moderately severe endogenous depressions respond best, while severe depressions do better with ECT. Depressions accompanied by much neurotic symptomatology or by hypochondriasis give poor results. Depressive moods in organic cerebral conditions were reported responsive to tricyclic antidepressants by some workers but not by others.

1. *Imipramine (Tofranil)*

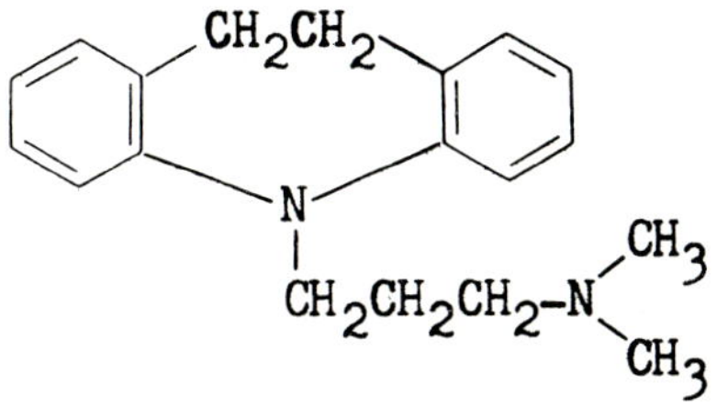

Imipramine (5-(3-Dimethylamino-propyl) - 10,11 - dihydro-5H-dibenz[b, f] azepine) has maintained its place among the antidepressants unchallenged since its clinical efficacy was first described by Kuhn in 1957.

The original findings by Kuhn have been confirmed again and again in subsequent reports. Since imipramine acts primarily on the melancholic dysthymia, it has also been called a thymoleptic. Aside from its mood changing effect, its action consists also in increasing drive and initiative. Therefore, it has a special therapeutic place in retarded depressions. Imipramine is equally effective in endogenous depressions of all types including involutional melancholia. It not only influences depressive mood and loss of drive but also the special characteristic of depression which has been described as "vital sadness." When psychotic depressions are associated with anxiety, the anxiety is reduced by imipramine in some cases. However, the anxiety can also become more intense, and the patient may feel driven by anxiousness or even experience severe agitation.

The majority of the numerous uncontrolled clinical investigations of imipramine as surveyed by Klerman and Cole, came to the conclusion that imipramine leads to favorable results in 60 to 80 per cent of all depressions. Double-blind studies present a similar picture; but they also reveal that placebos alone have already a beneficial effect on one third of all patients with depression.

Most workers report high percentages of what they call improvements or favorable results. Freyhan rightly defines an optimal result as the total disappearance of depressive symptoms which he found only in about one-third of endogenous depressions. Many of these cases had required ECT in previous episodes, and it is beyond doubt that imipramine can qualify as a true therapy for endogenous depressive psychoses. Results are more contradictory in some conditions with associated depressions. Kiloh et al. made a factor analysis on imipramine results. Age over forty, a qualitative difference of subjective experience of depression from normal being depressed, loss of weight, insidious onset, duration of less than a year, and sleep disturbances with early awakening were positively correlated with a good outcome. Self pity, irritability, subjective retardation, inability to concentrate, hypochondriasis, hysterical features and restless sleep make for poor results. Angst demonstrated the importance of genetic factors, blood relatives having identical treatment results. Friedman et al. found imipramine most useful in the treatment of moderately severe endogenous depressions, but of little value in severe depressions. It is less effective in the reactive than in endogenous depressions.

Such differences in outcome explain why therapeutic results largely depend on the composition of the patient material treated, and that various investigators, even in methodologically well planned double-blind studies, reach the conclusion that imipramine is not more effective than a placebo. Thus, Roulet et al. found no clearly identifiable difference between imipramine and placebo, when clinical criteria alone are judged; only some psychological tests revealed a superiority of imipramine over placebo. Bassa and Vora, in a double-blind study, concluded that imipramine is no progress in treatment of depressions. Robin and Langley, in another controlled trial, saw only slight initial superiority of the drug. Such results often neglected variables like patient material and criteria for evaluation. Even though the literature on imipramine includes a relatively large number of double-blind studies with negative results, it is quite apparent that of all the available antidepressants imipramine is one of the most effective ones (Klerman and Cole). The best indications, since the observations by Kuhn, are still the retarded endogenous depressions and involutional melancholia. In ambulatory patients Abraham et al. found imipramine in neurotic depressions equally effective as in endogenous depressions. Comparing ECT and imipramine in a large, carefully planned study, it was found that imipramine was comparable to ECT in results, although the effect of the drug is slower. In some follow-up studies imipramine also came out equal to ECT (Kiloh and Ball).

Therapeutic results with imipramine are less good in patients with a mixed symptomatology. Thus, the presence of paranoid symptoms in depressed patients often leads to a poor response (Hordern et al.). Already Kuhn noticed that the prognosis in depressions was considerably less favorable if they were complicated by schizophrenic features or if the depression was only one symptom in the course of a schizophrenic process. He saw some spectacular results in the relief of catatonic stupors, but in the majority of his schizophrenic cases the drug had no effect at all or the patient became more agitated. In all acute schizophrenics, particularly those in whom hallucinations are prominent, imipramine in our opinion, must be considered as contraindicated in view of the psychiatric complications from the drug. In patients with so-called anergic schizophrenia, Feldman was able to reactivate the patient even in chronic cases. Heinrich believes that this symptom provocation in schizophrenics by imipramine and other antidepressants can be therapeutically utilized. After such provocation of a florid symptomatology, previously treatment-resistant schizophrenics may respond well to subsequent neuroleptic therapy. The diagnostic significance of this symptom provocation is doubtful because also organic depressions can respond to imipramine with schizophreniform symptoms (Helmchen and Hippius). Depressed patients with chronic physical diseases respond well to small doses (Fryer and Timberlake). Physical complaints which are symptoms of a depression, may also clear up (Paulson) as does any type of "latent" depression.

In geriatrics Straker and Roth found imipramine ineffective and thereby confirmed the impression of others that the depressive mood of organic brain disease does not respond to imipramine. However, Schmied and Ziegler obtained very satisfactory results not only in typical depressions of the old age group, these probably being true endogenous depressions occurring in old age rather than depressions in cerebral arteriosclerosis or senile dementia, but also in those with hypochondriacal and neurasthenic complaints. Many patients with quarrelsome and nagging dissatisfaction who were constantly irritated became friendly and sociable and gained a new outlook on life. In patients with reduced physical resistance, mainifestations such as cachexia and decubital ulcers appeared to improve with the increase in their vitality. Staehelin suggests trials with Tofranil combined with psychotherapy in psychosomatic and allergic conditions. Several reports, particularly from the Italian literature (C. Trabucchi et al.), mention that obsessive-compulsive patients were improved. In these cases, according to Geismann and Kammerer, long-term medication with high doses of up to 375 mg. daily, are necessary. Those obsessive-compulsives who are afraid of doing harm to others, respond best (Tellenbach). In patients with episodic agoraphobia who did not respond to neuroleptics and ECT, the attacks subsided under imipramine after 3 to 14 days.

Some rather unexpected results in cases with varying psychopathology are probably explained by the fact that quite different syndromes may be caused by a depression without a depressed mood being recognized. This is true for some recurrent neurotic syndromes and psychosomatic conditions. Kuhn mentions complete cure of an impotence of two years' duration after four weeks of medication, and he emphasizes the great practical significance in many accident cases in which injury had led to obstinate pain and depression. While the therapeutic results in such diversified conditions must be expected to be unreliable, since they depend on many different factors, the anti-depressant effect in endogenous depressions remains the primary indication for Tofranil.

There are a few psychopathological studies all of which show that imipramine is not a stimulant and does not have euphorizing effect per se but rather a sedative effect. It must be assumed that it has a direct effect on the pathophysiological changes believed to be the basis of depression. When Gruenthal gave the drug to normal individauls he found a blunting of emotions without loss of initiative. Schmitt tried to study the psychopathology of this drug by investigations on himself. He did not feel sleepy as after barbiturates but, following a short phase of pleasure relaxation, he noticed a feeling of inner harmony and increased vitality which, however, was not identical with the urge for action felt with the amphetamines. In an attempt to single out those endogenous depressions that respond from those that do not benefit from the drug, he observed that those responding experienced their depression as a physical ailment accompanied by impairment of sleep and appetite. Apparent causal relationships with preceding physical ailments were frequent in these patients. Freyhan speculates that depression represents a variety of psychobiological disturbances with different therapeutic requirements. The degree and the rapidity of the effectiveness of electric convulsive therapy for depressed states remains thus far unchallenged, but in comparison with other anti-depressant drugs, imipramine excels both in its range of therapeutic applicability and its mode of clinical effectiveness.

Imipramine has some indications other than depression. One is enuresis which was first mentioned by McLean whose report was followed by many others. While some investigations were negative (Hicks and Barnes; Abrams), recent double-blind studies proved beyond doubt that imipramine together with psychotherapy and milieu therapy is very useful (Bindeglas et al.; Thomsen et al.; Poussaint and Ditman). The apparent effect of imipramine on the muscles of the bladder has also been used in organic bladder conditions (Epstein and De Quevedo), and by Schunzelaar in the treatment of encopresis. Attempts by Italian authors to use imipramine as an anti-parkinsonian drug (Dobrina; Antonini et al.) were confirmed in other countries. Whittier et al. improved the mood disturbances in patients with Huntington's chorea, but the hyperkinesias became worse. Akimoto et al. used imipramine sucessfully in narcolepsy. Finally, it can be used for intractable pain (Hugues et al.; Daxelmüller) as has also been done with neuroleptics in order to reduce the need for opiates and other analgesics.

MODE OF ADMINISTRATION AND DOSAGE: The drug can be administered orally and by intramuscular injection. Many hospital psychiatrists prefer to start with intramuscular injections, because the drug is excreted rather rapidly—following with oral administration and tapering off the parenteral medication concomitantly. The daily dosage averages between 75 and 250 mg. or more, and should be increased slowly. Clinical results usually become noticeable towards the end of the first week. This makes the drug superior to the monoamine oxidase inhibitors with their slower effect. The danger of suicide in depressions makes an early drug effect imperative. In geriatric patients the dose must be lower, and psychoorganic symptoms suggest caution, when the dosage has to be changed. In enuresis of children under 10 years of age 25 mg., over 10 years 50 mg. are given at bedtime.

2. *Desipramine (Pertofrane, Norpramin)*

Desipramine or desmethylimipramine (5-(3-methylaminopropyl)-10, 11-dihydro-5H-dibenz [b, f] azepine) is the monodesmethyl or nor-compound of imipramine.

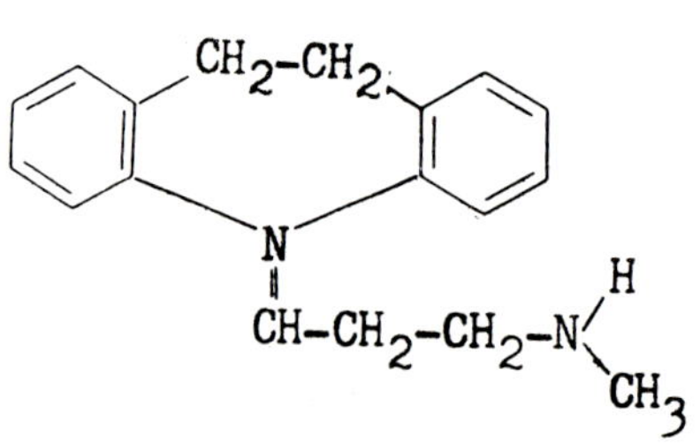

Expectations with regard to this antidepressant were based primarily on theoretical grounds. Salser, Watts and Brodie had shown that desipramine is a metabolite of imipramine in the organism differing from imipramine in the absence of one N-methyl group. Since this monomethyl derivative of imipramine has a quicker action in some experimental tests such as tetrabenezine- and reserpine-reversal than imipramine itself, it was assumed for some time that desipramine is actually responsible for the antidepressive effect of imipramine (Battegay). However, in clinical use the shorter latency in the effect of desipramine in comparison to imipramine could not be conclusively ascertained. Various double-blind studies did not prove differences in the effect of desipramine nor a quicker onset of its action. (Waldron and Bates; Edwards; Rose and Westhead; Hollister).

Overdose and acute poisoning may become dangerous through cardiovascular complications (Bucher and Stucki). Aside from being an antidepressant, desipramine is also used in the treatment of narcolepsy (Hishikawa et al.).

MODE OF ADMINISTRATION AND DOSAGE: All medication ranges between 75 and 200 mg. Parenteral application by intramuscular injection should not surpass 125 mg. daily. In case of sleep disturbances the last desipramine dose is preferably given sometime in the afternoon.

3. *Monochlorimipramine (Anafranil)*

Monochlorimipramine (7-Chlor-5-(3-dimethylaminopropyl)-10, 11-dihydro-5 H-dibenz [b, f] azepine) is the chlorine substituted analogue of imipramine.

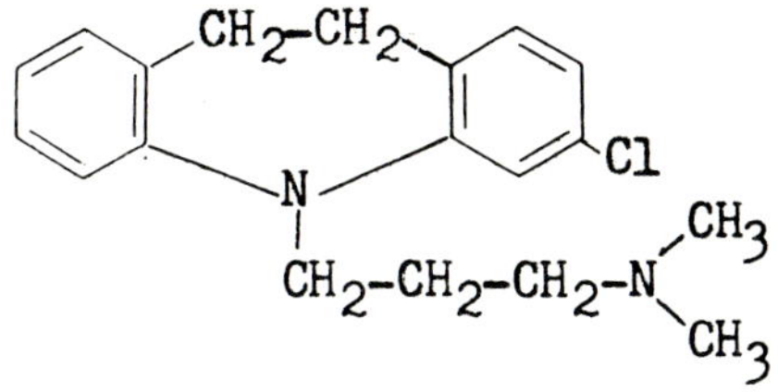

Clinical reports available so far have shown that monochlorimipramine and imipramine are of equal value as antidepressants. A first report was published by Brandner in 1964, and at the World Psychiatric Congress in Madrid in 1966 several studies were presented. A double-blind study by Symes showed that basic differences in the action of the two drugs do not exist. Like desmethylimipramine, also monochlorimipramine was expected to have a stronger action with shorter latency period; but this hope was not fulfilled. Piret et al. emphasize as an advantage that the anxiety-producing effect of monochlorimipramine is minimal.

MODES OF ADMINISTRATION AND DOSAGE: The main reason for the acceptance of monochlorimipramine was that it is particularly recommended for intravenous application by means of drip infusion. In otherwise treatment resistant cases these continuous drips sometimes lead to surprising results which are explained not so much by the superior antidepressant action of the drug but by the faster attack of this mode of application. Monochlorimipramine is given by Cordoba and Lopez-Ibor Jr. in obsessive-compulsive neuroses with isotonic glucose solution in daily doses of 100 to 200 mg. with an additional 100 mg. by intramuscular injection or orally. In general it is sufficient to give 50 to 75 mg. in 250 to 500 ml. as continuous drip within one to three hours. However, doses up to 300 mg. daily have been tried. In cases of mood variations during the day the infusion should be given at the time of the lowest mood. All doses are somewhat lower than with imipramine, usually 50 to 150 mg. daily.

4. *Trimepramine (Surmontil, Stangyl)*

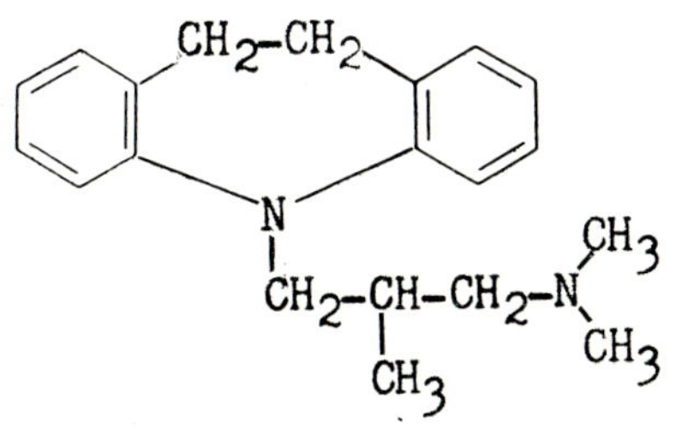

Trimepramine (1-(3-dimethylamino-2 - methylpropyl) - 10,11 - dihydro-5H-dibenz[b,f]-azepine) has, as, for example, laevomepromazine of the phenothiazine group, a branched aliphatic side-chain. It is quite possible that the strong sedative-inhibitory effect of both these drugs is related to this branched side-chain.

Since trimepramine combines an antidepressive action with a sedative effect, this drug has a particularly broad range of indications. Lambert and Guyotat who gave one of the first reports on this drug, point out that, in contrast to imipramine, trimepramine can also be given in anxious depressed patients. This difference in the sedative effect of the two drugs was later confirmed by English authors in controlled studies (Burns; Salzmann).

Tablets of 25 mg. are available for oral use. In severe depressions 400 mg. can be given, and French authors gave up to 600 mg. daily. In ambulatory treatment a 4 per cent solution (one drop contains 1 mg. of the active substance) permits a more individual adaptation of dosage. Trimepramine can also be given by intramuscular injection.

5. *Amitriptyline (Elavil, Tryptizol, Saroten, Laroxyl)*

Amitriptyline is 5-(3-dimethylaminopropylidene)-10,11-dihydro-5H-dibenzo [a,d]cyclopheptadiene.

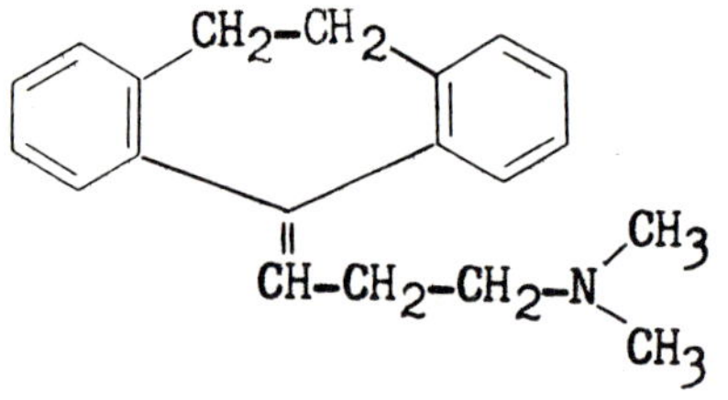

Amitriptyline was introduced four years after imipramine, and they are the two most widely used antidepressants. Contrary to imipramine, amitriptyline does not augment drive but is rather a sedating, calming antidepressant. Therefore, it has a broader spectrum of application than imipramine.

Already the first investigators in 1960 found amitriptyline more reliable than imipramine in anxious and depressed patients (Dorfman), and Ayd emphasized its good tolerability. The subjectively unpleasant vegetative side-effects of imipramine are less intense and less frequent with amitriptyline. At a symposium in 1961, Ayd, comparing amitriptyline, imipramine and three MAO inhibitors, found the two tricyclic antidepressants definitely more effective and better tolerated than the MAO inhibitors. Barsa and Saunders prefer amitriptyline to imipramine in depressive syndromes of schizophrenics because it is less apt to activate schizophrenic symptoms than imipramine and the MAO inhibitors. It was seen early that agitated depressions which had not, or even unfavorably responded to imipramine and the MAO inhibitors, benefited the most (Arnold and Foitl). Angst, comparing amitriptyline and imipramine, found amitriptyline significantly superior to imipramine in agitated depressions, while amitriptylne was significantly inferior in retarded depressions. In hypochondriacal depressions both drugs show identical results. Bente et al. found the effect of amitryptyline on anxiety and restlessness related to its sedative side-effects, and the effect on other symptoms of depression related to the vegetative side-effects. The superiority of amitriptyline in agitated depressions was confirmed in double-blind studies by Skarbek and Smedberg. In placebo studies Hollister et al. gave the placebo group atropine so that the amitriptyline group should not recognize the amitriptyline from its atropine-like side-effects like dry mouth. They claim that amitriptyline contrary to imipramine, is also effective in depressive guilt feelings. Some authors like

Browne et al. concluded that amitriptyline is also valuable in reactive depressions. In a very well planned investigation Hordern et al. judged amitripyline to be the presently best antidepressant, and limit the use of ECT to delusional depressions. However, amitriptyline must be taken for at least six months, and maintenance doses reduce the relapse rate even more than ECT. In a similar comparative study between amitriptyline and imipramine Sandifer et al. explain Hordern's contention of a superiority of amitriptyline with too low doses of imipramine and with the inclusion of older patients with depressive delusions. In the latter group of patients Hoenig and Visram also found amitriptyline superior to imipramine. They as well as Snow and Rickels emphasized that amitriptyline acts faster. The usefulness of small doses in senile depressions between 72 and 94 years of age was demonstrated by Hader and Madonick.

Comparisons between amitriptyline and ECT remained contradictory. L. Rees and Davies found ECT clearly superior. A control study by McDonald et al. using four groups of patients, found amitriptyline and ECT superior to simulated ECT and placebo. It might be mentioned that the drug effect is not dependent on an intact anterior hypophysis-adrenal regulation; therefore, patients with adrenalectomy can be treated with amitriptyline, and ECT be avoided (Rudberg-Lindquist and Lindquist), although the osteoporosis of such patients is actually no longer a contraindication to ECT.

In chronic depressions Skarbek saw that amitriptyline can also be useful, and Gerry and Leonard had good results in one third of a group of chronic depressives who had been unresponsive to ECT. In these chronic patients the results must be stabilized by continuous medication. Ayd found long-term medication with amitriptyline particularly indicated in chronic depressions with obsessional personality or with marked obsessive symptoms, while patients with cyclothymic or hypomanic features in their basic personality did not react so well. In long-term therapy the hypnotic effect of amitriptyline is often disturbing, although, according to Ayd, this side-effect becomes more apparent only when the patient has already recovered from his depression.

In patients who are depressed as reaction to a hopeless physical disease like hemiplegics with aphasia, amitriptyline was found to be very helpful (Pressman and Weiss). In child psychiatry Poussaint et al. used amitriptyline for enuresis in the same way as imipramine.

Mode of Administration and Dosage: Ambulatory patients receive slowly increasing amounts of 50 to 200 mg. daily. In hospital patients 300 mg. can be given. The optimal dose for maintenance therapy is 70 to 100 mg. (Ayd). Acute conditions can be handled with intramuscular injection (Dorfman). In older patients low doses are preferred (30 to 100 mg.). Side-effects are avoided by slow increase and slow discontinuation of the drug. If a sleep-producing effect is wanted, the entire daily dose can be given in the evening, or 100 mg. injected intramuscularly.

6. *Nortriptyline (Aventyl, Allegron, Nortrilen, Acetexa)*

Nortriptyline is 5-(3-methylaminopropylidene)-10,11-dihydro-5H-dibenzo [a,d]cycloheptene.

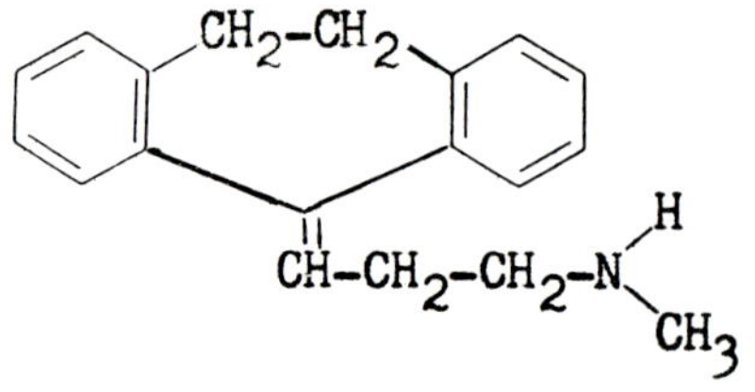

In analogy to the corresponding iminodibenzyl-compounds desipramine and imipramine, it was to be expected that nortriptyline compared to amitriptyline is superior in increasing drive and initiative. Clinically this was confirmed, giving nortriptyline an intermediate position between amitriptyline and imipramine (Ropert and Berges; Kielholz). First reports suggested that nortriptyline, aside from being an antidepressant, can also be used as a minor tranquilizer (Bennett). Geriatric patients and those with psychosmatic disorders responded well. So did hostile, paranoid, irascible, anxious and tense individuals. Apathetic chronic psychotics became activated (Barron et al.). The anxiolytic effect of nortriptyline was confirmed by Hughes and Forney in psychological experiments. Anxiety and disturbances of performance after delayed audiofeedback were diminished after nortriptyline. On the other hand, like other activating antidepressants, this drug may intensify anxiety in depressed patients (Petrilowitsch). There is still some contradiction in reports on nortriptyline. In one of the few controlled studies Chestrow et al. found it effective in anxiety, apathy, depression, irritability and hostility. It was particularly valuable for the relief of the depressive component in anxiety states. Leahy and Martin comparing nortriptyline with amitriptyline and using the Hamilton Rating-Scale, did not find a difference between the two drugs. In treatment-resistant psychotic children Kurtis found nortriptyline helpful for hyperactivity, aggressiveness, destructiveness, depression and autism, whereby also urinary and fecal incontinence were favorably affected. In disturbed mentally retarded patients nortriptyline had an antidepressant and tranquilizing effect which was not superior to sodium pentobarbital or chlorpromazine (Carter). The anxiolytic effect of nortriptyline was used by Seid in anxious patients before urological interventions.

MODE OF ADMINISTRATION AND DOSAGE: Nortriptyline can be administered orally and parenterally in doses of 30 to 250 mg. daily. In ambulatory patients 30 to 75 mg. are recommended if it is used as a minor tranquilizer with antidepressive effect. In parenteral application side-effects are particularly negligible (Lang).

7. *Noxiptyline (Agedal)*

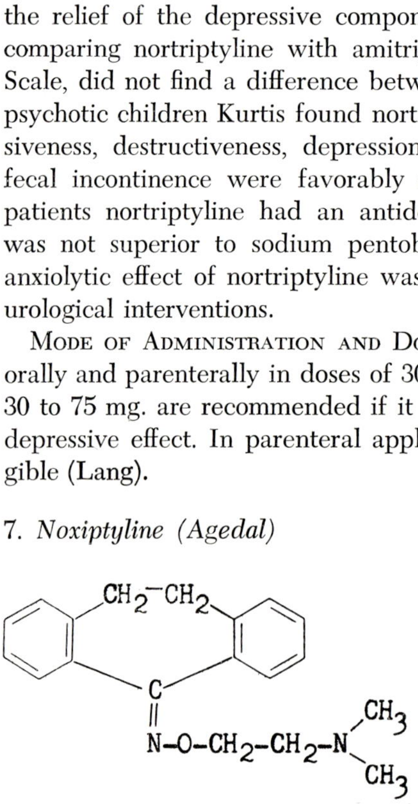

Noxiptyline (- 5 - Dimethylaminoaethyl-oxyimino 5H-dibenzo a,d cyklohepta-1,4-dien hydrochloride), used mostly in Germany, is an antidepressant with the advantages of a broad range of indications and good tolerability (Bente et al.; Himwich et al.). It has a less hypnotic effect than amitriptyline and a less central-anticholinergic effect than imipramine, amitriptyline and trimepramine.

Mode of Administration and Dosage: In the beginning parenteral use is recommended (three injections of 50 mg.); oral dose ranges between 150 and 450 mg. daily.

8. *Protriptyline (Vivactil, Triptil, Concordin, Maximed)*

Protriptyline is 5-(3-methylaminopropyl)-5H-dibenzo[a,d]cycloheptene.

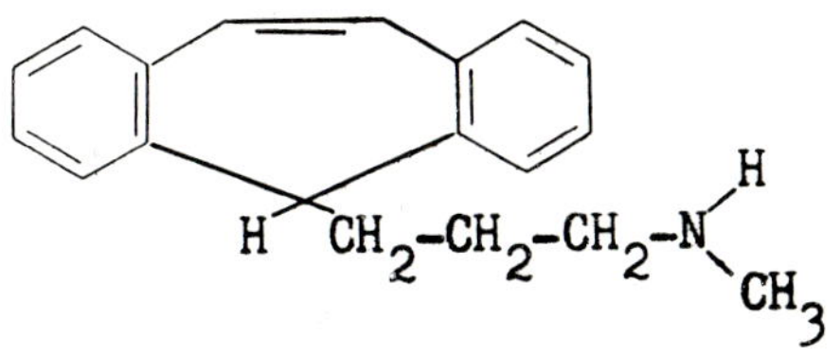

Like all N-demethylized tricyclic psychopharmaca, protriptyline is an activating antidepressant and, therefore better suited for retarded than for agitated depressions (Angst and Pöldinger). It is a fast acting antidepressant (Arnold and Kryspin-Exner; Straker et al.). Opinions differ regarding its tolerability. Goldman saw minimal side-effects, while Arnold emphasizes that because of pronounced side-effects like restlessness, sleep disturbances and tachycardia protriptyline should be started in the hospital and only after adaptation of the organism, continued on an ambulatory basis. Feldman uses the activating effect of protriptyline for the treatment of anergic schizophrenics. If in depressions the activating effect is too intense, particularly in the presence of anxiety, combination with a minor tranquilizer is recommended (Krakowski). In a double-blind study by Brick et al. who compared protriptyline and amitriptyline in anxiety and depressions, the target symptom "depressed" favored protriptyline; but if anxiety and restlessness were present, a tranquilizer had to be added.

Senile depressions, according to Ambrozi and Birkmayer, responded well to small doses because, contrary to amitriptyline, there is no tiredness, and the activating effect is beneficial in these patients. Lack of drive in the morning suggests that the total daily dose be given in the morning. Vaisberg also sees the main indication of protriptyline in old age depressions, and Rickels et al. found in a control study on neurotic depressions that the older age group did best.

Mode of Administration and Dosage: Protriptyline is available only for oral medication. The dosis is lower than for other antidepressants. In moderate depressions 10 to 25 mg. and in severe depressions 60 mg. are recommended. In geriatric patients 20 mg. should be the maximum. An experimental injectable protriptyline has a hypnotic effect, quite contrary to the activating effect of the orally given drug.

9. *Dibenzepine (Nevoril, Noveril)*

Dibenzepine (5-methyl-10-β-dimethylamino-ethyl-10, 11-dihydro-11 oxo 5-dibenzo [b, e] [1,4]-diazepin) was readily accepted in Switzerland and Germany as a well tolerated antidepressant. Compared to imipramine, it gives fewer vegetative symptoms and, thus fewer subjective side-effects. Dibenzepine also has a far less sedative effect than amitriptyline (Bente et al.). Also there are fewer anticholinergic side-effects. The comparatively few side-effects makes this drug suitable for ambulatory treatment of depressions (Angst and Kind)

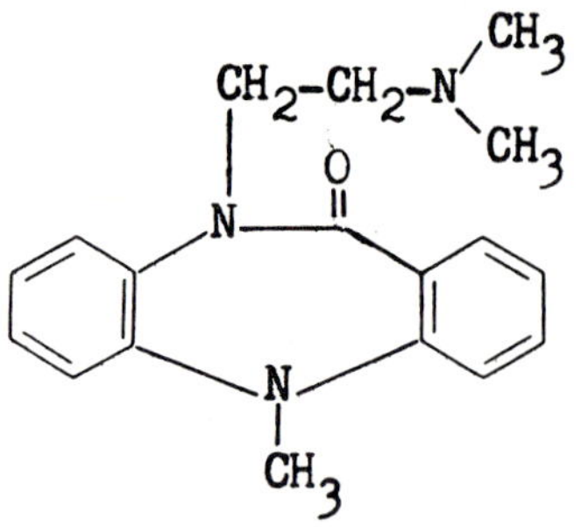

and for geriatric patients with organic depressive states (Baron). Its therapeutic action resembles that of imipramine but has a lesser drive inducing effect.

MODE OF ADMINISTRATION AND DOSAGE: The dosage must be higher than in all other tricyclic antidepressants. Oral medication is started with 160 to 200 mg. daily and, according to the severity of depression, can be increased to 320 or 640 mg. daily. After improvement sets in, the dose can be reduced to 120 to 360 mg. which is recommended as maintenance dose for several weeks or months after disappearance of the depressive symptoms.

10. *Opipramol (Ensidon, Insidon)*

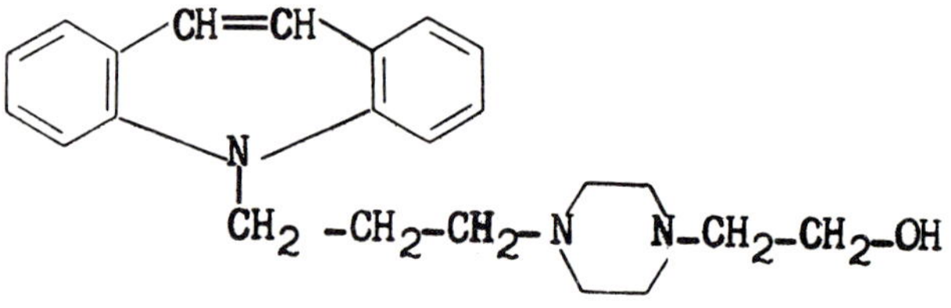

Opipramol, 4-[3-(5H-dibenz[b,f]azepine-5-yl)propyl]-piperazine-ethanol, occupies chemically a middle position among tricyclic psychopharmaca. As an iminostilbene derivative, it is related to imipramine and also to protriptyline, while the side chain corresponds to that of perphenazine. Also, clinically, opipramol has a position between several groups of psychotropic drugs, and simplifying one could call it "a minor tranquilizer with antidepressive properties" (Pöldinger). Because of its relationship to imipramine Azima et al. and Kristof et al. first studied its antidepressant effect which turned out to be inferior to that of imipramine (Kiloh et al.). However, it was superior to imipramine in anxious neurotic depressions because of its stronger sedative effect (Schmitt et al.; Angst). Since it was well tolerated, it was recommended in ambulatory patients. A joint study by 21 general practitioners defined as its best indications non-psychotic dysthymias, anxiety, vegetative symptoms and menopausal complaints (Junkenitz and Schäffer). Restlessness, tension and anxiety respond first, followed by mood elevation and stabilization of vegetative regulatory functions. Animal experiments indicate that these effects are due to a strong inhibition of limbic structures related to regulation of such autonomic functions as ACTH secretion and intestinal motility (Hernandez-Peon and Naranjo). Opipramol being more a minor tranquilizer than an antidepressant, it was compared by Grosser and Ryan in a double-blind cross over study with another minor tranquilizer, chlordiazepoxide. They found the two drugs equally effective in nonpsychotic anxiety and thereby confirmed earlier results by Gradwell.

Mode of Administration and Dosage: An average oral dosis of 150 mg. daily was augmented by some up to 300 mg. daily. The initial hypnotic effect can be kept at a minimum by starting with 50 mg. in the evening and increasing slowly.

11. *Dimethacrine (Istonil)*

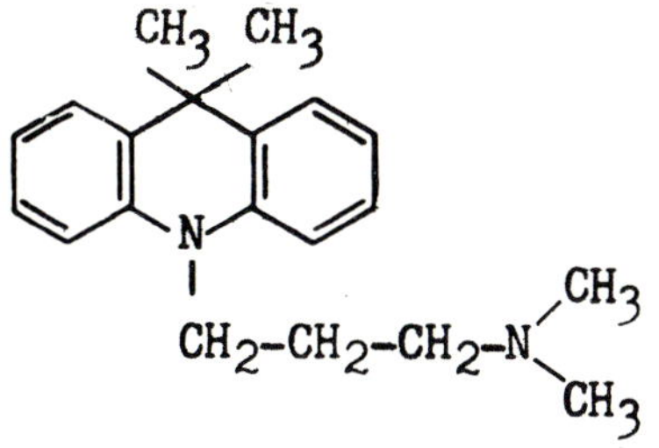

Dimethacrine (9,9 dimethyl-10-dimethylaminopropyl-acridan) like melitracene represents a group of tricyclic antidepressants which, contrary to imipramine, amitryptiline and all other tricylic antidepressants has a six-member central ring in its molecule.

It appears from the few available clinical reports that pharmacological action and treatment results are similar to those of imipramine (Taen and Pöldinger). No control studies have yet been made, but it seems that the therapeutic effect sets in within three days, when used intramuscularly or intravenously (50 mg. three times daily), according to Gut and Hoffmann.

The oral dosis is between 50 and 200 mg.

12. *Melitracene (Dixeran, Trausabun)*

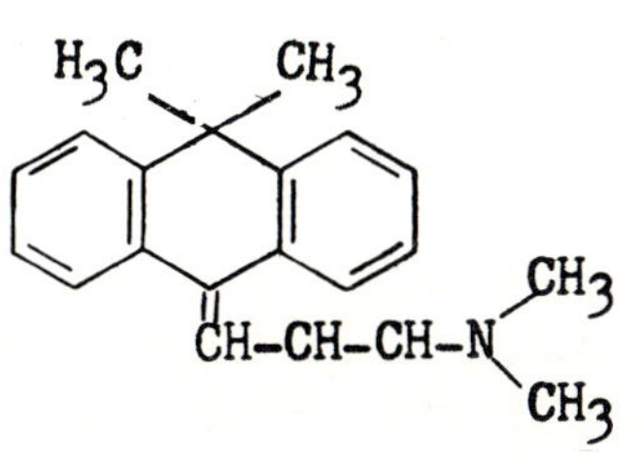

Melitracene (9-(3-dimethylaminopropyliden)-10, 10-dimethyl-9, 10-dihydroanthracene), a diphenylamine-derivative, is the chemical analogue to the diphenylamine-derivative dimethacrine. The two pharmaca are related in the same way as chlorprothixene and chlorpromazine in the neuroleptic group.

The therapeutic effects resemble those of other tricyclic antidepressants. While, within limits, the antidepressant effect does not depend on the dosage, low dosage is more antidepressant and activating, and larger dosage more drive-attenuating and sedative. Therefore, low doses are useful in retarded depressions, while larger doses are effective in agitated depressions (Bente et al.; Glatzel). Melitracene had been introduced because of its broad spectrum and the low frequency of side-effects which make it useful in ambulatory treatment, particularly in geriatric patients.

Mode of Administration and Dosage in retarded depressions and geriatric patients is 30 to 50 mg. daily; in agitated depressions up to 200 mg. daily. The effect can be accelerated by beginning with injections (40 to 60 mg. daily). It is better tolerated, when started with low doses and slowly stepped up.

13. *Iprindole or Pramindole*

Iprindole or pramindole is a tricyclic pharmaca with an indole structure (5-(3-dimethylaminopropyl) - 6,7,8,9,10,11-hexahydro - 5H - cyclooct-(β) indole). Although its chemical structure deviates widely from other tricyclic antidepressants, such cholinergic side-effects as visual disturbances, dryness of the mouth and constipation are rare. Therefore, it is well tolerated by geriatric patients. Its efficacy was proven in double-blind studies with placebo (Daneman) and imipramine (El-Deiry et al.). The dosage is lower than for imipramine (60 to 120 mg.).

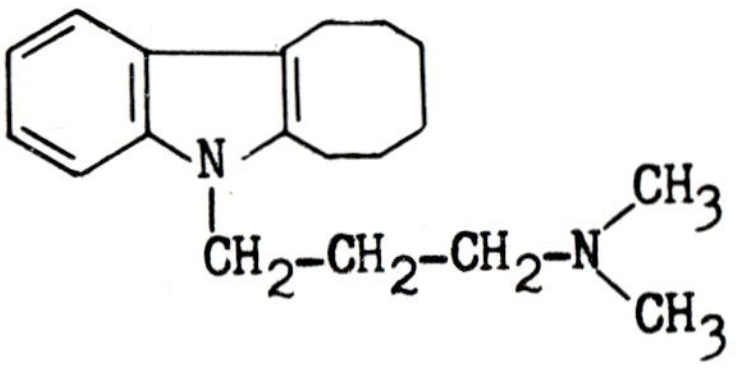

Side-Effects and Complications of Tricyclic Antidepressants

The side-effects of tricyclic antidepressants do not differ in principle from those of the tricyclic neuroleptics. Contrary to the neuroleptics vegetative side-effects predominate. There are differences within the group, e.g. imipramine having primarily vegetative side-effects, while amitriptyline has more anticholinergic effects such as dryness of the mouth. Also intensity and frequency differ e.g. dibenzepin has comparatively few side-effects. Basically they are so similar that, like those of the neuroleptics, they can be discussed together for the whole group of tricyclic antidepressants.

Disturbances of Somatic Functions

1. Vegetative Side-Effects: The signs of vegetative irritation are identical with those already described for the neuroleptics. However, while the neuroleptics produce more parasympathicotonic phenomena, antidepressants in low doses affect more sympathicotonic functions (Hollister; Wagensommer; Kähler). As demonstrated in animal studies, this is due to the characteristic anticholinergic and noradrenaline-potentiating effect of the antidepressants (Klerman and Cole). Dry mouth, disturbances of accommodation, tachycardia, constipation, urinary difficulties, perspiration and occasionally a fine vegetative tremor usually become less troublesome after some weeks of treatment. These vegetative side-effects are mostly harmless but uncomfortable for the patient who may refuse to continue the medication.

Circulatory effects, although less pronounced than with neuroleptics of the chlorpromazine type, can affect the treatment considerably. Orthostatic hypotension may lead to collapse, when the patient gets up from his bed, particularly in older patients and those with hypertension. Subjectively, unpleasant tachycardia may occur with and without blood pressure changes. Palpitations can be due to tachycardia but also due to drug-induced auricular fibrillations (Morehead and Knox). Occasionally, blood pressure rises occur. Severe hypertensive crises on the one hand, and collapse on the other hand, have been observed, when a tricyclic antidepressant was preceded by a MAO inhibitor. Harrer et al. demonstrated the effect of antidepressants on blood pressure regulation by showing how antidepressant medication affects the cardiovascular reactions to noradrenaline and sympatol. The gradual blood pressure rising effect during the first week of treatment is followed by a decrese which may lead to a paradoxical effect. Therefore, one cannot postulate a general incompatability of tricyclic antidepressants with MAO inhibitors. Gradual increase of the tricyclic antidepressants does permit combination with MAO inhibitors. Like Sargant, Horwitz combined MAO inhibitors and tricyclic drugs, particularly tranylcypromine and amitriptyline without ill effects.

Postural hypotension as parasympathetic, and hypertensive spells as sympathetic overreaction are autonomic responses which Horwitz did not look upon merely as side-effects but as indications of the drug action. He considered the three "side-effects" of postural hypotension, urinary hesitancy and visual blurring as the physiological responses which most closely parallel clinical improvement. If they do not occur, he felt that the particular drug is not active for that patient at that time which applies particularly to chronic depressed patients who were the main subject of Horwitz' study. In the responsive patient the mood improves as the signs of autonomic drug activity appear, or within several days thereafter. He measured blood pressure in the lying, sitting and standing position before and throughout the treatment period. The more chronic the patient, the higher the homeostasis must be. He also found that most patients do not respond to the same drug in a subsequent episode but may respond to another drug, or have to receive ECT which then again may be followed by drugs. The hypotensive effect can be increased by diuretics, whereby in older patients precautions against falling are necessary. According to Cornu, sudden falls due to weak spells without unconsciousness are not caused by change in blood pressure.

Special attention was recently given to cardiac effects of the tricyclic antidepressants. They are identical to those described for the phenothiazines. Imipramine and amitriptyline produce these changes in the electrocardiogram with particular regularity (Lehmann and Ban). Although not studied systematically in other antidepressants, isolated observations suggest their occurrence also in other antidepressants, like desipramine. The cardiac effects of antidepressants can be reproduced in animal experiments (Evreux). The changes such as arrhythmias and widening of the QRS complex with S-T shift are so typical that in unidentified intoxications the EKG changes permit the diagnosis of poisoning by tricyclic antidepressants (Barnes et al.).

Gastro-intestinal symptoms such as constipation are often noted. Diarrhea, lack of appetite, nausea and vomiting occur (Wagensommer). Paralytic ileus is rare.

Urinary disturbances, are pollakiuria, difficulty to urinate and even complete urinary retention (Childers). These incidents are especially frequent in older men with hypertrophy of the prostate gland, when the bladder is distended during sleep. Secondary complications like urinary tract infection (Johnson and Boucher) require proper medication or catheterization.

Dryness of the mouth is more frequent than in neuroleptics because the antidepressants have a stronger parasympathicolytic effect. Some authors consider absence of a dry mouth prognostically equally unfavorable as Horwitz assumed for the absence of circulatory reactions. Dryness of the mouth is sometimes accompanied by intense thirst, unpleasant taste and a coated or black tongue. It can also lead to small ulcerations of the mucous membranes and, in rare cases, even to stomatomycosis (Dally).

Visual disturbances: Blurred vision and disturbance of accommodation are a frequent anticholinergic effect which contraindicates these antidepressants in patients with glaucoma. Sometimes glaucoma manifests itself for the first time under antidepressant medication (Hordern et al.).

2. Endocrinological Side-Effects: They also largely correspond to those described for the neuroleptics. Thus, Klein et al. saw galactorrhea, and Greenberg erection without ejaculation during treatment with imipramine in 5 per cent of male patients usually after three weeks of medication, at a time when vegetative side-effects diminish. Gain of weight after long-term medication, parallel to that seen in the neuroleptics, is also seen in the antidepressants, more often with amitriptyline than with imipramine (Arenillas). Antidepressants do not seem to affect function of the pancreas. In diabetes Kaplan et al. noted a decrease of glycosuria in mildly diabetic patients.

3. Hemopoietic Side-Effects: They also do not differ essentially from those of the tricyclic neuroleptics. Blood changes like leucopenia were noticed after several months of medication by Denmark. The differential blood count often shows eosinophilia, occasionally up to 60 or 80 per cent (Wilson et al.; Joynt and Clancy). Agranulocytosis may also occur (Anatko et al.; Rothenberg and Hall; Gault), as well as aplastic anemia (personal communication by R. Abrams).

4. Disturbances of Liver Function: Jaundice, disappearing after withdrawal of the drug, has been reported in isolated cases by Lehmann and Kuhn and by Hoaken. If these reports mostly concern imipramine, this is explained by the fact that it is the drug used for the longest time (Hollister). Recently identical observations were made with amitriptyline (Biagi and Bapat; Cunningham).

5. Dermatological Side-Effects: Allergic skin manifestations due to imipramine are relatively frequent and consist of pruritus, urticaria, erythemas which may be generalized (Kähler). Amitriptyline and related drugs lead rarely to allergic skin conditions. Photosensitivity does not seem to occur (Degkwitz).

6. Neurological Side-Effects: Tremor is frequent after larger doses, especially of imipramine and other antidepressants of the imipramine type. There is no evidence that this tremor is a beginning Parkinson syndrome. Imipramine seems to have rather an anti-parkinsonian action, and only in very high doses it may aggravate a preexisting Parkinsonism. In lower doses Sigwald et al. established that akinesia which, contrary to rigidity and tremor, is not relieved by anti-parkinsonian drugs or surgery, responds remarkably well to imipramine and related compounds.

Paresthesias, both visceral and peripheral, which the patients describe as burning sensations substernally and in forearms and hands, occur early in the treatment. Disturbances of coordination and muscular weakness may contribute to the sudden falls with possible fractures (Foster and Lancaster). Combination with dampening drugs like chlorpromazine can lead to various neurological symptoms (Kane and Taylor).

An important complication of antidepressant therapy are convulsions, usually only after high doses (Leon). Convulsions seem to be more frequent due to antidepressants than to neuroleptics. Harrer explains the lower convulsive threshold with fluid retention due to the antidiuretic effect of imipramine. Kiloh et al. confirmed the epileptogenic effect of imipramine by means of EEG studies. Convulsions were also seen with amitriptyline either in the beginning of medication, or when the dosis is increased (Betts et al.). Davison even used amitriptyline, 30 mg. intravenously to elicit EEG changes for the diagnosis of epilepsy. While in epileptics paroxysmal activity in the EEG was precipitated or aggravated, depressed patients showed only unspecific changes.

Psychiatric Side-Effects

Psychiatric complications during antidepressive medication are more frequent than with neuroleptics but have the same characteristics. Therefore, the psychiatric side-effects of all tricyclic psychopharmaca have been dealt with together in some surveys (Helmchen and Hippius). Like the neuroleptics, the antidepressants may lead to disturbances of vigilance which are due to an effect on sleep regulation. Amitriptyline and trimepramine have a sedative-hyponotic effect similar to that of the neuroleptics. Also, patients on imipramine, during the first days of treatment, may sleep a lot. Later, the sedative effect recedes, but may persist with amitriptyline for a longer time. Antidepressants of the imipramine type like desipramine as well as protriptyline may cause sleep disturbances and even complete insomnia which is often associated with restlessness.

Hypomanic and manic states may manifest themselves during antidepressive medication (Schorer). It is difficult to decide whether they are a direct effect of the drug, or the change from a depressive to a manic episode as seen in spontaneous remissions as well as after other treatment for depressions like ECT. The swings to manic states are more frequent after drugs than after ECT, probably because ECT also affects manic states. The probability that such a manic state is due to the antidepressant drug as such, is greater when the patient has had several previous episodes with purely depressive symptomatology (Helmchen and Hippius). Some patients experience acute anxiety and panic states which may be premonitory signs of a developing delirious or confusional state.

Paranoid-hallucinatory pictures or merely some paranoid symptoms may also be caused by the drugs themselves. These long known schizophrenia-like syndromes during antidepressive medication, were first considered as activation of a latent schizophrenia. They even were interpreted as differential diagnostic evidence that such patients were actually schizophrenics. This "symptom provocation" (Heinrich; Newman and Fisher) is, however, nosologically unspecific because any symptomatic psychosis characterized by depression, may be changed by drugs to a schizophrenia-like syndrome. This occurs particularly in such acute brain syndromes as encephalitis, while depressive symptomatology in slowly progressing brain damage like cerebral atrophy can be treated quite successfully with small doses of antidepressants without producing schizophrenia-like symptoms.

While delusional hallucinatory syndromes frequently leave the question open whether they are drug effect or activation of the basic disease, visual hallucinations are almost always side-effects of the medication (Klein). Sometimes such hallucinations are of the hypnagogic type and connected with dream activation which is particularly frequent in antidepressants (Kramer et al.; Whitman et al.).

The most striking psychiatric complications are deliria and confusional states which are much more frequent with antidepressants than with neuroleptics. This is probably due to the more intense central anticholinergic action of the antidepressants. Also the degree of sedative-hypnotic effects which change with the different antidepressants has an influence on the frequency of pharmacogenic deliria. Therefore, they are more frequent (approximately 8 per cent) with amitriptyline than with imipramine and newer antidepressants like dibenzepin and melitracene, where they occur in approximately 2.5 per cent of the cases (Helmchen and Hippius). Immediately after a delirium abates, the depressive symptomatology may show an impressive improvement. These observations led to attempts to produce deliria as a method of treatment for depressions (Grahmann and Peters). This had already been done with ditran, but since any pharmacogenic delirium is difficult to control and may even have a fatal outcome, such methods are not advisable. In predisposed persons like older patients with cerebral damage or a history of pharmacogenic or alcohol deliria, the manfestations of a delirium may be prevented prior to antidepressant medication by giving dihydroergotamine (Bauer).

Overdosage

It was to be expected that antidepressants would often be used for suicidal purposes because the suicidal, depressed patient frequently uses the last drug prescribed for him by his physician. Therefore, most cases of overdosage were suicidal attempts. Other recent cases were unintended intoxication in children.

Most reports are on imipramine and amitriptyline as the two most widely used antidepressants. Observations on opipramol poisoning were reported by Angst et al., and on desipramine by Bucher and Stucki. The clinical picture is similar for all these tricyclic antidepressants.

Fatalities due to imipramine were reported in adults by Loo et al. after intake of 2500 mg., and in an eighteen month old child after 575 mg. by Thiemann et al. Fatalities due to amitriptyline were seen by Davies and Allaye in a 70 year old woman after 950 mg., by Im Obersteg and Bäumler in a 25 year old man after 1250 or 2500 mg. and by Sunshine and Yaffe in a 15 month old child after 1250 mg. In view of the relatively large therapeutic latitude of antidepressants the outcome is usually not fatal. A patient of Foster and Lancaster who took 1500 mg. of imipramine had no discomfort for 45 minutes and then fell asleep. He woke up with involuntary movements of the extremities and head with inability to articulate words. His sensorium was clear and after an hour the movements were superseded by paresthesias which persisted for another hour. Tremor, over-alertness, and tachycardia lasted for three days. The depression was not influenced and he was later cured with ECT. Tremor and paresthesias seem to be the most frequent symptoms of overdosage. A patient of Broke and Weatherly who took 800 mg. developed an anxiety state, myoclonic movements, and finally a grand mal convulsion. Convulsions were also seen by Delay et al. in two cases, one of whom developed a status epilepticus. Both these patients had received more than 350 mg. of imipramine. Severe intoxication leads to anuria, mydriasis, myoclonic movements, reflex changes, convulsions, cyanosis, hypotension, cardiac complications with EEG changes, and finally also to coma (Longmire and Davis; Scharfetter).

Monoamine Oxidase Inhibitors

At the same time as imipramine was introduced as the first tricyclic antidepressant, the first promising reports on the antidepressive effect of the monoamine oxidase inhibitor (MAO) iproniazid were published. Iproniazid was a step beyond the tuberculosis drug isoniazid and, like this, was also originally used for the treatment of tuberculosis. During the treatment of tubercular patients with these two hydrazine derivatives of the isonicotinic acid it had been noticed that they induced euphoria, greater initiative and increased appetite. Therefore, they were tried in psychiatric patients, first in anergic schizophrenics and later in depressed patients (Loomer et al.; Crane). The therapeutic results were promising and aroused special interest in connection with the pharmacological properties of iproniazid. Zeller had already found in 1952 that iproniazid has an inhibitory effect on the enzyme monoamine oxidase. Based on the hypothesis that the therapeutic action of iproniazid in depressions is due to the inhibition of monoamine oxidase, extensive studies on the MAO inhibitors were undertaken. One of the goals of these investigations was to find new antidepressants, particularly when iproniazid proved to be too toxic for practical use. The second goal of this research was the clarification of the biochemical cause of depressive mood. Even though original hypotheses regarding the MAO inhibitors later turned out to be erroneous in many respects, the research impulses originating from the MAO inhibitors led to a thorough study of the role of the biogenic monoamines in the central nervous system for the causation of depression. Today, the MAO inhibitors are therapeutically less important than the tricyclic antidepressants, but their theoretical interest remains unchanged. It is strange that in the area of the neuroleptics reserpine, and in the area of the antidepressants iproniazid gave the decisive theoretical impulses for erroneous hypotheses on drugs which today play a minimal role in practical therapy.

Biochemical, Physiological and Pharmacological Properties: Substrate of the monoamine oxidase are numerous physiologically significant amines for which different relative metabolic rates have been found (Pletscher et al.): Dopamine, tryamine, 3-methoxytyramine, tryptamine, 5-oxyhydrtryptamine, noradrenaline, adrenaline and many others. In most investigations about the action of the MAO inhibitors most attention was paid to 5-oxyhydrtryptamine (serotonin) and the two catecholamines noradrenaline (norepinephrine) and dopamine. We refer to Ajuriaguerra, symposium on monoamines and central nervous system in Geneva 1961.

It has been observed experimentally that the administration of reserpine releases both serotonin and catecholamines from the brain. The level of these brain amines falls and depression is induced, the brain amines level being found to correlate with the behavioral changes observed.

However, if certain drugs, such as iproniazid, are given prior to reserpine, there is apparently a blockage of the enzyme monoamine oxidase which normally destroys the amines. Therefore, although they are still released, they cannot be broken down; and, instead of depression, marked excitation ensues with no change in the total amine level in the brain. However, when iproniazid is given after reserpine, the normal action of the latter is exerted before the enzyme can be blocked; and so the brain amines fall.

The monoamine oxidase inhibitors raise the brain levels of amines when administered alone (Pletscher). A correlation has been found for several of them between the rise in the norepinephrine level and the development of psychomotor activity.

In addition to effects on the central nervous system the MAO inhibitors possess cardiovascular actions (Biel et al.). They are hypotensive agents and relieve the pain of angina pectoris. Zbinden et al. have discussed the theories of the mode of production of this effect. The ideas postulated include a central psychostimulation raising the pain threshold, coronary artery dilatation, which, although demonstrated experimentally, is unlikely because the drugs are more efficacious in advanced arteriosclerosis, ganglionic blockade, analgesic activity (the drugs have analgesic effects similar in strength to codeine), or a direct oxygen sparing effect on the myocardium. It has also been suggested that coronary dilatation may be brought about by the blood serotonin, the level of which is raised by the MAO inhibitors, or that there is decreased norepinephrine sensitivity due to an inhibition of catecholamine release.

In pharmacological tests three main actions of MAO inhibition can be demonstrated: First, increase of biogenic endogenous amines; second, counteraction of reserpine or tetrabenazine-induced depletion of amines; third, potentiation of actions of exogenous amines and their precursors. These biochemical effects are the basis for all known pharmacological and physiological actions (Pscheidt). They characterize both the group of hydrazine MAO inhibitors, and the group of nonhydrazine MAO inhibitors (Biel et al.; Zirkle and Kaiser).

Nonhydrazine derivatives are:

1. Iproniazid (Marsilid)
2. Pheniprazine (Catron, Catroniazid)
3. Nialamide (Niamid)
4. Isocarboxazide (Marplan)
5. Phenelzine (Nardil)
6. Phenoxypropazine (Drazin)
7. Mebanazine (Actomol)

Hydrazine derivatives are:

8. Tranylcypromine (Parnate, Parstelin)
9. Etryptamine (Monase)
10. Pargyline (Eutonyl)

1. *Iproniazid (Marsilid)*

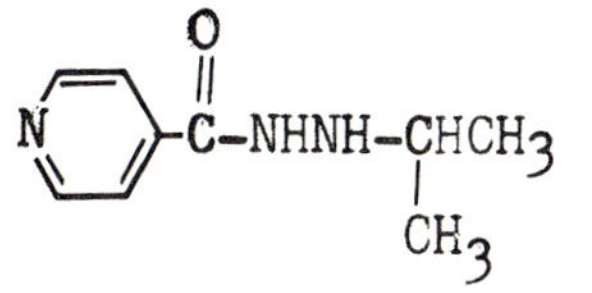

Iproniazid is 1-isonicotinyl 2-isopropylhydrazine. This drug, the first MAO inhibitor to be used as antidepressant (Loomer et al.) was withdrawn from the market in the USA and some other countries. In Great Britain it is still used (Dally). Soon after its introduction, the enthusiasm over the favorable results reported was somewhat dimmed in view of its side effects. Further, and somewhat surprisingly considering the enthusiastic reports of the efficacy of the drug in reports by Joel and many others, a controlled trial by Cole et al. showed that in a group of hospitalized depressed patients there was no significant difference between the response to each of three therapies—iproniazid, placebo or psychotherapy—to which the patients were randomly assigned.

An attempt has been made by some investigators to predict which outpatients will respond to the drug. West and Dally considered that those patients who improved on iproniazid were predominately neurotic with phobias, had a tendency to become depressed toward evening, had often demonstrated a poor response to ECT, and showed relatively small evidence of guilt feelings. On this basis, they tried to select a group of patients whom they considered would be iproniazid responders, and they found that among these 19 out of 28 were improved by iproniazid, while only 1 out of the 28 controls responded to the placebo. Gallinek has observed that retarded depressions with many somatic complaints and a chronic neurotic background respond best. These patients obviously fall into the "atypical group," described by West and Dally, in which Kalinowsky also obtained his best results with marsilid. Some authors claimed good results in endogenous retarded depressions. It is ineffective in agitated depressions. The "atypical group" includes patients with schizophrenic features who do not show a deep depressive affect but are rather listless. They may respond temporarily to ECT but relapse again and again in the same way as do chronic depressions of the older age group with hypochondriacal ideas and a resentful attitude. Such patients may respond surprisingly well to iproniazid, although more florid schizophrenic or manic pictures may occur. Kline and Stanley in their report at the Neuropharmacology Congress in Rome reported results superior even to ECT in manic-depressive and involutional depressions.

Iproniazid, like the other MAO inhibitors, was used in withdrawn and regressed schizophrenics with limited success. It may, however, reactivate psychotic symptoms. Contrary to Kline and Stanley who used iproniazid as a "psychic energizer" in burnt out schizophrenics, Freymuth et al. found no essential differences between iproniazid and placebo in these patients.

Some authors are still of the opinion that iproniazid is one of the most effective antidepressants. However, the increasing number of reports on liver damage (Zimmerman et al.; Popper) led to withdrawal of the drug, although cause and relation of this serious side-effect is not fully understood (Pletscher et al.).

MODE OF ADMINISTRATION AND DOSAGE: Since iproniazid is still available in countries like Great Britain, remarks on its administration are in order. An initial dose of 50 mg. had been originally recommended but Kline stated that, to be effective, a daily dose of 150 mg. is advisable. It was only after serious toxic effects on the liver had been reported that a maximum daily dose of 75 mg. was postulated. Kline even mentions daily doses of up to 250 mg. in resistant cases. The drug can be increased slowly over a period of two to six days, depending on the response; and the maximum dose should be reached by the end of two weeks. Alternatively, it has been suggested by Robie that, where there is no history of a manic state, the initial dosage may be 150 mg. daily, gradually reduced after two weeks to a maintenance level.

There is usually a delay of three to four weeks from the beginning of therapy before the drug's full effect is obtained, but in some cases a much earlier response is seen. As with all anti-depressant drugs, medication should be maintained for a long period of time because, contrary to ECT, the drugs suppress the depressive syndrome but do not necessarily shorten its duration. Attempts to withdraw medication may be made, but often it is necessary to reinstitute the drug and to maintain the patient on medication for the same period as his untreated depression would last.

2. *Pheniprazine (Catron, Catroniazid)*

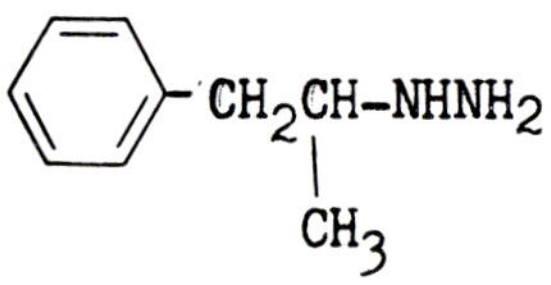

Pheniprazine is (1-methyl-2-phenyl)-ethylhydrazine. This drug, a relatively potent MAO inhibitor, was regarded by Lemere as comparable to iproniazid. When cases of fatal liver necrosis became known, the drug, like iproniazid, was withdrawn from the market. Another side-effect of pheniprazine was red-green color blindness (Frandsen).

3. *Nialamide (Niamid)*

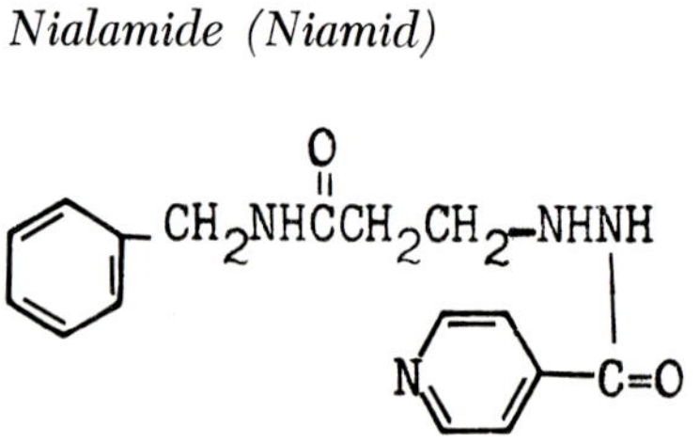

Nialamide, 1-[2-(benzylcarbamyl)ethyl] -2-isonicotinoylhydrazine.

RESULTS OF CLINICAL INVESTIGATIONS: Nialamid possesses a fairly wide margin of safety, its toxic effects, particularly its hypotensive-action, being less marked than in the other MAO inhibitors so far developed. However, a number of comparative studies have also indicated that, together with this decrease in toxicity, there is some decline in clinical effectiveness, nialamide being less potent than the other MAO inhibitors. But favorable reports have been made.

Nistri and Sgambati found that, it patients who were going to benefit, a clear improvement was noted at the end of the first week; and that, in general, two weeks' treatment is sufficient to ascertain whether response will take place. They found that, of a mixed group of depressions, a total remission was produced in 38.4 per cent, the best results being obtained in neurotic depression and psychotic depression of endogenous type. A combination of nialamide with chlorpromazine was useful in cases with anxiety, since in some patients the anxiety appeared to be resistant to nialamide alone.

Aside from chronic depressions, there are reports on improvement also in chronic withdrawn schizophrenics with only a small number becoming excited and violent as has been reported with some of the other MAO inhibitors. However, a number of other workers, such as Mendes et al., have reported aggressive behavior with an exacerbation of psychotic symptoms in schizophrenics given nialamide, and they regard it as contraindicated in this condition. They also draw attention to the fact that suicidal tendencies may be increased under the drug, because of the improvement in speed of psychomotor activity and thinking. This is indicative of the need for close observations of patients with suicidal ideas, particularly when they begin to improve.

Van Reeth, emphasized that in severe endogenous depression nialamide does not produce as many remissions as are obtained with ECT and opinions differ as to whether the drug reduces the number of ECT necessary in patients who require it. The majority of observers agree that the best results with nialamide are obtained in endogenous depressions of the retarded type. Where there is considerable agitation, this may be increased. There is less unanimity about neurotic depressions, some workers reporting good results while others found little response. This may be partially due to discrepancies in diagnostic criteria, some of the neurotic depressions probably being of the endogenous type with accompanying neurotic symptomatology. Depressions in the senium, involutional melancholia, and the depressions associated with organic disease have all been reported as responding, although to a lesser degree.

Nialamide has been used in the treatment of various types of mental defectives. In some patients, notably mongols, who were retarded in motor movements, a considerable increase in motor activity resulted so that they were able to stand or walk freely (Rett). Davies found the drug efficacious in improving the social and emotional control of a mentally defective group. He quotes the interesting case of a mongol, previously mute, who began to talk to a limited extent following nialamide medication. Despite the anti-convulsant action of the MAO inhibitors, no decrease in the incidence of epileptic fits was observed in this group or in various psychiatric patients with seizures. Combination of nialamide with phenothiazine was recommended by Feldman in chronic schizophrenics to prevent exacerbation of psychotic symptoms. Ayd et al. also used phenothiazines and barbiturates with nialamide in depressions with marked paranoid features, anxiety, agitation, anorexia, and insomnia. They did not find that nialamide potentiated the effects of these other drugs, nor were there any complications from its use in association with ECT. All clinical investigations emphasized that nialamide is particularly well tolerated. This is probably the reason why nialamide is also used in neuroses with hypochondriacal symptoms. In these patients who react badly to the subjective experience of any side-effects, Leyrie reports good results.

Mode of Administration and Dosage: Nialamide may be administered orally in two ways: either commencing with an initial dose of 100 mg. daily, increasing to 300 mg. or more over a period of 2 to 4 weeks and then reducing to a maintenance level of 50 to 100 mg. daily, or commencing with a high dosage of 300 to 500 mg. daily which is progressively reduced as soon as improvement commences. It is claimed that the latter method reduces the latent period before response to the drug becomes apparent, although agitation and confusion are more common at this dose level.

Dunlop pioneered in the intravenous use of nialamide. Without risk of side-effects, nialamide can be given intravenously to treatment-resistant depressions. According to Gann, this administration shortens the usual latency period for the therapeutic effect of MAO inhibitors from approximately twelve days by one half. Barek et al. following the suggestion of intravenous nialamide therapy, injected 1 gr. daily for ten days without seeing essential advantages of this mode of application. Also Eilenberg came to disappointing results but confirmed the good tolerability of intravenous administration. In a careful placebo-controlled study Nussbaum et al. confirmed these observations, when they gave 500 to 700 mg. daily as 1,000 ml. infusion intravenously. Pare and Jenner found that the blood level for nialamide is not greater with intramuscular injections than with oral medication.

4. *Isocarboxazide (Marplan)*

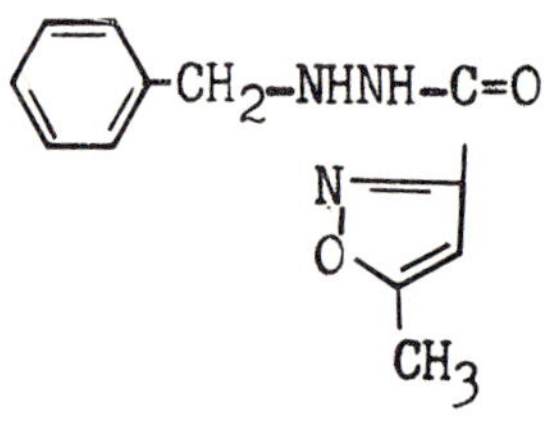

Isocarboxazide, 1-benzyl-2-(5-methyl-3-isoxazolyl-carbonyl)-hydrazine, has a higher potency than iproniazid in vitro and in vivo.

Results of Clinical Investigations: Isocarboxazide was introduced by the same firm that manufactured iproniazid in an attempt to market a less toxic MAO inhibitor. There is no doubt that it is less toxic, and, although opinions have varied as to whether it is as effective as iproniazid, Azima et al. found it valuable in a carefully controlled study; and Dally and Sargant regard isocarboxazide as being almost as effective as iproniazid. Rothman found that psychotic depressions remitted on the drug very quickly. Some patients developed schizophrenic symptoms, but their depressive features were alleviated. Thus, it appears that the drug is able to relieve all types of depressions.

Oltman and Friedman observed that results were good in involutional and psychoneurotic depressions. They were poorer in the depressive phase of a manic-depressive illness as well as in the "circular" type of this disorder. However, a number of patients had to be taken off the drug before its efficacy could become apparent, and were given ECT because of the suicide risk. These workers noted that males responded less well than females, as did Freyhan for imipramine. Patients over 70 had more unfavorable results, but concomitant organic brain disease as such did not seem to worsen the prognosis. There was a tendency for patients to swing over into mild hypomanic reactions as with the other antidepressant drugs. The authors emphasize the necessity for continuing with the drug even after apparent complete remission until the depressive attack has "run its natural course." Rothman et al., comparing isocarboxazide with placebo in a double-blind study, found the drug effective. Joshi obtained the best results in agitated depressions of older patients. Neurotic depressions responded best, when associated with obsessive-compulsive symptoms or anxiety. However, contrary to these mixed depressions, endogenous depressions did not improve.

In a broad comparative study Greenblatt et al. compared isocarboxazide with phenelzine, imipramine, ECT and placebo. Isocarboxazide turned out to be the least effective of all treatments investigated in this study. Kurland et al. trying to find an explanation for the contradictory opinions on isocarboxazide, undertook a study in two different set-ups, and found favorable results only in a small research ward; in the other setting, where the patients were scattered over a number of wards, there was no difference between the drug and placebo.

Mode of Administration and Dosage: The initial dose is usually 20 mg. daily, increasing to a maximum of 40 mg. within two weeks, with a reduction to a maintenance dose of 10 mg. daily. Its action is usually seen within 10 days but may not become apparent until the third or fourth week. Ayd believes that a higher dosage of up to 90 mg. daily may be necessary to achieve the maximum benefit.

5. *Phenelzine (Nardil)*

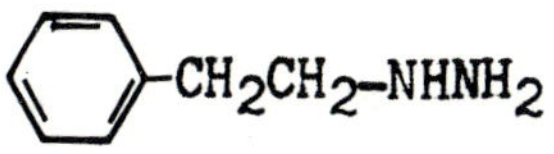

Phenelzine is β-phenylethylhydrazine.

Furst found that this drug approaches the effectiveness of iproniazid and that it is less toxic. It produces less effect on the autonomic nervous system than some of the other MAO inhibitors. Apparently, phenelzine has less monoamine oxides inhibiting effect in the liver and more in the brain in comparison to iproniazid which inhibits the enzyme equally in both organs. The latter drug appears to accumulate in the liver, but phenelzine easily passes the blood-brain barrier, and this may account for its rather speedier action.

Results of Clinical Investigations: Favorable results in depression have been reported by a number of observers. Sainz observed an 80 to 90 per cent response in endogenous depression and regarded these results as comparable to those with ECT; Thal obtained similar figures and only 55 per cent response with iproniazid in the same type of case. Kruse and Hoermann have reported that in manic-depressives who respond, improvement is noticed within 1 to 3 weeks of commencing therapy and sometimes as early as the fifth day. Response is slower in schizophrenics, the maximum benefit often not becoming apparent until the second month of treatment. They recommended a higher dosage, up to 90 mg. daily, for schizophrenics. The first two symptoms to remit in depression, according to Hutchinson and Smedberg, are the inability to sleep and early waking, followed by a gradual disappearance of the other depressive manifestations. Middlefell, who reported good results in endogenous depressions, claimed a lower relapse rate than in ECT. Involutional melancholia also responds well. Depressions occurring as part of a schizophrenic illness, with conversion reactions or accompanied by delusions, hallucinations, and numerous somatic symptoms, react less well, according to Thal who, contrary to Sainz, found a beneficial effect also in psychoneurotic depressions. Rees and Davies, who conducted a double blind trial comparing phenelzine to a placebo, found that the improvement obtained with the drug as compared to the placebo response was statistically significant, and the therapeutic efficacy of the drug was born out by the observation that those patients who had responded to phenelzine relapsed when they received the placebo. Rees and Davies found that depression, anxiety, tension, agitation, guilt feelings, and self-deprecation were the symptoms which were significantly improved by the drug. In about 10 to 15 per cent of patients there was some increase in agitation, but less so than with many of the other anti-depressants. He recommended amylobarbitone and levomepromazine.

Sainz has revealed a lack of correlation between monoamine oxidase inhibition as measured by the increase in catecholomine levels in blood obtained from the jugular vein, and remission with phenelzine. He regards this as an argument against the idea that monoamine oxidase inhibition is the primary cause of the action of these drugs in reversing depression. There are a number of sceptical reports which question the therapeutic efficacy of the drug altogether (King; Stanley and Fleming). However, since phenelzine is well tolerated, it has become one of the most widely used MAO inhibitors after the withdrawal of iproniazid and pheniprazine.

Mode of Administration and Dosage: The initial dose is usually 30 to 45 mg. daily in divided doses, reaching a maximum of 60 mg. and then reducing to a maintenance level of 15 to 10 mg. When the drug is given by intramuscular injection, a burning sensation, but without subsequent abscess formation or induration, is produced and lasts for a few minutes.

6. *Phenoxypropazine (Drazine)*

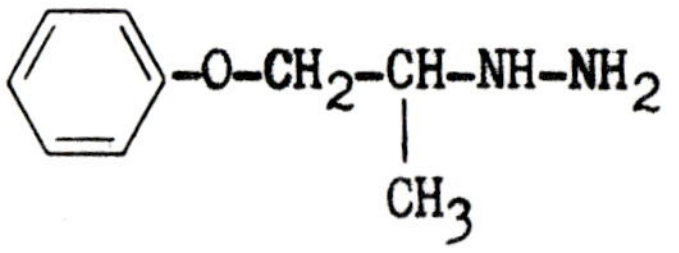

Phenoxypropazine is (1-methyl-2-phenoxyethyl)-hydrazine. The drug is not available in the USA or on the continent, and has only been introduced in Great Britain. Although there, too, it was withdrawn for a while, some British reports published in the USA suggest that phenoxyprozine is a well tolerated MAO inhibitor with antidepressive action (Leahy et al.; Imlah). It is effective in very low daily doses of 5 to 10 mg. (Dally).

7. *Mebanazine (Actomol)*

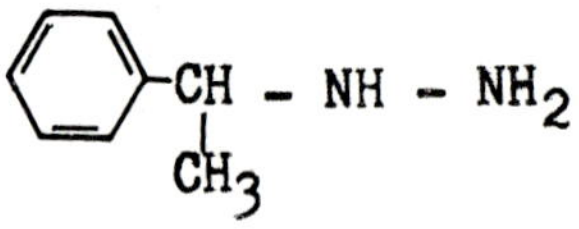

Mebanazine is (1-methyl-3-phenylmethyl)-hydrazine. The drug was introduced in Great Britain only recently, but appears to be no more effective in depressions than its predecessors. Cooper and Keddie soon noticed such severe side-effects that they warned against its use in older patients because of the possibility of circulatory collapse. They also observed an insulin-like effect, and Cooper warned against the danger of hypoglycemic shocks, Keddie notes the possibility of circulatory collapse. They also observed an insulin-like effect, and came to negative conclusions about the drug. Later, controlled studies by Gilmour and Barker et al. arrived at a more favorable opinion. The daily dose is 10 to 30 mg.

8. *Tranylcypromine (Parnate)*

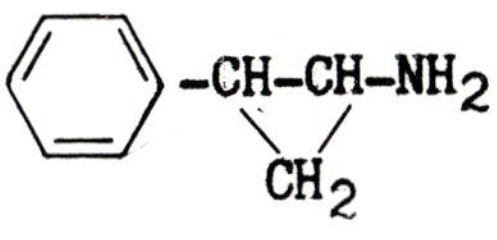

Tranylcypromine is trans-2-phenyl-cyclopropylamine. This drug, unlike other MAO inhibitors, is not a hydrazine derivative. Structurally it is similar to amphetamine. Pharmacologically it is related both to amphetamine and the MAO inhibitors (Zirkle and Kaiser). Like amphetamine, tranylcypromine causes "group toxicity" in mice and induces EEG alerting reactions. Like the MAO inhibitors, it potentiates the action of exogenous amines and reverses the reserpine effect. The onset of action—pharmacologically as well as clinically—is very rapid. It is possible that it combines the MAO inhibitor action with the direct stimulating effect similar to that of amphetamine.

Results of Clinical Investigations: Petersen and McBrayer emphasized the rapid onset of action which makes the drug superior to all other MAO inhibitors (Lemere). After a number of uncontrolled trials reviewed by Atkinson and Ditman, some controlled studies were published. Bartholomew demonstrated a significant superiority of tranylcypromine in reactive depressions, but no significant difference between the drug and placebo in severe endogenous depressions. Gottfries, in a double-blind trial could not verify the rather good results of some other studies. Overall et al. compared tranylcypromine with dextroamphetamine. Both did better in anxious and hostile depressions than in retarded depressions. Self-ratings by the patients showed that tranylcypromine was only slightly superior to dextroamphetamine. The possibility of addiction to the drug cannot be excluded (Le Gassicke).

The most serious complication is the occurrence of hypertensive crises and cerebral hemorrhage which will be discussed in the section on side-effects of the MAO inhibitors. It was this complication that led to the temporary withdrawal of the drug in the USA. Later, it was reintroduced with the recommendation to limit its use to hospitals.

Mode of Administration and Dosage: Initial dosage of 10 mg. twice daily increasing to 40 mg. daily is necessary. It has been claimed that, as compared to iproniazid, the cumulation of the drug is much less, the effect of tranylcypromine lasting for only 48 to 72 hours after withdrawal, while that of iproniazid persists for up to two weeks.

Tranylcypromine, particularly in England, used extensively in combination with neuroleptics, particularly with trifluoperazine under the trade name of Parstelin. Schiele found this combination especially valuable in pseudoneurotic schizophrenics. Barsa and Saunders investigated the therapeutic value of such combinations of a MAO inhibitor with a neuroleptic in chronic schizophrenics. Trying both tranylcypromine and pargyline, they found tranylcypromine for such combined treatment in chronic schizophrenics more suitable. Schiele et al. concluded, however, that the favorable results of combined tranylcypramine and trifluoperazine in chronic schizophrenics is due to the trifluoperazine. In a double-blind study the neuroleptic, when given alone, did equally well as the combination.

9. *Etryptamine (Monase)*

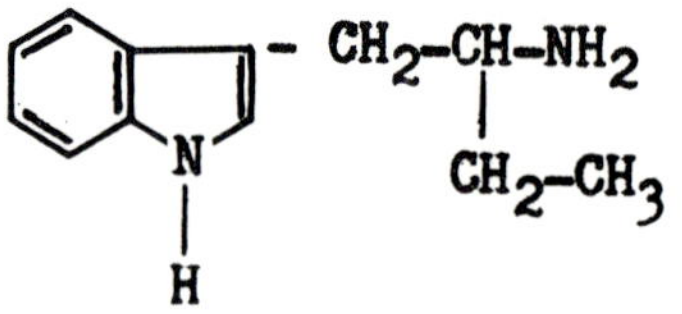

Etryptamine is 3-(2-aminobutyl)-indole. Reports about the efficacy of the drug in depressions were presented in a symposium in 1961. However, it was withdrawn in 1962, when it appeared unduly liable to cause agranulocytosis (Shepherd et al.).

10. *Pargyline (Eutonyl)*

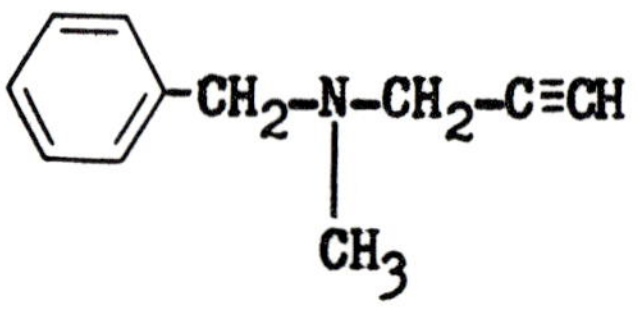

Pargyline is N-methyl-N-2-propynyl-benzylamine. The drug was marked as a hypotensive agent with MAO inhibitor action. Some authors believe that pargyline is an effective antidepressant (Oltman and Friedman; Ayd). In a controlled study Jacobs and Pillard showed that it is significantly more effective than placebo in non-psychotic but chronically ill patients with depressive mood. Turner and Merlis tried to increase the therapeutic action by simultaneous administration of dopa, but several patients developed deliria.

Side-Effects and Complications of MAO Inhibitors

1. *Postural hypotension* is the most frequent side-effect. In elderly patients it has caused falls resulting in fractures. Dizziness and vertigo are symptoms of hypotension.

2. *Other effects on the autonomic nervous system* are vascular headache and exacerbation or occasionally amelioration of migraine, decreased sweating and increased warmth of the extremities, constipation, difficulties in micturition, and dry mouth.

3. *Edema of the extremities,* particularly the ankles, is a frequent side-effect which usually responds to diuretics. Goldman recommends large amounts of vitamin B complex including pyridoxine.

4. *Acute liver necrosis* is most common with iproniazid, with which the incidence is about 1 in 4000 with 20 to 25 per cent fatalities (Scherbel). The new MAO inhibitors are less toxic, except perhaps pheniprazine. Kline mentions 33 liver deaths which may have been due to iproniazid. Transient elevation of serum transaminase has been found in a number of patients on the amine-oxidase inhibitors, but this returned to normal with no impairment in liver

function tests despite continuation of the drug. A persistent elevation is indicative of early disturbance of hepatocellular functioning and is an indication for stopping the drug immediately. Scherbel reports that there is evidence that this complication is associated with either overdosage or previous or present liver disease; Floody et al. found that, with iproniazid, cases can occur at a dose of less than 75 mg. daily.

The histopathology of the liver necrosis resembles a more severe form of that found in acute infectious hepatitis of viral origin; and Floody, noting that the incidence of the two conditions was similar, has suggested that the drugs may increase the severity of intercurrent attacks of viral hepatitis, rather than produce independent liver damage. In fact, it is still not clear whether the necrosis is due to a direct effect of the drug upon the liver or whether it is due to intercurrent viral hepatitis, the drug either increasing the severity of an attack or making, in some way, infection more likely. Robie has suggested that it is the hypotension with resultant hepatic anoxia that gives rise to the liver necrosis; but, in fact, one would expect that more prolonged and severe hypotension would be required to produce such damage.

Toxic liver conditions were the reason for withdrawal in the USA of the two hydrazine antidepressants iproniazid and pheniprazine. According to a survey by Hollister hepatocellular damage was rare following other hydrazine derivatives such as phenelzine, nialamid and isocarboxazide.

5. *Blood changes*, leading to normocytic, normochromic anemia of unexplained etiology are found in about 6 per cent of cases. Scherbel suggests that, since these drugs are chelating agents, they may bind iron. Leucopenia has been reported with catron and niamid.

6. *Skin manifestations* include maculopapular rashes and dermatitis.

7. *Neurological complications*—neuralgia, polyneuritis as well as hyperreflexia—have been observed. Goldman regards them as due to vitamin B deficiency. Convulsions have been reported (De Smedt et al.).

8. *Color blindness* in the form of red-green blindness due to pheniprazine was seen by Gillespie. It was reversible as was also loss of color vision with other MAO inhibitors.

9. *Impotence*, but also increase in sexual activity have been mentioned.

10. *Weight* may be increased, possibly due to accumulation of fluids. Occasional anorexia has also been seen.

11. *Withdrawal symptoms* may consist of blood pressure rise with tachycardia and precordial discomfort (Ayd). Therefore, MAO inhibitors should not be abruptly withdrawn because of the danger of coronary thrombosis or cardiac failure.

12. A very important, well studied side-effect is sudden *hypertension* which was soon recognized as being related to the intake of cheese, and is, therefore, also known as "cheese reaction." This complication begins with severe headaches, often followed by a hypertensive crisis. Subarachnoid hemorrhage and death may occur (Blackwell and Marley). Most cases of this complication were attributed to tranylcypromine. De Villiers has reviewed reports on this problem, and was able to describe 16 patients who developed intracranial hemorrhage. After finding that these reactions often followed the ingestion of cheese,

Blackwell et al. were also able to identify many other food stuffs that were involved in this complication during treatment with a MAO inhibitor. The mechanism of these reactions was later elucidated. All food stuffs which contain tyramine and other pressor amines are able to precipitate such hypertensive crises in patients under MAO inhibitors (Blackwell and Marley). Therefore, patients on this medication must be warned against cheese, chicken livers, and pickled herring, among other foods.

13. *Psychiatric complications* during medication are also found. Development of hypomanic states in manic-depressives and, in our experience, also in patients with atypical psychoses are one of the most frequent and most unpleasant complications. Withdrawn patients of the schizophrenic group may become acutely deluded and hallucinated. Both hypomanic states and exacerbation of schizophrenic syndromes can be controlled by phenothiazines. Heinrich attributes diagnostic value to his activation in schizophrenic symptomatology in apparently depressed patients.

A true toxic psychosis with confusion has been reported by Kimbell and Pokorny. Goldman described a state of motor restlessness and confusion with irregular movements of the whole body which cleared up under triflupromazine. The mention of memory impairment by Harnhoff and Heller is interesting and in accordance with our own experience (LBK) of occasional similar complaints by patients on various types of antidepressant drugs.

THE PSYCHOSTIMULANTS

The Amphetamines

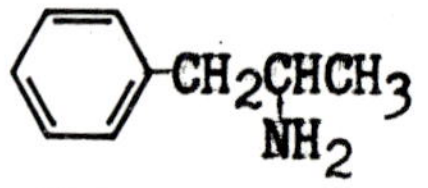

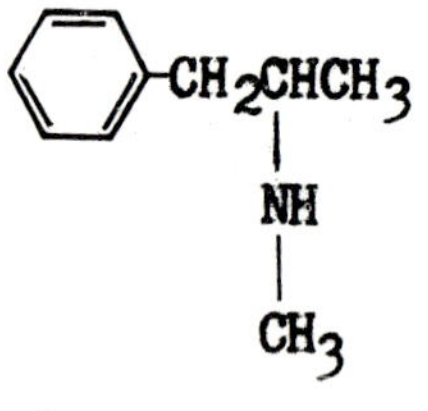

Mainly three compounds belong to this group of stimulant drugs:

1. *Amphetamine* (Benzedrine) which is the sulfate of dl-2amino-1-phenylpropane;

2. *Dextro- or D-Amphetamine* (Dexedrine, Elastonon), the sulfate of the dextro-rotatory isomer of amphetamine;

3. *Methamphetamine* (Methedrine, Desoxyn, Pervitin, Amphedroxyn), the N-methylated amphetamine as hydrochloride.

The upper formula is for 1 and 2; the lower formula is for 3.

Amphetamines are usually given in amounts of 5 or 10 mg. twice a day, preferably during the first half of the day to avoid sleeplessness.

All are known to stimulate mental activity and to give a certain euphoria to the normal person. It is obvious that these effects counteract in mild psychotics such symptoms as lack of concentration, loss of ambition, and depressed feeling. After Myerson had studied its effect on normals and neurotics, many others used it with psychotics. In schizophrenics, few favorable results have been reported. Some effect is obtained in early catatonics by the intravenous use of benzedrine. In child psychiatry, Bender and Cottington, while reporting favorably on its use in neurotic children and behavior problems, saw no effect in schizophrenia.

In deep depressions benzedrine is wholly ineffective, but, in slight depressions, its symptomatic effect is sometimes valuable. In mild depressive reactions which may be influenced by psychotherapy, benzedrine can be helpful. Sargant and Slater rightly point out that depressed patients "just hovering on the brink of invalidism can be carried over for a short time with the aid of benzedrine." Amphetamines are often used by general practitioners in depressed patients; but a recent controlled trial in which several practitioners were involved, showed that amphetamine 10 to 15 mg. daily is not better than placebo (Shepherd et al.). Psychiatrists often use amphetamines simultaneously with antidepressants to ease the patient's suffering until the slowly acting antidepressants take effect. Amphetamines are often combined with small amounts of amytal. Gottlieb gives maximal doses of sodium amytal and benzedrine by mouth, reducing the dosage of amytal if the patient becomes sleepy, and of benzedrine if he is too restless, until an optimal effect is obtained.

The favorable effect of benzedrine on some symptoms of a psychosis is not infrequently counterbalanced by such undesirable effects as increase of anxiety, tension, and aggressiveness. Schube et al., in a systematic study, reported no improvements but a number of patients who became worse. Dangerous tendencies in schizophrenics may be brought into the open by the stimulating effect of the drug. Agitated depressions may be precipitated. Even in patients who benefit the effect wears off quickly. In overactive, noisy and aggressive children amphetamine often has a paradoxical sedative effect (Zrull et al.).

Methamphetamine is apparently more effective than other amphetamines. The usual dose is 3 mg. compared to the 5 mg. dose of amphetamine. It also produces a temporary elevation of mood and is used in conditions accompanied by a general feeling of "depression," but in true depressions it is considered as unreliable. Methamphetamine intravenously (in ampules of 20 mg.) is used for psychotherapy in a way similar to that in which sodium amytal is used. It has the advantage that the patient is never amnesic about the session as he not infrequency is after sodium amytal interviews. Hoch and Polatin have shown that the drug has a normalizing effect on certain schizophrenic symptoms, most pronounced in the pseudoneurotic form of schizophrenia. Contrary to sodium amytal, which also has a normalizing effect, methamphetamine produces a state of positive well-being with increased alertness. Interesting although transitory improvements in severe depersonalization syndromes were reported by Davison. Delay et all described as "amphetamine shock" the reaction to a single massive dose of 30 mg. of amphetamine. Hypomanic states were transformed into frank manic states; mute schizophrenics became delusional and self-accusatory. No lasting therapeutic value was attributed to this "amphetamine shock."

In narcoanalytic work, Delay found that sodium amytal is more effective in revealing unconscious thoughts and in relieving amnestic states, while methamphetamine is more valuable in exploring thoughts already present but not expressed by the patient. Rothman and Sward used pentothal followed by desoxyn intravenously to obtain an optimal psychophysiological state for "pharmacological psychotherapy."

The therapeutic use of amphetamines has two serious dangers. It may lead to addiction, and a large number of cases of amphetamine psychoses were discovered in the German and Japanese armies; later also in civilian psychiatry. According to a monograph by Connell, these patients present an acute psychosis with ideas of reference, delusions, and hallucinations in a setting of fairly clear consciousness, which may be indistinguishable from paranoid schizophrenia.

Methylphenydate (*Ritalin*)

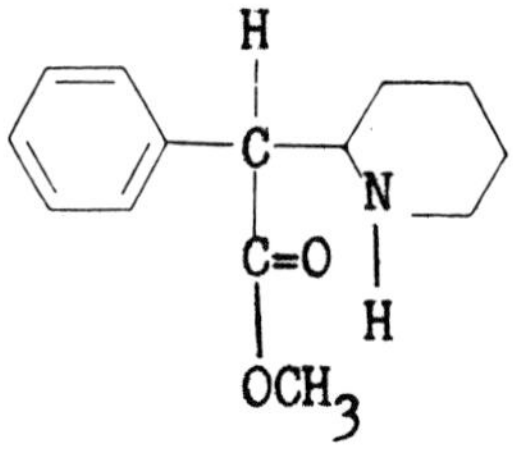

Methylphenydate is the hydrochloride of methyl-α-phenyl-2-piperidinacetate. It is a stimulant with properties similar to those of amphetamine. It is claimed, however, that the drug has no sympathetomimetic effects on the blood pressure, respiration, or heart rate, and, in fact, Darvill found a hypotensive action in some of his geriatric patients. "Jitteriness" and anorexia can occur as with amphetamine, and the drug does not alleviate anxiety. It antagonizes the sedative action of reserpine, a fact which has been utilized in therapy (Plummer et al.). It is liable to produce insomnia if given late in the day, and the usual dose is 10 to 20 mg. orally before breakfast and 5 to 10 mg. before lunch, with none being given later than noon.

Freed has used ritalin intravenously in doses from 10 to 15 mg. as a psychotherapeutic aid. He found that a rapid flow of speech ensued, but that this was associated with less emotion than occurs with methedrine or sodium amytal. There was a hostile rather than a euphoric affect. He found that in 10 to 15 per cent of cases headaches and a feeling of constriction in the chest followed the injection. Hartert and Browne-Mayers also used the drug intravenously in a similar dosage in alcoholics to overcome their resistance to psychotherapy, and Ticktin et al. in barbiturate poisoning. It was found to be of some value in moderate barbiturate depression, but relatively ineffective in deep coma. Ayd reported that the drug was also useful in overcoming the effects of over-sedation with chlorpromazine and reserpine in a dosage of 30 mg. daily. Over-stimulation of the central nervous system, with pressure of speech, over-activity, restlessness, insomnia, and anorexia may occur.

There have been a number of trials with ritalin in depressed patients and chronic apathetic schizophrenics. Carey et al. found it to be without demonstrable effect as compared to a placebo in chronic schizophrenics. They noted that some of the patients showed a loss of appetite and weight. In another controlled trial, Robin and Wiseberg found it to be ineffective in depressed out-patients. A more favorable though uncontrolled report was that of Natenshon, who treated a group of patients with reactive depression, including some on depression-producing medication. He found that stimulation without tension or tachycardia was produced, with alertness and minimal side-effects. There was no rebound depression, loss of appetite, or evidence of habituation. He regarded ritalin as contraindicated only in extremely nervous patients in whom hyperstimulation could occur. Neither Pargiter nor Bhaskaran and Kand found any evidence that it was of value in arousing chronic apathetic schizophrenics. Lytton and Knobel, was found improvement in disturbed children, were unable to correlate psychological, psychiatric, or electroencephalographic measurements of performance with the children's degree of responsiveness to the drug. Darvill, in a controlled trial, did not find any evidence that geriatric patients who were senile and retarded were helped by ritalin.

It appears that the efficacy of ritalin in psychiatric conditions has not been substantiated, except as far as its action in antagonizing the sedation effects of the neuroleptic drugs is concerned. It is possibly of benefit in mild reactive depression not associated with anxiety, which may be exacerbated; but there is no clear evidence that more severe depressions or other types of psychiatric illness are helped by the drug. Rothman as well as Ling and Buckman found methylphenydate to be a good adjuvant to psychotherapy in treatment-resistant neuroses.

Pipradol (Meratran)

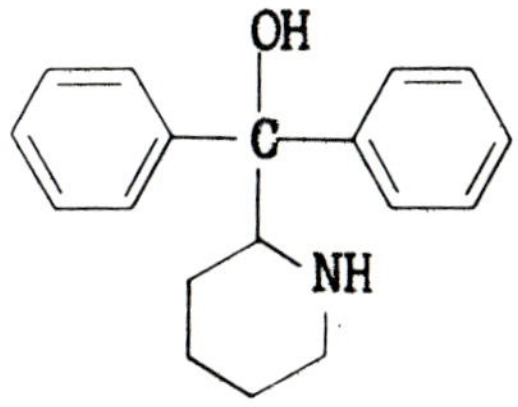

Pipradol, the hydrochloride of α, α-diphenyl-2-piperidine-methanol, has been described by Fabing as a true central nervous system stimulant. If the nervous system is "set" in a pattern of pathological overactivity, meratran will enhance the existing abnormal behavior. Thus, a manic becomes more excited and a paranoid patient more deluded. If the nervous system is "set" in a state of underactivity or psychomotor retardation, meratran appears to counteract this and to restore more functional level. Experimental evidence indicates that the reticular formation of the upper brain stem or the septal area or both are the primary sites of action of the drug.

The usual initial dosage is 1 mg. three times daily, increasing to 2.5 mg. three times daily after one week. A total daily dosage of up to 25 mg. has been given in depressed patients.

Fabing et al. observed good results in reactive depression and in endogenous depression. They also found the drug useful in epileptics who became depressed, dull, or tense when their seizures were controlled by anti-convulsants. Hoch, in the discussion of this paper, noted that in schizophrenics and depressions he had found no difference between the drug and a placebo, and patients had complained of insomnia, tension and poor appetite. Fullerton saw improvements in reactive depression and in depression secondary to senile change or to the neuroleptic drugs. It tends to exacerbate agitation anxiety, and delusions. Where improvement is going to occur, there is often an elevation of mood after the first dose of the drug, and the full beneficial effects begin to appear within 48 hours. During this initial 48 hour period a decrease in appetite is seen, but the anorexia disappears concomitantly with the commencement of improvement. There was a continuation of anorexia and loss of weight in those patients who did not respond to meratran. Martin et al. who found the drug useful in alleviating mild depression and emotional fatigue, recommended the use of reserpine (0.25 mg.) in combination with it in patients suffering from agitated depression.

A Russian paper by Fedotov et al. indicates that they have used meratran in schizophrenia, and they claim that it abolishes what they regard as the pathological cortical inhibition of the disease. Schut and Himwich also regarded the drug as beneficial in non-deluded depressed and retarded schizophrenics. It is contraindicated in patients with active delusions since it may activate them. Agitated depressions do not respond well, the agitation often increasing. Rosner et al., comparing the drug with frenquel in chronic psychotics, found that it seemed to increase social withdrawal and irresponsibility and did not decrease depression. Disappointing results were also reported by Houston in chronic schizophrenia.

The drug has also been used in chronic alcoholism (Bensoussan and Villiaumey), in depression with resultant periodic drinking (Proctor), in obesity or malnutrition due to depression (Cohen), to prevent depression when chlorpromazine is used as an anti-emetic in pregnancy, in narcolepsy (Talley), and in behavior disorders in children.

Side-effects are not serious but include nausea, rashes of macular type, over-activity, exacerbation of delusions, agitation and anxiety, pallor, tachycardia, and occasionally, with very high doses a psychotic reaction with anxiety, agitation, and sometimes hallucinations (Schou). Unlike the amphetamines, there is no pronounced cardiovascular action and little interference with sleep.

Schut and Himwich regard meratran as contraindicated in delusional, anxious patients, and disturbed arteriosclerotics. A case of accidental overdosage in a two and a half year old child who swallowed 15 mg. of the drug, has been reported by Fabing et al. The child became excited and overactive, ate voraciously, and developed stereotype activity accompanied by a rise in blood pressure and pulse rate for about 48 hours.

Dimethylaminoethanol (Deaner)

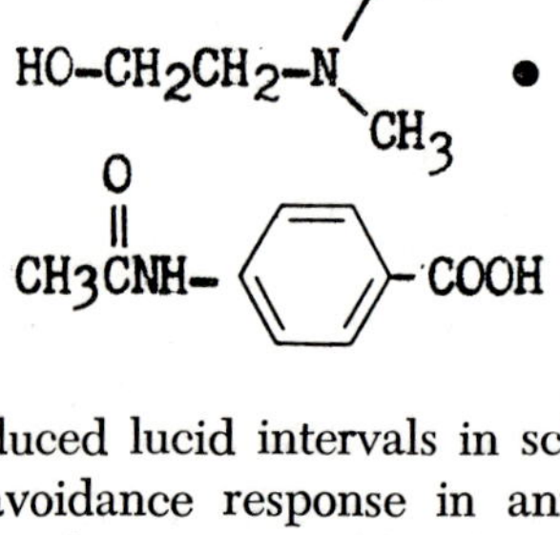

Dimethylaminoethanol or deanol has been regarded as a precursor of acetylcholine. The p-acetylaminobenzoate of deanol is known under the trade name: Deaner.

The development of this compound was the result of research into the possible role of acetylcholine in brain function and in the production of psychiatric abnormality. The fact that parasympathetic stimulation of the brain produced lucid intervals in schizophrenic patients and inhibited the conditioned avoidance response in animals (Pfeiffer and Jenney) led to a search for a substance capable of increasing the brain level of acetylcholine. Deaner is not only a precursor of choline but also, unlike choline and acetylcholine, will pass the blood-brain barrier. While it has been assumed that deaner acts by means of conversion to acetylcholine, Pepeu et al. have reported that experiments failed to show an increase in acetylcholine synthesized from deaner in rat brain slices.

The drug has been used in mild depression since its main effect in central nervous system stimulation with activation of the reticular formation. It is also claimed to be of value in chronic fatigue states and vascular headache (Moriarty and Mebane). In chronic schizophrenics it was found to be effective only in combination with one of the neuroleptic drugs (Barsa and Saunders). Portnow et al. found no change in the behavior of chronic schizophrenics treated with the drug as compared to a control group, and the ward personnel were unable to guess better than chance which patients were receiving the drug.

Greene believes that deanol is suitable for geriatric patients with chronic brain syndromes because, contrary to other psychotropic drugs, it has few side-effects; and in brain damaged old patients one should turn to drugs with few side-effects. The well tolerated deanol leads to increased alertness and greater cooperation, thus requiring less nursing care.

Centrophenoxine (Lucidril, Helfergin)

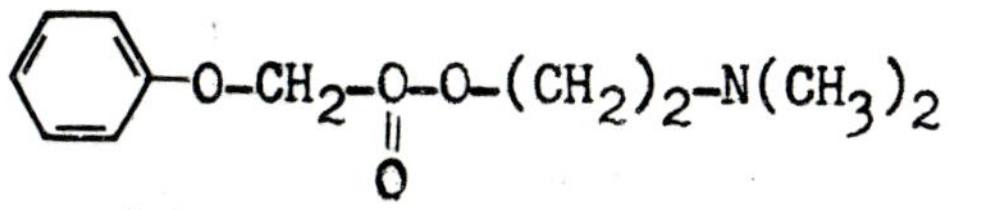

Centrophenoxine, another compound of dimethylaminoethanol, and therefore related to deaner, is the p-chlorphenoxyacetate of dimethylaminoethanol. The chlorphenoxy-acetic acid is a plant growth hormone from the group of the auxines. Esterization of dcanol with this auxine derivative was hoped to increase the stimulant effect of deanol because it was known that chlorphenoxy-acetic acid enforces the intensity and duration of the hormone effect (Thuillier et al.).

As Delay et al. already stated, its stimulant effect is most noticeable in disturbances of vigilance due to organic cerebral conditions. Gerstenbrand and Hoff confirmed this in posttraumatic disturbances of consciousness, organic dementias and organic psychotic brain syndromes. Kohlmann and Rett showed in a placebo-controlled study that centraphenoxine is effective in brain damaged children in motor-static retardation, increasing drive and improving test performance. Confusional states, delirious syndromes in alcoholics and senile patients could be controlled by intravenous administration of 1.5 to 3 g. daily for about one week (Fodor; Houillon et al.). Nickel et al. explain these therapeutic effects with improved glucose absorption in the brain, while dimethylaminoethanol alone does not influence the passing of glucose through the blood brain barrier. Nandy and Bourne have observed in animal experiments that prolonged administration of centrophenoxine eliminates lipofuscin, the pigment of old age, from the nerve cells. If this is so, centraphenoxine would be the first substance with an effect on the aging process in the brain.

Delay et al. investigated centrophenoxine in various psychiatric disorders. They found that, on the one hand, it can be compared to the tricyclic antidepressants, and on the other hand, to psychostimulants of the amphetamine type; but it did not prove its value in depressions or anergic schizophrenics.

Phenmetrazine (*Preludin*)

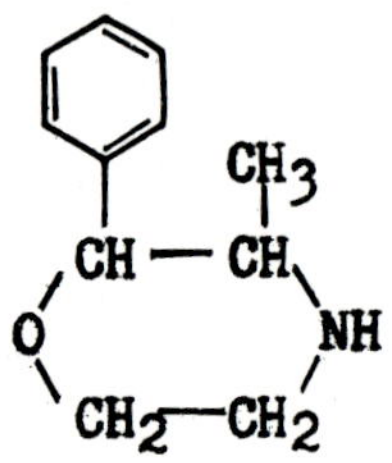

Phenmetrazine is 3-methyl-2-phenylmorphine. Introduced as a "safe" appetite suppressant, it produces weight loss, comparable to that obtained with amphetamines (Patel et al.). The appetite depressing effect is more accentuated, when the patient knows what to expect from the drug (Penick and Hinkle). In psychiatric patients and normals Spiegelberg found increased drive and reduced fatigability. But this therapeutic similarity between phenmetrazene and amphetamines is associated with the same danger of abuse and toxic psychosis (Randell, Kellner).

PSYCHOTOMIMETICS (HALLUCINOGENS) IN THERAPY

Drugs that are able to produce psychotic symptoms and which have been called psychotomimetics, and more recently, psychodysleptics, were also applied therapeutically. This was not the case with mescaline, but lysergic acid diethylamide offered itself for such use, probably because its influence on mood and a sense of well-being is more pronounced than with mescalin. Other drugs with hallucinogenic action were also used for "psycholytic" and other treatment in psychiatric disorders. This was most likely caused by the great psychopathological interest of these drugs. In this book their discussion will be limited to their therapeutic use.

1. *Lysergic Acid Diethylamide* (*Delysid*)

Lysergic acid diethylamide (d-LSD_{25}) was discovered as a drug with hallucinogenic action by Hofmann. There always was and there still is much disagreement about the therapeutic usefulness of this drug. The Swiss psychiatrist Stoll as well as Condreau, who first used lysergic acid diethylamide (LSD), gave up the therapeutic use.

In 1959 the Josiah Macy Jr. Foundation organized a large symposium on "The use of LSD in psychotherapy" which gave a good account of the present state of this therapeutic approach. It has been claimed that some of the patients become relaxed, communicate, and are in good rapport. However, as Hoch pointed out, many of these patients become blocked, and their sensory phenomena lead to a very definite anxiety which can be so much in the foreground that an interview is gainful neither to the patient nor the therapist. The general opinion that the drug has no addicting properties is also not fully established. Small doses of 25 to 50 μg. may be useful. Seventy-five μg. is the usual limit patients like to take, but doses of 100 to 150 μg. have also been given. Limitation lies in the fact that patients must be watched for the whole time of their abnormal state of mind, at least for eight hours. Therefore, Sandison in England used day and night hospital facilities for his administration of LSD in psychotherapy. Abramson in this country used LSD in psychoanalytical therapy. In his work unconscious material is produced under effect of the drug and then interpreted according to psychoanalytical principles.

Most psychiatrists use LSD as an abreactive drug for any form of psychotherapy. The intensified perception and decreased emotional control make it suitable for this purpose.

Spencer, who, in a special LSD unit in an English hospital, often combines LSD with intravenous methylphenidate (Ritalin), gives an extensive survey of his own and others' experience. In another survey of work in this area and its relationship with other adjuvants to psychotherapy, Cornu lists the great variety of neurotic conditions and psychopathic personalities who were successfully treated with the drug. Recently interesting results were obtained by R. Fox in alcoholics. Although Shagass and Bittel also found alcoholics and sexual deviates to respond favorably, they conclude that the status of LSD as a therapeutic agent remains uncertain and controversial. At the International Congress in Madrid, Delay also expressed scepticism about the therapeutic use of these drugs. Leuner, who is favorably impressed by the therapeutic value of "psycholytic" drugs, recently brought up the question whether the use of LSD for this purpose can be justified in view of the increased abuse of LSD which has been popularized by Aldous Huxley, and is in vogue in college and "hippy" circles. He, therefore, recommends replacement of LSD with the less controversial psilocybin.

The question remains whether LSD is a therapy in itself or whether it only facilitates psychotherapy in the same sense as sodium amytal, pervitin, or other drugs used in narcocathartic and narcosuggestive psychotherapy.

Such complications as suicide have been reported but might be avoided by proper handling. On the other hand, the danger of prolonged psychotic reactions is a very serious one, and will probably limit a more extensive use of this interesting drug for therapeutic purposes.

2. *Psilocybin (Indocybin)*

Psilocybin is 3(2-dimethylamino)-ethylindol-41ol dihydrogen phosphate. It is a hydroxytryptamine derivative, closely related to serotonin and contains an indole ring structure found in many hallucinogens. It is extracted from a mushroom Psilocybe Mexicana Heim which has long been known to Indian tribes of Southern Mexico for its psychological effects.

This hallucinogen has been studied extensively by Delay et al., and used by several groups therapeutically as a "psycholytic" drug in the same way as LSD. It is a hundred times weaker than LSD and can be given orally (3 to 40 mg.). Malitz et al. working with both, psilocybin and LSD, warn against any hallucinogen for psychotherapy in an out-patient setting, particularly because of possible development of "depression with the ever present risk of suicide." With psilocybin they saw the same pattern of autonomic reactions, perceptual disturbances and affective variations due to the toxic effect, and, on the other hand, specific responses of the individual according to his basic personality structure. Leuner who replaced LSD with psilocybin, found that patients treated with both drugs could not distinguish between them. The main advantage of psilocybin is that its effect only lasts five hours as compared to the 8 to 12 hours of the LSD effect. It also has fewer vegetative side-effects, and abuse is less probable because it cannot be as easily manufactured as LSD.

3. *Phencyclidine (Sernyl)*

Phencyclidine is 1-(1-phenylcyclohexl)-piperidine hydrochloride. Although it produces an immediate psychotomimetic effect with the added advantage of subsiding within an hour (Domino), it appears that it did not find application in so-called psycholytic therapy. Its psychotomimetic qualities were primarily used for experimental purposes in combination with sensory deprivation. Therapeutically Luby et al. reported that the drug was successful in controlling anxiety states, and it is of interest that they also noted remission in an acute catatonic schizophrenic. Davies reported good results with doses of 0.5 to 5.0 mg. in some obsessive states. Vegetative side-effects seem to have limited its therapeutic possibilities.

4. *Ditran*

Ditran, N-ethyl-3-piperidyl-cyclopentylphenyl-glycolate-hydrochloride, is a psychomimetic drug used in the treatment of depressions.

Meduna and Abood have investigated the 3-N-substituted piperidyl benzilates, which, in doses of 5 to 10 mg., are psychomimetics, producing visual and auditory hallucinations in normal individuals, with a delirium-like confusional state, followed by marked physical weakness for 10 to 24 hours. However, it was also observed that about 24 to 36 hours after the administration of the drug some of the subjects became euphoric with increased drive. This led to the idea of using such drugs in the treatment of depression; and ditran, in which both the hallucinogenic properties and duration of action are increased because of the substitution of one of the phenyl groups in benzilic acid by a cyclopentyl group, was tried by them in depressed patients.

Ditran is anticholinergic and produces an atropine-like action resulting in symptoms such as dryness of the mouth and dilation of the pupils in association with the psychiatric effects. The drug is given orally in doses up to 20 mg. and in about an hour's time produces a clouding of consciousness, bewilderment, restlessness, confusion, disorientation, hallucinations, illusions, and distorted thinking. The recollection of the patient of this episode after recovery depends upon the degree of clouding of consciousness. Some patients may develop an acute hallucinatory state in a setting of clear consciousness. The condition lasts for 2 to 6 hours and is followed by weakness. The atropine-like effects persist for about 18 hours, by which time signs of psychiatric improvement may be observed.

Meduna and Abood found that the drug is very effective in reactive depression, with only one treatment being required but psychotic depressions were not so responsive. The mode of action of the drug is unknown, but Meduna and Abood believe that it has a normalizing rather than a stimulating effect upon brain functioning.

A comparison of ditran and LSD was made by Wilson and Shagass. The changes produced by the two drugs differ markedly from one another. Ditran produced severe psychotic symptoms in all subjects, but LSD only in some. The ditran experience was usually not remembered, while the LSD experience was. Hallucinations were usually auditory with ditran, and visual with LSD. Pharmacologically ditran was studied by Bradley and Fink. Clinically it appears that ditran has never been used widely.

Additional Drugs

Further drugs are discussed under "Various Pharmacological and Other Methods" in Chapter VI.

CHAPTER III

The Convulsive Therapies

Von Meduna introduced convulsive therapy, choosing the pharmacologic provocation of convulsions. However, his method was never meant as a new drug treatment for mental diseases. Its primary object was to utilize the effect which convulsive seizures may have on the disease process. It, therefore, was a logical development when Cerletti and Bini replaced chemical convulsive agents with electric current. The advantages of this electric convulsive treatment are convincing, but the method should be understood essentially as a technical modification of the original convulsive treatment; again, it was not the electric current that was expected by Cerletti and Bini to have a therapeutic effect per se. The latest development is the discovery of a pharmacological convulsant "Indoklon" which is mostly used by inhalation.

The section on Pharmacological Convulsive Treatment will be limited to description of the techniques. Most clinical aspects of the various methods will be dealt with jointly in the section on Electric Convulsive Therapy. It is hoped that in this way repetition can be avoided.

Pharmacologic Convulsive Treatment

The provocation of convulsions by pharmacologic means has taken a secondary place since the electric method was introduced. However, knowledge of the pharmacologic technique remains important for many reasons. It is still used, principally in combination with insulin. There are workers who prefer it, and a comparative study by Bianchi and Chiarello even comes to the conclusion that results with metrazol are superior to those obtained with electric convulsive therapy. The main reason that the experience with pharmacologic convulsive agents cannot be ignored is that our present knowledge of many aspects of convulsive therapy is based on experience with pharmacologic methods.

Von Meduna, in his first group of patients treated with pharmacologic convulsive therapy, used 25 per cent camphor in oil injected intramuscularly. The initial dosage was 10 cc. (2.5 cc. of camphor). This could be increased to single doses as high as 40 cc. The injection was given before breakfast for nausea and vomiting were frequent complications. Other disadvantages were the impossibility of anticipating the time of the convulsive attack which could occur from fifteen minutes to three hours after injection, as well as the possible occurrence of several convulsions or failure to convulse at all.

Metrazol and Other Drugs

These disadvantages led von Meduna to the choice of the soluble synthetic camphor preparation, pentamethylentetrazol, known in the United States as metrazol (Knoll), in European countries as cardiazol or corvis or tetrakor. It can be injected intravenously and was first used in a 20 per cent aqueous solution which sometimes caused pain and coagulation of the vein at the site of the injection. As a result, it was later used in a 10 per cent solution although this increased the amount of fluid to be injected.

The convulsion sets in three to thirty seconds after injection of the drug. Quick injection is necessary to provoke a convulsion with a minimum amount. Differences in the rapidity of the injection may be responsible for occasional variations in the amount necessary for the same patient on different days. Friedman tried to lower the convulsive threshold to metrazol by alkalinization of the blood with appropriate diet and sodium bicarbonate by mouth. Fluid intake was limited for the same reason. None of these modifications became a routine procedure; their influence on the convulsive threshold is negligible.

The initial dose is usually 5 cc. (0.5 Gm.). If no convulsion takes place within one minute, subsequent injections are given. Such failures to produce a convulsion often lead to great discomfort on the part of the patient who may feel nauseated and apprehensive for hours.

One of the greatest drawbacks to pharmacologic convulsive therapy was that the patient does not lose consciousness as long as no convulsion takes place. In the interval between injection and convulsion he has what is described as a feeling of impending death and sudden annihilation.

Other convulsive drugs have been recommended, among them picrotoxin, coriamyrtin (Blackwinn et al.), and ammonium chloride (Bertolani). A greater number of studies were dedicated to cyclohexylethyltriazol known mainly as triazol or azoman (Mayer-Gross and Walk). Advantages over metrazol were supposedly the absence of severe discomfort and the smaller amounts of fluid to be injected. Triazol, particularly when injected intramuscularly, was introduced with much hope, but led to disappointment because of the delay in its elimination from the organism, sometimes leading to repeated convulsions. In the event of failure to convulse, repetition of the injections may produce status epilepticus. Several fatalities have been reported. Berg and Robbins experimented with a tetramethyl-succinimide (PM-1090). Like many authors who compared pharmacological and electric convulsion treatment they found the drug superior, but delayed convulsions occur. Bemegride, known for its use in barbiturate poisoning was used for convulsive therapy by Lüttke and Koch, and found superior to ECT. Metrazol has been used with succinylcholine by Komora and Padula. Intravenous use of Indoklon which is mostly applied as an inhalant, will be discussed later.

The convulsion can be described as follows (von Meduna): A few seconds after the injection, the patient becomes pale and rigid, makes a few clonic movements or escape movements and may cough. Only after this phase does he lose consciousness and go into a tonic spasm. At this moment he usually opens his mouth and keeps it open long enough to permit insertion of a mouth gag. The tonic phase repeats essentially the picture of decerebrate rigidity. At the end of the tonic phase slight twitchings take place which initiate the clonic part of the convulsion. The tonic phase lasts for about ten seconds, the clonic phase forty to forty-five seconds. A comatose sleep of not more than five to ten minutes' duration is followed by a period of confusion lasting half an hour or longer. The amount of the drug does not determine the length of the convulsion. Postconvulsive excitement states occur as they do after any convulsion regardless of the stimulating agent. The duration of the seizure varies in the individual patient with each treatment. Sal y Rosas stated that the length increased with subsequent convulsions, but this has not been confirmed.

The main difference between this seizure and a spontaneous epileptic seizure is the so-called first clonic phase which precedes the tonic phase. According to H. Strauss et al., the movements of this phase have a different rhythm from those of the clonic phase proper, suggesting a central mechanism peculiar to the "first" clonic phase. This initial phase is probably the expression of direct stimulation of motor cortical cells by the injected drug. The duration of the motor phenomena following metrazol injection seems longer than in electric convulsions, not only because of this "first" clonic phase but also because of irregular jerks at the end of the "second" clonic phase. An occasional second convulsion may be explained as due to particles of metrazol still circulating in the blood after the convulsion.

The patient has an amnesia for the convulsion, but unfortunately, he remembers the feeling of deadly fear which he experienced between injection and convulsion. If no convulsion takes place, anxiety, restlessness, and general discomfort may continue for hours. This is the most unpleasant feature of metrazol treatment and is one of the most valid reasons for the superiority of the electric method of producing therapeutic convulsions.

Today these subjective disadvantages of metrazol convulsive therapy can be easily overcome with barbiturate anesthesia and muscle relaxation as the usual routine in any convulsive therapy. If the superiority over ECT claimed by some clinicians for pharmacologically induced convulsions, were confirmed, metrazol treatment with premedication would be just as acceptable as Indoklon treatment as an alternative to "Electric Shock Treatment" in patients who refuse the latter procedure because of its name.

Inhalation Convulsive Treatment with "Indoklon"

In 1957, the pharmacologist Krantz and his co-workers studied aliphatic fluorinated ethers, one of which had found practical use in anesthesia under the name of fluoromar (trifluorethyl vinyl ether). A very similar compound, hexafluorodiethyl ether, turned out to be a convulsant in addition to having some anesthetic properties. Even such a small concentration as 29 or 30 parts to a million in the inspired air produced convulsions, while 6 to 8 per cent in the air were necessary to produce anesthesia. The drug was called "Indoklon." It produced convulsions in all animal species. Its use for convulsive therapy was first reported by Esquibil et al. in 1958.

Indoklon is a colorless, non-inflammable liquid. It is not metabolized in the human body, and leaves the body unchanged. It is applied by means of a mask and a vaporizer is loaded with gauze saturated with the liquid material. If the mask is closely applied, a convulsion occurs within 15 to 30 seconds. The patient loses consciousness, has some myoclonic movements similar to those seen in metrazol convulsions, and then goes slowly into the tonic phase followed by the clonic phase of a convulsion.

Our first experience with this method was based on treatment given without barbiturate anesthesia. In this unmodified application the convulsion was often followed by a second or even third seizure after an interval of one or two minutes, probably due to continued circulation of the gas in the blood. Today this is usually avoided by more careful dosage and perhaps due to the barbiturate anesthesia. Our original impression of less nausea and less confusion was not confirmed by our present experience with Indoklon modified by anesthesia techniques. Nausea is now so frequent that it became almost routine procedure to give Compazine, 5 mg. intramuscularly or intravenously. Confusion, too, seems to be at least as pronounced as in ECT which is of obvious theoretical interest and contradicts the concept that confusion in ECT is due to the passing of electric current through the brain.

One of the main disadvantages of Indoklon treatment is the difficulty to determine whether the patient really had a full convulsion. The often prolonged myoclonic movements prior to the convulsion must be followed by a clearly recognizable tonic phase with plantar flexion of the feet. Even the experienced therapist often remains in doubt whether the patient had a true convulsion, and we sometimes follow with an electric convulsive stimulus to make sure that the patient has the full benefit of a convulsive treatment.

Technique of Indoklon Treatment: The technique of modified Indoklon treatment was first described by Karliner and Padula and recently summarized by Karliner in accordance with our technique for electric convulsive therapy, developed with the anesthesiologist S. Dell'Aria.

Anesthesia is induced by applying an intravenous drip of 0.2 per cent solution of Brevital (methohexital sodium). When axis deviation of the eyes, nystagmus, yawning or the usual signs of unresponsiveness indicate that the patient is under complete barbiturate anesthesia, we switch to a bottle of 0.2 per cent of succinylcholine (Anectine) and again use the drip method for complete muscle relaxation. Usually the appearance of fasciculations in the neck and upper extremities marks the stopping point for the drip. Subsequently the lower limbs begin to fasciculate, and when the fasciculations stop, it can be assumed that the patient is fully relaxed. From the beginning of the succinylcholine drip a mask is applied to the patient's face. The mask is attached to a

5 liter bag and also to a special vaporizer. Respiration is assisted with a flow of oxygen, 9 liters per minute. When sufficient muscle relaxation is obtained, 0.25 to 0.5 cc. of Indoklon is injected into the vaporizer through a rubber diaphragm. The oxygen flow is now interrupted and the bag repeatedly squeezed, thus forcing the Indoklon mixed with the remaining oxygen into the lungs. Myoclonic movements soon appear, but squeezing of the bag must continue until the tonic phase takes place. The mask is now removed from the face, the Indoklon blown into the air, the oxygen supply resumed, and the patient ventilated until spontaneous respiration sets in.

Krantz was able to develop Indoklon for intravenous administration. As a solvent, polyethylene glycol (carbowax 300) is being used. Like inhaled Indoklon, the intravenous drug is also eliminated in the exhaled air as demonstrated by a mouse placed in a bag together with a dog. The mouse convulsed at the same time as the dog in whom an Indoklon convulsion had been elicited. In humans, convulsions occur after a latent period of approximately 20 seconds following injection of 0.2 ml/Kg. of Indoklon solution. Since the solvent is excreted through the kidneys, patients with renal insufficiency should not be treated with this method.

More clinical studies have to be awaited for a better appraisal, but there is little doubt that they will give further impetus to the use of this chemical for convulsive treatment. All the clinical evidence available so far confirms the expected fact that this modification of convulsive therapy is equally as effective as metrazol and electrically induced convulsions. This was convincingly demonstrated by a comparative study by Kurland et al. In spite of this Indoklon has not replaced ECT, and it is difficult to determine the reasons. Side-effects have been described by Dolenz in an otherwise favorable report. They consisted of confusional states and delirium which, however, hardly differ from the organic reactions of ECT. This author also warns against combination with MAO inhibitors because one such patient developed hypertension for a week. He also observed a nonfatal cardiac arrest. In our own experience we, too, had the impression that some patients had slight cardio-vascular difficulties which they did not have, when we changed them over to ECT. On the other hand, Rose and Watson prefer Indoklon in patients with cardiac pace makers, where one likes to avoid the electric current. Another technical advantage we saw is that in patients with loose teeth, the teeth are better protected because even in well relaxed patients under ECT the direct electrical stimulation of the jaw muscles leads to strong contractions of these muscles. This does not occur with Indoklon treatment.

We must agree with Biddy and Smith that Indoklon has mostly a place as an alternate technique for patients who reject so-called electric shock because of its name but who are in need of convulsive therapy and accept an "inhalation treatment" more easily.

Electric Convulsive Therapy

The use of electrically induced convulsions, introduced by Cerletti and Bini, replaced the pharmacologic method with metrazol chiefly because of the following advantages: (1) the method is technically simpler and cleaner than the repeated intravenous injections of a drug which easily lead to thrombosis of the veins; (2) there is an immediate loss of consciousness which spares the patient any discomfort; (3) failure to respond with the desired convulsive manifestations can be avoided.

The simple method of unpremedicated electric convulsive treatment has been replaced in most psychiatric facilities by methods using a muscle relaxant with or without a barbiturate. Some do not have anesthetists, and find it inadvisable to use an intricate anesthesia technique without an anesthetist. Others have serious objections to complicating a treatment with practically no danger to life with an anesthesia procedure which, in itself, undeniably presents a potential danger. It was, therefore, found advisable to describe electric convulsive therapy both with and without muscle relaxation. Most precautions to avoid fractures should remain routine measures for the simple reason that sometimes muscle relaxation is inadequate, and an unexpectedly strong convulsion can occur in spite of a muscle relaxant drug, even in the hands of the most experienced therapist.

Technique

The original machine for electric convulsive therapy (ECT) was built by Bini. A large number of modifications has been recommended since, but many of the machines used are still based essentially on Bini's design. It consists primarily of a stop watch for time regulation to fractions of a second and of devices for measuring and regulating the current. Alternating current from electric light circuits having a frequency of 50 to 60 cycles is used. A voltmeter regulates the voltage to be applied. The original machine had a second low-voltage current circuit for preliminary measurement of the resistance of the patient's head. An automatic time clock or various time relays from 0.1 to 0.5 seconds or more interrupt the current after the desired length of time. Several workers use machines which permit the setting of the actual milliamperage to be allowed to flow through the patient's head. The reliability of this development is a matter of controversy, however. All the various machines on sale serve their purpose to produce convulsions. The simplest models seem to be the best for they are not complicated by many gadgets which are clinically unimportant and a frequent cause for breakdowns of the machine. Modifications based on different types of current will be discussed later.

Several types of electrodes are in use. Metal strips or a meshwork mounted on a rubber sponge, were originally recommended because they permit the greatest adaptability to the shape of the patient's head, but simple metal discs may also be used. We still very definitely prefer Bini's forceps electrode in which the electrodes are mounted by movable articulations on a bearer system whose two arms act like the two blades of a large forceps. This type of electrode permits strong local pressure on the head and can be much more easily applied than electrodes fixed with rubber bands which slip off easily when the patient moves his head.

Von Braunmühl overcomes the difficulty of applying electrodes in disturbed patients by pressing them against the temples manually. Elaborate systems have been devised by Holzer. For instance, when it is impossible for the operator to stand behind the patient's bed, he recommends fastening the electrodes to a bridge which can be easily applied to the patient's head from the side. Bini has used a device in which the current flows through the head clamp only as long as it is pressed against the patient's head. This and other devices actually do away with the time measurement and let the current flow until the patient reacts with a generalized seizure.

Skin resistance is usually decreased by an electrode jelly such as is commonly used in electrocardiography or electroencephalography. Swabbing the temples with alcohol in which a small quantity of saturated saline has been dissolved is recommended by Hemphill and Grey Walter in order to remove the grease film and replace it with the conducting solution. Salt water alone is used by others.

A preliminary measurement of the patient's head-resistance can be omitted. The resistance varies as much as from two hundred to several thousand ohms with various workers; also, the individual worker will find wide variations in different patients, and even in the same patient on different days. There is a marked drop in resistance after the first passage of a stimulating current. No definite relation was found between preliminary measurement of the resistance and the amount of current necessary to produce a convulsion. Milliammeters which measure the current actually passing through the patient's head during the application can also be omitted. The time during which the current flows is so short that the needle of such an instrument easily overshoots, making exact measurement impossible unless an expensive ballistic milliammeter is used.

Amount of current: Potential differences of 70 to 130 volts for 0.1 to 0.5 seconds will produce a convulsion with the usual technique. The actual amount of current passing during the treatment was found to range between 200 and 1600 ma. Sogliani was the first to keep the voltage constant at 110 volts and to increase only the time of voltage passage if necessary. Strauss and MacPhail set a fixed time of 0.35 seconds and increase only the current. Others set the machine at a standard voltage and time reading which is sufficiently high to produce a convulsion in all patients, even those with high thresholds. In our own work we originally started with 70 volts for 0.2 sec. in the hope that the patient might have a delayed, slowly developing seizure which resembles the seizure of epileptics who are less prone to fractures. Since muscle relaxants are being used, we apply a maximum stimulus to assure an immediate convulsion. With some machines the desired intensity is reached gradually within 6 or 8 tenths of a sec. This gradual increase, called the "glissando" technique by Tietz, has found wide application. It was thought that thereby the patient would go into a more slowly developing convulsion and be less endangered by fractures, a problem which no longer exists.

Few reports deal with the electrophysiologic implications of ECT. Grey Walter discusses the spread of current in the cerebral tissue and comes to the conclusion that the electrical resistance network made up of scalp, skull, and meninges attenuates the brain potential approximately a hundredfold. Alexander and Loewenbach tried to determine the pathway of the current experimentally by tracing the vascular reaction in certain parts of the brain. However, only with doses above the therapeutic dose, both with regard to strength and duration, did they produce clearcut capillary anemia of the frontal lobes. Ewald and Haddenbrock suggest that the greater density of the current has to be assumed in the parts close to the ventricles. Hemphill and Grey Walter call the fear of high currents "superstitious," as the stimulating current spreads widely and its intensity is not great in any area of the brain. Hayes came to the same conclusion in a careful study of the distribution of the current through the simian head.

Page and Russel tried to improve the therapeutic effect by increased voltage and duration and, furthermore, by applying several aditional stimuli during the convulsion itself. This procedure of giving treatment with five additional stimulations was repeated up to three times on the same day, thereby reducing both failures and relapses to half compared with the usual ECT routine. We are inclined to believe that not the additional stimuli but the frequent convulsions explain their good results. An interesting observation by these authors was that the additional stimuli caused no intensification of the convulsion. We made the same observation; that no response occurs during and also for a minute or so after a convulsion.

Unidirectional and brief stimuli techniques: Various types of current have been applied in ECT. Friedman and Wilcox recommended unidirectional wave forms eliminating the alternating oscillation of the city current. They claim that in this way the amount of current necessary for provocation of a convulsion can be lowered, and that the memory impairment as well as the electroencephalographic changes following a course of treatments are less marked. These authors, however, use a longer total time of stimulation and, consequently, their claim that a lower voltage is required is doubtful in view of Hemphill"s and Grey Walter's findings that increasing the time lowers the voltage necessary whatever the current used. The duration of each pulse of the stimulating current used in the classical and in the unidirectional technique is considerably larger than the chronaxie of the cortical motor neurons. Liberson, therefore, replaces the 60 per second stimulation by a "brief stimuli" technique, individual stimuli lasting from one-sixth to one-third millisecond. Under these conditions convulsions are produced with at least twenty times less electrical energy as compared with the classical technique.

Our own experience never convinced us that any current or any machine give superior results compared to others. Much discussion has centered around the various currents used in the machines manufactured by Reuben Reiter. One of his most widely used machines delivers a series of spiked unidirectional pulses of 0.1 to 0.2 milliseconds. This machine has not only been used for convulsive treatment but also for non-convulsive methods. Wilcox recommends it for a very elaborate individualization of the electrical stimulation based on such factors as the type of awakening of the patient after the treatment. Impastato using the Reiter machine, recommended to maintain the current during the clonic phase, and L. Alexander, doing the same, reduces the current to a level where it works as a respiratory stimulant. Robie recommends the Reiter Electrostimulator for electric stimulation in his treatment of patients with barbiturate poisoning. Friedman using this machine, follows the regular convulsion with 3 to 5 minutes of as much current as will permit stertorous breathing; he prefers this in cases with severe anxiety. The so-called "Sedac High Frequency Stimulator" can be attached to this machine. When the current from the Electrostimulator passes through this attachment consisting of a neon-type filtering bulb, all the low frequency elements are filtered out, and only the very high frequency values pass through. The current in the lower ranges is almost painless and considered helpful for psychotherapeutic purposes, although it has been recommended for a variety of psychiatric and neurological conditions. In a survey Ulett et al. rightly come to the conclusion that claims by Eyres et al. are not convincing enough to change the negative findings by others regarding this type of current. The "counter-shocks" with non-convulsive stimulation after the convulsive treatment as a means to diminish amnesia as recommended by L. Alexander, was also questioned by others (Cronholm and Ottosson, Pulver and Jacobs).

Delmas-Marsalet uses a pulsating direct current, half-wave rectified 50-cycles, similar to the unidirectional current of Friedman, but with short duration of stimulus and high intensity. His experimental work leads to the conclusion that the appearance of the electric convulsion depends not on the quantity of electricity or on the wattage but rather on Lapicque's laws of iterative excitation of the nervous centers. Strauss and MacPhail's instrument for "electroplexy" stimulates with a condensor discharge which is interrupted by a high-speed oscillating vacuum switch. The initial stimulus is maximal and decreases during the condensor discharge, quite contrary to the "glissando" technique (see above). Larrogoiti tried to reduce the intensity of the current by interrupting the 60-cycle alternating current 900 times a second.

We cannot discuss here all the technical problems involved in wave form, pulse strength and duration, intervals between the pulses, polarity, and summation, and must refer to Spiegel's Progress in Neurology and Psychiatry with surveys by Wilcox, Ulett et al., and Smith and Biddy.

Unilateral ECT

The use of unilaterally applied current was first recommended by Thenon in Argentina in 1956. His reason was to reduce the area of the electrical impact. He already preferred the non-dominant hemisphere and found less marked confusion of the patient who recovers with perfect notion of time and place. Independently Lancaster et al. published the first report in the English language in 1958 based on the observation of many of us that focal fits with or without unilateral application lead to less confusion. A second reason for the work by these authors was the unsubstantiated fear of eye damage with bilateral stimulation. The authors used the non-dominant side of the skull assuming that damage of brain function on this side would be less significant. The lower electrodes were applied slightly above a line between the lateral angle of the orbit and the external auditory meatus; the upper electrode was placed 7½ cm higher. Slight deviations from these points are immaterial. Generalized seizures were obtained with this unilateral application. The authors found less memory impairment but, interestingly enough, they already had the clinical impression that bilaterally induced seizures had slightly better therapeutic results. Therefore, they recommended unilateral treatment for less serious depressions and for patients in whom memory impairment would interfere with their job.

It was only in 1962 that Cannicott took up this line of research. He came to the conclusion of less memory impairment and good clinical results, although some of his colleagues had the impression that unilateral treatment had to be given more frequently than bilateral in order to be effective.

Martin et al. and most subsequent workers claimed more unequivocally than the first two papers that therapeutically the results are identical which is contrary to our own personal experience (L.B.K.) No questions, however can arise regarding the amazing and not easily understood absence of memory impairment of unilateral ECT. Only McAndrew et al., on the basis of more elaborate tests such as the Finger Agnosia Test question the absence of organic signs in unilateral electrode placement.

Electroencephalographic studies demonstrated clearly the unilateral predominance of electroencephalographic changes which were of the type usually found over both cerebral hemispheres after bilateral ECT. The logical conclusion is that the current as such is responsible for the electroencephalographic changes as well as for the concomitant confusion and memory impairment. No explanation offers itself why this is so, when we consider that pharmacological treatment with the inhalant Indoklon leads to the same if not greater degree of confusion than bilateral ECT.

The importance of electrode placement on the nondominant hemisphere was tested by Zamora and Kaelbling who found memory impairment more significant in electrode placement over the dominant hemisphere, although it was still less pronounced than with bilateral placement. In a more elaborate study, Gottlieb and Wilson attributed some importance to the placement of unilateral electrodes over the parietal and temporal lobes compared to the frontal stimulation in bilateral ECT.

The decisive factor for the preference of unilateral over bilateral treatment is, of course, the therapeutic efficacy. Some of the papers published so far, did not really evaluate results in a convincing way. Others left some question marks. Thus, Impastato and Karliner admitted that more treatments must be given if unilateral ECT is applied, and that in disturbed patients bilateral treatment is more effective. On the other hand, the absence of confusion makes it possible to reduce the total treatment time by applying unilateral ECT daily as was done by Abrams, who was able to discharge a patient immediately without memory impairment even after 20 daily treatments. Two recent studies by Cannicot and Waggoner, and by Abrams and de Vito comparing unilateral and bilateral treatment, support previous results. Strain et al. who contributed very careful memory studies, caution that in high risk patients the more reliable bilateral treatment might be preferable because a greater number of treatments would also require more frequent anesthetic exposure.

Most original reports were based on schizophrenic material, where evaluation of results is known to be difficult. In endogenous depressions which always clear up under a few bilateral ECT, our experience (LBK) with unilateral ECT has been unconvincing. Before reporting this in more detail we should mention that just recently a single issue of the British Journal of Psychiatry contained three favorable reports on depressions treated with unilateral ECT (Zinkin and Birtchnell; Valentine et al.; Halliday et al.). We can unequivocally agree with the claim of considerable less memory impairment even in very old patients who in previous treatments had shown most pronounced organic reactions. However, our clinical results were unsatisfactory. Most informative was our experience with depressed patients who could be their own controls because we had treated them successfully in previous depressions over a period of up to 20 years. They did improve but in a less convincing way, and they relapsed early or remained moderately depressed. Two patients drew the dangerous conclusion after a few treatments that they had reached the point, where the previously successful treatment was no longer effective in their case, and, therefore, considered suicide. Others carried on their activities but had to return for bilateral treatment without having recovered completely. Attempts to combine the two treatments were made by removing the more serious symptoms of a depression with three bilateral ECT and then continuing with unilateral ECT. This led to several relapses and the need for a return to bilateral treatment with prolongation of the total treatment time. Multiple treatments within a single day are being investigated. At the present time we feel that the goal of recovery within a short period of time should not be jeopardized by relying on unilateral ECT which has the important advantage of less memory impairment but which has not yet proven its therapeutical efficacy.

Electric Narcosis

Attempts to replace convulsive therapy with an electrically induced narcosis for the treatment of mental illness represent a logical development. The aim of such attempts is to protect the patient against the violence of the muscular discharge with its imminent danger of fractures; it would also permit prolongation of the individual application of the treatment. Unconsciousness without the muscular phenomena was also induced by applying subconvulsive stimuli with the usual electric shock technique, but therapeutic results were disappointing. True electric narcosis has never been achieved, and therapeutic attempts, described in this chapter, actually produced modified convulsions which were of some interest but did not replace ECT.

Research along such lines was available since long before the shock treatment era. Leduc, in 1902, induced what he called "electric sleep" and general anesthesia by means of unidirectional pulsating current of high frequency applied to the nervous system. In the first experiments on animals the sleep-like condition was preceded by a convulsion, but later on, by using a rheostat to step up the current slowly, the convulsion could be prevented, so that the animal fell asleep gradually. The first human being to be treated in this way was Leduc himself. Respiration and pulse remained normal during the stimulation which actually produced "Electric Sleep" as used by Soviet psychiatrists (see next chapter).

Experiments, aimed at replacing ECT with electric narcosis, were made by Frostig et al. They used 60 cycle alternating current. Milliamperage of 250 is applied and maintained for thirty seconds; after that the stimulation is decreased to a level at which respiration becomes possible (45 to 90 ma.). The current intensity is then gradually raised again to a maximum of 125 ma. After seven minutes the current is interrupted. The patient responds to the initial current with a tonic spasm in which he remains as long as the full amount of current is applied. This phase is accompanied by arrest of pulse and respiration. When, after thirty seconds, the current is reduced, a few clonic movements take place. During the following minutes of slowly increasing stimulation, the patient is sometimes relaxed and does not move. More often he is in a rigid state with arms flexed and legs extended. The patient is left in this state for seven minutes. Some workers continue this "narcosis state" for a longer period of time. The patient may become quite restless and resist the treatment which he obviously begins to feel. The placement of the electrodes is said to be of some importance. Ordinarily they are placed 5 cm. anterior to the external meatus. Goldman advances them forward if the patient has respiratory difficulties, and uses a more posterior position if there is too much restlessness.

Several complications, especially collapses similar to those of traumatic shock, were observed by Garmany and Early. They also saw confusion which appeared related to cerebral anoxia. Since their results with electronarcosis were not superior to ECT, these authors as well as others advised strongly against further use of this treatment. Altschule reported fatal adrenal apoplexy under electric narcosis in a patient who had had 45 regular ECT without accident.

The physiological concomitants of electronarcosis, studied particularly by Rees, correspond closely to those observed in regular ECT, although blood pressure rise, salivary, bronchial and perspiratory secretion, blood sugar rise, and so on, are more pronounced. The fact that increased autonomic responses do not increase the effectiveness of the treatment and do not clear up a depression with a lesser number of treatments than ordinary ECT can be taken as evidence that autonomic responses are not the effective agent of these treatments.

It is open to dispute whether the term "electronarcosis" is justified for the technique described above. The initial tonic state apparently does not differ in any way from the tonic phase of a convulsion. This and the few clonic movements which become visible after the current is reduced make it appear that the treatment is actually an electrically induced convulsion in which the usual development of the clonic phase is prevented by the continued stimulation;

and that only when the stimulating current is decreased does the end of the suppressed clonic phase come through.

Thompson et al. originally claimed superiority of electronarcosis over ECT. Its therapeutic effect in schizophrenia was said to be similar to that of insulin treatment. However, in their original report they compared a series of patients treated routinely with 15 treatments with the unduly poor results of others who obviously had used a much smaller number of standard ECT. Goldman saw favorable results in the same type of patients responding to ECT. Tietz, Paterson Monro, and Geoghegan consider it to be better than ECT and safer than insulin. Medlicott saw no better results than with ECT except for anxiety, hypochondriasis, and in paranoids. Dax gave it up after an extensive trial.

Our own two years' experience with electronarcosis did not convince us of its superiority over standard ECT. It is cumbersome, and many patients become apprehensive if they happen to feel the current toward the end of the treatment. The best evidence that the effective part is the initial convulsion only is the need for an equal number of electronarcosis treatments in depressed patients as they had required with standard ECT in previous episodes. The same observation was made in an extensive and critical study on electronarcosis therapy by Bowman and Simon. These authors also found that electronarcosis is no better than ECT in manic-depressives and schizophrenics.

Electric Sleep

Electric sleep treatment as introduced by Giljarowskij and co-workers is one of the features of Soviet psychiatry that attracted the greatest interest in the United States. Yet, it seems to be used very little in psychiatric centers in its country of origin. Giljarowskij's contention that it has a cerebral effect is questioned by most of the others. What is emphasized as being therapeutically useful is the rhythmic nature of a peripheral stimulation which indirectly produces sleep even when the electrodes are applied to the legs. The usual technique consists of applying one electrode to the occipital region and the other to the root of the nose with extensions to both eyes. The patient is placed in a dark room and told that he will fall asleep within less than half an hour. The current may be left on for two hours, and the patient usually continues to sleep after the current has been turned off. A group of several patients can be treated with several leads from the same machine. Electric sleep is also used in insulin treatment during the precomatose state to facilitate sleep. The main indications for electric sleep are not the psychoses but neurotic conditions of various kinds including nervous exhaustion and neurotic depressions.

These remarks are based on impressions by Kalinowsky during a visit to some psychiatric facilities in the Soviet Union. The original work by the late Giljarowskij and his co-workers is best available in a German translation of his monograph that appeared under the title "Elektroschlaf."

More recently some reports have appeared in the American literature about the use of electrosleep in psychiatric disorders. Miller and Mathas treated various patients with a commercially produced machine applying the current

30 to 50 minutes several times a week. Only a small fraction of the patients actually fell asleep. Neither these authors nor Woods et al. in another report were able to establish a therapeutic effect in any disease groups treated. It is even doubted whether currents of the magnitude employed, would penetrate the cranium in sufficient intensity to produce the changes which the Russian originators of the method assume. The EEG can show a sleep pattern of reduced alpha amplitude in patients who sleep but also in some who did not sleep.

Examinations Prior to ECT

Little preparation is necessary prior to ECT, and there is no uniformity of opinion as to what examinations should be made. In addition to the usual routine examinations of the chest organs, blood pressure, and so on, a number of special examinations have been suggested. Most of them have limited importance, as the findings obtained with them rarely have produced contraindication. In hospitalized patients a general medical work-up is customary in every patient at the time of admission. In emergency ECT such work-up can be dispensed with. It is also unnecessary to delay ambulatory treatment, or to burden such patients with the expense for tests which are non-contributory to the decision regarding ECT.

Electrocardiograms were not routinely done in unpremedicated ECT. The use of barbiturate anesthesia made electrocardiographic examinations more important, and the demonstration of myocardial damage might suggest avoidance of the barbiturate anesthesia even when muscle relaxation is administered. Soon after the introduction of ECT it was pointed out that in agitated psychotics even severe myocardial damage is not a contraindication for ECT. We treated our largest series of institutional patients before the advent of anesthesia techniques without an electrocardiograph at our disposal, and we had no accidents. Like X-rays of the chest, an electrocardiogram is a desirable procedure in patients over 40, but it is not indispensable and should not delay treatment or increase the financial burden for the family.

Electroencephalograms are not necessary prior to ECT. In rare cases it might be interesting to find a convulsive brain pattern prior to treatment as demonstrated in our rare instances of such patterns or convulsions after ECT (Pacella et al.). If present, however, a convulsive pattern does not preclude treatment.

Lateral x-ray of the spine was recommended by Smith et al. as a control for later post-treatment films to check on previous compression fractures for medico-legal reasons. Since muscle relaxation is used, such X-rays have become valueless. Osteoarthritic and other changes of the spine were not considered as precluding ECT even without muscle relaxation.

Pathological conditions should be known to the therapist prior to ECT, and the risk weighed against the risk of the psychosis. The later sections on Complications and Contraindications endeavor to enable the psychiatrist himself to select the patients and to be aware of possible risks.

Preparation of the Patient

Each individual treatment requires little preparation of the patient. If treated in the morning, the patient should have no food. If treated after mid-day, he may have a light breakfast consisting of coffee or tea, and one slice of toast at least four hours prior to the treatment. Otherwise, nausea is frequent, and vomiting during the treatment is particularly dangerous in premedicated ECT, when the gag reflex is absent due to muscle relaxant medication. The patient should void the bladder shortly before the treatment.

Dentures are a special problem. While plates are usually removed in anesthesia, we prefer to leave partial dentures in place because often oddly spaced teeth may easily break or fall out in spite of muscle relaxation. They are better protected, when the partial plate is left in. If such patients are carefully watched, partial dentures are no danger during the short anesthesia. It is known that in otherwise completely relaxed patients the jaw muscles still contract strongly enough to endanger weak teeth. The explanation seems to be the direct muscular stimulation of the jaw muscles by the electrodes. This can be eliminated by pharmacological convulsive therapy, and we, therefore, prefer Indoklon to ECT in patients with loose teeth.

Chewing gum, of course, should be removed, but we are sure to have inadvertedly treated patients with chewing gum without having encountered untoward effects. Hair pins and other metal objects are often removed, although there are no reports of accidents, when this is not done. If the patient does not wear a nightgown or pajamas, tight clothing should be loosened.

All medication should be omitted in the morning because of the requirement of an empty stomach. Sleeping medication can be given during the night before the treatment. Sedatives for the purpose of alleviating fear of the treatment have little value, but they are not harmful. More problematic is the question of psychotropic drugs in patients under ECT given with barbiturate anesthesia. Most psychotropic drugs lower the blood pressure which also tends to fall under intravenous barbiturates as well as during a convulsive seizure. It is, therefore not surprising that the Rauwolfia derivatives led to serious hypotension and even fatalities during ECT. The same danger has been claimed for phenothiazines, but some experienced workers like Sargant combine phenothiazines and ECT without apparent trouble. Anesthesiologists are more hesitant to give barbiturate anesthesia to patients under phenothiazines. Koupernik advises to discontinue all hypotensive drugs 72 hours before ECT and wait in patients under reserpine as long as two weeks. Gonzalez and Imahara conclude that phenothiazines, contrary to reserpine, can be combined with ECT. Our own present opinion is that the combination of ECT with phenothiazines and antidepressant drugs is not as dangerous as it was originally thought to be. However, we rarely use this combination because there is no proof that it is more effective than ECT alone. In our ECT work we still prefer to delay treatment in patients under high doses of phenothiazines for a day or two in order to reduce the blood level at least to some degree. We, like most workers, always omit all neuroleptic drugs on the morning of the treatment and prefer barbiturates for the sedation of patients scheduled for ECT.

The same precaution is taken with antidepressants because of their hypotensive effect, although no untoward experiences became known with these groups of drugs in connection with ECT.

Nausea after the treatment can be prevented with 100 mg. dramamine by mouth before the treatment or by intramuscular injection after the treatment. Even more effective and apparently safe is intramuscular injection of Compazine, 5 mg., which can also be injected intravenously—although this appears to be less harmless—after the convulsion into the tubing which we use routinely in premedicated ECT (see section on Present Technique of ECT). If patients wake up with post-treatment excitement—an occurrence which is not less frequent since barbiturate anesthesia is used—the same tubing can be used for a very slow drip infusion of the barbiturate for a period of 20 min. after the next treatment. Hypnosis used for anesthesia by Weinberg et al. was not found by us to be reliable. Various other aspects of hypnosis and ECT were discussed by Maholik and Wartentin, and by Bowers and Berkowitz.

Premedication with cardiovascular stimulants is usually limited to individual cases. For patients who have shown respiratory difficulties in previous treatments, metrazol was recommended prior to the electrical stimulus. Injection of 5 cc. of coramine intravenously was recommended by Fabing for patients with psychotic excitement. This method gives good results comparable to metrazol convulsive therapy which, in excitement states is considered by some to be superior to the electrical method. Fabing explains the efficacy of this combined chemical and electrical stimulation as an "ultramaximal stimulus" in the sense of Pavlow with the resulting state of cortical inhibition; Jacquel et al. confirmed the good results, explaining them in terms of vasomotor cerebral changes.

Atropine is given routinely by many therapists. In vagotonic patients with a history of "vagal" crisis Larragoiti first recommended it. It became widely used after the introduction of barbiturate anesthesia and muscle relaxant drugs. Vagal stimulation during ECT is considered the main factor causing cardiac arrest. Richardson et al. recommended 1/25 grain of atropine (2.4 mg.) as completely blocking the cardiac portion of the vagus nerve. Cropper and Hughes consider 1/45 grain (2 mg.) the minimal dose to be given intravenously just prior to the barbiturate, and state that the often recommended dose of 1/50 grain (0.4 mg.) half an hour before the treatment is inadequate.

Considering the doubtful evidence of efficacy of atropine prior to ECT, we have never used atropine in ECT and were strengthened in this attitude by some animal experimentation which showed a high percentage of fatalities in electrically induced convulsions in mice pretreated with a variety of atropinic substances (Sabelli). Prior to the introduction of anesthesia techniques for ECT we considered a convulsion such a natural occurrence that we hesitated to complicate the treatment with any drug. We also like to spare the patient the additional discomfort of dryness of the mouth from atropine. Although the anesthesia is an additional element in the treatment, our extensive experience did not suggest to us a change in our thinking regarding atropine, as an unnecessary premedication in ECT.

The Use of Muscle Relaxant Drugs

OLDER METHODS INCLUDING CURARE: A. E. Bennett has done pioneer work in the chemical prevention of fractures in convulsive therapy. After Hamsa and Bennett suggested metrazol treatment under spinal anesthesia, Bennett, in 1940, reported on the use of curare (extracted from Chondodendron tomentosum). Appropriate dosage will not paralyze the muscles completely but will "soften" their contraction sufficiently to prevent surgical complications. Curare was first used in the form of a concentrated aqueous extract known as "Intocostrin." Various curare preparations were later synthesized and were equally effective but, unfortunately, equally dangerous.

Phenomena very similar to myasthenia gravis are observed. Paralysis of the eye muscles (ptosis and visual disturbances) are first noticed; huskiness of the voice comes next. Difficulty in lifting the head is the best test for the progressive paralysis. The muscles of the legs and arms follow, and weakness of the respiratory muscles is last. Prostigmine 1 cc. injected intravenously, is a reliable antidote for the paralyzing effect of curare, but is apparently not able to prevent a probable central effect responsible for a great number of fatalities.

Fatalities were reported in some of the first investigations on convulsive therapy with curare (Charlton et al. in metrazol; Ebaugh et al.; Smith et al., Cash and Hoeckstra in ECT), and Impastato and Almansi stated as early as 1943 that an unduly large percentage of the fatalities reported in ECT had been treated with curare. Its use was discontinued after the number of reported fatalities increased steadily. Frequently fatalities were described as electroshock fatalities but were obviously due to the curare. This is particularly well illustrated by patients who died from curare before ECT had been applied as in the well documented case of Riggs and Schlomer. One of us (L.B.K.) had his first fatality after many thousand patients in a case treated with curare.

Many other drugs with curare-like action were recommended for use in convulsive therapy. Less toxic chemicals with moderate muscle relaxant effect were also given. Recently, Ekinoi et al. unsuccessfully tried diazepam (Valium) to prevent fractures. Actually this can be accomplished only with drugs paralyzing the muscles completely. Today all previous such drugs were given up in favor of succinylcholine.

SUCCINYLCHOLINE: Today the muscle relaxant of choice in ECT is succinylcholine. Premedication with this drug has been introduced in 1951 by Holmberg and Thesleff in Sweden, and at the same time by Arnold and Boeck-Greissau in Vienna. Succinylcholine iodide had been discovered in 1949 by the Nobel prize winner Bovet. It is broken down in the body by esterases probably into succinyl acid and choline, both of which are natural metabolites. This explains the short duration of the effect and the low toxicity. Even large doses have no effect on the circulatory system. There is no cumulative effect even with repeated doses, and while there are some differences in individual sensitivity, its action lasts only for a few minutes. It is administered intravenously, and relaxation is obtained within one or two minutes. The relaxation is preceded by muscular fibrillations and fasciculations. There is no antidote, but the rapidity with which it is broken down, makes an antidote unnecessary.

The convulsion will last somewhat longer which might be explained by the oversaturation with oxygen in a treatment given under constant oxygen supply (Holmberg).

Arnold and Boeck-Greissau injected a small test dose to determine the sensitivity. This is still being done by some workers but seems to be unnecessary. The normal dose lies between 0.1 and 0.3 mg. per Kg. of body weight. Arnold and Boeck-Greissau injected succinylcholine without barbiturate, which, undoubtedly, is less dangerous but unpleasant for the patient because he experiences respiratory distress from the paralysis of his respiratory muscles, and it appears also that the muscular contractions preceding the relaxation are painful. Holberg and Thesleff, even in their first report, recommended combination with a barbiturate. They slowly inject intravenously within 60 seconds a mixture of succinylcholine and 0.15 or 0.2 Gm. of pentothal. On account of the alcaline pH of the barbituric acid derivate, the succinyl choline is broken down fairly rapidly and should be drawn up only minutes prior to the injection, or, preferably, in a different syringe. Immediately after the injection has been given, oxygen is applied by insufflation. When the patient is relaxed, the convulsion is given; and, after the convulsion, insufflation of oxygen is continued until the patient breathes by himself after one to several minutes. Many modifications of this method have been recommended and were listed in a survey by Impastato and Berg. If the succinylcholine is injected in the same syringe with the pentothal the patient may have unpleasant sensations before he falls asleep. Therefore, most psychiatrists prefer to give the pentothal first, and the succinylcholine in a special syringe.

Present Technique of ECT

Our own technique developed by the anesthesiologist S. Dell'Aria is as follows: Realizing that some of the complications in the use of intravenous barbiturates are due to the concentrated solutions, we prefer the drip method using a 0.2 per cent solution of the fast acting barbiturate methohexital (Brevital) in 5 per cent dextrose solution after insertion of an 18 gauge thin wall needle with the container hung up at a level of about 40 inches above the patient. An average of approximately 40 mg. of Brevital are sufficient to induce sleep. Then the drip system is switched to the drip of a solution of 0.2 per cent succinylcholine chloride (Anectine) in 5 per cent dextrose solution. Instead of changing bottles, a three-way stopcock can be used. At this point we begin to oxygenate the patient, first by spontaneous respiration and then by assisted and controlled respiration. Fasciculations soon appear followed by almost complete muscle relaxation which is obtained with an average dose of 25 mg. The convulsion is produced, and the patient's respiration continues to be assisted until spontaneous respiration resumes. Only when the vital signs return to normal, the needle of the tubing is withdrawn because in case of complications emergency injections can be given through the tubing without delay.

A comparison between the above method and giving the solution by syringe has convinced us of the superiority of the drip method which permits oxygenation during the entire procedure, and limits the amount of the drugs used, to a minimum, rendering the treatment more innocuous.

We prefer to have the assistance of a fully trained anesthetist. Unexpected accidents may occur: One of our patients who had eaten a full meal without our knowledge, vomited, and the gastric content threatened to suffocate him because of the absence of the gag reflex due to the succinylcholine. Only the anesthetist's skill saved the patient; and we know of two similar instances, without an anesthetist, where death occurred in one and lung gangrene in the other. It is because of such accidents that we feel more comfortable with an anesthetist without claiming that his presence is a conditio sine qua non. There are still hospitals where preference is given to ECT without muscle relaxants. There is little doubt that the anesthesia techniques connected with ECT add to the dangers for the patient's life, while the dangers of unpremedicated ECT are bone complications which never endanger his life. The most decisive reason for the use of ECT with anesthesia are medico-legal considerations because of many successful malpractice suits against psychiatrists based on fractures in ECT. Today legal actions in connection with ECT hardly occur.

Although the managing of a patient during the treatment is different when muscle relaxants are used, the rules outlined for unpremedicated ECT should not be completely ignored because even in the hands of experienced therapists muscle relaxation may be incomplete at times. In such instances adherence to older established rules may prevent complications. The best way is to have the patient in a relaxed and unrestrained position. The shoulders are lightly held by a nurse in order to prevent extreme arm movements which would also displace the infusion needle. The legs do not have to be held because in unpremedicated ECT fractures of femur and acetabulum occurred from holding the legs tightly extended.

A subjective complaint in connection with succinylcholine was first reported by Baumer and Baumgartl, and confirmed by us: It is an unexplained pain in jaw and neck which is mostly experienced in the first treatment but not in subsequent ones. A few patients complain of generalized muscle pains which may be due to the first phase of succinylcholine action characterized by fasciculations. Actual dangers do not seem to be connected with succinylcholine. Oversensitivity with prolonged apnea is extremely rare and, with oxygenation, should not be any problem. It never was in our experience. In conditions like liver disease, where serum cholinesterase levels may be reduced, apnea after succinylcholine may be prolonged. According to Matthew and Consten, plasma and whole blood should be available for transfusion in such cases.

It was soon recognized that cardiovascular complications due to barbiturate anesthesia, are more frequent than in unpremedicated ECT (Baumer, von Baeyer, others). Some fatalities have been reported, and some are known to us from personal communications. More frequent are instances of patients becoming pale and pulseless. We have seen this in several patients who had withstood previous unpremedicated treatments without difficulty and again took the treatment very well when it was continued without premedication. We also know of a number of patients with previous coronary thrombosis who suffered new attacks shortly after treatment with premedicated ECT, an occurrence which is exceptionally rare in unpremedicated ECT. We had three such cases in our own material but none in our much larger series of unpremedicated ECT. There is little doubt that the muscle relaxant succinylcholoine is not responsible for such accidents, but that it is the intravenous barbiturate, although Robinson and De Mott reported a fatality with succinylcholine probably due to a preexisting liver damage. Shorter-acting barbiturates than pentothal were recommended. Fatalities due to pentothal are known to all anesthetists. In the psychiatric literature, Maclay mentioned 9 anesthesia deaths where pentothal had been used for mostly minor procedures in mental patients. Anesthetists are also familiar with the fact that accidents occur even in younger people but with greater frequency in patients with cardiovascular diseases when intravenous pentothal is used. Although it has been claimed, contrary to our own opinion, that the pentothal-succinylcholine medication makes the treatment safer for cardiac patients, other psychiatrists must have had similar experiences and accidents. Lieser warns against succinylcholine when ECT is used in pernicious catatonia or patients in cardiac or respiratory distress. Impastato recommended a technique that omits the barbiturate and makes the patient unconscious by means of a subconvulsive stimulus. He gives $\frac{1}{50}$ gr. atropine 30 minutes prior to treatment. 10 mg. succinylcholine are injected intravenously, and 10 seconds later a petit mal or subconvulsive stimulus is given. This is followed 20 seconds later, or whenever the patient is relaxed, with a full convulsive stimulus. Whereas 20 to 40 mg. are necessary to produce relaxation in a barbiturized patient, 10 mg. are usually sufficient, when a petit mal is used for anesthesia. We have used this technique extensively but found two disadvantages. It is difficult to establish the proper amount of current for the petit mal response. If the current is set too low, the patient feels the "electric shock" and becomes frightened; if too much current is used a convulsion rather than a petit mal may ensue before the succinylcholine has become effective. We, therefore, limit this technique to patients in whom cardiovascular, respiratory or allergic conditions make barbiturate anesthesia inadvisable.

Today the faster acting barbiturate methohexital (Brevital) is generally preferred to penthotal. The patients wake up faster, and side-effects including nausea seem to be less frequent. However, neither Brevital nor other barbiturates prevent the occurrence of postconvulsive excitement nor do they seem to make the treatment experience more acceptable to the patient. This clinical impression by us was confirmed in a double blind study by Huggins comparing barbiturate-modified and unmodified ECT.

Another attempt to avoid barbiturate anesthesia was made by Weinberg et al. They used hypnosis to make the patient unaware of the injection of succinylcholine and the subsequent respiratory distress. This method worked well in a number of cases, but in others the patients became extremely fearful because their hypnotic state was not sufficiently deep to mitigate the respiratory discomfort.

A sponge inserted between the teeth usually offers sufficient protection for the teeth, but tongue bite is more safely prevented by a loop-like mouth gag made of rubber tubes; this also prevents biting on the more precious incisors.

If the patient has partial dentures resting on irregularly spaced teeth, it is much safer to leave the partial dentures in, for reasons given in the section on Preparation of the Patient.

After the convulsion the therapist's attention should continue to be directed to the patient's respiration. After the treatment the patient must be watched so that he does not get out of bed. Straps or sheets to tie him to the bed should be available in case he becomes assaultive in the post-convulsive state. Even if this may increase his panic, it is unavoidable, when help is limited. No patient should get up until he is able to answer simple questions satisfactorily. Even when this is the case, the patient may still misinterpret the situation and become dangerous.

Discomfort after the treatment is not infrequent with complaints of headache, dizziness and nausea. These symptoms occur more often, when anesthesia is used. Intramuscular injection of Dramamine and other antiemetics is often necessary, and patients are not encouraged to eat for one or two hours after the treatment.

Spacing of Treatments. Regressive ECT. Prophylactic ECT

Convulsive treatment was originally applied by most workers twice a week, and later three treatments a week became the more commonly accepted procedure. Daily treatments lead to confusional states. The first three treatments given within five days, remove the most acute symptoms as, for instance, the danger of suicide in depressions. In Germany the "Bloc" of three treatments on subsequent days is frequently used for this purpose; but it is our experience that this leads to unnecessary confusion, especially in older patients. After the most disturbing symptoms have been removed, further scheduling of treatments will depend on whether the patient is in a hospital, where confusion would be less disturbing, or whether ambulatory treatment is given, in which organic symptoms should be avoided as much as possible. In depressions, for instance, it became our routine to give three treatments the first week, two the second week, and one more a week later. Recently, however, Blachly and Gowing gave 4-8 bilateral ECT in a single session without any regression and with amnesia and confusion usually seen after 1-2 treatments.

In very acutely disturbed patients such as catatonic excitement states (Pernicious catatonia) three treatments given within the first day are well tolerated and often a life-saving procedure. Poor physical condition or fever, not infrequent in these cases, are definitely no contraindication for such active treatment.

Sogliani has shown that electrically induced convulsions may be repeated within a few minutes after regular respiration is obtained and the patient begins to regain consciousness. In this way he has given as many as five convulsions within ten to twenty minutes. He applies this procedure in all patients who fail to recover with the usual treatment. As many as eight treatments a day have been given by Jacobs and Gilson. We agree with Valentine that it is not possible to reduce the total number of necessary convulsions by using such intensive treatment. Such summation treatment (Heuyer et al.) was also called "regressive" treatment by Kennedy and Anchel, and "annihilation" treatment by Bini. He, and independently, Milligan recommended it primarily for psychoneuroses. Glueck et al. are in favor of replacing regular ECT with regressive treatment because of the frequent relapses after standard courses of ECT. They describe the technique of three treatments a day in several hours' intervals for several days a week until "regression is complete." This requires an average of 34 treatments, and in some patients even up to 65. A state of regression is reached when the patient is incontinent in both bowel and bladder function, has dysarthria or muteness, and requires spoon feeding. The patients regress further after treatment is discontinued. They also have neurological findings such as rigidity, increased reflexes and Babinski sign. Emergence from this state takes 7 to 10 days. No lasting damage occurs as evidenced by psychological tests in 50 patients. Also the electroencephalographic changes clear up completely. Temporary disturbed behavior in the sense of organic reactions can be controlled with neuroleptic drugs. The authors consider this treatment as superior to both standard ECT and insulin coma treatment, and request a trial with this method in all schizophrenics under consideration for psychosurgery. They see the main indication in catatonics and paranoids among the group of chronic schizophrenics. Cameron and Pande use intense electric shock treatment combined with prolonged sleep lasting 30 to 60 days. The sleep technique used is the one recommended by Azima combining chlorpromazine and a combination of a short- medium- and long-acting barbiturate. After 10 days ECT is started. Complete "depatterning" is achieved after about 30 ECT, then both sleep and ECT are slowly reduced. After a month the patient leaves the hospital, but the rehabilitation plan, including one ECT a month, is extended over two years during which time supportive psychotherapy is given. This method was particularly recommended for paranoid schizophrenics. Sagebiel warns against regressive ECT in cases complicated by alcoholism, a combination which led to two fatalities. In other cases he finds it of great therapeutic value. No superiority of regressive over ordinary ECT was found in a comparative study by King who also had an unexplained fatality in the regressive group.

Prophylactic ECT can be given successfully in patients with episodic psychoses. It was first recommended by Geoghegan and Stevenson who used it in manic-depressive psychoses once a month and convincingly prevented the occurrence of both manic and depressive episodes. After one or two years they reduced this prophylactic treatment to one every two or three months. In our own experience this method gave highly satisfactory results in well selected cases. It continued to be important after the advent of pharmacotherapy because preventive antidepressant medication easily leads to manic exacerbation, and neuroleptics given after a manic phase, may elicit depressions. Recent experience with Lithium carbonate makes prophylactic ECT rarely necessary.

In schizophrenic patients with frequent relapses prophylactic ECT remained disappointing. However, there are patients with frequent catatonic withdrawal, who do not respond to available drugs and in whom symptomatic or "maintenance" ECT still has indications.

Hospital and Ambulatory Setups

Hospital setups will depend on local conditions. It is highly desirable that a patient neither see nor hear another patient during or after treatment. The ideal hospital setup includes a treatment room with a table on roller casters by means of which the patient is removed after treatment to a single room for at least fifteen minutes. From there he can later be taken to a rest room with beds for several patients.

In every large mental hospital a centralized treatment unit for active therapy should be set aside and staffed with specially trained doctors and nurses. Psychotic patients with a reasonable chance to respond to therapy should be sent to this centralized treatment unit. Here, facilities for all treatments must be available, with an experienced therapist in charge of the whole unit in order to avoid competition between various procedures. The therapist must remain independent in his decisions on choice of treatment and their combinations. Patients who are able to leave the hospital should leave from this unit, and a physician from this unit should participate in after-care clinics, where such patients are followed.

Treatment facilities, in addition to the centralized treatment unit, should be available also in the admission building. Provisions must be made for patients in urgent need of immediate treatment so that they can be given ECT as an emergency measure to prevent any further aggravation of their illness, or in order to prevent psychotic exhaustion or to counteract suicidal or homicidal danger. In such cases, an emergency staff consultation is desirable to ascertain the diagnosis before ECT changes the clinical picture to a point where a proper diagnosis may no longer be possible. In spite of the great strides made by pharmacotherapy, ECT facilities also must still be available in every chronic ward. Only in this way tube feeding, restraining measures and oversedation can be successfully avoided.

It is easy to establish a pleasant atmosphere in ECT units if those administering the treatment are aware of this problem. What we see in many treatment centers contrasts strangely with the opposite extreme of providing music as an aid to the patient in his experience with shock therapy (Price and Knouss). We are not opposed to such efforts, but the most important requirement is to avoid observation of the treatment by patients who are not only frightened themselves but through their reports contribute to the opposition against the treatment by others.

Treatment in general hospitals is frequently denied by the hospital administration to the disadvantage of patients when such treatment would be strongly indicated. In obstetrical, surgical and medical cases in whom drugs have failed or are too time-consuming a few electric convulsive treatments may enable the treating physician to proceed with surgical or other therapeutic measures in a setting which is usually more appropriate than it would be if the patient had to be removed to a mental institution. The establishment of psychiatric wards in general hospitals received great impetus from the introduction of treatment procedures which so considerably reduce the hospital stay of many cases.

The possibility of treating ambulatory patients with ECT in a hospital was recognized by Bini. However, little systematic use of ambulatory treatment has been reported from hospitals. Mental institutions in the United States in general have no set-ups for ECT in their clinics. Ambulatory ECT is applied on a large scale in English mental hospitals. If patients are treated in the out-patient departments of institutions, admission to the hospital can often be avoided. Such treatment clinics should also provide active treatment in their out-patient departments for those who have been discharged and show a tendency to relapse or who need maintenance treatment. It is obvious that many readmissions to the hospital can thus be avoided. Undoubtedly, the admission rate of mental hospitals can be lowered considerably if patients with recurrent depressions are treated on an ambulatory basis.

Ambulatory ECT has been widely accepted and applied as an office procedure. Strauss and MacPhail were the first to report favorable experience. Wender et al., who found extramural metrazol treatment unsatisfactory, reported favorably on extramural ECT. Office treatment should be given only where the patient can rest for hours if necessary. Postconvulsive excitement is the greatest problem in office treatment. Patients should be accompanied to the office, as no physician should take the risk of sending home alone a patient who may still be in the aftermath of a twilight state. Favre's suggestion that ambulatory patients be observed for at least twelve hours after the convulsion is worthy of attention, but only when the patient's psychotic condition or the treatment confusion require it is constant supervision indispensable. Treatment in larger intervals, and especially maintenance or preventive treatments are instances which show that any steadfast rules for constant supervision cannot be made.

The principal limitation of office practice is the difficulty of applying adequate shock therapy to patients who need a long course of treatments, such as schizophrenics or involutional paranoids. All too readily the usual initial improvement in such patients leads to premature discontinuation of treatment, and a long course is usually impossible because of the confusional state or even more dramatic organic psychotic reactions. The most suitable patient for office treatment is the depressive who usually requires only a few treatments, therefore does not become too confused, and in whom hospitalization and possible commitment would have serious social implications. The greatest danger in these cases is the suicidal risk, and constant supervision, day and night, must be secured from the relatives. Patients needing maintenance treatment in order to keep them out of institutions, are also suitable for office treatment. Office treatment of schizophrenics who require a full course should be initiated only after the family has been warned that completion of the course in an institution may be necessary should an organic reaction or an activation of the psychosis develop. One of the dangers of inadequate office treatment is that the patient, when later admitted to an institution, may receive no more treatment because he has already "failed" under shock therapy. One of us (L.B.K.) has treated episodic schizophrenic psychoses with very acute symptomatology in the office. They usually respond well to a few treatments, and we treated successfully several catatonic excitements of a patient who had spent decades in a mental hospital, although she had been symptom-free during the intervals.

Treatment in the patient's home is undesirable as it is always improvised, and because experienced post-treatment supervision is usually unavailable.

It must be candidly admitted that the greatest problem in ambulatory treatment is the supervision of the patient not just immediately after each application but on the intervening days and for at least a week after the last treatment. This problem is presented by the patient's increasing confusion during the course of treatment. We warn the relatives most carefully to keep the patient away not only from friends (who, seeing him in this confused state, might draw wrong conclusions as to his mental capacities) but from his business, where he might do much harm without realizing it. It is surprising that legal complications as a result of the confusional state of ambulatory patients are so rare. The only case known to us is one that was dealt with by the German Courts and was first published by Leibbrand and later by Fleck. On the day after the fifth treatment, the patient (a 61 year old man), signed a partnership contract. He later contested this contract and claimed that he had no recollection of having given his signature. The Court rejected the proof of incapacity because the claimant had been able to carry on a normal conversation. It is known, however, that this fact does not rule out later amnesia, and the case remains a warning example. The patients rarely have any insight into their shortcomings during the treatment, and as soon as their condition has improved they are especially anxious to take up their usual activities. It is the task of the responsible relatives to prevent this; they should also be warned against the patient's driving a car or taking up other activities where quick reactions are necessary.

On the whole, the disadvantages of ambulatory treatment are outweighed by its social importance provided it is limited by an experienced psychiatrist to carefully selected cases. In the office we consider the assistance of an anesthesiologist and of experienced nurses even more important than in a hospital setting.

Convulsive Threshold

The threshold in ECT is lower in male than in female patients. It is higher in older than in younger individuals. Those with the highest threshold are usually females in their fifth or sixth decade of life. The higher threshold in older people appears to be in accordance with the lower incidence of seizures in older epileptics and greater tendency to convulse in children. Dehydrated patients have a high threshold. Also, acute excitement apparently increases the threshold, a fact which Ewald and Haddenbrock explain as due to increased tone in the sympathetic system in agitated patients. Despite great variations of threshold, experience with ECT has demonstrated beyond doubt that every human brain is able to react with a convulsion. No patient fails to convulse if adequate current or several successive stimuli are applied.

Kalinowsky and Kennedy used various methods to increase and decrease the threshold. It can be decreased by producing water retention with the help of pitressin (McQuarrie test). In our endeavor to induce slowly developing convulsions with threshold stimuli we frequently provoke a generalized seizure by lightly slapping the face of a patient who shows only a subconvulsive response, or by applying other sensory stimuli. As soon as the patient blinks or shows any motor reaction at all, such "reflex" convulsion can no longer be obtained, and another electric stimulus must be applied. Bromides and hyoscine have no measurable anticonvulsive effect; barbiturates raise the threshold slightly if given orally, but sodium amytal does not increase the threshold to a degree which would interfere with the treatment when given intravenously shortly before the treatment. Only dilantin increases the convulsive threshold to a considerable degree, as was also demonstrated by Hemphill and Grey Walter.

There is a spontaneous increase of threshold after each seizure. This is equally true in chemically produced convulsions. When a minimum amount of current is used in ECT, it is necessary to increase it during a course of treatments, particularly after the first seizure. This spontaneous rise of the convulsive threshold is temporary, as seen in patients whose threshold was much higher at the end of a first course of convulsive therapy but who, after a lapse of a few months without treatment, responded again to the original low amount of current. According to Hemphill and Grey Walter, the threshold for metrazol as a convulsant may be low in patients who have a high threshold for the electric current, suggesting that the initiating mechanism in the two methods is not identical. Various authors have noticed that on certain days —in our experience on cold and dry days—a higher amount of current is required. Contradictory statements have been made regarding the variations in threshold when small electrodes are applied to different areas of the skull. It is generally claimed that the frontal adversive field (6a beta of Vogt-Brodmann's classification) has the lowest threshold.

Any subcomatose or comatose state increases the convulsive threshold remarkably. This is true for patients under the effect of large doses of sedatives. It is also true for patients who are still in a postconvulsive coma when a second stimulus is given, and those in hypoglycemic coma.

Convulsive and Subconvulsive Responses

The various responses can best be understood by describing the effect of increased amounts of current. Assuming that the time is kept at 0.2 second, potential differences of below 50 volts may not lead to unconsciousness; this response described by Cerletti and Bini as "shock mancato" (missed shock) is characterized by violent vertigo, nausea, and vasomotor phenomena, and should be avoided assiduously.

Currents ranging from 50 to 70 volts lead to unconsciousness without producing a convulsion. Such nonconvulsive responses may be short at 50, longer at 60 and 70 volts. If the current is further increased, the patient will first show the same response of unconsciousness, but followed after some time by a convulsion (delayed convulsion). By increasing the current still further, the period of unconsciousness prior to the convulsion becomes shorter and finally unmeasurable, so that an "immediate convulsion" results. In rare instances one-sided convulsions are seen. They are quite unpredictable and cannot be induced at will. Clinical experience suggests that they are therapeutically ineffective. Therefore, when "Jacksonian" seizures occur and are recognized as such, we immediately apply another electrical stimulus in order to transform the unilateral seizure into a generalized one. The same is done whenever an atypical seizure arouses our doubt whether we are dealing with a typical generalized convulsion. In general, experience with ECT suggests that the brain in its convulsive response follows an all-or-none law.

The electrically induced convulsion repeats the manifestations of a spontaneous convulsion. Even if the patient is treated with muscle relaxant drugs these manifestations should still be noticeable though in an alleviated form, and the sequence of tonic and clonic phase must be the same as in an unpremedicated convulsion. Even if only slight toe movements are noticeable they must last for the minimum duration of an ordinary convulsion, otherwise an abortive and thus ineffective response must be suspected. In this case the stimulus should be repeated. In premedicated ECT oversaturation with oxygen prolongs the convulsion (Holmberg). This confirms an old theory that anoxia terminates spontaneous convulsions. In anesthesia techniques of ECT it is wise to temporarily discontinue oxygenation if the seizure is unduly prolonged.

The ordinary electrically induced convulsion, if unpremedicated, is characterized by a tonic phase followed by clonic movements which in the beginning are fast and of small range and later become slower and more forceful, until they fade out after a total of thirty to fifty seconds for the whole seizure. The convulsion is accompanied by apnea. There are a few patients who lose urine, semen or, very seldom, feces. A patient who, in spite of having voided his bladder before the treatment, loses urine during the convulsion, will do so during each subsequent treatment. The same constancy of convulsive and postconvulsive behavior in the same patient can be noted in many other manifestations.

Some observers describe an occasional second convulsion. We have never seen this, and believe that such observations refer to half voluntary automatic movements of the semicomatose patient during the postconvulsive phase. The seizure is followed by a coma of short duration from which the patient wakens in a confusional state lasting from five to thirty or more minutes. Caplan, comparing spontaneous and electrically produced fits in epileptics, finds that this postconclusive confusional state is shorter in ECT than in spontaneous convulsions and that it is less frequently followed by headache.

NONCONVULSIVE RESPONSE: This response, often described as petit mal, analogous to the corresponding phenomenon in epilepsy, is essentially characterized by mere unconsciousness accompanied by apnea. Toman et al. feel that subconvulsive responses resemble the seizures of psychomotor epilepsy more closely than petit mal responses. This response does not have any therapeutic effect comparable to what is seen in treatment with generalized convulsive seizures. During a petit mal response, most patients flush momentarily, and after the initial mass movement they usually become immobile. Others show uncoordinated automatic movements. Some articulate senseless sentences;

others scream. The patient usually repeats his pattern in subsequent petit mals. It should be considered an epileptiform response, and it could be demonstrated in epileptics of our observation that artificially produced nonconvulsive responses may repeat the pattern of the patient's spontaneous petit mals. The motor phenomena which initiate a petit mal response do not lead to the surgical complications seen in convulsions. This petit mal response has no parallel in metrazol treatment where unconsciousness does not occur if the injection does not lead to a convulsion. Kalinowsky et al. have shown that this response is inadequate for therapeutic purposes and should therefore be avoided. Ziskind et al. come to the same conclusion. The recommendation of some authors that nonconvulsive treatment be employed in weak, elderly and otherwise physically impaired patients is unjustified, for this therapeutically ineffective response is accompanied with particular frequency by cardiovascular complications. It is also followed by confusion. Fatalities in apparent connection with subconvulsive responses have been repeatedly mentioned (Folksom, Moore, Cropper and Hughes).

Electrostimulatory Nonconvulsive Treatment

Various means of electric stimulation had been tried long before convulsive treatments were introduced. After the discovery of ECT came the first attempts at nonconvulsive treatment with subconvulsive stimili leading to unconsciousness but not to a convulsion ("petit mal response"). Hirschfeld's "electrostimulatory treatment," was preceded by Berkwitz' "faradic shock treatment." In most non-convulsive methods this electrical application is only one part of the treatment, the other consisting of intravenous injection of pentothal or sodium amytal to produce a narcotic effect. Since the electrical phase of the treatment does not differ from electrical applications used in former times by physicians for all kinds of nervous symptoms, it is probable that beneficial effects of this treatment should be attributed to the barbiturate narcosis rather than to the electrical treatment. Encouraging results were claimed in various psychotic conditions, particularly in toxic-organic psychoses. Thompson, who made a controlled study, apparently without use of barbiturates, states frankly that no cures were obtained but that the treatment sometimes controlled destructiveness. He discusses the possibility that such favorable effect on some patients is "due to the associated discomfort." Hirschfeld has treated certain mental disorders with nonconvulsive electric stimulation by means of the spiked, unidirectional current developed by Reiter, but later achieved the same effect with other machines. He described this method as electric stimulation of the diencephalon and applied the electrodes bitemporally rather than bifrontally, placing them one inch above the ear. An average current of 5 milliamperes is used. The patient feels the current as a painful sensation which necessitates the administration of sodium amytal in a 5 per cent solution prior to the treatment. Dilatation of pupils, flushing of the skin and moderate perspiration during the treatment on the one hand, and emotional outbursts immediately following stimulation on the other hand, suggested a possible diencephalic irritation because these symptoms did not seem to occur when the electrodes were applied to the frontal lobes. In one of our own patients treated in this manner we saw something resembling such an emotional storm of supposedly diencephalic origin. The patient showed the same response, however, when we applied the electrodes one next to the other on the forehead in such a way that the current could not go through any brain tissue at all. Hirschfeld noticed a relation between affective outbursts during the treatment, autonomic reactivity and clinical improvement. Individuals with flattened affect and poor prognosis did not show any of these responses. The treatment is recommended for anxiety states, paranoid schizophrenia, late schizophrenia and psychosomatic conditions but not in depressions.

L. Alexander continued Hirschfeld's work by using unidirectional current 1½ to 5 milliamperes with spikes up to 60-200 milliamperes. The current was applied for from 30 seconds to 6 minutes. He found that the use of nonconvulsive "counter-shock," given after convulsive treatment, had a modifying and alleviating effect on memory loss, on post-treatment anxiety, and on the spontaneous hyperactivity which, in his experience, frequently remains after ECT. He therefore changes freely between convulsive and nonconvulsive treatment in the same patient according to the latter's response to the treatment. In a very careful study with controls Pulver and Jacobs proved convincingly that nonconvulsive electrostimulation actually has no effect on the various side-effects of ECT.

An attempt to stimulate the diencephalon was undertaken by Breitner who used a small electrode placed through the patient's nose at the retropharyngeal wall with a second large electrode over the cortex. Under pentothal anesthesia 4 milliamperes of unidirectional current were applied for several minutes. Results similar to those with ECT are claimed.

Monopolar stimulation is used by Epstein who applies a monopolar electrode to certain regions of the head, and the indifferent electrode to the right forearm. Unilateral convulsions have been purposely induced by Impastato et al. in an attempt to reduce memory impairment or electroencephalographic changes. In our experience unilateral convulsions were ineffective. On the other hand, localized stimulation of the brain can be used for generalized convulsions (see Chapter on Unilateral ECT). Negrin uses a technique placing the electrodes surgically through trephine openings into the brain. His procedure which has remained experimental, allowed the electrodes to be left in the brain of chronic patients for repeated convulsive stimuli.

There is reason to believe that the therapeutic benefit from nonconvulsive electroshock is due solely to stimulation of peripheral nerve pathways. This assumption was stated by Jones and Shanklin who obtained good results in a variety of psychiatric conditions when they applied electric stimuli of 15 to 20 milliamperes to the legs. They speculate that this may stimulate the reticular activating system. Our skepticism regarding any effect of nonconvulsive treatment was supported by the recent work of Ottosson which seems to prove conclusively that a generalized convulsion or the accompanying changes in the brain are necessary for any therapeutic effect.

Combined Insulin-convulsive Treatment

Pharmacologically and electrically induced convulsions are used in combination with insulin coma treatment. Georgi introduced a combined insulin-metrazol therapy on the basis of theoretical considerations, and because of sudden improvement in insulin-treated cases after the occurrence of "spontaneous" hypoglycemic convulsions. The main object of combining the two large groups of shock treatments is, of course, the hope of achieving an aggregate of the effect of the two methods.

The classical method of "summation" recommended by Georgi consists in effecting a convulsion during the second hour of hypoglycemia when the lowest blood sugar values have been reached; this is also the time when most spontaneous hypoglycemic convulsions occur. Others induce the convulsion during the time of deepest hypoglycemic coma. Since the introduction of ECT we gave electrically induced convulsions at the time of the deepest hypoglycemic coma with the aim of intensifying the therapeutically effective coma and the underlying pathophysiologic events in the brain.

It is customary to terminate the hypoglycemic coma after the convulsion. Müller states that after a convulsion, hypoglycemic patients usually come out of the coma sufficiently to be able to drink the sugar solution. Shepley and McGregor have demonstrated an increase in the blood sugar of about 15 mg. per cent after electrical convulsions. Although hypoglycemia is said to reduce the convulsive threshold for both metrazol and electric current (Sandison and McGregor), this is reversed in deep coma. Here, in our experience, the response to the electrical stimulus is not infrequently an atypical or incomplete convulsion. The clonic phase of the convulsion is often shortened or barely noticeable. In a few instances of very deep coma with loss of corneal reflexes, no convulsion could be elicited with the highest available current. Fernandes and Polonio found the insulin-metrazol combination more effective than insulin-electric shock; so does Georgi and some others.

There is no evidence that the combination of insulin and convulsive therapy increases the danger of treatment. The mortality rate in von Braunmühl's material, treated chiefly with the combined methods, was 0.37 per cent, which corresponds to the lower average for insulin fatalities. Fractures are rare if the convulsions are induced during hypoglycemia when the patient is relaxed. Since in deep hypoglycemic coma succinylcholine can be applied without pentothal its use with proper oxygenation should not be dangerous. The less frequent occurrence of fractures in spontaneous hypoglycemic convulsions led Kant et al. to attempts to elicit hypoglycemic convulsions by giving sodium chloride in addition to forcing fluids.

There are many ways to combine insulin and convulsive therapy. Most clinicians will add convulsions twice a week during insulin treatment. Another way to administer combined insulin-convulsive therapy is to remove the most disturbing psychotic symptoms with convulsive treatment, after or during which insulin treatment is instituted; more convulsive treatments may be given either at certain regular intervals or when clinical improvement under hypoglycemic therapy alone has reached a stalemate. In the U.S.S.R. Vassilyeva et al. start quite arbitrarily with either of the methods, later apply the alternative, and when both have failed, combine the two. Von Braunmühl claims that a number of hypoglycemic reactions must precede any combination with convulsive therapy. At the International Congress in Paris in 1950, Sakel gave detailed recommendations for combined treatment in certain clinical pictures and requested avoidance of convulsions in others. We agree with Mayer-Gross, who commented on Sakel's report and was unable to follow these detailed recommendations. He sees the usefulness of convulsions in insulin therapy (a) to achieve the cooperation of resistive, negativistic, restless, excited and stuporous patients, (b) to induce a coma in patients where it is otherwise difficult to produce it, (c) to combat affective admixtures in the schizophrenic picture, (d) to speed up recovery in patients who, after initial improvement, remain on the same level for three or four weeks without further progress.

At present, since insulin coma treatment is available only in very few centers, electric and other convulsive treatments will always be tried first. Only in failures with these methods insulin treatment will be considered and, in order to intensify its effect, it should be given in combination with convulsive therapy.

Combination of Pharmacotherapy and Convulsive Treatment

Since the introduction of modern pharmacotherapy combinations of the newer drugs and convulsive therapy, particularly ECT, have been recommended. This will be discussed in the chapters on treatment results of the various psychiatric conditions. As a whole, it has hardly been proven that the simultaneous use of the two methods has any advantage. On the other hand, the question of adding to the danger of convulsive therapy by the simultaneous use of the drugs has been stressed. Neuroleptic drugs are hypotensive and mention has been made of some complications in patients under ECT, when chlorpromazine was added. The danger is definitely greater with Rauwolfia drugs which even if the patients receive them for high blood pressure, should be discontinued for several days before ECT can be started. Many psychiatrists have maintained patients on chlorpromazine and other phenothiazines when they started ECT. Nevertheless, an experienced anesthesiologist will have some misgivings about such a procedure because both ECT and neuroleptic drugs have a hypotensive effect which adds to the hypotensive effect of barbiturates used in anesthesia, and this adds up to a potential danger of serious fall in blood pressure during the treatment. Most hospitals will at least avoid neuroleptic medication in the morning of the treatment. We avoid the combination all together, and if the patient needs sedation during the treatment, we prefer barbiturates for this purpose. There is some reason to assume that pharmacological convulsive therapy makes it easier to combine convulsive treatment and neuroleptic medication. Most convulsants are analeptics, and Nahunek prefers convulsive medication with pentazol rather than ECT, when neuroleptic drugs are given at the same time.

Psychotherapy, Occupational and Social Therapy during Convulsive Treatment

There has been much discussion about the role psychotherapy should play in patients under ECT. Opinions differ according to the basic orientation of the therapist.

Levy and Grinker combine convulsive therapy and psychotherapy systematically, the latter being usually of the reassuring or loving type, taking advantage of mother transference. In another paper Grinker and MacLean show how psychotherapy during convulsive therapy may uncover dynamically significant conflicts. When a few convulsive treatments are used by psychotherapists for the specific purpose of releasing the patient's resistance to psychotherapy, the role of organic treatment merely as an adjunct to psychotherapy is obvious. The questionable point is the degree of psychologic treatment necessary in order to achieve favorable results in the usual type of psychotic patient benefiting from convulsive treatment.

Schilder recommended taking advantage of the transference situation set up by the completed course of convulsive therapy. A different question is that of the usefulness of psychotherapy during the convulsive treatment itself as practiced by a great number of psychiatrists. There are some who feel that the physician giving the shock therapy and the psychotherapist should not be the same person. In our experience psychotherapy during convulsive therapy has often been impossible because of the patient's confusion. Even in the beginning of treatment it is not very promising, as either the patient cannot concentrate sufficiently or he forgets the details of the psychotherapeutic interviews. A survey of the literature yields little objective information as to how much simultaneous psychotherapy influences the outcome of a course of convulsive therapy. One of us (LBK) had the opportunity to treat 2 series of patients in two different hospitals, one in a large institution where the patients were seen individually only on shock treatment days; the other in a hospital where most patients were under constant simultaneous psychotherapy by another physician. The results were far superior in the institution, i.e., the first group. This, of course, is not due to the lack of psychotherapy but to the more favorable material found in the mental institution; but the experience shows that optimal results may be obtained in psychotics with no attempt at psychotherapy. This should in no way discourage psychologic interest in the patient's problems, but when this is impracticable, its absence does not adversely affect the outcome. This applies only to psychotic material. The necessity for combining psychotherapy with convulsive therapy in the few neurotics where convulsive therapy is indicated, will be discussed in the section on the psychoneuroses. A great value in clearing up depressive elements interfering with psychotherapeutic efforts has been attributed to ECT by Linn and Rosen, who discuss the best ways to integrate the two approaches. Binswanger tries to outline the type of psychotherapy which should be given after ECT. He assumes that shock therapy produces fear and thereby attempts new repression, whereas psychoanalysis tries to uncover repressed material. Therefore, reassurance and discussion of the future rather than of the past (as in analysis) is indicated.

The problems which shock therapy presents to the occupational therapist have been discussed by Kalinowsky. Occupational therapy should assume an even more active role in the therapeutic program with the advent of the various somatic treatments. The occupational therapist must be acquainted with such features of ECT as the organic reactions, during which the patient's activities should be limited to very simple tasks. After the treatment is over, occupational therapy has a great psychotherapeutic value in making the patient more interested in some kind of work. The occupational therapist can, furthermore, facilitate the patient's vocational adjustment together with the social worker, and thus contribute much to the improvement of the results of a shock treatment unit. On the other hand, while C. Schneider feels that any somatic treatment of schizophrenia should be started with occupational therapy, Lopez-Ibor finds this unnecessary, although he, too, considers occupational therapy a useful adjunct to shock therapy—so is, of course, work therapy. Today the great variety of social psychiatric measures including rehabilitation will be applied to any patient who terminates a series of convulsive treatments. Pharmacotherapy will further contribute to the success of such measures. The combined use of these various methods has to be adjusted to the needs of the individual patient.

Medical Observations

Medical observations of patients under convulsive therapy, especially ECT, are surprisingly scarce. Rarely are systematic studies found, and even statements on such simple observations as pulse rate, blood pressure, and so on, are contradictory. Observations in ECT are of particular interest for problems of epilepsy. In metrazol therapy the effect of the drug itself makes the evaluation of the effect of the convulsion more difficult. Where not otherwise mentioned, findings refer to unpremedicated convulsive therapy. In more recent investigations it is often not clear whether anesthesia and muscle relaxation had been used. A monograph on cardiovascular aspects of ECT was prepared by Perrin.

The largest number of studies is dedicated to cardiovascular phenomena. In ECT, Accornero from Cerletti's staff, noticed in increase in the heart rate of about twenty to thirty beats beginning with the clonic phase; transient arrhythmia or extrasystoles were occasionally noted. On the other hand, Hemphill and Grey Walter found bradycardia during and after the convulsion. Hadorn, quoted by Müller, noticed tachycardia in generalized convulsions but bradycardia in nonconvulsive responses. The radial artery often appears pulseless after the end of a convulsion; but Fleischhacker was able in such cases to feel the pulse of the abdominal aorta. In metrazol, according to von Meduna, convulsions are followed by tachycardia. Schmid observed tachycardia in some patients, arrhythmia in others, whereby the same patient always maintains the same type of response. Epstein states that the heart rate may show a precipitous decrease, or an increase, or a mixed response. More reliable than palpation of the pulse of the radial artery during a convulsion, however, should be observations under the fluoroscope, as made by Abramow and Kopeliovic. They saw that the heart stops during the tonic phase. The clonic phase is accompanied by tachycardia, fibrillations and arrhythmia.

Electrocardiographic changes are negligible in ECT. Bellet et al., who found noteworthy changes in two thirds of all cases under insulin and less severe ones in metrazol treatment, noticed very slight changes in ECT. The most usual were minor arrhythmias. Once, and that following a delayed convulsive seizure, they found an inverted T wave; the only case of a serious type of arrhythmia was seen after a treatment combined with curare. Hadorn also found arrhythmia the most frequent electrocardiographic change in both ECT and metrazol therapy. He points out that in spontaneous epileptic seizures such arrhythmias are absent. Sinus tachycardia up to 250 is usually followed, after a few minutes, by arrhythmia and auricular extrasystoles. The nonconvulsive response is accompanied by bradycardia. Bellet et al. showed that there is no relationship between the amount of current or the length of the seizure and the severity of the electrocardiographic changes. Most changes were interpreted as vagus stimulation effect. Bradycardia in nonconvulsive responses points in this direction, and tachycardia after a generalized seizure may be a secondary effect of the muscular effort in unmodified ECT.

Several studies of electrocardiographic findings in ECT were performed by Altschule and his co-workers. They confirm the findings of vagal hyperactivity and list as symptoms pronounced sinus arrhythmia, periods of sinus brachycardia, frequent auricular tachycardia. It is not clear whether their increase in vagal tone results from stimuli from the brain, from reflexes activated by the cardio-respiratory changes induced by the convulsion, or from the potentiation of acetylcholine from acidosis due to the high carbon dioxide levels. Increase in the size of P-waves, also seen in a similar study by Holzer and Polzer, is probably a sign of dilatation of the auricle due to increased venous pressure and venous return. In two patients with serious cardiac difficulties during the treatment, Altschule demonstrated an abnormally sensitive carotid sinus mechanism. Atropine sulfate 0.8 mg. given before each succeeding treatment prevented further difficulties.

The consensus seems to be that slight temporary myocardial changes may occur and are best explained by the apnea and anoxemia occurring during the seizure, but that in the long run no electrocardiographic changes are caused by ECT. This is in accordance with the absence of clinical signs of myocardial damage due to or aggravated by ECT. In pharmacologic convulsive treatment Hadorn attributes some of the changes to the drug rather than to the convulsions; Guttmann and Reitman disagreed.

The systolic blood pressure, according to Accornero, increases about 50 to 60 mm. of mercury, while the diastolic pressure barely rises. The blood pressure returns to normal within thirty minutes. In animals this rise is preceded by a short drop in blood pressure for a few seconds (Bini and Puddu). Such initial fall was also seen by Deshaies and Renault. The following increase is greater for the systolic than for the diastolic pressure, thus leading to pronounced changes in the pulse pressure. A careful study of intra-arterial blood pressure changes from the femoral artery showed a rapid rise in the tonic phase, a rapid fall in the clonic phase, and a continued fall under the pretreatment level after the end of the clonic phase. Muscle relaxants cause a more gradual rise and fall of the blood pressure, but the maximum rise was as high as in unpremedicated ECT.

Respiration follows a rather typical pattern during treatment. Bini and Puddu observing animals, and Accornero, men, noticed a sudden strong inspiration followed by apnea. The apnea lasts forty to sixty seconds and is followed by short inspirations which become deeper and stertorous. This phase is followed by a period of hyperpnea up to forty respirations a minute. It is noteworthy that in dogs, section of the vagus nerve does not change the respiratory pattern. During the apnea, according to Altschule et al., the patients perform maximal forced expiration (the Valsalva maneuver). This resemblance between electrically induced convulsion and the Valsalva maneuver with increased intra-abdominal and intrathoracic pressure including arterial, venous and spinal fluid pressure was also found by the Swedish workers Nyman and Silfverskiöld.

The length of the apnea varies considerably even in the same patient and is apparently independent of the duration of the muscular discharge; it usually lasts longer than the convulsion. However, when a long latent period with apnea precedes the convulsion, respiration sometimes returns before the clonic phase of the convulsion has ended. Barbiturates increase the length of the apnea (Challiol). Friedman and Barry demonstrated in pneumographic studies that some respiratory movements with passage of air occur in the clonic phase of the convulsion even though no respiratory movements are seen.

Hematologic findings after pharmacologically and electrically induced convulsions are divergent. The white cell count shows leukocytosis after pharmacologically induced convulsions. Von Meduna tried to correlate the degree of leukocytosis and clinical improvement. Neutrophile leukocytosis was seen in metrazol whether or not a convulsion had been obtained. In ECT Felici found lymphocytosis which lasted thirty to forty-five minutes, setting in five minutes after the seizure. This is contrary to findings of decreased lymphocytes following metrazol convulsions. The lymphocytic response to stress situations is usually a lymphocytopenia, but psychotics, especially schizophrenics, are defective in this response. In a thorough study, Parsons et al. observed an abrupt 50 to 100 per cent increase of lymphocytes. The neutrophiles also showed a consistent 50 to 80 per cent rise. Within thirty minutes both types of cells had returned toward the preshock level. After two or three hours the lymphocytes had reached a minimum of 45 to 70 per cent below the initial figure, after which they returned to the normal level within five or six hours. The polymorphs usually remained above the normal level. Rees, who studied the same feature in electronarcosis, explains the early lymphocytosis by the muscular activity, while the later lymphopenia is perhaps attributable to increased adrenocortical activity. Stern et al. relate both leukocytosis and lymphocytosis to autonomic stimulation. An eosinophilia described in metrazol was not seen in ECT by these authors but was occasionally reported by later investigators. Altschule et al. found a constant decrease of eosinophiles, independent of the type of patient treated or the outcome of the treatment. A decrease of red blood cells after a certain number of convulsions was noted by Centini and

Bandettini di Poggio. Carse and Slater saw violent fluctuations in the number of neutrophiles but a constant rise of lymphocytes, more marked in schizophrenics than in others. Walther found the thrombocytes to be increased about 35 per cent, returning to normal within a few hours. The sedimentation rate is usually increased but the findings have not been uniform. The coagulation time is lowered 50 to 60 per cent, and its return is synchronous with thrombocyte values. Increase of blood hemoglobin of 7 to 20 per cent and increases of serum protein were seen by Parsons et al. immediately following treatment but these returned to normal in less than an hour.

The possible relationship between changes in the blood constituents and the response of the adrenal cortex to the body's reaction to shock and stress led to several studies on the effect of convulsive therapy on the excretion of cortins and ketosteroids. Ashby, in a thorough study on the response of the "sugar-active" cortins, the "reducing" cortins and the 17-ketosteroids, found a brisk outpouring of adrenal cortical steroids during the first few days of ECT but a return to normal even when treatment was continued. The greater the outpouring, the greater the tendency to clinical recovery. The 17-ketosteroids, however, in most cases show no changes in their excretion rate, as had been previously noted also by Simon et al. It should be mentioned here that some biochemical changes seem to relate to the disappearance of individual symptoms which had caused them, such as anxiety or depression. There is also some reason to believe that the biochemical changes described in ECT are more pronounced in affective psychoses than in schizophrenics, who are known to be more inert in many physical reactions. Finally, many of the findings reported in convulsive therapy were due to the muscular contractions and are not necessarily present in ECT under muscle relaxation. It can be assumed that recent investigators usually treated their patients with muscle relaxation without mentioning it (e.g., Ito et al.). These authors found that not only ACTH but also urinary gonatropin excretion is increased in ECT. Since this was more pronounced in acutely disturbed patients, it is probably not due to simple stimulation of the pituitary gland but by helping the sick organism to restore its physiological equilibrium in terms of endocrine functions which are especially sensitive to emotional stress. Many biochemical findings in older studies are probably explainable by the muscular contractions. This is exemplified by Reichlin and O'Neal who found that increase in plasma concentration of PBI, labeled thyroxine and labeled triiodothyronine following ECT in man is eliminated, when muscle relaxation is used.

A hyperglycemia of 20 to 40 per cent above normal is a constant phenomenon after convulsions. The maximum is reached fifteen or thirty minutes after a convulsion; return to normal takes place approximately one hour later. Nonconvulsive metrazol responses fail to show a definite hyperglycemia. However, electrical petit mal responses which, unlike metrazol failures, are accompanied by unconsciousness and are therefore epileptiform in type, do lead to hyperglycemia. This increase of blood sugar in the nonconvulsive response suggests that the hyperglycemia is not caused by mobilization of muscle glycogen during the motor phenomena but by central stimulation. Ewald and Haddenbrock found the hyperglycemia to be higher and of longer duration in metrazol than in electrical convulsions.

The cholesterol content in the blood shows contrasting results in petit mal responses and generalized seizures (Katzenelbogen et al., Kalinowsky et al.); in the latter it is increased, and in petit mal it drops in most cases. Cholesterol studies are known to be contradictory, and it should be mentioned that Simon et al., studying cases under electronarcosis, did not find an increase in blood cholesterol or any change in the excretion of 17-ketosteroids after electric shock or electronarcosis. Georgi attributes special importance to changes in the lipoid metabolism during shock therapy.

Various other chemical constituents of the blood have been studied, particularly by Georgi and Strauss in metrazol, and by Katzenelbogen et al. in ECT. The latter authors point out that the apnea and, therefore, the anoxemia are extremely short and that the subsequent hyperpnea makes it even more appropriate to speak of hyperoxemia rather than of anoxemia. An initial alkalosis of the blood during the tonic phase appears to change into a strong acidosis during the clonic phase (Selbach). An increase of the calcium level in the blood after ECT was found to be limited to the nonultrafiltrable part of the calcium (Salomon and Gabrio). In studies on calcium metabolism in depressions Flach found that convulsive therapy is accompanied by a significant decrease in the urinary excretion of calcium in those depressions which respond well to the treatment. Klaus and Wenzel found an increased plasma concentration of 5-hydroxy-tryptamin, tryptamin and tyramine. Reports on serotonin level were contradictory. An increase was found by Garattini et al. Kety et al. found that like drugs which ameliorate depressions, ECT has a significant effect on norepinephrine in certain regions of the brain. In the same laboratory Schildkraut et al. found that electrically induced convulsions given to animals that had received norepinephrine although cisternially, lowered the level of norepinephrine in the brain of these animals more than in the controls. This suggests that electric convulsions increase neuronal discharge of norepinephrine in the brain.

Water metabolism and renal function also show changes. Kreienberg and Ehrhardt found the diuresis to be considerably diminished and noticed that even in the case of heavy fluid intake before ECT, the normally expected diuresis is delayed for approximately two hours. This is in accordance with our clinical observation that patients who remain in the office for about two hours after the treatment, hardly ever urinate. A change of the urine concentration does not take place, and, therefore, the diuresis is only delayed. Altschule and Tillotson, studying the same problem of water metabolism, found a decrease of the plasma volume and an increase of the hemoglobin content of the blood. These changes seem to depend on the muscular contractions because they were fewer after premedication with curare.

The urine shows increased acidity as well as increased content of ammonia and phosphates. As a whole, the changes in the urine can be considered insignificant. Investigations of gastric secretion and gastric contractions during electrically induced convulsions suggested increased vagus activity (Fetter, Fetter and de Jong).

The spinal fluid shows no significant changes in convulsive therapy. Chemical and cell content and the permeability of the meninges are unchanged in pharmacologic as well as electric convulsive therapy. While the pressure is decreased following a convulsion, a temporary increase of pressure during the tonic and part of the clonic phase has been observed. This is quite understandable in view of the maneuver of raising spinal fluid pressure during lumbar puncture by voluntarily contracting the abdominal muscles. The venous stasis observed on the open skull during the later part of a convulsion and the resulting increase of brain volume also explain the temporary increase of spinal fluid pressure. The downward trend begins with the clonic phase in large oscillations and equilibrium is re-established six hours after the treatment (Deshaies and Renard). There was only one study, by W. Schulte, in which a greater cell increase after electrically induced convulsions was reported. Slight increase in cells and protein was noted by Ulrich, who also saw changes in the pneumoencephalogram.

An interesting approach to understanding the physicochemical changes in the brain during a convulsion by studying the spinal fluid was undertaken by Spiegel and his group. It was shown that ECT influences the ultraviolet absorption of the cerebrospinal fluid (initial decrease followed by increase). Enzymatic substances apparently belonging to the groups of nucleases and desaminases increase in the CSF following electroshock convulsions. Lipases are much less affected by electroshock convulsions than are the nucleases. They found that the electrolyte content of the cerebrospinal fluid as indicated by its conductivity, the total interferometric values and the ratio of the interferometric value of non-electrolytes to that of the electrolytes was increased. There was a distinct increase in the potassium and phosphate content. Both electrolytes and non-electrolytes were increased after convulsions, the latter even to a higher degree than the electrolytes. Neither abnormal permeability of the blood-brain barrier nor abnormal content of glucose and protein were found to be responsible for the increase of non-electrolytes. In spectrometric studies, some breakdown of nuclear substances under the influence of convulsions of the blood-brain barrier was found to be markedly increased following a series of electrically induced convulsions by Aird, and he is inclined to see the effect of ECT related to this phenomenon. Mann et al. found an increase of cerebrospinal oxalacetic acid transaminase in patients receiving electroconvulsive therapy and in neurological diseases. Findings in experimental animals cannot be listed here, but so far have not contributed to our understanding of the mode of action of the treatment.

Two important expressions of definite *neurovegative-endocrine* effects of convulsion therapy are increased weight and menstrual changes.

Increase of weight is the most frequent physical change observed during a course of convulsive therapy as well as in insulin treatment where it had been explained as an effect of the insulin itself. In ECT, where a similar gain in weight takes place even faster, it can no longer be explained by drug effect nor by the fact that with improvement the patient eats more. Observations have shown that the increased amount of food does not explain this phenomenon. The patient gains weight after a few treatments and continues to do so for some time after the whole course. Kalinowsky showed that in both manic depressive and schizophrenic episodes, the clinical manifestations are often preceded by loss of weight, and the clinical improvement by a beginning gain of weight. Neither electric stimulations nor the convulsion as such seem to be responsible for the gain of weight, which occurs as well in spontaneous improvements. The only exception is seen in "regressive" treatment, when patients lose weight during the treatment but gain in a few days after it. Altschule et al. demonstrated that body weight and extracellular fluid parallel each other in their increase during the first few electric shock treatments. Later, only the gain of weight continues.

Menstruation is equally affected, although less definite rules can be established. Menstruation often ceases during a long course of ECT. In these patients as well as in those in whom amenorrhea already accompanied the psychosis prior to treatment, normal function usually returns about two months after successful treatment. This is likewise true in many cases of so-called involutional psychosis at the age of between 45 and 50, when menstruation had ceased but returns. Those patients who become amenorrheic only during the treatment but regain their regular cycles sometime after, demonstrate that the psychosis alone does not explain the endocrine disturbance, but that the treatment itself probably influences the diencephalic centers for these endocrine functions. It may be added that amenorrhea during ECT is not limited to psychotics alone but is seen in neurotics as well. An analogous change in the sex hormones of the male was assumed by Michael on the basis of clinical observations of impotence during ECT. Westman obtained normal ovulation in rabbits during ECT. However, the relation between ECT and menstruation is quite contradictory, and E. Schneider failed to see any effect on the amenorrhea of psychotics. Michael demonstrated that the resumption of menstruation is increasingly delayed in proportion to the number of treatments.

The endocrine concomitants of ECT were investigated extensively by Reiss. In particular, thyroid function and ACTH were studied, and the contradictory results summarized in a 1950 paper.

There are more symptoms of possibly diencephalic origin like variations in the sleep mechanism. They usually parallel the loss of weight at the onset of a psychosis, or even precede it. Under ECT normal sleep often returns later than the gain of weight but earlier than irregular menstruation. Rises in temperature after each treatment are rare, but in patients in whom this symptom occurs, it is quite constant during the course of treatment. This fever was explained by Pakesch as due to muscular contraction, but we see it even more frequently in ECT under anesthesia and muscle relaxation, and we assume that in some cases it might be a reaction to the intravenous barbiturate. Most authors like Donnadieu and Hauser, and Delay who observed it sometimes only six hours after the treatment, explain it as a neurovegetative derangement of diencephalic origin. Lunn explains the raise in skin temperature immediately after a convulsion as due to opening of arterio-venous anastomosis.

Prognostic Tests for ECT

Various attempts have been made to predict the outcome of ECT. These attempts were not very successful. The best known work in this area is the

FUNKENSTEIN TEST: A systematic attempt was made by Funkenstein et al. to understand the mechanism of shock therapy in terms of autonomic responses. They studied the response to epinephrine chloride and mecholyl. Electric shock increases the systolic blood pressure response after epinephrine and lessens the response to mecholyl. Varying responses as well as anxiety and chills occurring after mecholyl were also thought to have prognostic value. Those patients who have more than a 50 mm. Hg rise in systolic blood pressure after intravenous injection of 0.5 mg. of epinephrine and a fall of blood pressure after 10 mg. of mecholyl intramuscularly with failure to return to their usual blood pressure within 25 minutes, have a good prognosis for ECT. The same is true for those who respond to the mecholyl with chills. Details regarding the various groups of responses and their prognostic significance have to be studied in the original papers on the so-called "Funkenstein Test." Ploog and Selbach tested sympathetic reactivity in ECT patients with Sympatol which leads to blood pressure oscillations in favorable cases but no changes in patients with poor prognosis such as chronic hebephrenics.

A more recent survey on the various papers by Funkenstein et al., and other reports on their test, was made by Ramapura et al. These authors as well as Geocaris and Kooiker conclude that too small a rise of systolic blood pressure after epinephrine also makes for a poor prognosis. They discount the contrasting findings of Pasquarelli et al. because the latter authors used smaller amounts of epinephrine than recommended by Funkenstein. The prognostic value was found in a survey by Feinberg to be inconclusive ten years after its introduction. Today nobody would exclude patients from treatment on the basis of this test.

Another way to prognosticate the response of manic-depressives to ECT, was given by Faure et al. They injected ACTH prior to ECT and found that the less abnormal the response of 17-ketosteroids, leucocytes and other ACTH reactions were, the better the prognosis for ECT-treated manic-depressives. The work by Fink and his co-workers (Kahn et al.) who use an amobarbital test to prognosticate clinical improvement, is mentioned elsewhere. They as well as Roth et al. correlated barbiturate induced electroencephalographic changes with prognosis. According to Shagass et al. a high sedation threshold in depressed patients makes for poorer therapeutic results than a lower sedation threshold.

Thorpe in a survey of all these tests questions their practical value. In a recent attempt to predict the outcome of ECT on the basis of the mecholyl-adrenaline test, psychological tests and clinical psychiatric interviews Gonda showed that the psychiatric interview gave far more reliable prognostic information than the other methods.

Psychopathological Observations

The patient's psychologic reaction to ECT is different from that seen in metrazol treatment where his attitude is determined by the deadly fear which he experiences before each convulsion. In ECT fear is not attached to some painful, definitely related experience. The patient loses consciousness immediately and has an amnesia for the whole treatment procedure. There is little discomfort after the treatment, and postconvulsive excitement and panic reactions are always covered by amnesia. Those patients who fear the treatment do so because they dislike being unconscious or are afraid of not waking up after the treatment. Various psychologic attitudes toward ECT have been described by Millet and Mosse. Gallinek has analyzed the various types of fear in connection with ECT. In spite of some statements to the contrary, it is our experience that the use of anesthesia techniques has not diminished this problem, and the fear increases with each subsequent treatment.

We agree with Schwab and Riechelmann that fear of the treatment is not more pronounced in patients with psychotic fears. After several treatments, when the patient is much better, he develops an increasing fear for which he is unable to account. This late and quite intense fear is not explained by any discomfort from the treatment, nor by the psychotic fears which have usually disappeared, at least temporarily, by this time. Interviews with patients suggest that this fear is connected with the experience of waking up and being unable to become oriented. In the German literature (von Baeyer, R. Jung, Schildge, in der Beek and Schmidt, Salm) this question has been studied extensively. "The agonizing experience of the shattered self" (Schildge) is the most convincing explanation for the late fear of the treatment, and the patient becomes aware of this only a week or two after the first application because of his slowly disappearing amnesia for this experience. Another explanation given is the recollection of noises during the treatments and the sight of other patients being treated, but in our experience treatments applied to individual patients in a sound-proof room did not prevent the occurrence of this fear.

Apprehension can be connected with unpleasant experiences during abortive (petit mal) shock treatments, in which feelings of electricity and various sensory manifestations are not infrequent. Whereas patients after generalized convulsions never remember an aura comparable to the aura of epileptics, those with abortive shocks do. Schildge describes sensory auras which were mostly of vestibular type, sometimes associated with optic, rarely with acoustic manifestations. All the sensations of abortive seizures are more frequently seen in brief stimuli and unidirectional treatment, where lower intensities of current are applied for a longer period of time. The painful experience of a stimulus that does not produce immediate unconsciousness increases the fear of patients treated with such modifications. Description of patients' psychological reactions to the treatment as given in "self-observations of a physician" (Bersot) and by a patient of Salm, are of great psychological interest, but the hope that they might be helpful in finding an explanation for the curative effect of the treatment in psychological terms has not been fulfilled.

The patient's behavior while awakening is of interest. L. H. Cohen described it for metrazol; Loewenbach and Stainbrook for ECT. In patients in whom metrazol and ECT were alternated, the pattern of the awakening was exactly alike. Hemphill described the various stages in the return of consciousness from a more neurological viewpoint. Variations in individual behavior are wide ranging, but the pattern in the individual patient is extremely uniform, repeating itself with each treatment. Some patients wake up terror-stricken, others are quiet. Again, some will mumble or always sing the same song; when spoken to, their answers will be inadequate. Some will ask questions in an attempt to become oriented, and failing to understand or retain the information given to them, will reiterate the question. The practical importance of establishing the patient's true orientation lies in the fact that if inappropriate answers are accepted, the therapist may be surprised when later the patient, who is still in a twilight state, unexpectedly misinterprets the situation and becomes assaultive. This can be equally as dangerous as the twilight state of an epileptic. It occurs in spite of barbiturate narcosis.

Elderly patients take longer to regain full consciousness. Patients who are confused from previous treatments need a longer time to become oriented with each subsequent treatment. Lunn and Trolle found that name and marital state are easiest to remember, while the concept of age seems very vulnerable. Orientation in time is more vulnerable than information on space. In Bersot's self-observation, after a single treatment a vague euphoria during the first day was followed by a depressed feeling and lack of concentration which lasted for weeks. Zubin describes an apparent loss of familiarity. Everything about the patient seems strange and new to him. When he is shown material he has seen prior to the treatment, he will protest that he never saw it, but when urged to guess, he will guess correctly more often than could be expected by chance. Zubin feels that loss of familiarity plays a role in the therapeutic process of ECT, and thinks that it may have a salutary influence on those perceptual causes in the patient's environment which evoked his anxiety.

Sensory perception is always impaired during ECT. Many patients complain that they cannot see well. This is obviously the general effect of mental "blurring," which makes it difficult for the patient to concentrate and to perceive clearly. Such explanation of this phenomenon was well illustrated by Michaux et al. in a recently blinded patient who complained of what could be described as "second blindness," because he temporarily lost the memories on which he relied for his orientation. After three weeks these difficulties completely subsided.

An unpleasant experience in ECT is occasional postconvulsive excitement immediately following the convulsion, which may last from a few minutes to one-half hour. Some patients, particularly males, become dangerously assaultive, develop enormous strength, try to escape, run around and injure themselves, and may strike anyone who attempts to control them. This reaction is not specific for ECT; we have seen it every time in a patient having twenty consecutive convulsions produced partly by metrazol, partly by electric current. Individuals who show this response often have had similar experiences after general anesthesia during surgery or when they were intoxicated. Some workers have attributed diagnostic importance to the postconvulsive behavior. Sargant and Slater felt that the true depressive generally remains quiet and pleasant, while the unrecognized schizophrenic may show suspicious and aggressive behavior. We cannot confirm this and feel that post-convulsive excitement bears no relation to the type of psychoses, but that personality traits and preformed patterns play definite roles. The most severe excitement was seen in a very good-natured patient who was a wrestler by profession and who, therefore, was accustomed to fight even in a half-conscious state. In ECT under anesthesia post-treatment excitement is only somewhat less frequent.

Convulsive treatment is followed by amnesia which first includes a long time-period before the treatment and gradually diminishes to the events immediately prior to the treatment. Stengel demonstrated how the retrograde amnesia shrinks only very gradually, while Mayer-Gross, who studied this symptom experimentally, saw surprisingly short retrograde amnesia. This is more in accordance with our own experience. Something quite different is the patient's frequent amnesia for the entire psychosis (Bodamer) or for one single delusion (Delay, Delmas-Marsalet). Observations regarding amnesia for the psychotic content are not uniform, and no conclusion of general validity can be drawn from it. Animal experimentation has contributed little to the study of amnesia after ECT. If Luttges and McGaugh claimed permanent retrograde amnesia in animals, this is contrary to anything seen in man during 30 years of experience with ECT.

Psychopathological studies were undertaken, in the German literature, by Von Baeyer and Grobe and by Weitbrecht. Von Baeyer realized the impossibility of interpreting the entire ECT effect by analysis of partial observations. In spite of this, many observations in the original work of Von Baeyer and Grobe are interesting for a psychopathology of ECT. They stressed the importance of the organic psychotic changes which will be discussed in more detail in the next section. They especially demonstrated the euphorization of the patient, and the influence which euphoria, increased and decreased impulses, increased reactivity to the environment and restriction of mental activities have on the symptoms of the psychiatric disorder being treated.

Such psychiatric observations appear to have greater importance than some psychodynamic interpretations which are occasionally presented without actual contact with clinical material. Yet, it should be realized that this psychopathological material, though of great interest, does not contribute to our understanding of the treatments. The same must be said regarding the material presented by Weitbrecht, who stresses the possibility of observing changes in the course of psychoses which, in the pre-shock era, could not be easily anticipated and watched. One of his essential conclusions is that not only are the reactive secondary schizophrenic symptoms influenced by shock treatments but that also the so-called primary or basic psychologically unexplainable symptoms may disappear under shock therapy. This is contrary to Von Baeyer and Grobe, who had previously arrived at the conclusion that convulsive treatment does not act on the more deep-seated primary symptoms. Weitbrecht also points out that cases refractory to treatment do not necessarily have an unfavorable prognosis, as exemplified by patients who later come to a spontaneous remission. It is necessary to differentiate between prognosis regarding symptoms and prognosis regarding deterioration. This opinion is in agreement with our own observation that patients who do not deteriorate (such as late paranoids or pseudoneurotic schizophrenics) are singularly refractory to treatment in spite of the frequent absence of primary symptoms. Weitbrecht differentiates between the effect on the total psychosis and a splitting up of units of symptoms. In paranoid reactions, for instance, the consolidation of a paranoid system can be prevented by interrupting the dangerous production of the system by means of repeated convulsive treatments. The fragments of the psychosis then lose actuality for the patient by means of such mechanisms as repression, amalgamation and objectivation. In case of relapse, the symptoms are often more colorless and have less psychotic content, and less affective charge than previously.

Another interesting problem is the patient's insight after the treatment, whereby distinction should be made between insight into the fact of having been sick at all, and insight into individual symptoms of the sickness. The concept of schizophrenic defect states which cannot be influenced any more is, according to Weitbrecht, not tenable since the introduction of active therapy; they cannot be compared with a scar because a process may be still going on. Cyclothymic depressions have many parallels to the schizophrenics as far as the response to shock treatment is concerned. Here, too, we can see a disappearance of the symptoms in toto, a dissolution of symptom-units and a change of symptoms. An essential difference is that relapses of manic-depressive cases are stable, uniform and not as different as the colorless symptoms of a schizophrenic relapse. A study by Gerstaker on the disturbances of thought in schizophrenics under convulsive therapy shows how the treatment isolates from an entirely disorganized thinking a rather resistive nucleus of thinking disorder which may be hardly noticeable but remains untouched. Such psychopathological studies on patients whose symptomatology can be changed at will by the treatment are a promising new approach.

Psychopathological aspects of the "post-electroshock" state were studied extensively and described in a monograph by Ebtinger. Most of the previous studies had been limited to the return of consciousness after one single treatment. This author follows the post-shock manifestations of an entire series of treatments and studies the parallel course of events in level and content of consciousness. Among other things he shows that memory is restored not simply from past to recent, but that lapses remain, particularly regarding the pathological period. When the treatment leads to a radical change of the clinical syndrome this always starts at the time of the return of consciousness. If there are no changes in this period the treatment has little chance of succeeding. Symptoms of acute psychosis usually show a complete change in the post-shock state, while symptoms of chronic psychosis remain unchanged. Ebtinger distinguishes three phases in the reconstruction: an excitation phase, a depressive phase, and the third phase in which consciousness is sufficiently restored to recognize and correct its own disturbances. It is certainly correct that the electric shock offers experimental conditions to study psychopathological changes, and we agree with the author that it is an important means to come to a better understanding of relations between organic pathological and psychopathological mechanisms.

Organic-Psychotic Reactions; Activation of the Psychosis

Different from the manifestations following each individual treatment are those organic mental symptoms which are caused by repeated convulsions.

They can be observed in practically every patient, although in widely varying degrees. They have been described as "organic-psychotic reactions occurring during ECT" (Kalinowsky). Korsakoff-like pictures are frequent. Some patients become bewildered, others show severe psychomotor excitement aggravated by delusional fears and hallucinations. Signs which differentiate these organic reactions from the patient's original psychosis are organic "blurring" of consciousness, greater emotional lability, more flighty delusions, more vivid hallucinations, and so on. These syndromes occur in neurotics as well as in psychotics. The pretreatment personality plays an important part in the determination of symptoms, as has been demonstrated in organic-psychotic reactions of varying etiology.

The correct recognition of these organic syndromes is of great practical importance. Therapy is often continued unnecessarily when an organic reaction is mistaken for residual symptoms of the original psychosis. Patients who have already improved from a depression may later show uncertainty and bewilderment of an organic type; if this is taken as a sign of depression, the patient may be subjected to further treatment, which only delays his recovery. Psychotic symptoms following a period of improvement, but still occurring during treatment, are usually an organic manifestation. Actual relapses seldom occur earlier than several days after discontinuation of treatment. Another frequent mistake is premature discontinuation of treatment because of an organic reaction which is taken for an aggravation of the patient's original psychosis. Interruption of therapy because of acute organic syndromes is unwarranted, particularly as further treatment usually leads to a less dramatic condition which may be characterized as temporary organic dementia. Whatever the degree of this organic reaction, it will disappear approximately a week or ten days after the last treatment. There are patients in whom, a few days after the course of treatment is terminated, a quiet confusional state is still followed by an acute delirium with vivid hallucinations and delusions, these being quite different in type from those of the original psychosis. If mistaken for relapse, these syndromes may lead to unnecessary reinstitution of treatment; if left untreated they subside spontaneously in a few days. In many instances they require great diagnostic scrutiny and are a difficult problem for the therapist.

It is not always easy to differentiate these organic-psychotic reactions from activation of the patient's psychosis, the latter apparently a much rarer occurrence. Activation of the psychosis can be best recognized when a quiet, blocked schizophrenic after the first treatment becomes acutely disturbed, actively delusional and hallucinating. We agree with Osgood that such change of symptoms, although impressive, should not be considered an aggravation of the patient's condition. More frequently an apparent depression clears up during the first few treatments, but is then replaced by the appearance of acute schizophrenic symptoms. In these instances, the superficial layer of "depression" has been removed by the treatment, and the underlying schizophrenic symptoms become overt. Halpern reports such instances under the title of "electroshock as a diagnostic aid in schizophrenia." The same is seen, when the depressive overlay of a schizophrenic psychosis is removed with antidepressive drugs.

Psychological Investigations

Convulsive therapy has stimulated psychologic research primarily regarding the question of impairment of memory function. No evidence has been brought forward to indicate that permanent mental sequelae are caused by the treatment. The question has received undue attention in the lay press and by those objecting to organic treatments on theoretical grounds. Many overlook the fact that we are treating mental disorders which imply a much greater danger to the personality than the treatments employed for their cure. It should not be forgotten that in many of the cases treated the disease progresses toward deterioration; and if it does so, it is not because of but in spite of the treatment. Only a few instances of intellectual impairment lasting for several months or longer have been claimed (Dynes with metrazol, Levy et al., Brody, and others with ECT). Neurotics with hypochondriacal tendencies complain more often than other patients of not remembering names and places, of difficulty in concentrating, or of forgetting more easily. Stone, who found a general impairment of cognitive functions, including comprehension, arithmetical computations, tasks involving abstraction, and so on during ECT, noticed a frequent rise beyond the pretreatment scores during the weeks after the treatment. This is probably explained by a removal of the emotional distress which interfered with the patient's intellectual performance during his illness.

Only part of the psychological investigations that have accumulated in the literature on ECT can be listed here. As a whole, they have brought convincing evidence that no lasting intellectual impairment occurs in ECT.

Wittman and Russell have stated on the basis of studies performed with a battery of psychologic tests that no substantiation of memory defect following metrazol therapy can be found. They stress that if such memory defect occurs, it is more than compensated for in their test results by improvement in interest, attention, and social responsiveness. In ECT Zubin and Barrera tried to obtain objective evidence of the degree of memory impairment by teaching some of our patients at the Psychiatric Institute a series of paired word associates composed of one familiar and one nonsense word. The normal saving in the number of trials when material is relearned was lost after treatment. Recognition memory is hardly touched. Some impairment of both learning and retention was noted but both returned within three weeks after treatment to a level as good or better than the pre-treatment status. ECT affected personal memories in about the same way as implanted memories. This was also seen by Janis, who tested the recall of a series of life experiences before and after the treatment. The hypothesis that the patient recovers because his memory for adverse events or situations is wiped out is hardly tenable since no evidence of permanent destruction of memory traces is available. Carter finds that unpleasant memories are selectively forgotten. The reversible nature of memory loss after ECT was demonstrated by Huston and Strother; Sherman et al.; K. W. Wilcox. Rabin showed the absence of permanent organic patterns in Rorschach tests even after 100 and more treatments.

Animal experiments using the conditioned reflex technique have been reported by Kessler and Gellhorn. They caused certain conditioned responses to be extinguished and noticed that when such animals were subjected to convulsive therapy, the conditioned responses reappeared. They concluded from this that the treatment may eliminate inhibitions, but it seems that a retrograde amnesia for the time in which the extinction was accomplished may explain equally well the return of the conditioned response. The same explanation can be applied to the findings of Masserman and Jacques. In their interesting investigations in animals with an experimentally induced neurosis, they observed a marked disintegration of neurotic paterns. Most of the effects on normal and "neurotic" animals were temporary after a few, and more permanent after a greater number of shocks. No enduring effect of ECT on the adaptive behavior was seen by Winkler and Frank, when the animals were decorticated.

Bunch and Müller found no impairment of relearning after metrazol convulsions; Siegel also failed to see any impairment after electrically induced convulsions. That in experiments by Duncan, relearning was impaired in terms of trials, errors, and time during relearning, is not surprising since relearning was tested only one day after thirty daily convulsions. The same author reported other interesting experiments which seemed to show a "habit reversal." The theory that convulsive therapy is effective because it produces a reversal to older habits was first presented by Rodnick in experiments with schizophrenics who were taught two incompatible habits; under metrazol treatment, the more recently acquired habit was "repressed and extinguished." This parallels clinical observations on patients who temporarily lose the last acquired of several languages. It has been stated by some clinicians and substantiated by Scherer that such techniques as brief stimuli therapy do not affect adversely memory, abstraction capacity or Rorschach responsiveness, showing again that memory impairment is not necessary for clinical improvement. Masserman et al., however, gave their findings on experimentally neurotic cats the interpretation that the effect of ECT on neurotic patterns corresponds to the degree of disorganization of both normal and neurotic behavior. We agree with H. E. Meyer that amnesia has no importance for the therapeutic results. Therefore, techniques for which absence of memory impairment could be proven, should be welcome. As far as lasting memory loss is concerned, the most convincing evidence that such does not occur, was given by Perlson's psychological testing of a patient who had had the unusual number of 248 convulsions. No intellectual or emotional deterioration was disclosed in a great variety of tests.

Also Löwenbach and Stainbrook using Wertheimer's Gestalt figures found that results closely approach the performance given prior to treatment. The same authors also studied the immediate Rorschach responses after ECT.

Piotrowski examined a group of our patients with the Rorschach technique before and after ECT. Definite psychologic differences were found to exist between those who improved and those who did not. The Rorschach prognostic signs devised by Piotrowski and discussed in the chapter on insulin have the same validity for ECT as for insulin. The correct prediction of the outcome of treatment was 87 per cent in ECT; this is about the same percentage as in insulin-treated schizophrenics. No such prognostic value was seen in the Minnesota Multiphasic Personality Inventory (Pacella et al.). The steady increase of the organic syndrome during ECT was studied in the Rorschach test by Lindner, who sees the actual therapeutic effect in the organic syndrome. Piotrowski points out that the Rorschach findings substantiate the view that both ECT and insulin have a curative effect on the secondary or compensatory personality changes but not upon the primary regression of the schizophrenic process.

Most of the psychological investigations on humans as well as on animals are interesting scientifically, but they only confirm what has been seen by the clinician. The same can be said about various other psychological techniques to demonstrate organic brain changes due to ECT, for instance the reduction of figural fluctuation frequency (Cesarec and Nilsson). Some psychological investigations like the one by Hardi on changes in writing and drawing after ECT are of interest for both, the temporary brain dysfunction and the changes due to the disappearance of abnormalities caused by the disease. There were also attempts to use such psychological tests as the Minnesota Multiphasic Personality Inventory for prognostication (Gonda), but their prognostic value was inferior to the clinical judgment.

Clinically important research was done by the Swedish psychiatrists Cronholm and Ottosson. They rightly pointed out that patients who after ECT are freed from their emotional distress, seldom complain of memory disturbances. These authors differentiated between the "subjective memory change" reported by the patient and the "objective memory change" measured by a memory test battery. One of their findings was the effect of ECT on learning which was judged quite correctly by the patient, while he is not able to judge forgetting. When a depression is relieved, learning ability dominates the patient's experience over the simultaneous impairment of retention. If therapy was not successful, learning is still poor and, with retention also being impaired, the patient realizes his poor memory. This inability on the part of the patient to judge his memory impairment properly, makes it impossible to rely on his own verdict in estimating his actual memory impairment which depends primarily on the degree of improvement of his depression. Some theoretical aspects of the work by these Swedish authors will be discussed in the chapter on Theoretical Considerations.

Neurological Observations

Neurological observations during convulsive therapy have been reported in ECT by Vattuone, Kino, Kalinowsky, Fleishhacker, Klein and Early and others; in pharmacologic convulsive therapy by Birkmeyer and by Hemphill, who studied especially various motor phenomena during and after an induced convulsion.

No reflexes can be elicited during the convulsion. Babinski sign was observed by Kalinowsky in not more than one-fifth of all cases, and, according to Savitzky and Karliner, it is always preceded by the absence of plantar reflexes. Shortly after the fit, the deep reflexes are increased. There is a first phase of flaccidity after the convulsion which, with a three-to-ten-second lapse, is followed by a phase of muscular hypertonia lasting for twenty seconds to two minutes.

It is during this phase that pyramidal signs appear in some of the cases. Kino, in his elaborate study on reflexes, points out that unlike the Babinski, a Rossolimo sign and fanning phenomenon could never be elicited. The pupils do not react during the convulsion and, later, often change repeatedly between rigidity and reflex activity. Klein and Early described some unusual pupillary phenomena. In general, it can be said that the corneal reflexes return first, followed by the pupillary reflexes, the Babinski sign disappears, and that the skin reflexes return last. Absence of Mayer's metacarpophalangeal joint reflex is the most contant reflex anomaly, lasting for six to nine minutes. A grasp reflex can be elicited three to six minutes after the convulsion for one to three minutes. However, we agree with Kino and Thorpe that it does not have the aspect of forced grasping and groping; these latter phenomena observed in prefrontal lesions in fully conscious patients were never elicited by us after convulsions. Also, Magnus-de Kleyn reflexes could not be elicited by Kino but were occasionally obtained by Fleischhacker.

Postconvulsive motor phenomena vary with each individual, and there is no reason to believe that they are different from those following a spontaneous epileptic convulsion. The same holds good for a phenomenon preceding the muscular discharge, i.e., constriction of the retinal vessels observed by Milch in several of our patients immediately before the onset of an electrically induced convulsion. Cavka saw it in metrazol convulsions, and Hemphill describes pallor of the whole fundus and disc which only in the second half of the clonic state is followed by hyperemia. Such findings are in accordance with observations by Foerster and others of vasoconstriction followed by vasodilatation on the exposed brain during convulsions. Kreineberg and Ehrhardt noticed that if the usual occlusion of the vascular supply to the brain is missing, only an incomplete seizure takes place.

Hemphill and Grey Walter syringed one ear in order to study the effect on the asymmetrical onset of seizures. They noticed that the seizure seemed to start on the side of the ear that had been syringed. Other workers who tried to localize the point of origin of the seizure concluded from the vegetative symptoms, which are more prominent in the nonconvulsive response and in the tonic phase, and from the preconvulsive wormlike "jumping jack movement" (Ewald and Haddenbrock), that the convulsions seem to originate in deep centers around the third ventricle with the cortex appearing only in the clonic movements. Kalinowsky and Kennedy reported on observations in ECT which seemed to be of some interest for various problems of epilepsy. Spontaneous and electrically induced seizures in epileptics appeared to be identical, including certain postconvulsive automatisms and manifestations during petit mal attacks.

The more complicated disturbances of cortical function were also studied. Finger agnosia and other symptoms of Gerstman's syndrome, difficulty in recognizing actions on a picture (described in brain lesions by Wolpert), and other difficulties in recognizing a "whole" in the sense of "Gestaltspsychologie" were described by Juba. Gallinek noted distortions of gnostic function which may involve perception of the face or other parts of the body but more often create either a feeling that everyone, including strangers, looks familiar or, to the contrary, that familiar faces or objects look unfamiliar or distorted. Disturbances of body image, including the feeling that the face is ballooned, fingers elongated, and so on, were seen. Also objects touched by the patient's hand might feel unfamiliar. There was a striking differentiation between subjective and objective perception and the patients stated that "the fingers do not feel as they look." This group of disturbances presents an interesting opportunity to study cerebral symptoms, although it does not permit localization of the symptoms in definite cortical areas.

Electroencephalographic Findings

Convulsive states are one of the main fields of interest for electroencephalography. It is, therefore, not unexpected that the possibility of inducing convulsive states in human beings was widely used for electroencephalographic investigations. Actually, the results have been somewhat disappointing, inasmuch as the main problem in research on epilepsy is not the convulsion itself but the cerebral state leading to the convulsion; it is obvious that artificially induced seizures cannot contribute much to the solution of that problem. In contrast to the seizures of an epileptic patient, the loss of consciousness in electrically induced convulsions is immediate; in metrazol treatment the patient experiences severe anxiety which in itself modifies the electroencephalographic pattern.

Following metrazol (cardiazol) injections, Cook and Walter have observed small six per second waves over the whole cortex. When a convulsion follows, there is a sudden increase in size and decrease in frequency in the frontal region; from this focus, which corresponds to area 6a beta and is considered particularly "epileptogenous" in man, the slow waves spread over the whole cortex. When the convulsion ends, no activity is seen until consciousness returns.

The observation of electrophysiologic phenomena accompanying an electrically induced convulsion offers greater difficulties. Grey Walter, the first to study electroencephalographic patterns in ECT, found that the strong electrical stimulus transforms the head into something resembling an electric battery. A continuous sequence of large spikes with a frequency of three to ten per second was noticed during the tonic phase by Lowenbach and Lyman in electrically induced convulsions in rabbits. There is little agreement on the electrophysiologic events taking place during the convulsion itself. Much greater interest, as far as electroencephalographic findings in convulsive therapy are concerned, lies in the events following convulsive treatment, and especially with regard to the influence of a series of treatments on the electroencephalographic pattern of the individual. Determination, on the basis of a pretreatment electroencephalographic pattern, of the type of patient who may respond to treatment, cannot be expected until typical electroencephalographic abnormalities are established in the psychotic syndromes treated with convulsive therapy.

The electroencephalogram after convulsive treatment resembles the pattern seen after spontaneous convulsions, as evidenced in pharmacologically induced seizures by Cook and Walter, Strauss and Rahm, and in ECT by Golla et al. and many other investigators. The material treated at the New York State Psychiatric Institute was routinely studied with the electroencephalograph (Pacella et al.) and the following observations were made: The electrically induced generalized convulsion is immediately followed by slow waves of 0.5 to 2 cycles per second which appear fairly equal on both sides over the entire cortex. When respiration becomes more normal, 2 to 4 cycles per second waves predominate. When the patient regains consciousness, and sometimes before, alpha waves reappear; the frequency of slow waves gradually increases. In general, an approximately normal state is resumed within five to thirty minutes after the seizure, with the frontal regions returning last to their normal rhythm. The amount of voltage applied for the treatment bears no relation to the degree of abnormality.

This return to normal within thirty minutes after the convulsion does not occur after several treatments; at this stage the record remains abnormal between treatments. This more lasting abnormality consists essentially of the frequent appearance of 3 to 6 cycles per second waves of moderate to high voltage. They persist first in the frontal area and only with subsequent treatment extend over the other areas of the cortex. Sudden bursts of continuous slow high voltage waves for a period of one to five seconds resemble the typical convulsive pattern, occurring in spontaneous seizures. This activity takes place simultaneously on both sides. The severest change of this kind usually appears between the sixth and twelfth treatment, if treatment is given three times a week. The abnormal slow waves disappear within one to five weeks in patients who receive six or less convulsions, one to three months after seven to twelve convulsions, and two to six months or even later when more treatments are given. After the slow potentials have disappeared, an unusual high voltage alpha rhythm often persists. However, the cerebral dysfunction after ECT as expressed in the electroencephalographic record is largely reversible. This has also been reported by Levi et al. Klotz noticed in several patients an improvement of the electroencephalogram after a course of ECT as compared with the pretreatment electroencephalogram, and explain this as being due to a decrease in anxiety and tension.

An extensive study of the electroencephalographic pattern in animals treated with electrically induced convulsions was presented by R. Jung. The interest of this study lies in the fact that the electric pattern was not only taken from the cortex but also from the striatum, thalamus, mesencephalon and cerebellum. Fast discharges of 40 per second are seen in cortex and thalamus as early as the latent period. In the tonic phase, all the areas—including the cortex—discharge, which contradicts the assumption that only the brain stem convulses in the tonic phase. The clonic rhythm is apparently an alternating stimulation between cortex and striatum. In a generalized seizure, all parts of the brain convulse, while the abortive shock is primarily a brain stem seizure. The intensive activity of the Ammon's horn was another interesting finding. In the same hospital Meyer-Mikeleit studied the electroencephalogram in ECT of humans. He avoided interference from muscular contractions by using curare.

In the latent period, alpha waves started in the frontal lobes and extended within a few seconds toward the parietal area; he found that when this area is reached, the tonic phase sets in. During this phase discharge of the various areas are not synchronized but become uniform during the clonic phase. After the seizure, every electrical activity ceases for 25 to 40 seconds.

Turner et al., and some others, tried to correlate pretreatment electroencephalogram and clinical improvement. Opinions on this point vary. Liberson found that the best clinical improvements are seen in patients with the least electroencephalographic changes. Kennard and Willner considered severely abnormal records as evidence of a severe and long-standing psychosis. Moriarty and Siemens failed to find any significant difference between the records of recovered and unrecovered patients.

Another question studied repeatedly is the relation between the organic side-effects of convulsive therapy and electroencephalographic changes. It appears that the onset of psychological and electroencephalographic changes goes parallel and that both set in earlier when treatment is given daily than when it is applied two or three times a week. However, the disappearance of the two types of symptoms does not seem to be correlated. It has been our constant experience that the memory impairment clears up much sooner than the electroencephalographic changes.

It may be mentioned that muscle relaxants do not modify the electroencephalographic pattern. When intravenous sodium amytal is given prior to electric convulsive therapy, the electroencephalogram, according to Impastato et al., returns more quickly to normal. The claim that special types of current produce slighter degrees of electroencephalographic alterations has already been discussed in the section on various types of current used in ECT.

The localized abnormalities over the one hemisphere in the electroencephalograms of patients treated with unilateral ECT, and the interesting implications of the differences in the EEG in unilateral and bilateral ECT have been mentioned in the chapter on Unilateral ECT. A recent comparison between electroencephalograms of metrazol and electric convulsions was made by Schulz et al. who eliminated muscular artifacts with muscle relaxants. There was no greater cerebral dysfunction in ECT than in pharmacologically induced convulsions. Another interesting finding was the regularity of focal temporal changes, predominantly on the left side. EEG changes after Indoklon convulsions are also not different from those in other forms of convulsive therapy.

Studies on petit mal seizures show that following this response in ECT slow potentials occur only if unconsciousness is long and deep. These slow potentials disappear after a very short time and, even when a series of such treatments is given, the preshock record has always reappeared within less than twenty-four hours. The "spike and dome" wave pattern described as typical for the petit mal attacks of epileptics was not observed in our material (Pacella et al.), whereas Levi et al. show this pattern in subconvulsive treatments. A comparison between electroencephalographic changes in pharmacologically and electrically induced convulsive and non-convulsive responses was undertaken by Cremerius and Jung. They found a much greater intensity and longer duration of electroencephalographic changes in abortive metrazol treatments, although contrary to the petit mal response in ECT, consciousness in abortive metrazol treatments is not impaired. Altogether, they observed less marked changes after ECT than after chemical convulsants; Davis and Sulzbach found the latter changes to last sometimes over a year.

Clinical improvement in convulsive therapy usually takes place before the electroencephalogram becomes abnormal. Relapses may occur while the electroencephalogram remains abnormal or following its return to the pretreatment pattern. To draw the conclusion from an abnormal electroencephalographic record that the patient should receive no more treatment, as done by Mosovich and Katzenelbogen and some other workers, is not justified. In our post-ECT material, Taylor and Pacella failed to see the development of convulsions in any of over 1000 patients with normal pretreatment electroencephalogram. In a group of 56 cases with definitely abnormal electroencephalogram, prior to treatment two patients had post-treatment seizures. There is general agreement that the abnormal electroencephalogram during convulsive treatments sooner or later returns to normal. On the other hand, many clinicians believe that ECT which leads to severe confusion accompanied by the most severe electroencephalographic changes is particularly successful. In recent years this view could be confirmed in extensive studies by Fink and Kahn. They found a significant relationship between the early appearance of delta activity as well as other signs of organic changes, and a favorable therapeutic response to ECT. Studies by Fink also tried to correlate biochemical, particularly cholinergic mechanisms with EEG changes.

Equipment with which to monitor electroencephalographic and electrocardiographic changes during ECT was used by Blachly and Gowing in connection with their method of giving multiple electric convulsive treatments at one sitting. One of their findings was that EEG evidence of seizure discharge persisted long after muscular evidence of seizures had stopped.

Complications

Today complications in convulsive therapy are rare. They are still overemphasized by many psychiatrists. The recognized concept of *nil nocere* remains the basic concept for every physician, but it is not meant to lead to therapeutic nihilism. The surgeon does not refuse a necessary operation because of its impending risks. Since active therapy is available in psychiatry, it should be used for the benefit of many patients even though a few may develop undesirable complications. Fortunately, fatal complications in convulsive therapy are extremely rare.

We agree with Sargant and Slater's statement that mental disorders are as destructive as a malignant growth and far more terrible in the suffering they may cause. Risks are therefore justified. It is gratifying that the Pennsylvania Department of Justice, quoted by Overholser, expressed an opinion to the effect that ECT is of recognized value and, therefore, may be applied to mental patients without the consent of the patient or his family. No court decisions on negligence for not applying shock therapy, where it is indicated, are yet available, but K. Schneider reports on a decision implying that early treatment would have improved the chances for remission in a schizophrenic. The legal implications of the treatment were recently reviewed in a German paper by Schönke. As to malpractice suits following fractures, the Supreme Court of Tennessee ruled that electric shock therapy is a scientifically accepted procedure in which fractures occur even if the treatment is properly applied. Today fractures have been practically eliminated, and malpractice suits in connection with ECT have disappeared from the list of legal actions against psychiatrists. The last suits had been mostly concerned with the question whether fractures must be prevented with muscle relaxants and barbiturate anesthesia in spite of the fact that such anesthesia technique introduces a new element of danger to the patient's life. A British Court (Ref: Medico-Legal Correspondent) returned a verdict for the psychiatrist after a psychiatric expert from another hospital mentioned four deaths in ECT with barbiturate anesthesia and succinyl choline but only one due to straight ECT. Most psychiatrists by now have accepted the use of muscle relaxation and anesthesia as routine procedure in convulsive therapy. Some still disagree. It is for this reason and, particularly because muscle relaxation may be inadequate in an individual case, that psychiatrists must still be informed about these potential complications. Therefore, a discussion of possible fractures as they were frequent in the past, cannot be eliminated from this chapter.

FRACTURES AND DISLOCATION: The most frequent complications in convulsive therapy were fractures caused by muscular contraction. The types of fractures occurring in metrazol and in ECT are essentially the same and, therefore, will be discussed together. They have in common the fact that they seem to occur during the first sudden muscular contraction when many observers have reported hearing the first cracking of a bone. The frequently sudden onset of artificial convulsions may explain why fractures occur in this treatment but are seldom seen in epileptics who customarily go slowly into the tonic phase of the convulsion. This is also substantiated by the fact that with the more sudden and lightning-like onset in metrazol convulsions, fractures are more frequent than in ECT. The delayed electric convulsion should, therefore, be the least likely to produce fractures, but delayed seizures are difficult to obtain due to inability to estimate the necessary dosage. Lately, we have made every effort to use threshold stimuli even if we have to repeat the stimulation two, three or more times in succession, in the hope of obtaining a slowly developing seizure. The application of a petit mal response, followed immediately by a second convulsive stimulus, is another useful measure as in this way the patient goes into the convulsion with a relaxed musculature. This procedure is especially desirable if the patient is very tense or struggles against the treatment. However, the value of none of these attempts has been proved to our satisfaction. The often made statement that elderly people are predisposed to fractures, has never been proved. Schmieder has shown that the fracture rate decreases in older age. No predisposing factor of any kind could be singled out. In cases where fractures have occurred it was never possible to determine any predisposing cause in the patient. The statement remains valid that the fractures are entirely unpredictable.

In the following paragraphs the most frequent types of fractures will be discussed. They have typical localizations, and fractures in other parts of the skeletal system are practically nonexistent.

Fractures of the femur: There seems to be a difference in the occurrence of this complication in muscular, younger individuals and in elderly, particularly emaciated, chronic patients. Complete "rupture" of the head of the femur seems to occur only in young muscular individuals when tight restraint of the hip joint is applied. In elderly people impacted fratures are more frequent. Sogliani saw a fracture of the greater trochanter. Considering the rarity of fractures of the femur in convulsive therapy, it is remarkable that bilateral occurrence during the same convulsion was reported several times in pharmacologically as well as in electrically induced seizures (Somers and Richardson, and many others). Lanzkron mentions a hip fracture in a patient with an amputation stump.

Fractures of the acetabulum: This otherwise rather rare type of fracture was not infrequently seen in ECT. It can be explained only by the sudden contraction of muscles which pull the head of the femur toward the pelvis. The fracture is perhaps more likely to occur in elderly people when the head of the femur perforates a weakened acetabular cavity and is pushed into the pelvis. The mechanism of this fracture seems to be the same as that of fractures of the neck of the femur. The impact of certain adductor muscles either compresses the femur so that it breaks, or, if the acetabulum is not strong enough to resist, it is fractured and the head of the femur is driven into the pelvic cavity. Abnormalities of the pelvis may be a contributory factor as described in a case of Haines which disclosed an *Otto pelvis* (deep acetabular cavity with a thin inner wall). In spite of the rarity of this complication, several instances of bilateral acetabular fractures have been reported. Linley and Robbins reported three bilateral fractures in a material of 230 patients. One of us (L.B.K.) saw acetabular fractures twice bilaterally, and both times during the first treatment. The younger of these two patients had a fracture of the femur on the one side and an acetabular fracture on the other. This shows that the mechanism must be the same in fractures of the femur and acetabulum.

Fractures of the arm: Fractures in the upper extremities were localized principally in the neck of the humerus. Here again, complete rupture between head and shaft was seen mainly in young, muscular men. In elderly patients there are sometimes impacted fractures with favorable prognosis. Tight restraint as a precipitating rather than preventive factor in fractures of the humerus seems less clearly established by clinical observation than in those of the femur. The only predisposing feature we were able to establish in patients who suffered fractures of the humerus was muscularity combined with adiposity. Osteoporosis was never seen. In a number of patients with complaints suggesting a fracture of the humerus, a bursitis with calcification was found as the cause of the rather severe pain. In other cases rupture of the tendon of the supraspinatus was diagnosed.

Fractures of the scapula: These are rare but were perhaps often overlooked, being very unusual in type. A triangular fragment is torn off the lower scapula, a fracture type which is almost unknown otherwise and which, in one of our patients, was recognized only after repeated x-ray examination. Functional impairment, aside from pain, is insignificant.

Fractures of the spine: There was a great disproportion between the clinical importance of the type of vertebral fractures occurring in convulsive therapy and the emphasis given them in medical literature. That their clinical importance is not very great is evidenced by the fact that only after several years of application of convulsive therapy were they recognized. Single cases were reported by Stalker and by Wespi. Polatin and others were the first to examine systematically their metrazol-treated patients and found more or less definite x-ray changes in 43.1 per cent of all cases. The frequency of positive findings will largely depend on the degree of scrutiny of x-ray plates before and after treatment, which explains the range of percentages given for their occurrence.

Hyperextension of the spine was recommended because the spine seems to bend forward during the convulsion. An important attempt to clarify this problem was made by Flordh, who demonstrated under x-ray control that the vertebral column during the treatment is not bent forward but compressed in a longitudinal direction. This mechanism would suggest that no position can diminish the danger of fractures.

Vertebral fractures in convulsive therapy are localized exclusively in the mid-dorsal region between the fourth and eighth vertebrae and are frequently multiple. The fifth thoracic being the weakest vertebra of the entire spine according to Fick, it is most easily crushed experimentally (Furst). X-ray examinations show all reactions from slight impression of the surface of the vertebrae with enlargement of the intervertebral space over chip fractures of the superior anterior edge to definite compression fractures. Easton and Somers found that pre-existing pathologic changes do not increase the tendency to fractures, and that calcium deficiency, held responsible by some, is not a contributory factor. Back pain during respiratory movements and, less often, local tenderness on deep pressure are the patient's complaints. The pain usually does not last longer than a few days or weeks. Often, there is no relation between severity of pain and fracture, and some patients remain without any discomfort. Polatin and Linn, in a ten-year follow-up of their original group of vertebral fractures, confirmed the general experience that no serious sequelae of an orthopedic or neurologic nature occur. Worthing and Kalinowsky point out that fractures in the mid-dorsal region, although occurring in tetanus convulsions, do not seem to occur in epilepsy. Cook and Sands, and Moore et al. found vertebral fractures in epileptics in other than the mid-dorsal region; here they were seen only by Reed and Dancy.

Special treatment of these vertebral fractures is not indicated and will frighten the patient unnecessarily. Originally, orthopedic appliances were recommended but they are superfluous. Schmieder found that when ECT is continued, compressed vertebrae are more resistant to new damage than are healthy ones. We continued such patients and we have sometimes seen even the pain disappear during subsequent treatments.

Dislocation of the arm: This is a rare occurrence. It is the only injury which is more frequent in the uncontrolled spontaneous convulsions of epileptics. It is probable that this is usually avoided in convulsive therapy by guiding the movements slightly, thus avoiding wide excursions of the arm. Dislocations combined with fractures have been reported.

Dislocation of the jaw: This was frequent in unpremedicated ECT. It is practically always reducible during the latter part of the convulsion when the muscular contractions become less frequent and are separated by periods of muscular relaxation.

COMPLICATIONS IN THE RESPIRATORY SYSTEM: A distinction should be made between those complications of the respiratory system which are of central origin, such as respiratory distress or arrest following a convulsion, and disease processes in the lungs caused by convulsive therapy. The first group is of greater practical importance.

Apnea is a physiologic phenomenon in any epileptiform seizure. It sometimes persists considerably longer than the seizure. Cases of long respiratory arrest were described in metrazol treatment but, apparently, they are more frequent in ECT where the pharmacologic effect of the respiratory stimulant, metrazol, is absent. According to Müller, respiratory difficulties are more frequent after subconvulsive responses than after generalized seizures. Wright points out that a probable cortical respiratory center in Brodmann's area 6a beta lies directly in the path of the electric current. He, therefore, alters the position of the electrodes posteriorly, while Frostig et al. finds that occipital application interferes with respiration most. Brill and Kalinowsky, reporting on the incidence of a long respiratory arrest, point out that both depression of the respiratory center and airway obstruction due to collapse of the pharynx and tongue together may bring about dangerous respiratory difficulties. When anoxemia persists, the patient may go into an extensor spasm, but only the next stage of general muscular flaccidity is the true danger signal.

Application of oxygen by a mask is now standard procedure. The use of muscle relaxants makes the application of oxygen a necessity in any treatment. Prior to the use of muscle relaxants artificial respiration had usually been sufficient. The patient's head should be bent backwards until he breathes regularly. We often saw that respiration stopped again when the head was bent forward, and returned immediately, when the head was extended. This experience in unmodified ECT can occasionally be seen even in modified ECT. Prolonged apnea due to succinylcholine is much rarer than can be assumed from some remarks in the literature. With proper oxygenation we never found it to be any problem. An uncontrollable cough with subsequent dyspnea and near collapse was seen once in a patient who, unknown to us, was allergic to barbiturates; the patient survived.

Bini and Puddu have pointed out—and we can only agree—that chemical respiratory stimuli, such as metrazol and alpha lobeline, appear to be of no value when apnea persists. They may, however, be used prophylactically. Clearing the airways and counteracting the collapse of the tongue with a rubber or metal airway today are standard procedures to prevent respiratory distress.

The development of pulmonary diseases during treatment is rare in ECT but was quite frequent in metrazol therapy. Here, pulmonary abscess and gangrene were originally explained as due to aspiration of foreign bodies or septic material while the cough reflex is absent, or by direct action of metrazol on lung tissue (Giannelli and Sani). Another explanation is the formation and later mobilization of thrombi on the site of the metrazol injection (Beckenstein; Zeifert). Pulmonary embolism from pelvic thrombosis has also been observed. The early literature on ECT contained only one case of pulmonary abscess which might have been accidental (Kalinowsky and Worthing). Kwalwasser et al. noted lung abscesses as a complication of ECT in 1 per cent of the total number of cases treated. Analysis of this institutional material shows that 22 of the 25 patients had been untidy and 7 had to be tube-fed. However, except for a few isolated cases, pulmonary abscess remained a rare complication in ECT.

Activation of latent pulmonary tuberculosis has been reported in metrazol cases (Bulley and Greene). Will and Duval give a survey of scattered reports on activation of tuberculosis in ECT. It should be realized that activation is frequent in any institutional material of tuberculosis. Several reports indicate that complications in the treatment of tuberculous patients are rare. In the Ontario Hospital (E. A. Clark) only 3 out of 49 patients with active tuberculosis died one to thirteen months after termination of ECT. In a report by Jentoft on 56 tuberculous patients treated with ECT, 12 became worse but in only 3 cases could a connection with the treatment be assumed. These 12 cases are certainly balanced by 9 cases where the pulmonary findings improved and 35 cases where the pulmonary lesion remained unchanged. The largest report by Pleasure also comes to favorable conclusions.

Cardiovascular complications: In metrazol treatment, cardiovascular complications, especially auricular fibrillation, were occasionally encountered. The toxic effect of metrazol itself was thought to damage the myocardium. This is doubted by Hoffmann et al. in view of the transient nature of the electrocardiographic irregularities and the absence of significant T wave changes; they believe that auricular fibrillation occurs as the result of an excessive central nervous system stimulus. Serious myocardial collapse occurs in metrazol in 0.06 per cent of all cases treated, according to Meduna and Friedman's survey. On the other hand, many reports are available on patients treated successfully in spite of severe cardiovascular conditions.

In ECT, reports on cardiovascular complications are even rarer. There are a few reports of patients with chronic endocarditis and myocarditis who collapsed or died after the convulsion. If in such cases cardiac dilatation occurs, the muscular exertion of the convulsion was held responsible (Jetter). In a few instances coronary death has been reported hours or days following a convulsive treatment, and it is a matter of speculation whether or not such an occurrence is due to the therapeutic procedure. In Moore's large material of cardiac patients treated with ECT, only one case with many previous myocardial infarcts had a new infarct after the third treatment. Auricular fibrillations were observed by Linn and Ottenheimer. In a similar case of Craddock and Gilbert this complication did not repeat itself in subsequent treatments. Cardiovascular complications have been reported in individual cases, but their number remains rare even after the introduction of anesthesia techniques. This is true, although the percentage of patients with severe cardiac disease prior to ECT is, at least in our own experience, increasingly high. In some of the reported cases of ill effects the causal relationship remained doubtful. The most convincing connection between ECT and myocardial infarction was a recent fatal case of Hussar and Pachter with two infarctions in the only two treatments the patient had three months apart. The treatments were given with barbiturate anesthesia, and the fact that the patient was in congestive failure already prior to the first treatment, raises the question whether avoidance of the intravenous barbiturate injection might have prevented the accident. In two fatal coronary occlusions, reported by Heggtveit, also treated with barbiturate anesthesia, there had not been any previous evidence of myocardial damage.

Cardiac arrest was described by Cropper and Hughes in a young patient with mitral stenosis. We had a similar difficulty in a patient of the same age of 29 in whom mitral stenosis was present but not recognized until the patient had recovered. However in the case reported by Cropper and Hughes three stimuli were given but no convulsion had occurred which make this case of particular interest. There are some other instances of cardiac arrest reported in the literature, and the question arose to what degree psychiatrists using ECT, should be prepared for such occurrences. Thoracotomy was performed after cardiac arrest in a case of Arneson and Butler, but the patient died 12 hours later. The availability of a cardiac pacemaker and defibrillator is recommended by Barron and Sullivan.

A rare cause of cardiovascular collapse has found little attention but is of definite potential danger. Baumoel mentioned a patient who suffered a circulatory collapse during a severe postconvulsive excitement state from which he was revived. The same, with fatal outcome, was seen by Hoch in a case reported in the section on fatalities. The possible relationship between cardiovascular complications and anesthesia techniques used in ECT has been discussed in the chapter on muscle relaxants and will be dealt with again under "contraindications."

NEUROLOGICAL COMPLICATIONS: Aside from symptom aggravation of brain tumors which will be discussed under contraindications, neurological complications are extremely rare. Shapiro and Goldberg reported on two fatalities in patients with previous cerebrovascular accidents. Although many patients with agitated depression suffering from hypertension are treated, we have never seen cerebrovascular accidents even in patients with previous cerebral thrombosis or hemorrhage. Halpern et al. saw a hemorrhage after a treatment that had not resulted in a convulsion; and Larsen and Vraa-Jensen found a subarachnoid hemorrhage after several failures to produce a convulsion. Müller describes a patient who, one hour after a petit mal, had several spontaneous convulsions followed by a hemiparesis. Olsen has reported on a 73 year old patient with low blood pressure who, after a treatment with unilateral convulsion, had twitchings and a brief hemiparesis of the affected side. The rarity of serious vascular accidents in convulsive therapy is in accordance with the fact that such complications are also unusual in spontaneous epileptic convulsions. The rare occurrence and temporary nature of cerebrovascular manifestations in hypertensive patients was also reported by Accornero and Guerra. A case by Riese and Fultz of a death, several days after a treatment, under signs of tetraplegia can hardly be related to ECT. A case of transient hemiparesis during ECT which cleared up and did not recur in subsequent treatments, rather supports the view that cerebrovascular accidents are not a complication of ECT.

An undiagnosed cerebral disease was aggravated by ECT in a patient of McKegney and Panzetta; the patient died two months later. Equally unclear is a case by Matthew and Constan with various intracranial bleedings.

Convulsive therapy does not lead to epilepsy. In pharmacologic shock treatment, status epilepticus has been reported, more often with triazol than with metrazol. In ECT we saw it once in a patient treated several years after a lobotomy. Epilepsy as a complication of ECT does not have to be feared. A few convulsions have been reported by Pacella and Barrera in two patients who had definite convulsive patterns prior to convulsive therapy; they stress the fact that no patient with a normal electroencephalogram seems to develop any seizures. A patient of Terruwe developed weekly seizures which were later limited to the menstrual period, and after a year or so disappeared entirely. Other cases were described by Schumacher. The largest group (6 patients) with epileptiform seizures following ECT was reported by Hedegaard and Hjerrild in cases with a relatively large number of treatments. Müller noticed a greater tendency to convulsions during insulin coma among those patients treated with combined insulin and ECT. The vast number of patients treated with ECT have not shown epileptiform symptoms. The practical absence of such reports suggests that the figures for this complication are rather lower than should be expected in view of the fact that the incidence of epilepsy in the general population has been reported as high as 5 per 1,000. This would appear to be sufficient proof that spontaneous epilepsy as a consequence of ECT does not occur. We never saw it in 30 years of work with ECT.

An unusual neurological complication has been reported by Holzer et al. who saw a neuritis of the right plexus brachialis with motor and sensory findings, subsiding within two weeks. Peroneal nerve palsy was seen by Mason as well as Elpern and Chodosh. We also saw an unexplained slight weakness of the peroneal muscles after a treatment. A patient suffering from periodic paralysis and hyperkaliemia, reported by Wharton, developed paralysis lasting three days but no hyperkaliemia, after ECT given with succinylcholine.

Other complications: Some rare complications prior to the introduction of muscle relaxant drugs could probably be attributed to sudden contraction of the abdominal muscle during a convulsion. Maclay mentions a patient who died from peritonitis after intestinal rupture. Our own attention was directed toward the possibility of abdominal complications by the observation of a case of rupture in diverticulitis leading to peritonitis during a course of ECT. Bleeding from a gastric ulcer was seen by Norman and Worthington, and by Ziegler. A fatal gastric hemorrhage from an ulcer occurred less than an hour after a metrazol convulsion in a patient of Levy's who had previous ECT. Tuta and Balko report a death from a perforated duodenal ulcer five days after a metrazol convulsion; similar occurrences reported by Moore and Friedman nine and seventeen months after metrazol therapy are of doubtful relationship to the treatment. A case of fatal hemorrhage into the thyroid gland is reported by Napier who points out that such hemorrhages may occur during any sudden strain. Various hemorrhages from the small dilated veins of the nose and throat, from the external ear, and from incompletely healed abrasions are observed occasionally. Subconjunctival hemorrhages are not infrequent; continuation of treatment does not hinder their absorption. We observed petechial bleedings around the neck during each convulsion in a patient who was treated simultaneously with dilantin which probably was a contributing factor. Some reports on renal complications are available. A case of oliguria after the first electric shock treatment, followed by anuria and leading to fatal renal failure within seven days, was reported by Clute and Fitzgerald. Two cases of lower nephron nephrosis, both dying in acute renal failure with uremia were observed by Goodman. He feels that the evidence of a connection was not conclusive in these cases, one of which had had a severe leukocytosis prior to the treatment. Renal insufficiency reported by McNichol as "crush syndrome" was obviously due to fractures of both femurs with massive muscle destruction, a complication which is hardly imaginable today. A case of acute renal failure with dehydration two days after a treatment, reported by Selzer et al., appears unclear in its causal relationship, and studies of kidney function and ECT by the same group of workers (Selzer and Inderbitzin) remained negative. No instances are reported, where a known renal disease was aggravated by ECT.

Ruptures of vessels and of intestines are rare in unpremedicated convulsions, and are no longer a hazard where muscle relaxants are used. Also mechanically explained is a fatality by Sediac and Cernik due to rupture of adhesions of the pleura followed by mediastical emphysema and rupture of the subclavian artery. A most unusual complication reported by Wassing in a personal communication concerned a patient who became amaurotic after the first ECT due to pre-existing cranial arteritis affecting the ophthalmic artery.

Fatalities: We do not wish to minimize the potential risk of fatal accidents when we state that fatalities in convulsive therapy are extremely rare. Kalinowsky reported in 1949 on ten years of experience with ECT applied to many thousands of patients without a fatality. A later death occurred in a case treated with curare and reported above in the section on this drug. Kolb and Vogel, in their survey of all American hospitals, found a death rate of 0.06 per cent for ECT and 0.1 per cent for metrazol, as compared with 0.6 per cent for insulin; Impastato and Almansi found 0.8 per cent in their Survey of the literature. The largest study including 16,685 patients made by Deshaies and Pellier quotes a mortality rate of 0.08 per cent. Some surveys probably include many deaths which on closer study would not be attributed to the therapeutic procedure. In their monograph, Sargant and Slater call the risk of death negligible and compare it with the risk of giving a general anesthetic. We would think that, in unpremedicated ECT, it is even less. In metrazol treatment cardiovascular complications, pulmonary embolism, and (in a case of Nightingale and Meyer) cerebral fat embolism have been reported as direct causes of death. Pessin and Reese found edema with herniation of the cerebellar tonsils, and they mention similar findings in epileptics who had died following a convulsion. Several deaths in status epilepticus were caused by overdosage of intramuscular triazol (Wyllie).

It has already been mentioned that the number of fatalities in ECT combined with curare was high considering the relatively small number of hospitals where curare was used routinely. A detailed survey of fatalities in electroshock was given by Will et al. After reporting the death of a patient who had received curare they list 33 cases from the literature; in the majority death occurred so long after the treatment that the connection appears doubtful. The cases of immediate deaths from Ebaugh's group had all received curare. In a report by Eyman and Morris on three fatalities, two of them, in which the causal relation between ECT and death was obvious, had also received curare. In England, Napier reported five fatal accidents, of which one occurred immediately after the treatment (hemorrhage in the thyroid gland spreading down into the mediastinum); in another, myocardial damage was found, and death followed half an hour after a convulsion; in a third, the patient died six hours after treatment. Two cases in which a causal relationship also seems clearly established have been reported by Jetter. These patients, both of them rather elderly, died in circulatory collapse. Of two cases reported by Riese, one who died immediately had received curare. The second case, who died suddenly two days after a treatment following a bath, was hardly connected with the treatment. A very unusual fatality was observed by Hoch in the first treatment of a 50 year old man with a depression. The patient had an uneventful convulsion followed by a postconvulsive excitement state. After a few minutes of psychomotor excitement, the patient collapsed and died. There had been a normal electrocardiogram but some arteriosclerosis of the aorta. The autopsy confirmed the aortic changes; in addition, arteriosclerotic changes of the coronary vessels were found.

Coronary occlusion has been found in some fatalities as the cause of death. In an unusual case reported by Gaitz et al. death occurred due to cardiac tamponade from a laceration in the left ventricle from previous myocardial infarction. Rupture of the heart has also been reported by N. Malamud and Zhendlin. A unique fatality was seen by Drake and Ebaugh in a patient in whom autopsy revealed a pheochromocytoma of the left adrenal.

The most extensive study was done by Maclay whose position on the Board of Controls of mental hospitals in England and Wales afforded the opportunity to study all deaths from treatment in those hospitals. Of 62 deaths, some of which were probably coincidental, three died from intracerebral hemorrhages and two from pulmonary embolism due to thrombosed veins. At a time, when only a small percentage had been treated with the muscle relaxants curare or Flaxedil, 28 of the 62 fatalities had received a muscle relaxant, and four had died after the injection and prior to the convulsion. Five had been given electric narcosis. Half of all fatalities had occurred in the first treatment. Maclay closes by quoting studies by Slater and by Polonio showing several times as many deaths in untreated than in treated groups of patients. In the majority of ECT fatalities the cause of death remains unclear, but if Eyres assumes in three cases the death wish as a possible cause, this can hardly be accepted in view of the death wish and death anticipation of so many psychotic patients.

It appears to us that fatalities in unpremedicated ECT are extremely rare. In twenty years we had no fatality in unpremedicated patients. On the other hand, we know of many published and unpublished cases of death in ECT when premedicated with pentothal alone, pentothal with muscle relaxants, and in patients under medication with neuroleptic drugs when receiving ECT. It is our opinion that electrically induced convulsions are not more dangerous for life than any epileptic seizure, but that various medications add to the hazards of the treatment. Even so, fatalities remain extremely rare and do not contraindicate a treatment which—for instance in cardiac patients with severe psychotic excitement—is life-saving. Aside from a curare death, we saw only two myocardial infarctions with later fatal outcome, both after we began to use anesthesia techniques. The incidence of such cases remains minimal considering the large number of patients with previous coronary infarctions we have under ECT at all times. Large statistics with higher rates of fatalities undoubtedly contained cases where death was unrelated to the treatment. If a patient of Merli suffered a sudden circulatory collapse 15 hours after ECT, no conection should be assumed. Such cases have not infrequently been added to statistics on fatalities in ECT.

Contraindications

At the beginning of the shock treatment era, those engaged in this work were reluctant to submit bad physical risks to the new methods. Certain contraindications were tentatively enumerated, but on the basis of accumulated experience it is now possible to be more liberal in the selection of cases. Smith et al. recommend that each patient be considered individually, balancing the advantages to be gained by a possible psychiatric recovery against the additional risk imposed by existing physical disease. Everyone will agree with this statement. It should be borne in mind that convulsions in epileptics hardly ever lead to aggravation of other diseases. Consequently, the actual rarity of complications from artificially produced convulsions is not too surprising. Whereas in metrazol treatment the injection of large amounts of a toxic substance adds to the risk of the treatment, the electrically induced convulsion is the truest imitation of a spontaneous seizure.

AGE: This should not exclude patients from the benefit of the treatment. We have treated a number of patients with senile depressions in the eighth and ninth decade of life. Evans reports on a group of elderly patients treated for various conditions without untoward results explainable by their age, although many of them offered physical abnormalities aside from being old. The same was convincingly shown by Mayer-Gross. Gallinek, whose oldest patient was 84, treated many cases in the old age group, even in the presence of marked neurological pathology due to cerebral arteriosclerosis. The most impressive material has been presented, still after the introduction of the neuroleptic drugs, by Wolff. This author used maintenance ECT in geriatric patients with great success. One patient, 82 years old, had 242 such maintenance treatments over a period of four years. As a side-line, the author mentions the low incidence of fractures in these cases compared to other fractures on the same ward. Today the choice between ECT and pharmacotherapy is an important problem in clinical work. We can only agree with Pauleikhoff that the side-effects of drugs on the circulatory system makes one feel much more comfortable with ECT in older people who are known to tolerate this treatment extremely well. In our experience patients in their seventies and eighties in whom a functional rather than an organic psychosis can be diagnosed, showed most gratifying results.

YOUTH: This is usually not considered a contraindication; no ill effects have been reported with convulsive therapy in children. Cottington used metrazol, Heuyer et al. ECT. Gurewitz and Halme, by means of a battery of tests, confirmed that intellectual efficiency in children is not impaired by the treatment. The largest group was treated by L. Bender. In a follow-up study she rightly stressed the importance of convulsive therapy to make education, socialization and psychotherapy possible, factors which are especially important in children. Hemphill and Grey Walter probably had the youngest patient, an epileptic aged 3, whom they treated with ECT.

PREGNANCY: In epileptics, pregnancy does not result in abortion or premature birth of the child. Many workers have treated with ECT in various stages of pregnancy. Even in a patient treated by us practically at termination of pregnancy, the convulsions did not induce labor pain or rupture of the membrane. Boyd and Brown surveyed the literature on ECT in the gestational and puerperal periods and found mention of vaginal bleeding and temporarily impaired fetal circulation but no serious damage to mother or child. Fifteen children whose mothers had received ECT during pregnancy, were studied by Smith and found to be physically and mentally normal. A similar follow-up of several years was done by Forssman. Absence of damage to the fetus was again proven by Sobel.

CARDIOVASCULAR DISEASE: As far as pre-existing diseases are concerned, the most frequent problem arises in regard to patients with cardiovascular disorders.

Hypertension is unfortunately a frequent reason for rejecting patients for ECT. This is particularly unjustified in psychiatric conditions where hypertension is partly caused by the mental condition. The close interrelation between emotional factors and blood pressure is known, and in psychotic conditions such as agitated depressions, where the blood pressure is raised by the mental condition, the hypertension, instead of being a contraindication, is a definite indication for ECT. The subsidence of the agitated depression after a few convulsions will be accompanied by a definite decrease in the high blood pressure and by improvement in symptoms caused by the hypertension. This is well demonstrated in a patient of Kennedy and Wiesel in whom not only did the blood pressure drop considerably but retinal hemorrhages disappeared during successful ECT.

Myocardial disease must be carefully weighed against the seriousness of the mental condition to be treated. However, the experience of practically all workers has shown that cases with myocardial disease can be treated. Where psychotic agitation represents a constant strain on a diseased heart, the cardiac condition does not preclude ECT, and treatment of the mental condition is definitely indicated. Cardiac complications are so rare and unpredictable that application of ECT should not be excluded even though electrocardiographic changes reveal a diseased heart. In several cases where cardiologists had postulated a contraindication against ECT, we were forced by a serious psychotic state to ignore this contraindication, and in none of these patients did we encounter any difficulty. The danger of suicide and psychotic exhaustion, well emphasized by Ziskind and Somerfeld-Ziskind, together with the unfavorable influence of the abnormal mental condition on the heart, will in practically all such cases lead to a decision in favor of treatment. Cardiac medication, discussed in detail by Bankhead et al., is sometimes given in patients with heart disease but should not delay unduly urgent ECT all the more as Plice and Pfister found many cases with pre-treatment EKG abnormalities, and normal EKG after the treatment.

Before muscle relaxants were available we considered aneurysm of the aorta an absolute contraindication. However, Wolford reported on a patient with a large aneurysm who had unpremedicated ECT until days before the aneurysm finally ruptured in a treatment-free period. Such cases will now be treated with succinylcholine. A more frequent and complicated problem is the question of administering ECT in patients with coronary thrombosis. It has been claimed again and again that the introduction of succinylcholine makes it possible to treat these patients who formerly could not be treated. Such statements are based on two mistakes. Anesthesia, particularly with pentothal, adds to the danger of the treatment as seen in several cases of our own experience. We may mention one of several cases, namely a man in his seventies who had very well tolerated a series of unpremedicated ECT in spite of a preceding coronary thrombosis. In a new depressive episode the patient almost succumbed to a first treatment with pentothal and succinylcholine. He was then continued with unpremedicated ECT without any difficulty. We also had the first instance of a coronary thrombosis within an hour after ECT in a patient treated with pentothal and succinylcholine. In unpremedicated ECT our own large experience and Moore's report on 238 cases treated in spite of cardiac disorders, present sufficient evidence that coronary disease is no absolute contraindication to ECT. Brevital as anesthetic is preferable to pentothal, and we now begin to use Valium (diazepam) intravenously which anesthesiologists tried even in cardioversion. The safest way in severe myocardial damage is to omit barbiturate anesthesia and to use succinylcholine with a subconvulsive stimulus for anesthesia. After a very recent coronary infarct ECT might be delayed for a few weeks if the psychiatric condition permits.

Heart surgery has also been proven not to be a contraindication. Many individual reports of such cases treated with muscle relaxation bear this out. The shortest interval between heart surgery and ECT was two months in a case reported by Weinstein and Fischer who treated a patient with rheumatic valvular disease after replacement of the aortic mitral valves by protheses. Three patients with aortic valve prothesis were treated and observed electrocardiographically by Blachly and Semler with their method of multiple-monitored electric convulsive therapy.

In summarizing, our attitude regarding cardiac disease as a contraindication to ECT is that we might be hesitant to give convulsive therapy to patients with a questionable psychiatric indication but that we never exclude a patient in definite need of this treatment on account of a simultaneous cardiovascular disease.

Respiratory diseases: Tuberculosis as a frequent occurrence in young schizophrenics is no reason to exclude such patients from the treatment of a mental condition which in itself has a deleterious influence on the tuberculosis because of feeding and other difficulties in the care of the patient. It has been shown in the section on complications that activation of latent tuberculosis is rare. Close saw improvement of the tuberculosis in x-ray controls during ECT. We have treated tuberculous patients in whom mental symptoms such as refusal of food, were considered as a more dangerous factor for the tuberculous process than the convulsive therapy. One such patient doubled her weight after ECT, from 68 pounds to 130 pounds. Pleasure's experience in the largest unit for mental patients with tuberculosis in New York. proved conclusively that tuberculosis is no contraindication in ECT. Pneumothorax has also been shown not to interfere with treatment. Pulmonectomy due to cancer (personal communication by Wassing) or other lung diseases also did not present any difficulties. In such cases as well as in severe emphysema we avoid barbiturate anesthesia.

Diseases of joints and bones: There is no reason to withhold ECT in any patient because of "osteoarthritic changes of the spine." Actually, no complication has ever been reported either in pharmacologic or electric convulsive therapy which could be related to osteoarthritic changes of the spine. Neither increase of pre-existing complaints nor special predisposition to vertebral fractures has been noticed in such patients even prior to the use of muscle relaxants. Experience has also shown that osteoporosis is no contraindication. Neither are laminectomies a contraindication. Interesting in this connection is one of our patients who had an extremely painful herniated disk between L_5 and S_1; convulsive treatment without relaxations did not aggravate the pain, nor was there any difficulty when ECT had to be continued a week after operation of the disk. Recent fractures must be treated in deep muscle relaxation with larger amounts of succinylcholine (80 or 100 mg.) than usually given.

Organic brain disease: This is frequently considered a contraindication. There is no evidence that this is justified in chronic neurological conditions. Heilbrunn and Feldman have reported on cardiovascular and respiratory difficulties in patients with meningovascular syphilis. In the meantime, many general paretics have been treated for their more acute psychotic symptoms without any untoward results. Kalinowsky and others reported on various neurological conditions treated for a simultaneous emotional disturbance. In such patients the neurological condition was never aggravated; in most cases impaired function was even improved to a surprising degree. Cases of Parkinson's disease have often been treated without harm, when complicated by a depression or other psychotic episode. Aggravation of the neurological symptoms of Parkinson cases by the psychosis often cleared up simultaneously with removal of the psychotic symptoms by ECT. Also treated were patients with poliomyelitis, cerebral palsy and other chronic conditions. We treated cases of multiple sclerosis with psychotic episodes without untoward results (Gallinek and Kalinowsky).

Cerebral hemorrhage in an epileptic during one of his attacks is practically unknown. Parallel with this experience, vascular accidents are almost unknown in convulsive therapy. Any patient with a history of subarachnoid hemorrhages due to aneurysm nowadays should be treated under complete muscle relaxation. The only definite contraindications in ECT are brain tumors. They may simulate symptoms of an endogenous psychosis. In one of our patients who had had two previous manic-depressive episodes, the first convulsive treatment for a new depression was followed by astereognosis which led to the discovery of a brain tumor. Marchand and Guirand saw a fatality in the last treatment of a patient with a tumor of the 4th ventricle. Brain tumor and other conditions of increased intracranial pressure are absolute contraindications. The change in the brain volume during seizures may have been responsible for fatal accidents in patients in whom death occurred during ECT, and an unrecognized brain tumor was found. Successfully removed space-occupying lesions do not seem to contraindicate ECT as illustrated by a case of the Indian psychiatrist Doongaji (personal communication) who gave ECT for an acute schizophrenic psychosis two years after removal of a large tuberculoma.

OTHER DISEASES: A number of other diseases have been considered as relative contraindications in the past. Exophthalmic goiter and Graves' disease always imply certain dangers, but such patients have been treated without untoward results. Absence of adrenal glands did not interfere with ECT in a patient of Crisp and Roberts. In acute infections with psychotic syndromes ECT has been used successfully, but today pharmacotherapy would be preferable. Jetter's case of a death from circulatory failure under ECT in a patient with acute glomerulonephritis is unique. Several reports indicate that mild infections can be aggravated, e.g. aggravation of a mild chronic otitis media in a case of Hemphill and Grey Walter. The same authors warn against convulsive treatment during vaccine therapy. Chapman reported on three cases of thrombophlebitis treated without complication, but today muscle relaxants should be used.

Fever as such is definitely no contraindication. This is a point of greatest practical importance in view of the frequency of fever of unknown, probably central origin in acute psychotics. One of the most important and, strangely enough, still rather neglected indications for ECT as a lifesaving procedure is the treatment of acute psychotic states with dehydration and high fever. Again and again we come across instances where a patient is considered hopeless because he is in a severe excitement state and threatened by psychotic exhaustion but, according to the treating physician, cannot be treated with

ECT because of simultaneous temperatures of 104° or more. If the patient is not yet in coma, we give in these cases two electric shock treatments within five minutes after premedication with 5 cc. of coramine, and follow this with a third electric shock treatment a few hours later. Almost invariably the temperature becomes normal the next morning, and the patient will be sufficiently improved to take nourishment. Neuroleptic drugs are less safe in these cases. Vasomotor collapses have been observed after the large amounts of drugs necessary to control a severe catatonic excitement. This has never been seen in ECT in such cases.

Peptic ulcer, which may hemorrhage during the convulsion, other gastro-intestinal conditions, such as diverticuli which may rupture, and patients with any type of hernia must be treated under muscle relaxation.

Diseases of the eye sometimes offer special problems. The most frequent questions that arise here are how far glaucoma and threatening ablation of the retina are contraindications for the treatment. As far as glaucoma is concerned, Ehrhardt reported that the intraocular pressure decreases during ECT. Extensive investigations by Küchle and Rohrschneider come to similar conclusions. While Manning and Hollander reported a case of glaucoma supposedly due to ECT, we treated many patients with ophthalmological complications including some with detachment of the retina and glaucoma as well as psychotic reactions following cataract operations, and never encountered any difficulties. Today all these cases are being treated with muscle relaxants. However, since succinylcholine is known to increase intraocular pressure we made it a rule to give Eserine prior to the treatment in patients threatened by glaucoma.

In conclusion, it can be stated that there are few if any contraindications to ECT. The seriousness of the physical illness and of the mental condition must always be carefully weighed against each other. Pre-existing physical disease should not be a reason to withhold ECT, where the treatment is indicated.

Neuropathology

The question of morphologic changes in convulsive therapy is far more controversial than it is in insulin treatment. Von Meduna published investigations on animals with convulsions induced by camphor prior to the application of this method in human beings. He described diffuse but mild changes in nerve cells. These findings of the originator of convulsive therapy were not confirmed by many other investigators who found negligible or no changes. Winkelman and Moore made a comparative study on the effect of insulin and metrazol and, contrary to their findings in insulin, saw little or no change after metrazol convulsions. Weil and Liebert noted histopathologic changes only in animals receiving unusually intense treatment. Small subarachnoid hemorrhages were seen by Strecker et al. in animals subjected to an unusually great number of convulsions, whereas others exhibited no changes. Whitehead et al. considered insufficient blood supply resulting from the convulsions the decisive factor in the pathogenesis of the various lesions. In addition to their findings on the brain, they observed mild tubular degeneration in the kidneys, scattered hemorrhages in the lungs, increased hemosiderin in the spleen, and generalized visceral congestion. In metrazol the possibility of a direct toxic effect of the drug on the nervous tissue must be considered. In monkeys, the best material for comparison with the human brain, Arieti found only very moderate acute cell changes and negligible vascular modifications of apparently functional character. Stender originally observed hemorrhages but recognized them as purely traumatic in origin and subsequently prevented them by keeping the animals in a padded box during the convulsions.

These experiments by Stender may offer the clue to the much disputed findings of one group of authors (Alpers and Hughes) on petechial hemorrhages in ECT. They discovered subarachnoid hemorrhages as well as punctate hemorrhages in various areas of the brain substance and in the meninges. Alexander and Loewenbach suggest that hemorrhages may be explained by excessive stimulation of the vagovasomotor centers of the medulla oblongata when the electrodes in the experimental animals are applied so that the current passes through the hindbrain. Hassin, discussing similar findings of Heilbrunn and Weil, points out that hemorrhages never occur in the meninges or in the brain tissue of electrocuted persons in spite of the much higher current applied. Cell changes but no hemorrhages have been found by Heilbrunn and Liebert in biopsy material from rabbits. Neuburger et al. have reported observing in their experiments with dogs slight vascular and nerve cell changes with some glia proliferation, especially in the pathway of the electrical current; the changes were less severe than those found by them after metrazol convulsions.

Much evidence has now accumulated that ECT produces no important morphological changes in the brain. The first investigation which came to this conclusion was made by Cerletti and Bini. They conducted extensive studies on dogs treated with varying intensities. In those given electric therapy comparable to that given to human beings, they found no destructive alterations of cells; some signs of edema but no disturbance of the architecture of the brain was observed. Our investigations on monkeys performed at the New York Psychiatric Institute (Barrera et al.) reached the same conclusion. Control monkeys included in this study and the group treated with electric shock revealed the same changes. Negligible changes were reported by Moore and, by Lidbeck; none by Fetterman. Globus et al. have observed no important pathology in studies on electronarcosis which they rightly consider a prolongation of electric shock. Ferraro and Roizin found some functional and morphological changes, mostly related to the vascular system, and neuronal changes of the reversible type. The histological alterations were more pronounced in the areas traversed by the current. This was also found in recent animal investigations by Quandt and Sommer who accuse the electric current rather than vasomotor changes. Contrary to most others they found extensive ganglion cell necrosis and increase of glia cells in the anterior part of the brain. Contrary to this, Siekert et al. found no alterations in the area between the electrodes or elsewhere. Histologic comparsion between experimental and control animals revealed no structural differences.

Reports on human material are scarce. It is difficult to evaluate the cases of Alpers and Hughes as they explained their findings of recent and old hemorrhages in patients who died as late as three and five months after ECT, respectively, as treatment effect. Ebaugh et al. have described an interesting case in which death occurred during the first convulsion. The changes present were almost entirely of a reversible type and, according to the authors, could not have interfered with brain function. Actually in most ECT fatalities no significant histological changes were found (Meyer and McLardy). Even in a carefully studied brain of a young patient, who had received the unusual number of 355 ECT, Heyck failed to find any pathological changes in the sense of a fall-out of ganglion cells. If Schulte and Dreyer found purpura hemorrhagica in the brain of a case complicated by barbiturate poisoning, such finding can be seen in so many different conditions that it cannot be attributed to ECT. A very extensive survey of histological changes was made by Corselli and Meyer who in patients with very large numbers of ECT found marginal gliosis over the surface of the hemispheres, and a moderate diffuse or perivascular proliferation of astrocytes in the white matter. Some pathological findings in the Ammon's horn were seen by Zeman. Widespread fat embolism was found in a case by Meyer and Teare.

An extensive experimental study and critical appraisal of the whole problem has been prepared by Alexander and Loewenbach. They show that even functional changes in the sense of arteriolar vasoconstriction and blanching are noticeable for less than half an hour within the path of the current only. Shock doses far beyond those used in ECT (1800 ma. for 5 seconds) are necessary to produce vasoparalytic stasis. Even this current brought about only reversible changes of the neural parenchyma which were still limited to the path of the current. The authors conclude that with shock doses wthin the range of the average amount of current used in electric shock therapy in man, no pathologic changes are produced which can be recognized with present day histologic methods. This is in accord with the results of our own and many other studies on this question. It does not exclude a temporary dysfunction of brain tissue as evidenced by psychologic and electroencephalographic changes. This dysfunction, however, is evidently a temporary one, and no neuropathologic or other changes occur which would explain a lasting disturbance of brain function.

Indications and Results

The various modalities of convulsive therapy are applied to the same groups of psychiatric patients. Indications and results will be discussed in the sequence of their clinical importance as it appears today after the introduction of the new pharmacotherapeutic agents. Some problems which are common to both types of "shock treatments" were first brought into the foreground when insulin coma treatment was introduced, and, therefore, such subjects as prognostic criteria, in spontaneous and treatment remissions, statistical evaluation and others relating to schizophrenia are partly dealt with in the chapter on Insulin Coma Treatment. The difficult subject of statistical evaluation of treatment results needs different criteria in the various treatments and, therefore, will be discussed separately in those chapters dealing with the various treatments.

AFFECTIVE DISORDERS: Since the introduction of antidepressant drugs convulsive therapy is no longer the only but still the most reliable treatment for depressions. It is the only method that can remove the depressive as well as the manic phase of a manic-depressive psychosis, a fact which is of considerable theoretical importance. Equally interesting is the fact that ECT is effective in retarded as well as in agitated depressions. In the present chapter the results of convulsive therapy will be presented. The question whether in a given patient pharmacotherapy or convulsive therapy should be given preference, is discussed in this chapter as well as in the one on antidepressant drugs. Attempts to establish the effect of ECT on the various symptoms of a depression were made first by Wilcox by means of a new rating scale. However, contrary to the action of pharmacotherapy on certain "target symptoms" all such attempts in convulsive therapy remained inconclusive except for the determination of prognostic factors.

It was not until several years after the introduction of convulsive therapy that its usefulness in the affective psychoses was recognized by Verstraeten, and stressed particularly by Bennett. It then became the treatment of choice for depressions. The responses of the various types of depressions are so similar that it is safe to assume a close relation or even the same underlying process in manic-depressive depressions, involutional depressions, senile depressions, and even so-called psychoneurotic depressions; they all react to approximately four convulsions. It is customary to give a few more treatments in order to stabilize the result, although the necessity for such additional treatments has not been proved. The total number of treatments given by most workers varies between five and ten; others discontinue as soon as the patient has improved. Treatments are usually given three times a week. They may be spaced more closely when the psychosis is very acute; on the other hand, treatments given only twice a week are equally effective and have the advantage of avoiding confusional states which are definitely not necessary for results in depressions. If a depression has cleared up after the third treatment, the last two or three treatments can be spaced in weekly intervals, during which the patient can already take up his normal activities. A frequent observation is that the depressed patient reports some relief of tension after the first treatment but that he is again uncomfortable after the second treatment and shows a real improvement from the third treatment on.

Recovery from a depressive episode after only four or five treatments, sometimes even earlier, is often helpful in differentiating between manic-depressive and schizophrenic psychoses. In schizophrenic patients, depressive symptoms as well as other acute symptoms also yield rather quickly to a few convulsive treatments, but often other psychotic symptoms previously overshadowed become more recognizable, or the removed symptoms return in a few days. On the other hand, in pure depressions no other psychotic symptoms are detectable after the depression is removed, and early relapses are rare. Failures in affective disorders amount to no more than 4 per cent in Bennett's and 5 per cent in Osgood's material. Unfavorable prognostic features appear to include various neurotic symptoms, irreversible brain changes, and schizophrenic features, in brief, symptoms which make the diagnosis of pure affective psychosis doubtful. Many feel that of all depressive syndromes those of later life react best.

Attempts to quantify many different factors of significance for the therapeutic effect of ECT were started by Hamilton and White as well as Roberts. Most of these studies confirmed previous clinical observations. Roberts found a pyknic body build important for favorable prognosis in female patients. Neurotic symptoms in Hobson's rating scale made for a poor prognosis which supports the general view of a different response to the two main types of depression. Carney et al., using in-patients rather than out-patients and thus having a larger number of severe cases, also used a rating scale on ECT-treated patients. Their findings showed that 77 per cent of patients classified as endogenous depressions responded to ECT, but only 15 per cent of those classified as neurotic depressions. Like Roberts, they confirmed the justification of distinguishing between endogenous and neurotic depressions. Factors predicting ECT results correlated fairly well with those suggesting a good response to imipramine. Milder depressions of the neurotic variety responded poorly to either form of treatment. Self-reproach and retardation were correlated with a good response to ECT, while neuroticism, hypochondriasis and hysterical features were associated with a poor response. In another similar study Carney et al. predicted correctly ECT responses in 87 per cent of the cases, and Mendels correctly prognosed 90 per cent of his patients. Ottosson, in a similar study, found cycloid personality traits the only factor clearly connected with a favorable outcome. He also suggests that the longer the interval since the previous course of ECT, the quicker the therapeutic response, and the greater the number of previous courses of ECT the less favorable the response.

The reliability of the response of depressions to convulsive therapy has remained without parallel in psychiatric therapy and was unfortunately not reached by the response to any of the available antidepressant drugs. Soon after the introduction of imipramine as the still most effective antidepressant drug Kiloh and Ball as well as Birkmayer and Danielczyk requested that after three weeks of unsuccessful drug therapy ECT should be instituted. Later Greenblatt et al., Bratfos and Haug, Fazio, Lauter and many others confirmed the greater reliability of ECT. Many psychiatrists still use ECT with what Ziskind called "backhanded reservation" which prolongs the sickness unnecessarily. In severe depression ECT must be used to reduce the danger of suicide and to prevent depressive states from lingering on indefinitely.

Manic-depressive psychosis: The rate of remissions in manic-depressive depressions in most reports varies between 80-100 per cent. Lower figures are given in some statistics including material from many different sources (Malzberg, Impastato and Almansi). These figures suggest that statistically collected material more than individually studied groups is likely to include inadvertently schizophrenics with depressive features who are treated under the preliminary diagnosis of manic-depressive psychosis.

The duration of illness has no bearing on the outcome. Untreated manic-depressive depressions which might otherwise last from a few weeks to one year can be cut short when treatment is instituted. It is in accordance with this clinical experience that Cerletti, in a personal communication, mentions that the average number of hospital days of manic-depressives in Italian institutions fell from 180 days to 31 days after the introduction of ECT. Oltman and Friedman found that 75 per cent of shock treated patients undergoing initial hospitalization for a depression were discharged within two months as compared with only 17 per cent of an untreated group.

Episodic recurrences of the psychosis cannot be prevented. The impression occasionally received that the symptom-free intervals between manic-depressive episodes are shorter following shock therapy than they would have been without such treatment is not yet supported by statistical evidence; should this prove to be true it would not diminish the value and the necessity for active treatment; an eventual subsequent episode may be treated equally well. A statistical approach to this problem by Oltman and Friedman showed that readmissions during the first year after discharge amounted to only 10 per cent in shock treated cases as compared to 25 per cent in untreated patients.

Prophylactic electric shock treatment has been introduced by Geoghegan and Stevenson. In all patients with two or more episodes they recommend single treatments at monthly intervals for the purpose of preventing recurrences. In a five-year-follow-up study they prove convincingly that in most cases this procedure will prevent the recurrences of manic-depressive episodes. After five years the intervals may be lengthened to two months, three months, and finally six months. Our own experience was equally favorable, although we found only few patients cooperative enough to accept such treatment program. In patients with usually long free intervals between their episodes we are reluctant to advise this prophylactic treatment. In patients with frequent episodes prophylactic ECT remains superior to prophylactic drug therapy. This was demonstrated by our own experience and by a patient of Hastings' who after five years of successful prophylactic ECT was tried prophylactically on several drugs, but relapsed each time, but placed again on monthly ECT had another five years symptom-free.

Frequently a depression clears up with the patient going into a moderately elated state. This is also noticed occasionally in spontaneous depressions, but it seems to be more usual in remissions after convulsive treatment. Closer studies of such cases suggest that the elation often has the euphoric tainting of an organic reaction, is accompanied by intellectual impairment, and clears up one or two weeks after treatment. True transition from a depression into a manic phase appears to occur only in patients in whom that pattern had also occurred spontaneously.

Patients with circular psychosis, constantly shifting from one phase to the other, offer discouraging results, except for a purely symptomatic removal of the most dangerous exacerbations of their illness. It is also questionable whether or not treatment should be given in patients with depressions which last regularly only from a few days to a week or two.

Other types of depressions related to the manic-depressive group, such as Myerson's "anhedonic states" and Kennedy and Wiesel's "manic-depressive equivalents" characterized by episodes of somatic complaints with only moderate depression of mood, have been reported as being equally good prospects for convulsive therapy. We were able to confirm this in many instances, and Gallinek describes similar cases as conversion depressions. Any neurotic syndrome of episodic character should be tried on ECT if other methods have failed. Grief reactions of unwarranted length, as defined by Myerson, also respond well. It is not necessary in such cases to produce a confusional state in order to erase the memory of the experience that had led to the depression.

Failures in manic-depressive depressions in our material have occurred for the most part in cases with doubtful diagnosis. Some papers limited themselves to the study of cases in which this almost specific treatment fails (Ch. Müller, Kalinowsky). Difficulties in differential diagnosis between manic-depressive psychosis and schizophrenia, neurotic reactions and other disorders are a frequent explanation for failures to which Müller adds debility, exogenous conflicts and a greater familial incidence of depression. Rickles and Polan make an attempt at delineating certain psychological conflicts as reasons for a poor prognosis. If Egsgaard et al. stress the poor response of postpartum depression, this is correct but probably explained by the schizophrenic nature of many of these syndromes. An interesting prognostic sign was mentioned by Sargant, who saw that depressed patients who go to sleep easily but wake up early and whose depression improves as the day goes on, have a better prognosis than those who fall asleep with difficulty and feel worse in the afternoon. The number of unfavorable reports (Kwalwasser, Kepner) is negligible. Reports by Campbell and others on ECT in manic-depressive children are also favorable.

The available reports on ECT in manic-depressive depressions are convincing enough to warrant the treatment in severe cases as soon as the diagnosis has been established. Any delay is unjustifiable because of the danger of suicide. Frequently overlooked is the fact that suicidal attempts are more likely in seemingly moderate depressions than in deeply retarded patients with complete loss of initiative. It has been shown by Ziskind et al. that the danger of suicide, as well as the danger of psychotic exhaustion in untreated cases, is definitely greater than the alleged risks of convulsive therapy. Robie tried to prove the effectiveness of ECT in preventing suicides on the basis of suicide statistics in the United States. It is known that in several hospitals the suicide rate has increased since the introduction of the antidepressant drugs, although the simultaneous liberalization of hospital management such as the open-door policy could also be responsible for some of these suicides. Already in 1961 Impastato demonstrated the dramatic increase of suicides in a large mental hospital, when drugs were substituted for ECT. His later experience as well as our own shows that even those of us who are aware of the danger of delaying ECT, had more suicides than before we had antidepressant drugs available. We can only agree with Engelhardt and many others that in suicidal patients antidepressant treatment must begin with ECT which then can be followed by antidepressant medication with drugs as a preventive measure.

Statistical figures for spontaneous remission rates in manic-depressive psychoses cannot be used for evaluation of the treatment. Granted that the final outcome of a manic-depressive episode is equally favorable in untreated cases, the patient's sufferings, the social implications of the illness, and the potential dangers are sufficient to stress the necessity of active treatment as soon as the diagnosis is made. Some psychiatrists object to the treatment because of assumed dangers, others object to any non-psychological treatment. Only few reports question the validity of the favorable statistics (Kargulla, Siegmann). However, everyday clinical experience invalidates such negative statistical findings beyond any reasonable doubt. At the present time this is borne out by a strong increase in the use of ECT as the treatment of choice in depressions.

Manic states respond to the neuroleptic drugs, especially to those reducing psychomotility like chlorpromazine. Yet, it will be shown in the chapter on neuroleptic drugs that failures do occur; and the therapist will still have to resort frequently to ECT in manic states. However, it is undeniable that the manic phase of the manic-depressive psychosis differs from the depressive phase in its response to convulsive therapy. Treatments given twice or three times a week are frequently ineffective in manics and led to discouraging conclusions. Treatments given at closer intervals have produced better results; our present routine provides for two or even three treatments in one day. In this way remissions have been obtained within two or three days (five or six treatments) in manics who in previous attacks had required twenty or more convulsions.

With this intense treatment the immediate remission rate almost equals that of the depressive phase. Slightly lower figures in some statistics again may be explained by the fact that certain manic syndromes are more difficult to differentiate from schizophrenia than the depressions. What has been said regarding shifting to the other phase of the disease and the failure to prevent future episodes is equally true for ECT of the manic phase. There have been some reports indicating that the very early stage of a manic attack is refractory to convulsive therapy (Cronick et al.). Patients in a manic episode are seldom cooperative enough to accept voluntary treatment. It is for this reason that prophylactic treatment is even more important in patients with many episodes than in those who only have depressions. Today, however, lithium salts are superior as a prophylactic treatment in these patients.

The same is true for the treatment of the individual manic episode since lithium has been found to be extremely successful in these patients in whom ECT never reached the results obtained in depressions. However, most clinicians using lithium, will agree that very acute manic excitement states are more quickly removed by ECT, and that the patient then be continued on the more slowly acting lithium salts. In less acutely disturbed manics treatment today will be started routinely with lithium.

Involutional psychosis: This disease offers spectacular results in convulsive therapy. The remission rate in pure involutional depressions reaches that for manic-depressive depressions. The necessary number of treatments is the same as in other depressions (five to eight). The results are equally good in deeply retarded and in agitated depressions. Failures are usually due to an admixture of paranoid or other schizophrenic symptoms. In pure involutional melancholia the prognosis is not influenced by the duration of illness, which in untreated cases may be much longer than in manic-depressive depressions. Therefore, the detection of such cases in the chronic wards of mental institutions produces very gratifying results and is a valuable means of decreasing the hospital population. Martin even made the unexpected observation that in this group patients with more than one year's duration of illness showed better results than earlier cases.

Senile or presenile depressions, i.e., depressions beyond the involutional age, respond equally well to convulsion treatment. Depressions are often still called involutional when they actually occur well in the presenile or senile age. The results in these old patients will depend on how far arteriosclerotic or senile brain changes have determined the depressive symptoms. The simultaneous presence of some arteriosclerotic brain changes in a patient with an affective psychosis does not exclude the possibility of favorable results. Bennett confirms this on the basis of a large group of such patients, the oldest being 83. We agree with Gallinek that arteriosclerotic changes are only one factor in the picture and do not always determine the prognosis. Although pronounced intellectual impairment, disorientation and other clinical expression of arteriosclerotic or senile changes make us reluctant to treat such patients in view of their post-treatment organic reactions, we do treat them when a true depressive affect is present. An observation by Krauss and also by von Baeyer that elederly men respond less well than elderly women is in accordance with our own impression. Patients in this group are too often diagnosed organic psychosis of the senile type, although no signs of intellectual impairment are present.

Donnelly showed that even organic signs such as confusion and carelessness in hygienic habits are often counteracted by ECT. In English mental hospitals scrutiny in the differential diagnosis between irreversible senile psychoses and affective psychoses occurring in old age has been stressed by Martin Roth; and we have our most spectacular successes in this group of old age depressions that had been diagnosed as organic psychoses.

Paranoid involutionals show a much less favorable response to convulsive therapy than patients suffering from involutional depressions. Consequently, the two groups have to be dealt with separately. Statistics combining the various types of involutional psychosis show extremely low figures (Malzberg). Kalinowsky, distinguishing between the two groups, found 86.9 per cent recovered and much improved cases in involutional melancholia and only 43.7 per cent in the paranoid group. This is even more significant in view of the fact that the latter group was treated with a minimum of twenty treatments, the former with only ten. Bianchi and Chiarello arrived at corresponding figures of 76.3 and 44.8 per cent. This entirely different response to convulsive therapy supports the long standing opinion that the paranoid type of involutional psychosis is more closely related to schizophrenia than to the affective disorders.

Unlike melancholia, for which even five treatments are usually sufficient, the number of treatments necessary in the paranoid group is ten to twenty, as in schizophrenia. Another similarity is that results in paranoid involutional psychosis, as in schizophrenia, are largely influenced by the duration of illness. Patients with a dramatic symptomatology show better results than those classified by Kraepelin as paraphrenia. A well preserved personality makes for a poor response to convulsive therapy. In many such cases the diagnosis of involutional paranoid psychosis and late paranoid schizophrenia is quite interchangeable. Paranoid involutionals with depressive affect and agitation have a better prognosis.

Prior to shock therapy the treatment of involutional psychoses consisted mainly of hormonal replacement therapy. The superiority of convulsive therapy has been demonstrated beyond doubt (Palmer et al., Bennett and Wilbur). The latter authors conclude that estrogenic hormones have no place in the treatment of psychiatric disorders except for symptomatic relief of vasomotor symptoms in the involutional age. Davidoff and Raffaele showed that only mild involutional symptoms without actual psychosis respond to hormonal treatment. Before the advent of antidepressant drugs ECT was the only means to shorten a depression. It still is the fastest method. In a twelve years' survey Halsbrook found a reduction in hospital stay from 126 days to 26 days after the introduction of ECT. The new antidepressant drugs are a valuable addition to the treatment of depressions, but the limited number of complete recoveries and the greater number of "improvements" tend to prolong hospitalization.

SCHIZOPHRENIA: Convulsive therapy was introduced as a treatment for schizophrenia, and for several years was used exclusively for this disease, but the spectacular results in the affective disorders have overshadowed its effectiveness in schizophrenia. Another reason why the value of convulsive therapy in schizophrenia is still considered controversial is that the importance of long and adequate treatment, postulated by most workers for insulin treatment, was not sufficiently emphasized for metrazol therapy. Cerletti, stressing Sakel's merit in recognizing the importance of consistently repeated application of comas in insulin treatment, applied this experience to ECT. He recommended as many as fifteen to forty convulsions. This requirement was difficult to fulfill in metrazol treatment, although Italian authors particularly (Petri-Canella and Levi) insist that only after thirty convulsions can the outcome be judged. In ECT such intense treatment can more readily be applied. The report by López-Ibor before the First International Congress of Psychiatry again stressed the need for long courses of convulsive therapy if results in schizophrenia are expected. Compliance with this request by some, and neglect of adequate treatment by others explain the contradictory statistics on ECT in schizophrenia. The relative value of pharmacotherapy and convulsive therapy in acute as compared to chronic schizophrenics has been discussed in the chapter on pharmacotherapy.

Reviewing the innumerable reports on convulsive therapy in schizophrenia, we must disregard those using figures from mixed material not separated into acute and chronic cases; high remission rates can easily be obtained by limiting treatment to acute cases, and unfavorable results are inevitable if chronic cases are in the majority. As to differences between pharmacologic and electric convulsive therapy, most workers who have employed both methods agree that their possibilities are the same and that, therefore, they may be discussed together. However, a dissenting opinion has been expressed by Bianchi and

Chiarelli who report favorably on both methods but find higher figures in metrazol treated cases. The same advantage of pharmacological over electric convulsive therapy was suggested in a large Italian study by Fasanaro. The opposite conclusion, that of the superiority of ECT, has been drawn by Malzberg in a purely statistical analysis. Superiority of Indoklon Inhalation Therapy over Electric Convulsive Therapy in some treatment-resistant or frequently relapsing schizophrenics has also been claimed but has not been proven.

The greatest amount of data on metrazol treatment was gathered by von Meduna and Friedman from 75 American and European hospitals. This study has the usual limitations of statistics from hospitals with different techniques and different reporting of results; but it gives much valuable information. The survey arrived at a remission rate of 60 per cent for cases of less than six months' duration, and 52 per cent when cases up to eighteen months of illness were included. An additional 20 per cent of cases with "great improvement" may be added to both groups. A steep decline in rate is seen in cases of more than eighteen months' duration of illness; only 10 per cent remissions and an additional 37 per cent improvements are listed. These figures demonstrate again the fact seen in insulin statistics that the remission rate remains rather steady for illness up to approximately one year's duration but drops sharply when the disease has progressed for more than one and a half years.

A compilation of metrazol statistics by Küppers listing 53 per cent "complete remissions" in cases up to one year's duration of illness even exceeds figures found by the same author for insulin treatment (39 per cent). This is contrary to the reports of most other authors, although actual comparisons between the two methods applied by the same worker in the same hospital are few in number. Hoch had practically identical results with the two methods in more acute cases; in chronic cases insulin and combined insulin-convulsive treatment yielded higher figures. Very similar are the figures given by Chase and Silverman for their material. Müller, pointing out that in a large survey of both methods the number of unimproved cases was almost identical, concludes that the two methods appear to have at least their limitations exactly at the same point.

Many workers realized early that a frequent reason for failure was the premature discontinuation of therapy because of the disappearance of all psychotic symptoms after four or five convulsions, as a result of which inadequate treatment symptoms reappeared within five to ten days. This accounts for the frequent statement that patients under convulsive therapy nearly always relapse. Gerhardt found that reinstitution of treatment after a relapse did not lead to the same favorable results as a long uninterrupted course of treatment. Reitman's statistic from many countries shows the highest figures (79 per cent in acute cases) in reports from Italian authors, probably because most Italian workers apply long courses of treatment.

The literature on ECT statistics essentially repeats what has been said about metrazol therapy. The value of ECT in schizophrenia has often been questioned and the superiority of insulin stressed, but actually most schizophrenics are treated at some stage of their illness with electrically induced convulsions.

A survey in the New York State Hospital System was made by Malzberg came to the conclusion that schizophrenics respond to electric shock better than to metrazol but not so well as to insulin treatment. The various tables of this report show the dissimilarity of the results in the different hospitals probably due to different material and different intensity of treatment. Another survey, by Impastato and Almansi, summarized the data from all available publications on ECT and compared the results with the New York State Hospital figures for insulin. This resulted in very similar figures for insulin and ECT; rates for full recoveries were slightly higher in insulin, those for all types of improvements higher in ECT.

An interesting comparative study of adequately treated material was presented by Danziger and Kindwall. They proved the far superior results in treated over untreated schizophrenics, and found that this is as true equally for electric shock-treated as for insulin-treated schizophrenics, even though the figures for insulin-treated cases are still higher. Danziger postulates a minimum of 30 ECT and 50 insulin comas as necessary for a satisfactory outcome. In his survey on the various shock treatments, López Ibor (with whom we fully agree) questions the general validity of the often made statement that convulsive therapy is the treatment of choice in catatonics, and insulin coma in paranoids. In catatonics, especially catatonic excitement, both treatments give equal results, and we have seen some paranoid schizophrenics respond very well to ECT alone. Therefore, any rigid approach to the problem is unwarranted, and the experienced therapist will achieve results with either method if he is flexible and, above all, persistent in his therapeutic efforts. Favorable reports come from workers who apply intense treatment, unfavorable results from those who give a lower average number of treatments. Physicians who treat their patients to the point of complete disorientation (Loewenbach, Glueck, Neymann) are highly satisfied with the value of ECT in schizophrenia. Such "confusional treatment" always uses many convulsions. However, Kalinowsky and Worthing, Gonda, and other workers have shown that intense treatment leads to good results whether the patient is purposely brought to the confused stage by daily treatment or whether avoidance of this was attempted by means of longer intervals between treatments; only a sufficiently high number of treatments was imperative. Unsatisfactory results have been reported by Bennett, also by Reznikoff whose patients were allowed to have only eight to twelve convulsions. Hemphill and Grey Walter also obtained a low remission rate in their own material but recommend a trial with ECT in all cases of schizophrenia; Smith et al. have had disappointing results, but admit that they have treated mostly chronic cases. Cook points out that there are surprisingly few suitable figures to draw upon in proportion to the large number of papers published, because most studies do not specify the duration of illness. Others fail to mention the number of treatments given. To state the average number of treatments for the entire group of patients leads to faulty conclusions, because a long course given in hopeless, chronic cases results in a high average which more than overbalances the average if the acute cases, who should receive many treatments, were actually given an inadequate number.

Material treated by the same physician in two different hospitals has been published by Kalinowsky who states that institutional material is more comparable in different countries than voluntarily admitted schizophrenics. This latter type of material usually contains a number of borderline cases whose diagnoses may vary with different schools of psychiatry. The author saw far less favorable results in his voluntary group; he attributes this to the fact that schizophrenics outside mental institutions more often present two features unfavorable for treatment, viz. insidious course and psychoneurotic symptoms in a schizophrenic psychosis. In a group of 275 institutionalized schizophrenics, all treated with a minimum of twenty convulsions, the remission rate (recovered and much improved) was 68.3 per cent in cases of less than six months' duration, 41.5 in those ill from six months to two years, and only 9.2 per cent in those ill more than two years. Patients with a longer history but with previous remissions have a rather favorable prognosis for the new attack (56.5 per cent remissions). In addition to those patients in whom a remission was obtained, a number of patients listed only as improved were also able to leave the hospital.

The figure of 68.3 per cent remissions in cases of less than six months' duration coincides with figures found by Cook for metrazol when he summarized reports from various countries on similar cases and came to 69.7 per cent remissions (43.4 per cent full and 26.3 per cent social remissions). Striking agreement in the total discharge rate is reported in two studies on two groups of patients in comparable hospitals in New York State, both of which received equally intense treatment with ECT and metrazol (Kalinowsky and Worthing, and Zeifert). The figures were 80.4 and 84.3 per cent respectively in schizophrenics ill less than six months. For cases of up to one year's duration of illness, remission rates may still reach between 55 per cent and 60 per cent, but they drop considerably if the patients have been ill more than one year.

Even though the question of how far results with ECT approximate those with insulin in schizophrenia remains undecided—in view of contrary statements and lack of comparative studies—the value of ECT in this condition is sufficiently assured. Cook, surveying all opinions, states that between 55 and 60 per cent of patients treated with convulsions in the first year of their illness may be expected to remit sufficiently to take their former place in society. This is considerably above figures for spontaneous remissions. A large survey from Norwegian hospitals, presented by Dedichen, arrives at 63.3 per cent remissions in cases of less than six months' duration, 30 per cent between six and twelve months' duration. In his comparison between 1459 treated and 969 untreated patients he found four times as many remissions in the cases up to six months, and twice as many in those of six months to one year's duration in favor of the treated group.

Statements as to the response of the various subtypes of schizophrenia to convulsive therapy are contradictory. Many authors feel that catatonics respond better than paranoids. The superiority of convulsive therapy in catatonic stupor, first stressed by Angyal and Gyarfas, is not confirmed in Kalinowsky's experience with ECT. It seems that the quick and spectacular breaking up of a catatonic stupor leads to the impression of a specific effect on this condition. However, it is this group particularly which in many cases relapses repeatedly so that the long-term results are disappointing. Neymann et al. have also had disappointing results with ECT in catatonic stupors and were surprised at the good results in paranoids. A more insidious course in paranoids makes results with ECT alone questionable and requires insulin or combined insulin-convulsive treatment. Patients with late paranoid schizophrenia, who develop their symptoms in the fifth or sixth decade of life and who have little or no tendency to deteriorate, show an extremely poor response to ECT. This is true for all patients with well preserved personality as exemplified by the negative response usually seen in the pseudoneurotic form of schizophrenia (Hoch and Polatin). In this latter group a symptomatic improvement by means of a few ECT can be obtained during depressive episodes or panic states. A lasting effect on the pseudoneurotic type of schizophrenia has never been seen. Most workers agree on the poor results in hebephrenics, but there are improvements, and therapeutic nihilism is not justified in these cases, all the more as here pharmacotherapy is quite ineffective. At the other end of the scale are the excellent results in catatonic excitements. In some of these cases, accompanied by high fever and poor physical condition (described formerly as "fatal catatonia"), convulsive therapy is a life-saving procedure when given in "blocs" of several treatments a day. In these patients the use of phenothiazines may be more dangerous and lead to vasomotor collapse. Several studies on neuroleptic drugs emphasize this point in acute catatonic states (Heinrich, Hoff and Hofmann, others).

Meduna, similar to Langfeldt, expresses the opinion that convulsive treatment is successful only in symptomatic schizophrenic states, but considers "endogenous schizophrenia" as refractory. He described the former group as "oneirophrenia." The outstanding subjective feature of these cases is a disturbance of the sensorium, with sensations of changes in one's body and environment. Oneirophrenia appears in two forms: a simple one, uncomplicated by hallucinations, and the deliroid form; both are responsive to convulsive therapy.

In childhood schizophrenia L. Bender reported very good results. She still considers ECT the most effective treatment if given adequately, and recommends 20 treatments on 20 subsequent days. Accornero and Anderson were less successful in the treatment of schizophrenic children. It seems to us that the prognosis depends on the same prognostic criteria as in adult schizophrenia.

Various statements have been made regarding the favorable prognostic significance of certain symptoms, such as psychomotor and affective manifestations (A. Kennedy), feelings of guilt (Pacella and Barrera), reduced physical health (Hemphill and Grey Walter). Rosal correctly generalizes that where emotional emptiness is visible, the schizophrenic disease process is rarely arrested by therapy. According to Mader, anxiety and compulsive features are definitely unfavorable. Most of these statements are valid for all shock methods. A detailed discussion of the prognostic importance of various clinical data in schizophrenia will be given in the part on insulin treatment. They are the same in convulsive therapy. In a study by Pfister, a positive sodium amytal test was in agreement with a favorable result of electric convulsive therapy in 75 per cent of the cases. Piotrowski's Rorschach studies were equally useful in insulin and in electric convulsive therapy.

Early relapses nearly always occur during the first two weeks after treatment. Therefore, no statistical conclusion should be drawn and no patient discharged less than two or three weeks after the last treatment. Kalinowsky found that of 111 patients who had been discharged after such a period of observation, only 13 returned within six months to two years. Patients who relapse after a good remission usually respond well to a new course of treatment. Studies on long-range follow-up in straight convulsive therapy are few in number. The statistical pitfalls are the same as in the other types of shock therapy. The difference between the final outcome in shock-treated and untreated schizophrenics may not be very striking, but the number of years spent outside the hospital is certainly higher in shock-treated patients. Early return to the hospital for retreatment would definitely improve the long-term results. This was pointed out by Feldman et al., who discuss the socioeconomic effects of shock therapy in schizophrenia and stress the need for more careful control of the discharged patients and for preparation of the family for immediate resumption of treatment when it is needed. Salzman's observation that untreated patients stay out of the hospital longer than the shock-treated ones only emphasizes the known fact that patients who have experienced early remissions before they receive treatment are the most favorable group. Another erroneous statistical conclusion is that shorter series of treatment lead to better results because patients responding to fewer treatments are necessarily those with better prognosis. The difficulty of demonstrating statistically what shock treatment does was well proved by one of our patients hospitalized permanently for recurrent schizophrenic episodes; she now receives a few treatments in the office for her episodes. Statistically she is relapsing, but she has now lived an almost normal life for ten years. Preventive treatment once a month can be considered in such cases, but results as reported by Stevenson and Geoghegan are less satisfactory in schizophrenia than in manic-depressive psychosis. A most negative statistical report on ECT by Karagulla has been criticized by Slater who pointed out that her untreated cases had not been treated for the very reason that they happened to have a better prognosis. In a comparison between brief psychotherapy, insulin coma treatment and ECT Gottlieb and Huston failed to find a significant difference in results during a follow-up period of one to four years. Bockoven et al, and many other statistical reports demonstrated the striking increase in discharges from mental hospitals since the routine use of somatic treatments, and particularly of the easily applicable electric convulsive treatment.

The manner in which insulin, convulsive therapy and pharmacotherapy should supplement each other will be discussed elsewhere; this section is limited to a survey of reports on the treatment of schizophrenics with convulsive therapy alone. The available material justifies the conclusion that convulsive therapy has an important place in the treatment of schizophrenia, particularly in early cases, where, as recently as 1967, Weise and Muhlbach confirmed the superiority of both, insulin and ECT in the number of remissions over the neuroleptic drugs which have their domain in chronic schizophrenia. Comparing the length of time drug- and ECT-treated patients spend in the hospital three years after the first admission, May and Tuma establish the superiority of ECT. The simultaneous use of pharmacotherapy and ECT is recommended by Kelly and Sargant as the best presently available treatment in schizophrenia. On the basis of our own extensive experience it is our opinion that in acute schizophrenia an attempt with psychopharmacology might be justified, but that after several weeks or a few months the drug should be tentatively discontinued, and in case of relapse convulsive therapy instituted. In early cases the goal must be a true remission rather than a symptomatic improvement. If this is not obtained with drug therapy, convulsive treatment is in order. Only if this also fails, maintenance drug therapy of long duration must be started in the hope that the patient continues on this medication indefinitely. Rehabilitation of a schizophrenic patient is still more promising in a true remission than in patients who must be kept on long medication with drugs which they might or might not be willing to take, results only in doses which lead to disturbing side-effects. In such individual cases maintenance ECT can still be a very useful therapeutic tool.

PSYCHONEUROSES: The application of ECT in the psychoneuroses was favored by its technical simplicity and the possibility of ambulatory application. However, results as a whole are disappointing. The difference in response between neurotics and psychotics is of particular interest.

A study by Kalinowsky et al. distinguishing between the various groups of psychoneurotics shows the following; patients with anxiety hysteria are the least amenable to ECT; most of them remain unimproved. Some felt temporarily relaxed and less tense, others were aggravated by the fear of the treatment or by side-effects, such as memory impairment and the feeling of unreality which is resented much more by neurotics than by psychotics.

Cases of conversion hysteria in the long run showed almost as unsatisfactory results. Occasionally, conversion symptoms were influenced in the same way as they are by any suggestive method. Patients who had been impressed by the improvement of others and had requested treatment were most likely to improve. Underlying depressive elements in patients with conversion symptoms make them more amenable to shock therapy: Instances of successful treatment of hysterical paralysis were reported by Cernaček as well as by Meggendorfer who explains them as a type of psychotherapy and essentially different from the effect of ECT in the psychoses. Cernaček cured hysterical paralysis by utilizing the patient's ability to move the extremities in the awakening period, which was done in the presence of witnesses. Amazing results were obtained by Parland with the same technique in acute hysterical manifestations of soldiers in the Finnish Army. In cases of pure simulation, the "surprise therapy," as Cernaček called it, failed. Simulated amnesia for identity was treated by Hemphill and Stuart, whose patient remembered his identity in the awakening period, forgot it again, but later admitted simulation. One of our cases of apparently true amnesia did not clear up under convulsive therapy. We did see favorable results in some individual cases of hysterical stupor, although the differential diagnosis in such cases often remains unclear.

As a whole, our own experience has made us very reluctant to treat patients with the characteristics of a "hysterical personality." More often than not hysterics present new symptoms during the treatment. Slight discomfort experienced after the treatment, such as muscular pain, dizziness, headache, etc., are elaborated on and may aggravate the patient's condition. It is not an infrequent occurrence to see hysterical gait disturbances, a picture resembling a Ganser syndrome or other hysterical manifestations of short duration developing immediately after a treatment in such patients.

Psychoneurotic depressions offer better results. They may clear up after a few treatments like any other depression. Most workers feel that psychoneurotic or reactive depressions respond less well than endogenous depressions. Our own results were quite unpredictable. Good response of reactive depressions even of long standing has been demonstrated by Myerson's study of "prolonged cases of grief reaction."

In obsessive-compulsive neurotics, results are uncertain. Most patients fail to show lasting improvement, but they do manifest some benefit temporarily. Even when compulsions and obsessions persist after the treatment, the emotional tension accompanying them is often lessened for a while and the patient is better able to adjust to his symptoms. Some patients become more accessible to psychotherapy at this stage. However, the symptoms in most cases return sooner or later with the same intensity. The same was seen by Delay and Maillard in the "neurasthenic" patient of the French terminology. Depressive states with obsessional trends, often respond well. According to Bennett, many anxiety states are affect disorders in which the picture is predominantly depressive. Convulsive therapy will break up the depression leaving anxiety which can then be treated with psychotherapy. If, however, in such anxiety state the anxiety prevails, psychotherapy is preferable. Also, in cases of conversion hysteria where results as a whole are poor, the affect present will determine whether or not the patient is likely to respond to convulsive therapy. There are cases where neurotic symptoms such as obsessive fears and severe anxiety have an episodic course. In such cases ECT is often successful and may be tried if drugs have failed.

There are a number of favorable reports. In psychoneurotics admitted to a private hospital, ECT was found by Hamilton to be a useful part of an over-all treatment program. It proved valuable in breaking up the pattern of neurotic symptoms. When such symptoms as insomnia, depression or obsessive phenomena were reduced, the patient developed greater confidence in the physician and became more amenable to suggestion. The patients had some psychotherapy in the hospital prior to receiving shock treatment, and the average period of hospitalization following the treatment was four months. Two favorable reports on psychoneurotic were based on regressive treatment; the "intense method" of ECT (Milligan) or "method of annihilation" (Bini and Bazzi). Our own as well as Stengel's results with intense treatment were disappointing, with the exception of a few obsessionals. Using regular ECT Moriarty and Weil gave a favorable report on a group of psychoneurotics treated in combination with psychotherapy. Flescher, Selinsky, and other psychiatrists find an occasional treatment useful in breaking through the patient's resistance to psychotherapy. In some special syndromes regarded as being of neurotic origin, results have been obtained. Thus, stammering has been treated successfully by Owen and Stemmerman after ECT had removed the tension of these patients. A number of psychosomatic conditions have been submitted to ECT with more or less success. Some of them will be mentioned presently under "various conditions." There is some evidence that ECT is often applied in neurotics for no other reason than that everything else has failed or because of its simplicity. Indiscriminate use in neurotics is particularly likely to discredit the method.

Non-convulsive electrostimulatory treatment was found to be valuable in psychoneurotics by Hirschfeld, and later by others. This had been preceded by Berkwitz' faradic shock treatment. In both these methods the pain connected with such stimulation was avoided by combination with intravenous injections of barbiturates. Therefore, the question remains unanswered as to what extent the electric current on the one hand, and the barbiturates on the other, are responsible for occasional improvements. We are inclined to believe in the latter explanation. A new and extremely active approach was recently taken in the treatment of apparently intractable tension states by Sargant et al. who used simultaneously light continuous narcosis, a combination of the supposedly incompatible antidepressants iproniazid and amitriptyline, and ECT stretched out over several weeks. The majority of these patients who had been sent to the authors for leucotomy, responded well, and only a few had to undergo psychosurgery after this intensive treatment program.

Study of reports on pharmacologic convulsive therapy applied in neuroses gives the impression that results are perhaps more favorable than with ECT (Cheney et al.). A systematic evaluation was attempted by Shapiro and Freeman who were favorably impressed. The more dramatic effect of metrazol treatment, with its terrifying experience for the patient, was used by Verstraeten, and others in neurotics with gross hysterical manifestations, and applied by British workers in war neuroses.

ECT in most types of psychoneuroses is symptomatic at best, and only few treatments will be applied except in obsessive-compulsives in whom intensive treatment often leads to a temporary disappearance of symptoms. There have never been many indications for ECT in the neurotic patient, and modern pharmacotherapy restricted its application in this group further.

Epilepsy: Treatment of epileptics with convulsive therapy seems illogical, but attempts were based on good reasoning. The raising of the convulsive threshold during any course of convulsive therapy led to the hope that such treatment might also raise the individual's convulsive threshold to the noxious agent in epilepsy. A pertinent observation was made by Hardon and Kraus who noticed that in combined insulin-metrazol treatment the metrazol fits inhibited the occurrence of spontaneous hypoglycemic convulsions. In epileptic patients Pozniak and Erb, and Sal y Rosas made practical use of the increased threshold by means of pharmacologically produced seizures; Kalinowsky and Kennedy applying ECT observed that in patients having spontaneous convulsions at regular intervals, e.g., menstrual epilepsy, an artificial convulsion offered some protection against a spontaneous fit which, occurring under uncontrolled conditions, might endanger the patient and jeopardize his social position. Failure of such attempts (Pacella and Barrera) may be explained by the withdrawal of anticonvulsive medication previous to treatment, which in itself increases the number of seizures in the sense of withdrawal convulsions. Convulsive therapy will never replace anticonvulsive medication, but Caplan has convincingly shown that when convulsions occur despite full doses of anticonvulsive drugs, convulsive therapy may have some value as an accessory treatment, even in institutional epileptics.

Another group of epileptic phenomena for which metrazol and ECT have been employed to some advantage by several workers are psychic equivalents (Treves, and others with metrazol, Kalinowsky and Kennedy, Guirand and Mallet with ECT). It is common knowledge that psychotic syndromes in epileptics frequently terminate in spontaneous epileptic convulsions. If such a seizure is produced artificially, the duration, especially of epileptic twilight states can be shortened at will. In our experience this represents the most promising use of ECT in epileptics. Repeated incomplete seizures of epileptics can also be terminated by one or two ECT.

VARIOUS CONDITIONS: Convulsive therapy has been tried in a number of other conditions, particularly in various organic psychotic syndromes. As far as these are short lasting, acute psychotic episodes, often associated with increased psychomotility, neuroleptic drugs became the treatment of choice. Formerly ECT had been used effectively, and it can still be used when drugs are ineffective or, as in some acute infectious conditions, considered dangerous because of their hypotensive effect possibly leading to vasomotor collapse. Favorable reports are available on the application in general paresis of both metrazol and ECT (Broggi, Ewald and Haddenbroock, Kenyon et al., Tomlinson). Many patients with general paresis have shown a quick disappearance of their most disturbing psychotic symptoms. ECT is also useful after fever or penicillin therapy if the antisyphilitic treatment has failed or, as it is not unusual, is slow in removing the psychotic symptoms. The value of convulsive treatment in disturbed paretics, for quieting the patient and improving his general condition preparatory to fever therapy, has been stressed by Jones and Pleasants, and J. H. Taylor. ECT has also been used in catatonic states after encephalitis (Ayaslioglu and Lange), in posttraumatic catatonia (De Natale and Paolozzi) and organic stupor due to head injury (Silverman). The disappearance of toxic psychoses due to bromide intoxication described by Arneson and Ourso, is not only of practical but also of some theoretical interest as discussed in the theoretical chapter of this book.

Reports by Fernandes and Polonio and some others are available on the removal of psychotic syndromes during pellagra, and in cases of pernicious anemia with hallucinations (Ende et al.). A number of observations on the treatment of psychotic complications of porphyria were made by Levy and Perry, Lemere and several others. Psychoses due to mepacrine, used in the treatment of malaria, as reported by Perk, cleared up with an average of four ECT. Delay mentions cases of uremic psychoses, and von Baeyer toxic psychoses from mushroom poisoning. Psychotic reactions in the course of treatment with ACTH and cortisone can also be removed with electrically induced convulsions.

Arteriosclerotic and senile diseases offer a difficult problem regarding indication for convulsive therapy. It is obvious that mental impairment, confusion and other reactions of undoubtedly organic nature do not offer any promise under ECT, which in itself produces the same type of organic reactions, though only temporarily. However, such brain conditions are often accompanied by manic-depressive or schizophrenia-like reactions which can be treated successfully with a few shock treatments. The agitation of some purely organic syndromes of old age could also be removed with as few as one or two ECT, but here the neuroleptic drugs are undoubtedly superior.

Depressions and paranoid reactions of episodic character occurring in Parkinson's disease offer an important indication for ECT. We have treated several episodes in the same patient with great success. These patients show an aggravation of their neurological dysfunction, while they suffer from emotional disturbances. One of our patients who walked fairly well became bedridden with severe rigidity of all four extremities with each psychotic episode. She was again able to walk quite well after ECT had cleared up the psychosis. The same was seen in many other neurological cases complicated by a depression or other psychotic disorders. Our material includes several hemiplegias, hemianopsias, aphasias, and two cases of multiple sclerosis. These experiences show that the amount of structural damage alone does not determine the degree of dysfunction in neurological disease.

Another neurological group in which treatment attempts were made concerns hyperkinetic manifestations such as tics and others (Kalinowsky). Here results were rather contradictory. Treatment with ECT for tics often aggravates the condition, because patients who had learned to control the involuntary movements for a limited period of time became unable to do so when their power of concentration was impaired by the treatment. In some other patients a temporary improvement was obtained (as also seen by Strauss and Macphail). In a case of Edwards bizarre psychogenic movements responded to regressive ECT after they had failed under regular ECT.

Other therapeutic possibilities arise from the utilization of some of the side-effects of ECT. The temporary emotional and intellectual "blurring has been used for various purposes; for instance, it is of value in preventing withdrawal symptoms in drug addicts (Kalinowsky). Metrazol has been used for the same purpose by Avery and Campbell. The desire for morphine is "forgotten," and withdrawal symptoms are not felt. It usually takes four treatments on succeeding days to make sudden withdrawal of the drug possible. Neuroleptic drugs often fail in the treatment of withdrawal symptoms, and their "epileptogenic" nature may, for instance in barbiturate withdrawal, precipitate convulsions, while ECT increases the threshold for withdrawal convulsions. The blurring effect of ECT is also used in skin conditions with severe itching. The spectacular improvements in patients with chronic eczema can only be explained by diminution of itching and consequent diminished scratching. This mechanism probably also explains the dramatic improvements in cases of probable neurodermatitis treated with ECT by Baur and Perrin. We saw similar good results, but also met with complete failure in a patient who gave up his usual effort to resist the temptation to scratch, and whose uninhibited scratching made the skin condition worse.

Individual cases, scattered through the literature, can be found in various conditions interpreted as psychosomatic. One condition, where original attempts looked promising, was asthma. As a whole, our results have not been much better than those of Cohen and Holbrook, who came to entirely negative conclusions. Peptic ulcer, often considered a psychosomatic problem, was treated with ECT by Corbella and Piredda; they reported lasting results after one or two series of 3 to 7 electrically induced convulsions in ulcer patients with hypersecretion and hyperacidity, but no results in those with hypacidity. They saw an advantage in such treatment even in cases with only temporary results, because improvement of the patient's general condition facilitated surgical intervention.

Anorexia nervosa has been often seen to respond to ECT. In some patients in whom psychotherapy alone had been tried unsuccessfully for years, ECT led to immediate improvement. In other cases no improvement whatsoever was obtained. In a paper on "controversial indications of ECT" Gallinek, too, lists good results. Similar experiences are reported by Italian psychiatrists, among others Balduzzi. All these authors stress the importance of following up the results with psychotherapy.

Pain can also be favorably influenced by ECT, but again the effect is usually limited to the period during which the sensorium is moderately blurred. There are, however, some reports claiming permanent relief. Complete disapperance of trigeminal neuralgia was seen by Janjigian. Disappearance of painful phantom limbs was observed by Pisetzky in a man in whom the amputation of both legs preceded an involutional melancholia. The depression as well as the painful phantom limbs had persisted for five years and disappeared simultaneously under ECT.

Cordoba et al. saw "vasomotor trophic neuroses" such as Raynaud's disease, acroparesthesiae, scleroderma and others improve remarkably when these happened to be present in patients undergoing ECT for a mental condition. They assume a favorable effect of ECT on the peripheral circulation, but the influence on the neurogenic mechanism of these "vasomotor neuroses" is also postulated.

In cases of psychopathic personality, ECT was tried without effect by Bennett and several others. Occasional results were obtained (Leggari). Two cases of psychopathic personality, described by Darling, had atypical features, one depressive and the other some schizophrenia-like symptoms. ECT does not change personality traits, and it is therefore not surprising that most reports on psychopathic personality are negative. This includes various forms of sexual psychopathy (Thompson). Ownsby reported on replacement of homosexuality with normal sexual desire, but confirmation of such results by others is missing. In sexual abnormalities, the question arises as to how far the homosexual trends or active homosexuality were preceded by a psychosis. Several of our manic cases with good heterosexual adjustment during the normal intervals became homosexual during their manic episodes. In such cases, the disappearance of the manic state under ECT restored the normal sexual behavior, but it would be misleading to value such results as a cure for homosexuality. Isolated reports on prison psychoses or similar psychogenic states can also be found in the literature. In metrazol treatment of prison psychoses the dread of the treatment has been considered as the healing factor.

Alcoholism has also been treated with ECT. Bennett has had some success in treating the prominent depressive and anxiety features in alcoholics. Failures have been reported by Petri-Canella and Levi in treating chronic alcoholism with metrazol, by Neymann et al. with ECT. Orenstein et al. have used metrazol with good results in acute alcoholic intoxications. We have treated one patient with dipsomania; after two or three convulsions given when the patient began to feel the tension preceding his bouts, his tension and the irresistible urge for alcohol were no longer felt. Many French psychiatrists, among others Thiebaux et al., report favorable results with ECT in delirium tremens. Also Lieser considers ECT as life-saving in acute delirium of any origin, and prefers it to chlorpromazine which may lead to sudden death in such cases.

ECT as a life-saving procedure is emphasized by Lieser also in other conditions like deep coma from hypoglycemia or barbiturate poisoning, and even comas from cerebral hemorrhage. In all these instances one to three convulsions revived patients who were already in cardiovascular and respiratory distress. Anesthesia techniques should be avoided in such severely ill patients. This author's experience shows that convulsive therapy as such is of minimal danger and even benefits patients in poor physical condition.

In patients who suffer from a serious mental condition including those with physical risks we are never reluctant to apply convulsive treatment. We are all the more hesitant to try it in psychosomatic and some of the other conditions mentioned in the last chapter, where results are unconvincing, and where other methods, especially psychotherapy and pharmacotherapy are the treatments of choice.

General Remarks

The quick and predictable therapeutic effect of convulsive therapy in depressions belongs to the most spectacular results obtainable in psychiatry. This explains why convulsive therapy, in spite of many objections, continues to be widely and, at present, increasingly used notwithstanding the advances in pharmacotherapy. Modern techniques make convulsive therapy easily applicable, safe, and sometimes better tolerated than drugs. We agree with Pauleikhoff and many others that the superiority of ECT is not limited to depressions but applies to many schizophrenic syndromes as well, particularly in acute cases. The same author rightly questions one of the objections often made against ECT, namely that it distorts the patient's personality. If so, this is a temporary effect which disappears entirely, while psychotropic drugs maintain a personality change often for a much longer period of time, when long-term medication is indicated. More disturbing are the purely emotional objections to ECT which influence many psychiatrists, and frighten the patients who are afraid of being "shocked" or even ashamed to have a treatment with this name. Kraines, summarizing a symposium on the unchanged need for ECT, suggests the term "cerebral stimulation." He feels that it is mostly the term "shock" that is responsible for the tendency of many psychiatrists to delay a treatment which, if applied early, can terminate the suffering of many patients in a much shorter time than most other forms of treatment.

CHAPTER IV

Insulin Coma and Subcoma Treatment

Insulin treatment as the first active therapeutic approach to the management of schizophrenia, had been wrongly considered a treatment of the past whenever new therapeutic agents were found. As soon as electric shock therapy was seen to be effective in certain cases of schizophrenia, the cumbersome insulin treatment was abandoned in many hospitals. The wave of enthusiasm and optimism which accompanied the introduction of the neuroleptic drugs immediately led to statements that insulin and other methods of the past had become obsolete. Yet, still today many clinicians with experience in all treatments of schizophrenia realize that insulin coma therapy continues to be a valuable therapeutic tool. In some countries such as the Soviet Union, it is more widely used than in others. The difficulty to staff an insulin treatment center with specially trained psychiatrists and nurses suggests that each geographical area should have one hospital at its disposal, where an insulin unit is maintained. Our own clinical experience gives sufficient evidence that many patients unresponsive to other forms of treatment, can still reach satisfactory remissions with this method. Its technical problems, its many interesting implications, and the enormous amounts of research it has stimulated, are adequate reason for a proper representation in a book on the somatic treatment approach. The excuse that insulin treatment is too difficult to administer is contradicted by a survey from Indian hospitals made by Vahia who found that 18 out of 21 hospital psychiatrists still continued insulin treatment ten years after the introduction of neuroleptic drugs.

Insulin was used in psychiatry before Sakel. Schuster, Steck, and Klemperer used it as a sedative for excited patients and in cases of delirium tremens. It was also used to overcome refusal of food and to build up run-down patients, but the dosage in these treatments was small, and, as Sakel rightly claims, only mild hypoglycemia was produced; the coma which is obtained only through marked hypoglycemia was avoided and even considered dangerous and unwarranted. The small dose insulin treatment and, as we shall see later, the so-called ambulatory insulin method has a definite place in therapy, but it is not insulin shock treatment. The term "insulin shock treatment" is so deeply ingrained in the literature that it is difficult to replace it, although deep hypoglycemia is not a state of shock, and the term "insulin coma treatment" is more appropriate.

Organization of Insulin Coma Treatment

Insulin coma treatment is a hospital procedure and requires a special set-up for its proper execution. It is advisable for hospitals to organize separate insulin shock units (Sakel, J. Wortis, Roemer, Jessner and Ryan). Worthing et al. describe the organization of a special treatment building set aside for insulin and other forms of shock therapy in a large institution. Sargant and Slater report successful treatments in general hospital wards among surgical and medical patients, but feel that, in most instances, it is preferable to give the treatment on psychiatric wards. If possible, a separate ward should be maintained. Male and female patients may be treated together if they are screened off from each other or placed in separate ward rooms. The room should be well ventilated, and kept warm at an even temperature. Heating the room on chilly days is important because of the patient's reduced temperature during hypoglycemia. In some hospitals the patients stay on the insulin unit all the time. In others they are returned to their respective wards each day after termination of the treatment. In the latter case, the personnel on the wards must be instructed in the manifestations of late shock in order that effective countermeasures may be taken. We prefer to have the patient remain on the same ward after treatment. In this way it is much easier to watch the effect of the treatment on the patient and to carry on psychotherapy by the same physician who treats the patient daily with insulin and is, therefore, in constant contact with the patient. It is also much easier to regulate the patient's diet, to pay attention to his eating habits, to organize his exercise and recreation periods. Separate rooms should be available in order to isolate disturbed patients and those who become noisy in the hypoglycemic state.

In some insulin wards, radio music during the treatment hours helps to cover the inevitable noises of patients under treatment. The atmosphere should be a pleasant one during as well as after the treatment. The importance of some kind of activity in the afternoons of treatment days has been stressed. Here occupational therapy is most valuable. Group therapy in a group of insulin patients has been described by Wender, and Scott tried to prove its value in a comparative study which showed superior results when group psychotherapy was applied. Interpersonal relations, so difficult to establish in schizophrenics, are already favored by the common treatment experience, and are further aided by group psychotherapy of the insulin treated patients. To this Laqueur added "conjoint family group therapy," whereby several families meet in weekly group sessions with their insulin-treated relatives to avoid breaking up of the family unit.

It has been suggested that a physician need be present in the treatment room only during the shock period of the treatment and for the termination of the hypoglycemia. We prefer that the physician be present during the whole time of active treatment as complications may occur even before the shock phase is reached; and symptoms displayed during the preshock phase are often indicative of advisable variations in the treatment procedure. Moreover, a physician should be on call during the entire day in order to take care of delayed reactions.

Nurses attending the patients should also have special knowledge of the treatment. One or more nurses should be assigned to the unit for an extended period of time in order to form the nucleus of a well conducted unit around which other personnel can rotate. This is expedient for the training of many nurses in the procedure. Usually one nurse is needed for every six patients for the first two hours of treatment, and another one should be on call during this period. During the coma and termination periods, however, the presence of more nurses is advisable.

The patient should always be in bed during insulin shock treatment. Beds with adjustable head parts should be used so that the patient may be raised or lowered as his condition requires. As patients can easily roll out of bed or jump up during periods of excitement, some restraining is often inevitable. Beds fitted with steel side rails or padded side walls are advisable. The patient should be kept warm all the time with an ample supply of blankets. After termination of treatment the patient should be dried as most of them are covered with perspiration, and before dressing they should receive a cleansing shower.

Insulin shock treatment is like an operative procedure. Just as the surgeon and anesthetist record their observations during operation, the physician and nurses should record their observations on the physical and mental changes that occur during and after hypoglycemia. The patient's temperature should be taken before treatment and every two hours during treatment, once in the afternoon, and again before bedtime. Pulse and respiration should be counted every thirty minutes during hypoglycemia and every fifteen minutes during the shock period. The patient's weight should be taken every week. In most hospitals a clinical chart is used for recording the following data: Name, age, sex, diagnosis, short description of the clinical symptoms of the psychosis and duration of illness, and entries of each treatment so that the exact number is kept, dosage of insulin, type of termination, amount of glucose given for termination, response of the patient to insulin (whether awake, in superficial coma, coma, deep coma, having epileptic convulsions or other complications), number of comas obtained, response of patient after termination (i.e., whether responsive, in good or bad contact with the environment, hallucinating) and finally the clinical attainment at the end of the whole course of treatment (recovered, much improved, improved, or unimproved).

Selection of Patients for Treatment

Every patient in reasonably good health is suitable for treatment. The most important contraindications are active pulmonary tuberculosis, acute or chronic kidney and liver disease, diseases of the pancreas, thyroid, or adrenal glands. Diabetes is also considered a contraindication, but, interestingly enough, it is a rare occurrence among schizophrenic patients. No patient should be treated during febrile disease of any kind. Müller's addition of pregnancy as a contraindication is supported by Gralnick. Damage to the fetus was reported by Sobel. Von Braunmühl warns especially against juvenile hypertension and lymphatic diathesis.

Most important is the exclusion of patients suffering from a cardiovascular disease. Hadorn and Schmid have shown conclusively the connection between hypoglycemia and circulation. Essential hypertension, angina pectoris, coronary sclerosis or occlusion, vascular heart disease, and myocarditis are all grave risks and should not be given treatment. Müller takes electrocardiograms before giving insulin and again during moderate insulinization. He has found that many patients who show no sign of electrocardiographic change without insulin manifest changes during mild hypoglycemia which require caution in the use of high insulin doses. He attributes the absence of mortality among 300 treated patients to his careful selection. On the other hand, most workers will agree that mild changes in the electrocardiogram should not be deterrent as a number of patients showing alterations at the beginning of treatment later adjusted themselves and showed normal electrocardiographic records. Electrocardiograms could probably be entirely dispensed with in healthy patients. Patients around 50 years of age do not tolerate insulinization very well and therefore should be treated only if their cardiovascular apparatus is in good functional condition. Under favorable circumstances, von Braunmühl is willing to consider treatment for patients up to 65 years of age.

The selection of patients from a psychiatric point of view has, of course, changed with the introduction of subsequent methods of treatment. Today insulin will be reserved for those patients who failed under other methods. This automatically makes for a less acute type of material. Laqueur in the U.S. and Arnold and Hoff in Vienna have shown that a longer series of comas than previously given can still be promising in patients with longer duration of illness. On the basis of our own experience we would add that this applies only to those patients of longer duration, who under other methods of treatment had shown at least a temporary improvement, but soon relapsed.

When insulin treatment is recommended for a patient, it is advisable to discuss the results and dangers with the responsible relatives. A written consent, as in surgical procedures, is required in most hospitals. The patient himself should be informed about the treatment. He should be reassured that the treatment is painless and without undue discomfort. The acquiescence or refusal of the patients has no influence on the efficacy of the insulin treatment as such, but his cooperation is valuable especially if he needs subsequent psychotherapy.

Technique of Insulin Coma Treatment

Before describing the technique of the treatment, it should be mentioned that there are patients who are allergic to insulin. In general, it is immaterial what brand of insulin is used, but there are patients who are allergic to one type and not to another. Insulin allergy, however, should not be confused with hypersensitivity to the drug. Where hypersensitivity is present, the patient responds in an exaggerated way to insulin; the hyperglycemic state is very rapid and profound.

The most common allergic reactions following insulin are local responses; the patient complains of an itching, burning sensation at the site of the injection, which becomes indurated and painful, and usually a small or large area of erythema appears which ordinarily lasts but a few days and requires only local treatment. Still less common are the generalized allergic reactions, mainly in the form of urticaria with considerable itching. This form of allergic response is apt to occur in a half hour or less after the insulin injection. Injection of epinephrine gives prompt relief.

Because of the danger of allergic reactions and hypersensitivity it is advisable to start treatment with small amounts of insulin, 10-15 units. Bond and Shurley test sensitivity and allergic response to insulin by giving all patients small doses of 5 units daily for a week before institution of insulin coma treatment. Müller deplores the suggestion to start with high doses; Wilder claims that insulin, even in therapeutic doses, may cause death in sensitive individuals even though glucose is given promptly. Rosendahl reports a fatality in a nondiabetic patient who received only 8 units of insulin daily for 4 days. In general, an initial injection of 10-15 units is well tolerated. It has been claimed that in schizophrenic patients insulin sensitivity is below normal. Meduna assumed that the schizophrenic patient has a special insulin inhibitory factor in his blood which he later limited to certain groups of schizophrenics. This anti-insulin factor may be identical with the glycotropic hormone of the anterior lobe of the hypophysis. Goldner and Ricketts did not confirm this, and Freeman found that the phenomenon of insulin resistance is not limited to schizophrenia but occurs in other types of psychiatric patients as well. Harris found in schizophrenic patients marked fluctuation in sensitivity to insulin. He observed variations in the amount of anti-insulin substances in the blood, which increased or decreased the activity of the drug, but found no correlation between the anti-insulin factors and the dose that produced coma. The nervous system of each individual shows its individual susceptibility to insulin, as it does to many other drugs. Sakel and Dussik originally thought that the coma dose of insulin was proportionate to the duration of the schizophrenic illness. Müller, however, has shown that this dose has no relation to the duration of illness or to the prognosis.

The opposite of insulin hypersensitivity, namely, insulin resistance, is much more common. Some schizophrenic patients are rather tardy in reaching hypoglycemia and even when given excessive amounts of insulin (1000 units in one of our cases), no signs of hypoglycemic shock appear. Lerman demonstrated the presence of substances in the blood of insulin resistant diabetic patients which protect animals against the hypoglycemic effects of insulin, and which show the characteristics of antibodies. It has been suggested that insulin resistance is brought about by these antibodies and that a return to normal insulin sensitivity is dependent upon their disappearance. Berson and Yalow differentiated serum anti-insulin factors into insulin antibodies and insulin antagonists demonstrable in the absence of a history of exogenous insulin administration e.g., insulinase. They believe that insulin resistance in the first few weeks of treatment is due to a contra-insulin hormone since insulin is a poor antibody producer. Resistance later in treatment may be due to the binding of insulin to gamma globulin which prevents rapid passage of the insulin through the capillary wall.

It is our impression that since most patients subjected to insulin had a previous series of electric convulsive therapy, the course of insulin treatments became more irregular. It is difficult or impossible to prove this, but it seems worthwhile to mention such clinical impressions. We also observed that one electrically induced convulsion is often a simple means to overcome insulin resistance, and to reach coma level on the next day with a dosage which had been insufficient before. Müller thinks that insulin resistance in certain individuals is due to constitutional abnormalities in the endocrine apparatus, particularly in the pituitary and thyroid glands. He has quite regularly found pituitary dysplasia and obesity in patients who have not responded to 300-400 units of insulin. Similar observations were made by Falta. Insulin tolerance increases with body weight (Oberholzer) and decreases with older age (von Braunmühl). Winkler and other German psychiatrists of the school of Kretschmer studied the relationship between body type and tolerance to insulin. They found that patients with pyknic body type have the highest tolerance, while the leptosomes need smaller amounts of insulin. These differences are not simply explained by the differences in body weight. The mixed body types showed a higher tolerance than the pure types. The various body types also show striking differences in their tendency to hypoglycemic convulsions, as will be mentioned later. Increased tolerance in anxious and antagonistic patients was seen by Fuhry. Müller as well as Patterson found that the patient's attitude towards the treatment was related to insulin resistance; those patients who thought favorably of insulin, had a lower resistance to it than those who were antagonistic towards the treatment.

Another illustration of psychological factors in the response to insulin are attempts in the Soviet Union to reduce the necessary amount of insulin by conditioning the patient to the injection. Serova was able to replace the insulin injection with NaCl solution. If not supported by some insulin such hypoglycemia by conditioned reflex can be maintained for only three to four days. According to Posnyakova, the first hypoglycemias on the basis of conditioned reflex occur after 8 to 10 repetitions, but become more marked after 20 to 30 repetitions. The blood sugar values do not drop as much as they do in regular insulin treatment, and it does not appear that this technique became a routine procedure.

The insulin injection should be given deeply intramuscularly and its site should be changed at each administration in order to prevent the development of local tissue changes, necrosis, or lipodystrophy. The injection should be given in the early morning to the fasting patient and food should be withheld for four to four and one-half hours. The treatment is applied five to six times a week.

The Various Levels of Hypoglycemia

The first or preshock or precomatose phase of hypoglycemia becomes clinically noticeable usually an hour after the injection or earlier. The progression of symptoms follows a certain general pattern but varies according to individual differences from patient to patient. Tables like the one by Frostig, reproduced here, are useful. They organize the symptoms so as to demonstrate the main stages of hypoglycemia. It must be borne in mind that these schemes are only roughly valid; many details depend on individual variations in response and are not always as clearcut as the tables indicate. The condition of the patient, especially the motor and vegetative mechanisms, fluctuates during hypoglycemia and, consequently, deviations from the expected are common.

Hypoglycemic symptoms observed in patients under insulin treatment are very similar to those seen in patients suffering from spontaneous hypoglycemia (Moersch and Kernohan). There are, however, hypoglycemic manifestations which are definitely due to the influence of insulin on the psychotic manifestations. At times it is very difficult to differeniate between these two sets of phenomena. Symptoms of the patient's psychosis are intermingled with mental symptoms of hypoglycemia during the first two hours of the treatment and again after awakening. If cortical activity is suppressed with high doses of insulin, the symptoms are more and more to be attributed to the release of lower brain functions and are the same in the psychotic and the nonpsychotic individual. The symptoms of hypoglycemia in the first hour include feelings of lassitude, somnolence, increased perspiration, and increased salivation; often there are complaints about hunger and thirst. In the second hour, these symptoms become more marked; consciousness becomes clouded and the patient is drowsy and frequently falls asleep. In other patients, however, there is excitement; they become restless, try to get up, turn and toss around, shout and yell, and demands for food are not uncommon. Some patients show alterations in perception; spatial and time senses are impaired; illusions are common. In most instances, there is an intensification of the hallucinations which the patient had before treatment. Sometimes patients previously free from hallucinations and delusions develop them. Emotional outbursts, such as laughing, crying, and aggressive behavior, are often observed. Many patients show disorientation and impairment of recent memory, at times reaching a true confusional state. Others are out of touch with the environment but respond to stimulation in "a quick, intensified and persevering way" (Jessner and Ryan). This so-called forced responsiveness is seen in many patients; on being touched, they forcefully move the arm or leg away or turn away, and repeated stimulation always evokes the same pattern of response. Many patients try to speak but are only able to make indistinct sounds; speech is often thick, dysarthric, and mumbling. At times aphasia and apraxia are present. The incoordination of speech, movement, and behavior is not specific for insulin but is similar to that which may

Hours	*Symptoms*		*Localization*
First	Latent Time Somnolences (97.2%) Hypotonia (97.4%)	 Perspiration (99.1%) Salivation (90.1%)	Suppression of cortical and cerebellar activity
Second	Clouded consciousness Fine tremor Aphasia Apraxia Agnosia Fall of temperature Diminished exteroceptive sensitivity	Perceptual disturbances Motor excitement Confusion Psychotic syndromes	
Third	Loss of consciousness (100%) Primitive movements (71.5%) Forced graspings (71%) Clonic twitchings (70.2%) Myoclonoid twitchings Choreiform, Athetoid, Hemiballistic movements (35.6%) Early torsion spasms	Motor restlessness Exophthalmus Dilated pupils Light reaction present Pulse rate increased Exteroceptive sensitivity increased	Release of the basal ganglia and hypothalamus
Fourth	Deepening stupor Increased tonus Coarse tremor Tonic spasms (82.6%) Tetanic postures Conjugate deviation of the eyes Late torsion spasms	Pupils small or large Pulse rate increasing or decreasing Signs of paralysis of the pyramidal functions Decreased exteroceptive sensitivity Increased interoceptive sensitivity	Release of the midbrain Suppression of pyramidal functions
Fifth	Tonic extensor spasms (34.1%) Posture reflexes Depression of tendon reflexes Deep coma Diminished sensitivity Lid and corneal reflexes sluggish Shallow respiration No corneal reflexes	Pin-point pupils No light reaction Pulse rate decreased	Release of the medulla oblongata

(After Frostig, *Am. J. Psychiat. 96:1186, 1940.)*

be observed in alcoholic or barbiturate intoxication or in the waking period after applications of convulsive therapy.

In the first two hours, some patients display "primitive movements" (Frostig). They lick their lips; they make sucking movements; forced grasping is also present. Slow undulating movements of the eyeballs or nystagmus is quite often seen. As the hypoglycemia progresses, many patients display hypotonia alternating with short hypertonic periods. Clonic twitchings, tremor, choreic, athetoid, and dystonic movements are observed. The majority of patients are somnolent, or a narrowing of consciousness is present when such motor manifestations occur, but they can be awakened or they awake spontaneously by their own motor stimulation. The psychiatric and neurological manifestations of hypoglycemia are very variable and will be discussed in detail in special chapters.

Some patients complain that they are chilly, and their temperature is often lowered. Respiration in this phase is unaltered or somewhat accelerated, especially in connection with the increase in motor activity. The pulse varies in frequency; usually it is well filled. Tachycardia and brachycardia sometimes alternate in quick succession.

The second phase, or *shock phase* is reached when the hypoglycemia is so marked that it produces loss of consciousness. If the insulin dose is adequate, this will occur at the beginning or during the early part of the third hour of hypoglycemia. This dose is highly variable from individual to individual.

There is unfortunately no agreement among insulin therapists as to the definition of coma. Von Braunmühl differentiates between half-coma or precoma, and coma. He believes that a half-shock or precomatose state is present if the patient shows clonic movements or is unable to drink due to impaired consciousness. We believe that this subdivision into precomatose and coma state is definitely useful for in many hospitals the precomatose state is considered as coma and in this way the patients do not receive deep enough insulin shocks and do not derive the maximum benefit from the treatment. As long as the patient is able to respond to stimuli, even though he is not able to drink, he is still in a state of precoma or superficial coma; in this phase some patients are quietly asleep but still respond to stimulation. The real coma phase is only reached when there is no response to outside stimuli.

The depth of coma to be aimed at is reached when the patient ceases to show any response to painful stimuli, this being most effectively tested by failure to respond to a needle or to supraorbital pressure.

Several authors have investigated the eyegrounds during hypoglycemia, with contradictory results. Reitman regularly found vasoconstriction and increased filling of the vessels. Schmidt, however, observed this phenomenon only in a small number of patients. The reactivity of the blood vessels as observed by ophthalmological observations as well as capillaroscopic studies during coma were used by Winnik et al. as a prognostic test.

Choreic, athetoid, and myoclonic movements become progressively less severe, finally changing into a generalized clonic tremor which is often interrupted by rigor. Sometimes hypotonia accompanies these motor manifestations. In many patients the motor manifestations become markedly increased if the patient is stimulated, for instance, by hearing a noise or by being touched. Vegetative nervous system changes, such as dilated pupils which still respond to light, increased pulse rate, and marked perspiration and salivation are induced in many patients, but some patients remain quite dry without perspiring (Sakel's "wet" and "dry" shock).

As the coma deepens at the end of the third hour or at the beginning of the fourth, spasms similar to those of decerebrate rigidity occur. The arms are often flexed and the hands are as in tetany; the lower extremities are in extension spasm and the feet in equinovarus position. Conjugate deviation of the eyes is common. The pupils do not respond to light; the pulse accelerates. Cyanosis and labored breathing are present. The spasms are interrupted by periods of hypotonia, during which the pulse rate drops to normal, or bradycardia becomes manifest, cyanosis disappears, and breathing is again normal. After a few seconds or minutes, a new spastic wave occurs with the same manifestations as mentioned above. Kino uses the abolition of the nasopalpebral reflex as a sign indicating a definite and yet not injurious coma. Another way to ascertain the depth of coma is Zimmermann's suggestion (also recommended by von Braunmühl) to blow on the eyelid, which normally contracts at such stimulation; this reflex is the last to disappear before loss of the corneal reflex. In the next "deep" coma level the patient remains in a state of hypotonia which is interrupted only occasionally by tonic spasms. The pupils now contract and do not respond to light; the corneal reflexes disappear. The pulse rate drops down to 50-60 per minute and respiration often shows Cheyne-Stokes or Küssmaul phenomena. This deep coma level is usually reached at the end of or during the fifth hour of hypoglycemia.

When the coma dose is reached, the patient should be kept in coma for only about fifteen minutes the first time. If no complications occur, the coma may be extended slowly up to an hour or longer. The "deep" coma level, as defined in the previous paragraph, should not be maintained longer than about fifteen to twenty minutes. Inexperienced workers are advised to extend the coma phase of the treatment no longer than one hour, and it is best for them to refrain from reaching the deep coma level. Experienced therapists, however, especially after they have studied the individual reactions of the patient, sometimes apply comas for longer periods up to one and one-half hours. Even then, the deep coma level should be kept for a maximum of one-half hour only because the limit of the safety margin may be reached at this point, and if over-stepped, irreversible coma results. As previously indicated, the shock dose of insulin should be regulated in such a manner that superficial coma is reached at the beginning of the third hour or in the early part of the fourth hour.

Adaptation of Insulin Dosage

The average coma dose is about 100-150 units of insulin. There are hypersensitive patients who reach coma with a smaller amount, and for them 40-50 units are sufficient. In these patients, it is not a rare occurrence for the coma to develop rapidly and in a precipitate manner in the second hour. In hyposensitive patients, on the other hand, much larger doses than 100 units are required.

Formerly, the insulin dosage was increased steadily until coma ensued, regardless of the amount. Von Braunmühl introduced the zigzag method of overcoming insulin resistance. For example, if 200 units does not produce coma in the patient on the first day of the zigzagging, we drop the dose to double the starting dose (if that was 15 units, we give 30 units). On the second day we give half the maximum dose (100 units), and on the third day the maximum dose of 200 units is given, the next day dropping to twice the initial dose (30 units). This zigzagging is carried out for five to six days until an adequate shock is produced.

Müller mentions another possible way to decrease insulin tolerance. He stretches the period of hypoglycemia by leaving a patient fasting for six to eight and a half hours after the administration of insulin if coma does not develop. Repeating this procedure for several days the hypoglycemia progressively deepens until coma is reached at the normal time. Nadeau & Rouleau proposed the administration of glucose before insulin in the management of insulin resistance on the basis that the initial hyperglycemia will produce a temporary inactivation of insulin antagonists so that the insulin can act without inhibition.

The enzyme hyaluronidase may also be used in conjunction with the insulin injection in order to facilitate the absorption of insulin (Keup). Alexander and Neander have reported that this method has no advantage over insulin administration alone with respect to average number of injections required to produce first comas, the number of coma reactions or the responsiveness of insulin-resistant patients. On the other hand, Gysin and Wilson reported that during the use of hyaluronidase there was a 35 to 50 per cent decrease in the dose of insulin required to produce comas, and both the induction and quality of the comas was smoother with a decreased proportion of second degree hypoglycemic reactions.

During coma the patient must be watched constantly. If irregularities of pulse and respiration occur, a wait of ten to fifteen minutes is permissible as in many instances these irregularities are only temporary. If, however, they persist and the pulse rate drops to 55 per minute or increases to 140 per minute, it is advisable to terminate. Peripheral circulation is a good indicator for interruption. If the patient is cyanotic and pale, a circulatory embarrassment is present and we should not wait longer than five to ten minutes before termination. The blood pressure is also used as an indicator of the condition of the cardiovascular apparatus. If the systolic blood pressure drops below 100, the patient should be watched; when it reaches 85, we terminate if the patient at the same time shows cyanosis or respiratory difficulties. Arrhythmias call for interruption only if the general condition of the patient appears to be unsatisfactory. Many arrhythmias abate after a while. Some patients show a respiratory embarrassment, breathing rapidly in a stertorous way and using the auxiliary muscles also for respiration. We usually introduce a nasal tube in such patients and often the respiratory difficulty ceases. If it persists, however, interruption of the coma is indicated.

Various complications of insulin coma will be described in a special chapter. If the patient experiences only mild complications, treatment should be continued the next day, and the insulin dosage should be increased or decreased as the patient's condition requires. In the event of a major complication, such as cardiovascular collapse, marked respiratory embarrassment, or prolonged coma, it is advisable to give the patient a day of rest, resuming insulin treatment a day or two days later. In most of these cases, it is also advisable to reduce the insulin dosage. If complications occur because the coma is too extended, it is obvious that in addition to reducing the insulin dosage, the duration of the coma should also be reduced. If a patient repeatedly develops serious complications even though the treatment technique is adequate, he should be considered a bad risk and no further treatments should be given.

Techniques of Termination

Hypoglycemia is terminated by giving an adequate amount of carbohydrates or by injecting the pancreas hormone glucagon. In most hospitals, ordinary sugar is used, dissolved in water, weak tea, or fruit juices. In a mild hypoglycemic state the patient is able to drink the sugar solution. Later he becomes unable to swallow even with much urging. In such cases it is unwise to force the patient or to pour the liquid into his mouth because of the danger of aspiration. Formerly, such patients were terminated by tubefeeding or intravenous injection. The main objection against routine intravenous termination is that daily injections of a hypertonic solution easily lead to thrombosis of the veins, and good veins must be preserved for emergencies. Tube feeding of sugar solution sometimes led to aspiration into the lungs with abscess and gangrene as complications. If such patients would not awake after 20 minutes 20 cc of a 33⅓ per cent glucose solution were injected, and if necessary, repeated after 10 minutes.

In recent years glucagon, a hormone discovered and named in 1923 by Murlin et al., is being used for the termination of insulin coma (Schulman and Greben; Esquibel et al.; Braun and Parker). Considerable experimental evidence points to the alpha cells of the Islands of Langerhans as a source of glucagon, and it is a substance which causes marked hyperglycemia in both normal and diabetic animals. Although it raises the blood sugar enormously, it is not an insulin antagonist in other ways since like insulin it assists in the peripheral utilization of glucose.

It has been used in doses of ⅓ to 2 mg. intravenously or intramuscularly, both to terminate insulin comas, and to treat secondary hypoglycemic reactions occurring later in the day. Awakening usually occurs in 10 to 20 min. and in general, doses of ⅓ to ½ mg. which might be repeated if the patient is not awake within 15 min., have been found to be adequate. Although it is extremely effective by intravenous administration, the main advantages of the use of glucagon are obtained by its intramuscular administration because of the damage to veins by intravenous interruption and saving of personnel. Glucagon produces a slow, gradual and smooth termination of comas. No side-effects or local reactions have so far been reported from its use.

Laqueur has used several intramuscular techniques of termination, and in double blind surveys has found glucagon to be the most effective, ⅓ to ⅔ mg. producing complete recovery from coma in 95 per cent of cases. He found a combination of adrenalin ½ mg. and 50 mg. thiamine to be effective in 80 per cent of cases while adrenalin ½ mg. alone was successful in terminating only in 46.7 per cent of cases, and thiamine 50 mg. alone was completely ineffective in all cases. In an extensive study by Ramirez et al. glucagon terminated successfully in 97.6 per cent of all comas, and the awakening was more tranquil than by glucose. It produced a decrease of glucose tolerance lasting 24 hours. Serial glucagon tolerance tests were used by Dussik et al. in an attempt to better understand the carbohydrate metabolism of schizophrenics.

In some patients it happens that a so-called after-shock appears several hours after termination of the treatment. The patient may complain of weakness, perspiration, feeling of hunger, or, if the condition is more marked, he may become drowsy or in some cases display an epileptic fit. This late shock occurs mainly in patients who have not eaten adequately or in whom the meal was arrested in the stomach. These conditions are easily controlled, and intravenous injection of 20 cc. of a 33⅓ per cent glucose solution is usually enough to terminate the after-shock; however, it is necessary, after the injection of glucose, that the patient also take carbohydrates in the form of food or liquid. Many workers avoid the use of high doses of sedatives in insulin-treated patients in order to be able to observe the appearance of such an after-shock.

Variations of Technique

Sakel described various termination procedures in different types of schizophrenia. He varies his terminations not so much according to the different subtypes of schizophrenia as according to different psychotic manifestations which may occur in any form of schizophrenia. He terminated those patients who show a paranoid symptomatology differently from those with catatonic stupor or excitement. Dussik, Cameron and Hoskins, and Marzynsky agree with Sakel. Müller and most other therapists, however, do not feel that Sakel's termination rules are sufficiently established. In his report before the International Congress in Paris in 1950, Sakel still individualized the treatment according to the type of schizophrenia treated.

Insulin treatment, according to Sakel's original method, is given six times a week with one rest day. In many hospitals, however, it is given five times a week with two rest days. The latter frequency is apparently sufficient in most cases. During the war, some workers applied the insulin three times a week only. In our opinion this is inadequate unless done in combination with electric shock or metrazol. Insulin shock treatment given alone two to three times a week is not very effective, for the action is cumulative and such application would therefore be insufficient.

Insulin treatment should continue as long as the patient shows a tendency to improve. Acute cases will require less treatment than chronic ones. Most workers apply 50-60 comas. This refers explicitly to coma days, not to treatment days as is frequently done. If the patient shows full recovery with a smaller number, it is obvious that the treatment can be stopped earlier, but even in cases of rapid recovery a minimum of 20 comas should be given to prevent relapse. Freudenberg states that the best results are obtained when the therapist aims at a total of 50 comas, even if the patients remit early in the treatment. If there is only a slight improvement, persistence is in order. Müller calls it a mistake to give up insulin therapy as unsatisfactory before the end of at least three months and he saw improvement of paranoid syndromes even after much longer treatments. If there is no improvement at all after 60 comas, it is generally believed that no change can be expected and treatment may be discontinued. If, however, after 50-60 comas the patient shows reasonable improvement, treatment should be continued. A very active approach is being used again more recently by the Viennese Clinic (Arnold). They consider the treatment-free Sunday a compromise, continue if possible during intercurrent infections, start from the beginning if an interruption of more than eight days had been necessary, and insist that the last 20 comas be given after the patient has become symptom free which, according to Arnold, can be temporarily achieved in practically all cases even if a lasting remission may not be obtained. He as well as Laqueur suggested 100 and more comas if necessary.

Since the introduction of insulin shock treatment, many variations of the original technique have evolved. The following modifications are so far removed from the technique in general use that they warrant special consideration.

TREATMENT WITH DIVIDED DOSES: Kronfeld and Sternberg reported a patient who would not respond to 100 units, but had a coma when 60 units were injected first and were then followed by additional 40 units. After this and similar observations Goldfarb, Yagdjoglon Kant et al. advise giving insulin in divided doses: one half at the usual time; the second half an hour later.

Recently Laqueur and LaBurt recommended the administration of multiple doses of insulin, and claim that their method reduces the danger and expenses of the treatment. After testing the patient's sensitivity with 5 units the first day they then apply the daily dose in three divided doses with intervals of 15 min. between injections. In this way they produce deep comas in most patients with total doses of 60 to 70 units of insulin. However, the patient goes into coma somewhat later than with other techniques, and the treatment time is prolonged to five or six hours. They combine this method with a dietary scheme in which the patients are given only two meals a day, breakfast at about 12:30 p.m. on awakening from coma plus a normal meal at about 5:30 p.m. This diet is supplemented by chocolate milk at 2 p.m. and a light snack at 8 p.m. The patients are allowed no food after 8 p.m. They claim that patients so treated do not gain excessive weight, and that the incidence of secondary hypoglycemic reactions in the afternoon and evening is greatly lessened.

TREATMENT WITH RAPIDLY INCREASING DOSES: Reese has tried to shorten insulin shock treatment by abbreviating its preliminary phase. Instead of starting with the normal 10-15 units, he starts with 60 units of insulin and increases the dose by 10-30 units daily until the shock phase is reached.

The method of rapidly increasing dosage has found wider application in American hospitals since Bond and Shurley have begun to use it routinely in the Pennsylvania Hospital in Philadelphia. They begin with 50 units, and increase the dose on successive days by the near-geometric progression of 100, 200, 400, 600, 800 and up to 1600 units. After deep coma has been reached, the dose is then dropped to determine the minimum coma dose. The main advantages are seen in the early induction of coma, rapid sensitization, and, most important, early change of mental symptoms. The authors warn against the use of this method by other than skilled therapists.

TREATMENT WITH DIFFERENT TYPES OF INSULIN: Protamine zinc insulin has been tried alone and in combination with ordinary insulin because of its prolonged action. Those who have worked with protamine zinc insulin advise against its use in insulin shock treatment (Goldman, Sandison and McGregor, von Braunmühl). The effect is not uniform and is not comparable to ordinary insulin. Shock symptoms are often delayed and are less predictable. Reese and Vanderveer furthermore have found that epileptic manifestations are more common than with ordinary insulin. Recently Laqueur has tried to adapt the type of insulin to the reaction of the patient. Slowly reacting patients go into coma at the desired time with fast "low zinc insulin"; fast, oversensitive patients are treated with slowly absorbed "lente insulin."

INTRAVENOUS INSULIN TREATMENT: The intravenous administration was first recommended by Ventriglia, who stressed the quicker occurrence of hypoglycemic symptoms with a 50 per cent smaller dose of insulin. In the United States and England, experiments have also been made in the intravenous use of insulin. Spencer reviewed the whole problem of intravenous administration and concluded that it offers insufficient advantages over intramuscular insulin to justify its use.

PROLONGED COMA TREATMENT: Soon after introduction of insulin shock therapy, it was occasionally observed that patients who went into a state of protracted coma quite often showed a remarkable improvement. Kraulis, impressed by these results, made an early attempt to utilize this condition for therapeutic purposes. He prolongs the insulin coma but at the same time feeds small amounts of sugar in order to prevent the occurrence of an irreversible condition, and has been able to leave some of his patients in insulin coma up to 9-12 hours, J. Wortis et al. up to 20 hours. Recently, Arnold recommended purposely protracted coma in patients who failed to respond to a long series of ordinary comas. The patient is being kept in coma once, or even several times, for four hours on the same day.

SUBCOMA (AMBULATORY) INSULIN TREATMENT

It has been mentioned before that hypoglycemia without producing coma was used in psychiatric conditions prior to Sakel. Sargant and Craske contributed to its revival when they recommended it in the therapy of war neuroses. Polatin et al. introduced this treatment in schizophrenics and claimed favorable results. The patient receives increasing doses of insulin until he shows signs of mild hypoglycemia, but then the insulin dose is not pushed further.

In order to obtain a good response Polatin et al. treated their schizophrenics for the same period of time as the psychosis had existed prior to treatment. Some patients have been treated for years. A larger group of 250 schizophrenics treated with subcoma insulin was reported by Tomlinson, whose results compare favorably with figures obtained by others for insulin coma therapy. More recently the value of subcoma treatment in many schizophrenic syndromes was shown by Greaves et al., but they kept their patients for almost an hour in a state of clouded consciousness, thus going beyond the usual technique of subcomas recommended for the neuroses, withdrawal symptoms, alcoholics, and so on.

Various combinations have been used of subcoma insulin with other somatic as well as psychological methods. It was used with electric convulsive therapy, but we were unable to see any convincing improvement of ECT results by this combination. In France, where colloidal gold and other colloidal solutions are used in the therapy of various psychiatric disorders, insulin subcoma was combined with these solutions (Doussinet and Thévenot).

According to Rennie, the administration of insulin in subcoma doses provides an effective method of sedation. Its specific action seems to be the alleviation of anxiety, and consequently the psychotic manifestations sometimes disappear rapidly. The method is said to be safe and far superior to that achieved by the usual methods of sedation. Brickner recommended this type of insulin treatment as an office procedure which is particularly useful in tension states.

It must be stated that not infrequently patients under ambulatory insulin treatment go into a deeper coma than intended. This makes it difficult to exclude the possibility that improvement in some schizophrenics may be due to these deeper hypoglycemic states. The often heard statement that subshock insulin is a less harmful procedure should not be overstressed in view of Malamud's communication of two fatalities. One of them died in a protracted coma on a day when two injections of small amounts of insulin had been given.

The use of subcoma insulin treatment in conditions other than schizophrenia, was widespread. Sargant and Slater have found the modified treatment useful in physically run-down psychoneurotic patients but unsuitable in other psychoneurotics. Patients with anxiety states and reactive emotional conditions, and some debilitated patients with hysteria, respond well to what is actually a modification of the original Weir Mitchell treatment. There are also some negative reports on the use of subshock doses of insulin in combat-induced psychiatric disorders. Thus, Teitelbaum et al. did not see any advantage of insulin compared to control groups treated with sodium amytal or with group psychotherapy without any medication. They were also unable to confirm the significance of gain of weight induced by insulin in combat-induced psychiatric disorders. Their technique as well as statistical conclusion was questioned by Sargant and Slater. The majority of reports on hypoglycemic coma alone or in combination with other methods, such as narcoanalysis in neurotics, is favorable but it must be admitted that the value of any therapy in neurotics is difficult to determine.

The ever increasing number of papers on the technique and the therapeutic value of subcoma insulin treatment in the most different psychiatric conditions makes it impossible to survey the whole literature on this subject. At the International Conference on Insulin in 1958, Bernath gave an up to date account of this treatment, and pointed out that the target symptom is anxiety, and that, although it does not cure anxiety, it is a useful adjunct in patients with different psychiatric conditions with anxiety. The usefulness of insulin in the withdrawal of morphine preceded the insulin shock treatment of schizophrenia (Sakel, Steck). Its value has been questioned by Wilder, who showed that a group of patients withdrawn without medication and another group withdrawn with insulin, had the same abstinence syndrome.

Based on experience with 1000 cases, Sargant reiterates his favorable impression of the treatment in selected cases but rightly warns against its use as a mere placebo for many unsuitable cases. In severe depressions it often makes the patient feel worse. Toxic confusional states may be shortened by insulin injections twice a day, an application which has been proved as valuable in delirium tremens together with glucose. Sargant and Slater have also found it beneficial in cases of mixed organic and psychogenic nature, especially in post-concussional states. We believe that subcoma doses of insulin can be used in anxiety states in order to make the patient more amenable to psychotherapy. Disturbances in the autonomic nervous system quiet down under insulin; the patient has a better appetite, sleeps much better, and gains weight. In the psychoses, however, this type of insulin treatment should not replace insulin coma or electric convulsive therapy.

Complications of Insulin Coma Treatment

In insulin coma treatment a variety of complications can occur. Most of them can be dealt with successfully. There is, however, a certain percentage of fatalities in insulin treatment. Mortality figures are generally higher in surveys covering large groups of hospitals than in statistics of individual workers with wide experience. Malzberg, in his survey of the first material treated in the New York State Hospitals, reported a death rate of 1.29 per cent. Kinsey reports 90 deaths from among more than 12,000 patients, which corresponds approximately with the death rate of .85 per cent as given by Kolb and Vogel in a survey of 305 hospitals. In both of these surveys hypoglycemic encephalopathy due to prolonged coma appears to be far the most frequent cause of death; pulmonary complications, second; and cardiovascular disturbances, third. Müller reported a mortality rate of less than 5 per cent. It appears that termination with glucagon has almost eliminated fatalities.

Cardiovascular Complications

During hypoglycemia many patients show an increased or decreased pulse rate, and in some cases arrhythmia and fibrillations are observed. The arrhythmias are usually not very important if the patient is in good general condition, not markedly cyanotic, and if the blood pressure does not drop rapidly.

There are two main types of more serious cardiovascular disturbances. The first is a myocardial failure (acute cardiac insufficiency); the second is a vasomotor collapse with or without cardiac involvement. Acute cardiac failure is not very common. In this state the patient is dyspneic and shows a gallop rhythm, and the veins of the neck bulge. In such a case Hadorn advises the use of strophanthin, 0.2 or 0.3 mg., together with caffeine, administered intravenously in order that it may act as rapidly as possible. In the event of vasomotor collapse, however, the patient is usually pale, the neck veins are empty, the pulse is thready and weak, the blood pressure is very low, and it is most important to raise the tonus of the blood vessels and to give medication, such as strychnine, caffeine, and particularly metrazol, or coramine in doses of 2-4 cc. intravenously, repeated every 10-15 minutes until the patient rallies. It is essential to mention that in cardiovascular complications the patient should not only receive medication for the heart but also the hypoglycemia be terminated instantly.

Prolonged Coma

The most important, and by far the most serious, complication during insulin treatment is the occurrence of a prolonged coma. Lester has calculated that a prolonged coma can be expected once in every 1877 individual treatments. Among 25 cases of prolonged coma he found a mortality rate of 16 per cent. The death rate due to this complication among a large series of insulin cases was 0.33 per cent. In a thorough study on post-hypoglycemic encephalopathy, Freudenberg reports an incidence of 2.7 per cent in his own material and quotes widely varying figures up to 30.1 per cent in the literature. As to the etiological factors, he found that the majority of protracted comas occurs in the first two weeks of treatment, that the more profound the hypoglycemia the greater the possibility of prolonged coma, that long duration of hypoglycemia (even if it is light) predisposes, and that post-coma confusion on one day is a warning sign that on the next day treatment may lead to protracted coma.

The origin of the prolonged coma is not fully understood. Some authors believe that prolonged coma occurs when the nerve cells become exhausted and are unable to utilize sugar even though there is an ample amount present in the blood stream (Georgi). Others believe that it is due to acidosis (Koch) or to vascular impairment (Kastein). Telatin assumes that it is caused by hyperinsulinism. Most workers agree that prolonged coma is not simply a state of hypoglycemia, but that some other alteration of the nervous system is present in addition to the changes seen in the hypoglycemic state. Freudenberg lists seven different theories: the vascular, anoxic, toxic-metabolism, aglucic, autonomic imbalance, increased combustion of protein, and deficiency of tissue-essentials theory.

Many authors have questioned the usefulness of further intravenous glucose in patients in whom the blood sugar has risen to hyperglycemic levels, but the brain is obviously unable to utilize the offered sugar. A great many suggestions have been made as to how to handle the situation. Vitamin B_1 administration has been advocated by many and rejected by others. Cortisone as well as ACTH have been suggested. Cleckley and Templeton believe that oxidation is disturbed and try to stimulate it by application of nicotinic acid, the efficacy of which has not been confirmed by others. Müller recommends oxygen-carbon dioxide mixtures. Inhalation of amylnitrate was attempted by Stendall because vasodilatation sometimes helps to terminate uncomplicated hypoglycemic comas. Glutamic acid was used in irreversible coma by Zeise. The same purpose was achieved with BAL (2,3-Dithiopropanol) 100 mg. given together with 50-100 mg. glucose. In patients with poor veins it has the advantage that it is injected intramuscularly. It is supposed to increase the synthesis of glutathione in the liver, and wakes the patient in normal insulin coma within 6 to 8 minutes. Stark and Barrera administer potassium in a 10 per cent solution in small fractions with a 1 cc. tuberculin syringe. They also deem it advisable to give potassium prophylactically before insulin treatment by means of potassium chloride, 2 grams four times a day, during the course of insulin therapy. The significance of phosphorylization in carbohydrate assimilation led Berenstein and Levi to the recommendation of adenosin-triphosphor-acid (atiphos) as a preventive against protracted coma. Intravenous injections of glutamic acid were tried successfully by Mayer-Gross and Walker. In a special study on this problem, Weil-Malherbe comes to the conclusion that the effect is due neither to a direct utilization of glutamic acid as fuel for the brain cells nor to its conversion into glucose, but rather due to adrenergic stimulation. Injection of adrenalin duplicated in every respect the effect of glutamic acid.

Dussik, Wortis and Lambert, Menzies, and others have used blood transfusions, giving the patient about 500 cc. of citrated blood with good results. Lately, the importance of maintaining adequate oxygen supply is more and more recognized, and there is a trend to secure the help of an anesthetist in the handling of prolonged coma. French anesthesiologists used "hibernation" therapy with chlorpromazine in the treatment of protracted coma (Campan and Parant). Another, more recent recommendation is the use of non-convulsive electrical stimulation. Peripheral electric stimulation of the legs was found equally effective as cerebral stimulation. Trephine opening of the skull has been successfully applied by Puech et al. in five out of six cases of protracted coma.

We agree with Müller that even though appropriate treatment of the protracted shock is very important, it is much more important to prevent its occurrence. Often a protracted shock appears as the result of faulty technique, especially if the sensitization of the patient to insulin is not taken into consideration. Frostig is of the opinion, and we subscribe to it also, that protracted coma will occur only infrequently if treatment is terminated shortly after the beginning of the medullary phase. If it is carried further, irreversible changes may take place.

Epileptic Attacks

It is debatable if the occurrence of epileptic fits during hypoglycemia is a complication or a desirable phenomenon. Sakel, in his first publication, warned against the occurrence of convulsions; later, however, he maintained that spontaneous epileptic attacks during hypoglycemia may be desirable; Winkler could demonstrate that the various body types differ in their tendency to hypoglycemic convulsions. Individuals of athletic body type show convulsive phenomena more often than both pyknics and leptosomes. The frequency of convulsions in those with athletic body type is three times as high as it is in patients with pyknic body type. Today we rather believe that the insulin convulsion is a complication, although we are inclined to agree with the conclusions of Hoenig and Leibermann who, more recently, again found that all epileptic phenomena occur more frequently in patients who recover. However, in those patients in whom we wish to provoke a convulsion, it should be elicited artificially by metrazol or electric shock. We cannot agree with Sakel who, in his report in Paris, considers infrequent spontaneous hypoglycemic convulsions harmless but warns against the dangers of artificially induced convulsions which he calls an "ineffective imitation method."

The investigations of Sakel on the time factor in connection with the occurrence of spontaneous epileptic fits in hypoglycemia are important. Some epileptic manifestations occur in the early stage of hypoglycemia, in the first and second hour, while others occur in the four and fifth hour in patients who are already in coma. Epileptic attacks which occur early are generally not dangerous while the less frequent attacks which appear late during the hypoglycemia are always dangerous and are usually connected with marked cardiovascular disturbances or with respiratory embarrassment. Status epilepticus is rare in the early phase of hypoglycemia. The convulsions appearing in the fourth and fifth hour, however, have a tendency to repeat themselves or to end in status epilepticus.

Many therapists do not interfere with those epileptic attacks which appear in the first and second hours of hypoglycemia, and some do not terminate the hypoglycemic state. Some patients come out spontaneously after the epileptic fits and are able to drink glucose. However, we feel that even though these epileptic attacks are not dangerous, they may be repeated or unwarranted cardiovascular manifestations may occur, and we, therefore, terminate. Late epileptic attacks should always be interrupted immediately.

There are patients who have a so-called epileptic pattern of hypoglycemia. They respond regularly to a certain dose of insulin with an epileptic attack. In such a case, it is best to try to suppress this tendency with 0.1 or 0.2 grams of luminal one to two hours before each insulin treatment, or 3-4½ grains of dilantin daily.

Neurological Complications

Palisa observed hemiparesis, hemianesthesia, hemianopsia, conjugate deviation of the eyes, sensory aphasia, dyslexia, dysgraphia, and astereognosis during insulin treatment. He was impressed by the fact that disturbances referable to the left hemisphere were more common than those to the right. None of these disturbances were permanent, disappearing after a few hours or days. Transitory hemiplegias and other focal cerebral syndromes, lasting not much longer than the coma, were described by Claude and Rubénovitch, also by Billet et al. We know of one patient in whom a permanant demented state developed after a prolonged coma. In a more recent survey of the literature Freudenberg lists the following neurological complications: confusion, stupor, aphasia, dysarthria, echolalia, apraxia, rotary movements, diplopia, facial paralysis, hemiplegia, and epileptiform seizures. Cerebral angiospasm, unilateral brain swelling, or the toxic effect of the insulin on the brain cells may play a part in the development of these focal neurological symptoms, but it is not likely that any one of these factors alone is exclusively responsible. Freed and Woffard described a subarachnoid hemorrhage during a hypoglycemic shock. The patient recovered, and no verification as to the diagnosis could be obtained.

Stern et al., in 10 out of 103 patients treated with insulin, observed disturbances of the cutaneous sensibilities. Five showed impairment of taste and smell. Patients complained about numbness or tingling sensation in the extremities. Only one patient showed objective sensory findings. Some maintained their complaints for several months. Some of Bückman's patients complained of itching of the fingertips and pain in the feet and calves. He found hyperesthesia in the fingertips for touch, pain and temperature, increased reflexes, and unsteady gait. He blames the rich carbohydrate diet and the lack of Vitamin B_1 for these sensory disturbances which he thinks are similar to those observed in mild cases of beri-beri. Accornero described a case of radial palsy developing during insulin coma.

Some of our patients in the older age group complained of severe pain in the legs for a few hours after treatment. No neurological signs were present, but the leg was pale and cold. These complaints may have been due to impairment of the peripheral circulation. Application of hot water bottles and injection of coramine during treatment eliminated the pain.

Mental Complications

Sakel, in his book on insulin treatment, describes the so-called hunger excitement, in which patients crave food and are noisy, abusive, and excited if they do not receive it. He advises terminating the hypoglycemia in such a state and increasing the insulin dosage the next day. Most of these hunger excitements, however, can be well handled by reassuring the patient or giving him some water to drink. In many instances, the hunger excitement is only a part of a generalized excitement which we usually interrupt if it lasts longer than twenty minutes, so as to prevent the patient from exhausting himself. Treatment should be resumed the next day with higher insulin dosage. The danger of giving heavy sedation in these excitement states was illustrated by White et al., who reported several patients who remained comatose and in critical condition when intravenous injection of sodium amytal was administered during hypoglycemia. The use of neuroleptic drugs seems to be even more dangerous. We know of a fatality after intravenous injection of chlorpromazine during a hypoglycemic excitement state. The danger in using this drug in hypoglycemia is also suggested by Dussik's observation of a patient who died following a hypoglycemic convulsion after premedication with 150 mg. of Thorazine.

Sakel also describes the so-called activation of a psychosis. This is a phenomenon seen in patients who, while under the influence of insulin, display hallucinations or delusions or excitement. This activation of a psychosis or reaction reversal is not uncommon. Its origin is not known. Müller believes that the hypoglycemia does not reactivate the original psychosis but may produce new mental symptoms in the sense of an organic reaction, which can also be seen in nonpsychotic individuals as well. We believe that more often we are dealing with a reactivation. We have made similar observations on patients who have received sodium amytal intravenously after the course of insulin or electric shock treatment was completed, and under the influence of the drug the psychotic material was again produced. It is important not to interrupt the treatment because of fear that the patient may be getting worse under treatment. We usually increase the insulin dose, and generally after a few days the activation disappears.

Memory defects, disorientation, and confabulation resembling Korsakoff psychosis have been described, and they frequently follow a protracted coma. Usually, the Korsakoff-like condition is present for only a few days or weeks, but Plattner has described cases which lasted six months. Similar cases have been described by Cortesi, and Müller. Polatin et al. found that this organic mental reaction lasted only a short time. In one patient, however, the electroencephalogram retained abnormal wave patterns, and even after some time the psychological test performance was decidedly inferior to the previous performance. It is possible, therefore, that in some patients permanent organic damage does result from the treatment. True dementia apparently can follow a protracted coma, although this is extremely rare.

Other Complications

Some other complications have been listed in the literature and may be mentioned here. An obviously rare occurrence was reported by Donnelly et al. They saw a case of thrombosis of the superior longitudinal venous sinus which they described under the name of thrombotic hydrocephalus. The authors made this diagnosis on clinical grounds in 3 patients. An initial hypoglycemic convulsion, impairment of consciousness, increased spinal fluid pressure and local signs, depending on the part of the cortex affected, are said to indicate this condition. None of the cases died. The authors feel that some of the insulin fatalities recorded as hypoglycemic encephalopathy have actually been caused by thrombosis of the superior longitudinal sinus. Müller, and also McGrath mention the appearance of diabetes mellitus after insulin shock treatment. Kautzky saw a 68 year old patient develop spells of hypoglycemia after insulin treatment with 20 mg. per cent blood sugar. These spells could be finally controlled with prophylactic doses of sugar. The patient died apparently from another cause. At autopsy a very slight pancreatitis was found.

In pregnancy Gralnick reported cases of stillbirths of women treated during the early part of their pregnancy. There is some evidence that the fetus is only injured in the beginning of pregnancy. Luban and Tuteur reported a case of insulin coma treatment during the later months of pregnancy without harm to mother or child. McConnell reported on similar cases. A recent study on the effect of the various somatic treatments on pregnancy suggests that insulin is the only treatment that might damage the child. Sobel found fetal damage in 35 per cent compared to a control group of 8 per cent.

Medical Observations and Laboratory Findings

Insulin treatment is an empirical procedure and although a great deal of research has been done on many of its phases, not a great deal of importance for the clinic has resulted; many of the basic mechanisms of insulin action are still obscure and need further elucidation. At the International Conference on Insulin Treatment in 1958, W. A. Himwich as well as I. F. Bennett gave surveys on research in this field. Although the main emphasis in this chapter will be on investigations of some clinical importance, an effort was made to include also studies instigated by this new therapy of schizophrenia but which have scientific importance beyond this particular treatment.

Blood and Spinal Fluid Sugar Content and Carbohydrate Metabolism

Sakel was the first to point out that the clinical manifestations of hypoglycemia are relatively independent of the blood sugar level. Since then many investigators have confirmed his observations (Zimmerman, Georgi, Erb, Bini). It is obvious that it is necessary that the blood sugar should drop to a certain level before hypoglycemic symptoms develop, but the severity of these symptoms is by no means connected with the blood sugar level. The depth of the coma, for instance, can not be appraised by blood sugar determinations. This explains the reason why calculation of the insulin dose in insulin shock treatment has to be done empirically, based on clinical manifestations. Coma has occurred in patients with a blood sugar level of 60-70 mg. per cent; on the other hand, the blood sugar of some patients has dropped to 30 mg. per cent without the patient's becoming comatose (Müller). Georgi and Dussik even found that the blood sugar rose at the start of coma. Bennett et al. in an experiment in which blood glucose levels were measured in 3 patients daily every 30 minutes from 7 a.m. to 10 a.m. during a 12 week period of a course of insulin coma treatment, found that in each subject it was necessary for the blood glucose to fall to approximately the same level each day for coma to occur, although the dose of insulin necessary to produce these levels decreased considerably. Thus it appears that changes in insulin sensitivity during treatment are due to an enhancement of the blood-glucose decreasing capacity of insulin rather than an increased sensitivity of the central nervous system to the concentration of blood glucose whereby patients become comatose at a higher blood glucose level after the initial stages of therapy.

Observations on the sugar content of the spinal fluid are not fully in agreement. Zeghauser and Erb have found that the sugar values in the spinal fluid fluctuate between 54-73 mg. per cent before coma, while in coma the values are 7-39 mg. per cent. They found that the severity of the clinical symptoms parallels the low sugar values in the spinal fluid. Dussik stated that a drop or increase of the sugar in the spinal fluid appears to be slower than that seen in the blood. Fischer finds no parallel developments between clinical manifestations and the amount of sugar present. Accornero and Bini have found normal sugar values in the spinal fluid during coma at a time when the blood sugar was already low, and deny that the change of consciousness during coma is related to the sugar content of the blood or spinal fluid.

Proctor et al. have investigated sugar tolerance in patients before and after insulin treatment. Pretreatment glucose tolerance curves reveal an abnormally prolonged interval before return to fasting levels. After treatment these authors find a direct correlation between clinical improvement and increased sugar tolerance, regardless of therapy; insulin administration was not a determining factor. Comparison with the group with complete remission and with the unimproved group showed a significant correlation in oral glucose tolerance tests; not so much in the intravenous tolerance tests. Patients remaining stationary or showing deterioration had an abnormally decreased sugar tolerance. The authors believe that the carbohydrate metabolism in schizophrenics with complete remission shifts toward the normal in the same way that Georgi found the fat metabolism does.

Blood

Observations of the blood of patients receiving insulin treatment show that leukopenia occurs in the first hour followed later by leukocytosis. In the first hour of treatment a relative increase of lymphocytes was found; in the third and fourth hours of the hypoglocemia the neutrophile leukocytes are in excess. Most authors believe that these changes in the white blood count are correlated with the presence of a relative acidosis or alkalosis during the insulin action: acidosis is linked with lymphocytosis and alkalosis with leukocytosis. The leukocytosis observed in insulin patients has also been interpreted as an increased action of the reticuloendothelial system. Patients who responded to treatment have shown a more marked leukocytosis than those who have failed to respond (Davidson).

Cardiovascular System

Blood pressure during insulin treatment reaches its highest altitude at the end of the second or early part of the third hour when it begins to drop. Both the systolic and diastolic pressure are raised, and the amplitude becomes more marked during this period. The patient looks flushed; the carotids pulsate. Not infrequently the increased blood pressure suddenly drops below normal in the third hour of insulin treatment and the patient becomes pale and cyanotic (Beiglbock and Dussik, Robinson). Georgi and Zimmerman believe that blood pressure changes occur simultaneously with changes in the blood sugar content. Jones, however, finds no correlation between the blood sugar content and the pulse rate or blood pressure.

The heart has been examined by a number of workers. Hadorn has found in 50 per cent of the insulin-treated patients a sinus tachycardia which he attributes to the increased amount of adrenalin circulating in the blood. One third of these cases show changes in the electrocardiogram similar to those seen in coronary sclerosis and myocardial lesions. The outstanding change in the electrocardiogram is a depressed T wave. These changes reverse when glucose is given. Hadorn believes, however, that prolonged insulin treatment produces a deprivation of glycogen content in the heart muscle which is not fully counteracted by the administered glucose; therefore, in some cases treated over a long period, myocardial damage is possible. Beiglbock and Dussik have found in many of their patients a flattening of the T wave, a widening of the QRS complex, and a disturbance in the conduction system of the heart. Administration of dextrose eliminates this syndrome.

During insulin treatment the output of the heart increases 30 per cent and the minute volume 50 per cent due to the fact that profuse sweating diminishes the amount of circulating blood. Farrell finds an increase in the fluoroscopic heart shadow in a number of cases, the maximum increase in one case being 22.6 per cent on the ninety-second day of treatment. It is interesting that this increase in the heart volume is seen principally in patients who respond favorably to treatment and who generally show improved circulation. For instance, patients who had a low blood pressure before treatment, show an increased pressure; when treatment is discontinued, the increased blood pressure and the increase in the heart volume go back to normal. Farrell explains these changes as being due to the stimulation of the sympathetic nervous system, which ceases when the treatment is discontinued.

Goldman has found abnormalities in the electrocardiogram of some patients even six moths after termination of treatment. Goldfarb and Bowman believe that the electrocardiographic changes are similar to those seen in cases of vitamin deficiency and that they can be reversed by giving Vitamin B_1. They attribute the cardiac changes to the large amount of vitamin-free glucose taken by the patients. We believe, however, that these irregularities are due to the hypoglycemia as they are also seen in patients treated only a short time or who in addition to their diet received adequate amounts of vitamins. Most authors did not see any serious electrocardiographic changes. A study by Bellet et al., who found the changes completely reversible within a few hours, was recently confirmed on a much larger material by Zohman and Russek. They noticed a striking absence of significant electrocardiographic changes in their 259 patients. Some patients with pre-treatment electrocardiographic changes revealed no further alterations after 60 or more hypoglycemic comas. They concluded that no cumulative injury to the myocardium takes place in insulin treatment.

Spinal Fluid

There have been many investigations of the changes in the spinal fluid during hypoglycemia. The spinal fluid pressure is apparently increased somewhat during hypoglycemia. No changes in the albumin-globulin ratio and no increase in the number of cells were reported until Kingsley and Freed found alterations in the volume of the cerebrospinal fluid and an increase in globulin. Nicolajev occasionally found increased permeability, of the hematoencephalic barrier when tested with Walter's bromide test, also observed by Georgi. Forstmeyer, on the other hand, saw no change in permeability. Ott found a decrease in permeability during coma. There is no agreement concerning changes of the hematoencephalic barrier.

Vegetative Nervous System

Domm and Gellhorn found that in schizophrenic patients when insulin leads to a fall in blood sugar below 50 mg. per 100 cc., a fall in the carbon dioxide tension occurs, probably due to central stimulation of the sympathetic nervous system. Restoration of the blood sugar levels leads to a rise in carbon dioxide tension. Gershberg and Long expressed the opinion that hypoglycemia activates the adrenal cortex by stimulating the pituitary gland to excrete its adrenocorticotropic hormone (ACTH). On the basis of extensive experimental work Gellhorn feels that the occurrence of a sympatheticoadrenal discharge in hypoglycemia is well established. Sympathectomized animals are hypersensitive to insulin, and adrenalin appears in the blood during hypoglycemia. Repeated insulin comas practically abolish the glycogenolytic effect of adrenalin. Gellhorn's theory that the common denominator in insulin and other types of somatic therapy of the psychoses can be explained by central autonomic discharges will be discussed in another chapter.

Gerard does not believe in the therapeutic effect of autonomic stimulation. Gellhorn expresses the opposite view, stating that hypoglycemia, like anoxia, stimulates the whole autonomic nervous system and that this stimulation is an important factor in therapy. Hofman concurs in this view. Tietz et al. found a rise in the blood adrenalin content during insulin coma which was retained in patients who recovered after insulin treatment. Several investigators have found increased sympathetic activity following therapy in those patients who exhibited clinical improvement. Gold using 15 mg. of mecholyl as a measure of sympathetic activity in 33 catatonic patients before and after insulin treatment, found that out of 66 per cent who showed increased sympathetic response after treatment, as indicated by a more rapid rate of recovery from the lowered systolic pressure in the mecholyl test, 75 per cent were improved. Shurley and Morris measuring the response of the autonomic nervous system to the insulin tolerance, adrenaline and mecholyl tests, prior to and following the termination of insulin therapy, found both that the nine schizophrenic patients tested showed a decreased response as compared to controls before treatment and that after the conclusion of treatment the increase in sympathetic activity was in proportion to the degree of clinical improvement. Cameron and Jellinek believe that in schizophrenic patients an impairment of the adrenosympathetic system is present prior to treatment and that the balance between the parasympathetic and sympathetic systems is restored in patients who recover, but not if the patient remains unimproved due to irreversible damage or constitutional malfunctioning of the vegetative nervous system. Fortuyn has found that both the parasympathetic and the sympathetic branches of the vegetative nervous system are stimulated by hypoglycemia. The increased gastric motility and secretion are suggestive of the stimulation of the parasympathetic; alteration of the blood pressure, increased pulse rate, and increased perspiration are due to increased action of the sympathetic nervous system.

Brain Metabolism

Dameshek and Meyerson found that the metabolism of the brain is reduced because the main food of the central nervous system, namely, sugar, is diminished during insulin hypoglycemia. Investigations by Wortis and Goldfarb on the arteriovenous oxygen content are important. Before insulin treatment they observed in schizophrenics no divergence from the normal. During coma, however, the arteriovenous difference was reduced. The arterial carbon dioxide content, raised during hypoglycemia, reverted to normal after administration of glucose. They also noted a marked rise in the carbon dioxide content before an epileptic convulsion. These authors concluded that during insulin coma the respiratory center is depressed and, consequently, its sensitivity to carbon dioxide, to which it is rather sensitive under normal circumstances, is diminished.

Himwich and his co-workers found no diminution of oxygen- or glucose-utilization in the brain if small doses of insulin were given, but when over 40 units of insulin were injected, most patients showed diminished metabolism of the brain which expressed itself in reduced utilization of oxygen. The alkali reserve of the blood was increased during hypoglycemia.

Beiglbock and Dussik found very marked alkalosis during hypoglycemia, as well as anoxemia which they believe is the basis of many of the symptoms seen during hypoglycemia. Kastein, however, thinks there is not enough evidence at present to accept or to reject the theory that anoxemia is responsible for most of the hypoglycemic symptoms. Many authors have tried to explain the clinical manifestations of hypoglycemia not on the basis of anoxemia but as a toxic effect of insulin on the nerve cells. This hypothesis is generally discarded today, even though Nobel and McLeod believe that intermediate metabolic products, like methylglyoxal, which appear due to the alteration of the carbohydrate metabolism, can be responsible for the symptoms of hypoglycemia. De Jongh and Laqueur, and Accornero, too, found no toxic substances in animal experiments.

There have been a great many investigations on salt metabolism and water metabolism in hypoglycemia. All authors agree that the salt metabolism is markedly disturbed during insulin treatment (Bini, Georgi). They find anhydremia almost always present during hypoglycemia and assume colloidal changes in the brain because the absorption of water during treatment is reduced. Unsubstantiated opinions that water is stored in the brain during hypoglycemia have also been expressed.

Beiglbock and Dussik found that movement of electrolytes is present during hypoglycemia: the so-called negative substances, such as sugar, urea, creatin, potassium, and phosphate, move away from the blood, while the so-called positive substances, such as sodium chloride, calcium, and magnesium, pass from the tissues towards the blood. These observations have been confirmed on animals. Kay and Throley also found a fall in serum potassium and inorganic phosphate consequent upon their movement with glucose from the extracellular fluid into the cell, together with an increased serum protein and sodium with decrease in serum chloride which they attributed to the profuse sweating and hemoconcentration produced during treatment. These investigators also found a significant decrease in bicarbonate which they believed to be linked with a failure of oxygen utilization in hypoglycemia.

Harris and Harris studied the metabolism of various amino-acids in insulin hypoglycemia. These findings indicated that pronounced changes in nitrogen metabolism, other than the uniform diffusion of amino-acids from blood into tissue, must occur during hypoglycemic coma. They also showed that the level in the blood of the total amino-acids and also of glutamine is sharply depressed during insulin treatment.

Ljunberg established that patients with reduced glutathione formation have low remission tendency, and he thinks that insufficient compensation of glutathione losses may be explained by a reduced activity of the liver. Gottfried and Willner found that the values for serum potassium, sodium, chlorides and magnesium, the blood levels of glucose and the total reducing substances of the blood were variable, being either low or high in a few cases before and after insulin treatment. Pyruvic acid was essentially normal. The lactic acid-pyruvic acid ratio had a wide range. Of the phosphate fractions, serum inorganic phosphorus was increased in a few patients before treatment, but was normal in all patients after treatment. Values for adenosine triphosphate phosphorus and the total organic acid-soluble phosphorus was somewhat increased after treatment, many of the pretreatment results being below normal before and after treatment. Olsen and Klein, during animal experimentation however, observed that the levels of glucose, glycogen, lactate, pyruvate and the energy rich phosphates in the brain all fell during hypoglycemia. The acetylcholine content of the brain is decreased in hypoglycemia (Crossland et al.), and Costa and Himwich demonstrated an increase in serotonin in the hippocampus, diencephalon and telencephalon. Himwich postulates that both these findings are consequent upon a decrease in the energy rich phosphates upon which both the acetylcholine synthesizing enzyme and the serotonin destroying enzyme are indirectly dependent for energy.

A study of changes of blood constituents was undertaken by Weil-Malherbe, who noticed a fall of inorganic phosphate two hours after the injection of insulin, but with a subsequent rise. Adenosinetriphosphate was unchanged after two hours, whereas serum citrate and serum calcium were decreased.

When the brain, as in profound hypoglycemia is deprived of glucose, it appears to be forced to break down its own structural materials for the production of energy. The findings of Geiger et al. on perfusing the cat brain with a glucose-free medium suggest that amino-acids, phospholipids and nucleotides are used which cannot be rebuilt in the continued absence of glucose. It has been suggested by Himwich that the beneficial effects of insulin hypoglycemia may be due to its destruction of newly formed schizophrenic behavior patterns stored in the brain as "chemical templates," thus allowing the reappearance or rebuilding of normal patterns. She believes that the efficacy of insulin therapy is dependent not upon the hypoglycemia itself but upon the effects of the consequent lack of energy on the hormones and enzymes of the brain.

Endocrinological Observations

The contra-insulin hormones adrenaline, thyroxine, ACTH, the growth hormone of the pituitary and the adrenocortical steroids have been the subject of much investigation in relation to both metabolic changes occurring during insulin therapy and the elucidation of the mysteries of insulin resistance.

The majority of investigators including Tietz et al., Holzbauer and Vogt, and Millar, who used the fluorometric estimation of adrenaline, have found an increase in plasma adrenaline level following insulin administration. Von Euler and Luft found an increase in urinary excretion of adrenaline following the intravenous administration of insulin to normal subjects. However, Weil-Malherbe and Bone using the differential fluorometric method studied both adrenaline and noradrenaline levels during insulin coma and found a rapid drop in adrenaline level reaching its lowest point thirty minutes after insulin injection. They considered that this was too soon for the fall in adrenaline to be attributable to hypoglycemia, while the blood sugar continued to fall after the blood adrenaline level became stable although at a lower level than normal. The noradrenaline concentration was unchanged. Experimental work on cats by Hökfelt demonstrated that the animal showed depletion of adrenaline from the adrenal medulla after insulin injection, but until the amount of insulin given was sufficient to induce hypoglycemic shock, the noradrenaline content remained unaltered.

Bowman and his co-workers studying the effect of insulin shock therapy on thyroid function with the aid of radioactive iodine found no significant change during treatment and no positive factors to correlate with clinical improvement. Both primary hypo- and hyper-thyroid activity are considered bad prognostic signs by Kay, the latter often increasing during insulin therapy due to the additional anterior pituitary stimulation with a resultant increase in thyrotropic hormone secretion. Where these thyroid changes are secondary to anterior pituitary disturbances, insulin therapy may correct them resulting in a return to normal functioning with associated clinical improvement. High thyroid activity secondary to excessive anterior pituitary activity may be diminished because of eventual exhaustion of thyrotropic hormone production under the stress of insulin therapy. The prognosis is also poor if previously normal thyroid activity, which is not usually influenced by insulin therapy, shifts outside the normal range consequent upon anterior pituitary stimulation.

Batt et al. related clinical improvement during the course of insulin coma therapy to observed changes in thyroid function and ketosteroid excretion rate. They maintain that for a successful treatment result both thyroid activity and ketosteroid excretion must come into and remain in the normal range, and where this is not so at the end of treatment relapse can be predicted.

During insulin hypoglycemia there is a fall in the eosinophile level most marked 4-8 hours after the commencement of treatment (Tsai, Dohan, Mann and Lehmann), indicative of adrenocortical stimulation. Bliss et al. demonstrated an increase in plasma 17-hydrocorticosteroids during insulin shock, while Marks and his co-workers in a study of a paranoid schizophrenic undergoing a course of treatment described a moderate increase in urinary 17-hydroxycorticosteroids being excreted with a gradual rise in the eosinophile count reaching a peak level during the sixth week. Freeman et al. reported in a three year follow-up study of patients after insulin treatment, that such an eosinophilia was a favorable prognostic sign. It appears that the contra-insulin hormones become exhausted by repeated insulin administration, their levels decrease with a consequent increase in insulin sensitivity so that smaller doses of insulin are required to produce coma.

As well as the contra-insulin hormones, other serum anti-insulin factors have been demonstrated, differentiated by Berson and Yalow into insulin antibodies and insulin antagonists, such as insulinase, found in the absence of exogenous insulin administration. The antibodies which develop following prolonged insulin administration are believed to bind insulin preventing its utilization with resulting insulin resistance. A dissociation of the bound insulin-globulin complex would result in a sudden break in resistance and a consequent severe hypoglycemic reaction. However, since insulin does not produce antibodies readily, it is more probable that the resistance encountered in the first few weeks of treatment is due to the contra-insulin hormones, while resistance later in the course might be due to the antibody formation. Berson and Yalow in their studies found insulin binding in all patients who had received insulin treatment for three months or more.

Psychiatric Observations

Studies of mental changes in schizophrenic patients undergoing insulin treatment are rather rare compared with the large number of papers on technique, physiological observations, and results of treatment. This is probably due to the fact that mental alterations in many patients are fleeting, difficult to define, and so varied that they preclude the systematization that is possible with many somatic findings. Even in mentally normal individuals who have received insulin treatment experimentally or in patients suffering from spontaneous hypoglycemia, the mental symptoms are not uniform. Some experience lassitude under the influence of insulin, others fear or apprehension; still others, irritability. In schizophrenics treated with insulin the same variations are present. In addition, their psychotic symptoms are modified differently by insulin, thus considerably complicating the appraisal of the mental manifestations. Studying normal persons under insulin, Wiedeking, in self observation, and Küppers describe a sensation of hunger, lassitude, irritability, inability to concentrate, and difficulty of recall. Müller believes that many mental phenomena observed in schizophrenics under treatment are not due to the psychosis but can occur in normal persons as well. Kepler and Moersch have observed in the insulin hypoglycemia of diabetics and in spontaneous hypoglycemia the same manifestations as those seen in schizophrenics during insulin treatment. Müller quotes several Russian authors who have investigated this problem more thoroughly. Vasilyeva as well as Sereijski and Geschelina differentiate between two groups of symptoms appearing during insulin treatment: the endogenous, due to alteration of the schizophrenic picture, and the exogenous, caused directly by the hypoglycemia in any person. The endogenous changes are characterized by accentuation of such schizophrenic symptoms as paranoid, hallucinatory experiences; in others, however, relaxation and diminution of paranoid, hallucinatory symptoms take place. Sereijski and Geschelina believe that 70 per cent of the psychic manifestations during insulin treatment are of exogenous origin.

We shall now describe in more detail the mental manifestations as they occur in various stages of treatment. Many patients feel relaxed, free, and even euphoric (Storch); others are apprehensive, fearful, and want reassurance. Some of them, at times, become frantic, very restless, and describe a feeling of being drowned or submerged (Shipley and Kant). Rubénovitch stresses the presence of anxiety which in our material was present in only about one-third of the cases. Von Baeyer also failed to see this anxiety to which Claude and Rubénovitch ascribe psychotherapeutic importance because anxiety supposedly leads to attachment and want for comfort. The combination with psychotherapy is undoubtedly facilitated by the patient's emotional state during the period of awakening. Levy and Perry underscore this preparedness of the patient to talk still further with narcosynthesis three times a week, immediately following insulin shock. Their technique is to terminate hypoglycemia in the usual way and, when the patient begins to respond, to inject sodium amytal intravenously until a state desirable for narcocatharsis is reached. Later on the same day, a psychotherapeutic session is held, during which the material obtained in narcocatharsis is used in developing insight.

In the precomatose state many patients show better contact with the environment, and they talk about their psychotic experiences. Their previously rigid or shallow affectivity is modified, and emotions are more readily displayed. They cry or laugh easily, or make obscene remarks. Most patients appear to be more lucid, more coherent, and more articulate. Later, perceptual anomalies are common occurrences. Benedek's investigations show that the patients often experience distortion of space, time, and motor sense, besides having optic and acoustic illusions. Objects are seen smaller or larger than they are in reality. The flow of time is slowed or accelerated. Minutes appear to be hours, and hours minutes. Similar observations were made by Orenstein and Schilder. Pisk described patients who felt that everything was speeded up: music was accelerated in tempo, people talked and walked very rapidly. Benedek pointed out that patients perceived movement in a decomposed manner, i.e., movements appeared to be jerky, sequence was not correctly perceived, and time sequence in which the movements occurred was altered. Intensification of color, sound, visual scenes, illusions, and hallucinations occur, similar to that observed in mescaline or LSD experiments. Weil, experimenting on himself, found that optic perceptions during hypoglycemia were similar to a primitive or archaic visual reaction.

There are few reports of experiences of patients during the coma phase. Guerra found that only 14 out of 30 patients volunteered information about their subjective experiences. Katzenelbogen reports a case in which the patient in each coma had the feeling of death and expressed joy that she was alive. This experience of impending death, however, is rare in our material.

The period of awakening from hypoglycemia is rich with observations of psychiatric import. Sakel states that "during the process of awakening one can actually see the return, level by level, of the progressively higher functions of the brain in almost phylogenetic succession. At first the less sensitive and apparently older and more primitive functional areas or centers are aroused." At first, according to Sakel, the reflexes reappear, then the motor functions become reintegrated. As the patient awakens, he recovers sensory perceptions and responds to stimuli. The last to return is normal speech function and ideational activity. Palisa and Flach found that motor functions, during awakening, do not reintegrate in the same sequence as they are abolished. In our opinion, the same is true in the higher psychic functioning.

Each patient has his own pattern of awakening which rarely changes. Usually the patient first responds to stimuli, makes spontaneous movements, turns around, or tries to sit up. Contact is not yet established. He does not speak in response to questions, but may mutter as if coming out of a heavy sleep. Later he begins to focus attention on the environment, the responses are more coordinated and directed to the source of the stimulus. Echolalia and echopraxia may be present. Then he begins to answer questions. Motor aphasia is often present, the patient being able to comprehend but unable to express himself. Even more common are amnesic-aphasic manifestations when the patient is unable to name an object but knows quite well what it is and can use it properly (Orenstein and Schilder). Shipley and Kant have described apraxias in this phase, especially that of swallowing: the patient is able to swallow when the pharynx is stimulated, but is unable to do so voluntarily. At this time the consciousness is still clouded; although the patient responds quite normally, he is often amnesic for this phase of awakening. Von Baeyer points out that certain dream-like experiences during the awakening period have no schizophrenic characteristics, but that the patient's later attitude towards such experiences is definitely schizophrenic in nature. He also points out that certain manifestations of symptom reduction appear first in the awakening phase and cannot be separated from the exogenous factor of hypoglycemia, as, for instance, Claude and Rubénovitch's "déblocage," where the patient talks more freely about his psychotic experiences but is still quite contradictory about them. Von Baeyer attributes great importance in the patient's cure to the toxic-exogenous change toward a more extrovert behavior.

Many patients, after awakening, show no sign of the previously existing psychosis. They appear to be relaxed, interested in their surroundings, ask for food, or start a conversation. They are in closer contact with reality, their affectivity is more vivid, and they show more interest in life and display more vitality. Preoccupation with themselves and with their mental content, characteristic of so many schizophrenics, is absent. Many have pointed out that the aggressive and suspicious behavior of paranoid patients is also absent. Some patients respond after awakening with a pendulum-like reaction from feelings of absolute unreality to an exuberant consciousness of themselves (Guerra). Euphoria and exuberance may be so marked as to present the clinical picture of a hypomanic state.

Shipley and Kant, describing patients with marked excitement and aggressiveness after awakening, believe that the patient's awareness of the futility and lack of direction of this uncontrollable motor discharge differentiates it from twilight states. It resembles the more organic twilight "driveness" found in certain diseases of the subcortical ganglia, such as epidemic encephalitis. We have seen similar excitement after awakening, though it occurs more commonly before consciousness is fully restored. The feeling of increased vitality is often linked to a certain lack of inhibition; some patients display an infantile behavior and bid for affection, in others erotization is noted (Ligterink) and sexual advances are not uncommon. Orenstein and Schilder, and Müller, found a tendency to homosexual transferences.

The lack of psychotic symptoms, the extraversion of the patient after awakening (Barison), the diminished autism, and the increased contact with reality persists in some patients only a short while after returning to consciousness. If the patient recovers, the period of well-being becomes more and more prolonged. Similar observations have been made on schizophrenics who were sick physically or were near death (Grotjahn).

The type of improvement in the insulin treated patient has been studied extensively. It has been found that the patient improves in all aspects of his personality—emotionally, socially, and intellectually. The gross psychotic manifestations are more influenced than the more subtle psychic background on which schizophrenic psychoses develop. Delusions and hallucinations are usually the first to yield after they have lost their emotional charge. In the same manner as recently described in treatment with neuroleptic drugs, voices become fainter, are less insistent, sound farther away, and become indistinct. The patients become able to shift their attention away from the delusional thought contents and think more freely. If the patient recovers, the delusions and hallucinations are discarded completely, and in many cases the content of his morbid experiences is corrected. He usually does not spontaneously gain insight into the dynamics of the mental symptomatology, but in most instances the recovered patient recognizes the morbidity and unreality of his delusions and hallucinations, as a delirious patient realizes the morbidity of his experiences.

Besides the elimination of hallucinations and delusions, many patients abandon the tendency to symbolization together with their involved dereistic mechanisms in thinking. Incoherence and illogical ideation are often markedly improved, even though the ideational impairment in schizophrenia is more persistent than the affectivity. The recovered patient usually retains the friendly, less autistic attitude seen after awakening and establishes better contact. This increased sociability is found even in patients who are only improved. Sensitivity and hostility are thrown off in the same way as infantile attitudes and many other regression mechanisms. The anxiety which is present in many schizophrenic patients, with regard to trivial life conflicts, is eliminated. Difficulties are approached in a more relaxed and optimistic manner. Patients report increased vitality after a successful treatment, i.e., they eat better, sleep better, and are free from disturbing bodily sensations and hypochondriacal preoccupations (Kronfeld).

Recoveries of insulin-treated patients have frequently been compared with those of spontaneously recovered patients. Spernau described three phases in the recovery of insulin-treated patients. At first the intensity of the schizophrenic psychosis becomes lessened, particularly the hallucinations and delusions diminish in intensity. In the second phase, the autism is broken through, the affectivity becomes more flexible, the patient realizes that he is sick, and reality is reappraised. In this phase the patient suppresses and represses the psychotic material. In the third phase, the patient "works out" the psychotic material, and repression of the conflictual contents is no longer necessary. Müller objects to this formulation, believing that in insulin recovery there is no repression or suppression of the psychotic content, but a conscious and rational elimination of it. Insulin recovery is characterized by the absence of a repression mechanism in contrast to the spontaneous remission in which the patient pushes aside the psychotic symptoms. Kronfeld has made similar statements.

Bond and many others feel that the quality of the insulin recovery is better than that of the spontaneous recovery. We are under a similar impression. Seclusive personality makeup, present in many schizophrenic patients prior to the psychosis, is not altered, even after successful treatment. It is our opinion, therefore, that the matrix in which the schizophrenic psychoses develop is not changed; only the superstructure of the psychosis is eliminated by shock treatment. At present, however, there is at our disposal no psychiatric therapy, somatic or psychotherapeutic, that can alter impressively the pre-psychotic personality makeup of the individual.

Psychological Investigations

Various psychologic studies have been made, some from a phenomenologic point of view, some in order to discover whether the patient has suffered any damage of the intellectual faculties through the insulin treatment, and some with a prognostic aim.

Orenstein and Schilder investigated the so-called *gestalt* functions during and after treatment. They found that the patient showed a slowed-down reaction time during treatment. In hypoglycemia, the patient had diminished perceptive ability, with difficulty especially in naming objects. A marked degree of perseveration was present and the visual-motor *gestalt* patterns were of a primitive type.

Psychologic examinations with the Rorschach method have been carried on by Helena Katz, Piotrowski, and Halpern. Katz reports that the Rorschach protocol usually corresponds with clinical findings during and after insulin therapy. However, there are exceptions to this general rule insofar as patients completely cured clinically may still show some schizophrenic signs in the Rorschach records. In a series of 15 fully recovered cases, only 5 were free of schizophrenic signs in the Rorschach protocol. The most common schizophrenic sign in the pretreatment protocols was poor form perception. Original answers and anatomic interpretations were also poor. Less frequently seen were marked qualitative differences in interpretations, frequent color interpretations, and detail answers. Fairly often definite delusional content was present in interpretations. Less frequent were inability to interpret some of the cards, abstract interpretations, and interpretation of the white spaces on the card instead of the figures shown. All the schizophrenic signs showed a gradual recession after insulin treatment. The movement interpretations changed very little, but the color interpretations which were prevalent in the untreated cases were greatly reduced with improvement. It is significant that delusions which appeared in the records of untreated cases remained unaltered, even though less distinct, in the so-called cured cases. Katz believes that delusions or the tendency toward them is retained as a special complex even in the cured patients.

Piotrowski, in his investigations of insulin-treated patients with the Rorschach method, focused his attention on the prognostic aid this test offers. He found that schizophrenic patients who remained unimproved after treatment showed Rorschach records characteristic for organic brain disease. He also has found that the Rorschach method distinguishes between emotional regression and intellectual regression, and only the emotional regression or fears can be alleviated by insulin treatment. Those patients who showed intellectual regression did not respond well to insulin shock treatment, while emotional regression did not affect the result. In some patients with an active emotional regression, the prognosis was definitely good. Halpern arrived at similar conclusions. Lipton et al. describe five positive signs in the Rorschach indicative of good prognosis with insulin treatment; productivity in more than twenty-five responses; a color sum of 2.5 or greater; a percentage of good form responses of 70 or greater; the presence of one or more human movement responses and of three or more sharply perceived whole responses. Negative signs indicative of a poor prognosis were three or more rejections in the Rorschach, and an I.Q. of less than 90 on the Wechsler-Bellevue test. Eysenck's objective test as a measure of psychoticism was used by Keehn, who did not find any relation between this measure of the severity of illness and response to treatment.

Bolles et al. used psychologic performance tests, so-called sorting tests, based mainly on the investigations of Vigotsky, Hanfmann and Kasanin, and Goldstein. They observed that usually no change in mental behavior occurred after treatment in patients whose performances were very poor. Zubin and Thompson, also using various sorting tests, arrived at similar conclusions. None of these authors mention impairment of the mental faculties of schizophrenic patients treated with insulin. Usually, the patients who did not do well before were those who also did not do well after treatment. Using the Minnesota Multiphasic Personality Inventory, Hales and Simon found that clinical improvement was clearly reflected in the profiles of patients responding to insulin treatment.

Wechsler et al. used five tests (Vocational Interest Blank, Counting by 3's Test, the Similarities Test, the Direction Test, the Word Meaning Test) on 20 schizophrenics before and after treatment. In contrast to other workers, they found that some patients who had received insulin shock treatment showed a lower score than before.

Neurological Observations

Insulin treatment of schizophrenia offers numerous possibilities for investigation of the nervous system in the hypoglycemic state. We have already described some of the neurological symptoms occurring during hypoglycemia and shall here discuss some special investigations in detail. Neurological complications during insulin treatment were discussed in the section on complications.

Golden divides neurological manifestations in hypoglycemia into two groups, the first occurring during the early hours of shock, just before or during the first part of the comatose state, and the second appearing toward the end of the hypoglycemic shock. The first group of phenomena appears slowly and last longer, while the second occurs abruptly. The first group comprises: (1) choreiform movements of the extremities and body and restless tossing of the head; (2) prolonged sucking movements; (3) pupillary dilation, flushing of the face associated with rigid extension of the extremities, and torsion movements, often in connection with labored breathing; (4) true defense reflexes; (5) positive Babinski in the somnolent stage, disappearing in deep coma; (6) absent corneal reflexes, clonus of the jaw, slow "trombone-like" tremors of the tongue, clonic movements of the eyelids and jaw, the so-called "frozen" athetoid movements in which the extremities remain fixed in the position of athetosis, and at times transitory hemiplegia and aphasia. The second group of sudden manifestations occurring at the end of the hypoglycemic state includes tremors, generalized seizures, small tonic pupils, flushed face, torsions, rigid attitudes, and respiratory changes.

De Morsier and Bersot describe similar neurological findings during hypoglycemia, but add that besides the motor phenomena there are manifold sensorial symptoms, for instance, auditory and olfactory illusions and hallucinations, as well as disorders of the vestibular apparatus, vertigo, sensations of gyration or levitation. In all cases disturbances of the vegetative nervous system are found, such as excessive perspiration, salivation, vasomotor imbalance, and so on.

Von Angyal has published several papers on neurological manifestations in hypoglycemia, expressing the view that there is a regular progression of events as the hypoglycemia attacks various parts of the brain in relation to their phylogenetic and ontogenetic organization. Thus, hypoglycemia affects successively the frontal pole, the premotor area, the precentral gyrus, later the basal ganglia, the extrapyramidal pathways, and finally the medulla. Talkativeness and psychomotor restlessness indicate beginning interference with the function of the frontal lobe. The next phase begins about two and a half to three and a half hours after injection, is characterized by somnolence, assumption of sleeping postures, and moderate hypertonus. These symptoms appear when a functional ablation of the frontal poles takes place. When the precentral gyrus and later the basal ganglia are affected, increased muscle tone, clonus, pathologic reflexes such as Babinski and so on, abnormal postures, sucking movements, and forced grasping may be observed. These changes are usually seen first on the right side in a right-handed person and later occur bilaterally. As the extrapyramidal apparatus is progressively involved, profound sleep, choreiform movements, and crossed tonus changes take place followed by general torsion spasms and periods of tremor. With deepening of the coma, these movements disappear. Deep coma produces an interference with the rubrospinal and tectospinal tracts resulting in increased muscle tone, diminution of reflexes, and the loss of pathologic reflexes, such as Babinski, which were present in the preceding phase. Finally, in very deep coma a complete areflexia sets in followed by cardiac and respiratory disturbances of bulbar origin. After termination of shock one sees a rapid reversal of these phases in regular order.

It is an interesting fact that patients receiving insulin therapy often show individual neurological patterns in their hypoglycemic states. If a patient presents jerkings of the head, tongue, and extremities simultaneously with auditory hallucinations, this combination will be repeated over and over again. Another may have recurrent epileptiform seizures, and yet another may regularly go into coma quietly without any motor or sensory manifestations. It may be that certain areas of the brain have an individual selective response to insulin or other agents leading to a slowly deepening state of unconsciousness. Thus, it is possible that not only do the higher functions of the nervous system show marked individuality, but that the lower ones also have individual characteristics (Hoch).

The superficial reflexes are the first to disappear in coma, particularly the abdominal reflexes. The deep reflexes follow, with individual variations. While the Babinski sign is usually present at the beginning of coma, we have only occasionally been unable to elicit it in deep stupor. It is interesting that although the Babinski sign occurs in coma, other pyramidal tract signs with similar significance, such as Rossolimo, Mendel-Bechterew, Chaddock and Oppenheim, seldom appear. The pyramidal signs of the upper extremities, such as the Hoffmann, Trömner, absence of Mayer's metacarpophalangeal joint reflex, and Leri signs may also appear.

Grasping appears when the patient is in superficial coma, no longer responds to questioning, yet still responds with a defense reaction to stimulation. Most of these cases show hypertonia and even spasticity. The term "tonic innervation" or tonic perseveration" used by Wilson and Walshe is probably better than "forced grasping," since the manifestation is an inability to relax a muscle group rather than a real grasping. We have also elicited real grasp reflexes in patients who showed no change in tonus.

Tonus changes are frequent and markedly variable. Some patients approaching coma become hypotonic; in others, hypertonia appears, especially in the muscles of the extremities, often accompanied by spasms. Incomplete pictures of decerebrate rigidity have been observed occasionally; the head and neck are often retracted, some opisthotonos is present, the extremities are rigidly extended and adducted, the hands overpronated, the wrists flexed, and the feet in equinovarus position. Fragmentary decerebrate rigidity, that is overpronation of the hand or an equinovarus attitude of the foot, is commonly noted. These postures in no way differ from those seen in certain midbrain lesions in which inhibitory pathways governing the vestibular and reticulospinal tracts are interrupted. Tonic neck reflexes (Magnus) have been elicited in certain patients, but were not clearcut in form. We have frequently observed both positive and negative supporting reactions *(Stützreaktionen)*, as described in diseases of the frontal and temporal lobes, the cerebellum, and the pons (Schwab). With respect to the righting reflexes, many patients emerging from coma display an infantile form of rising similar to that observed by Schaltenbrand in children or that seen in adults having a temporal or parietal lobe tumor.

Electroencephalographic Findings

If the supply of sugar to the brain is markedly reduced, the recorded electrical activity of the brain is slowed down (Berger). During coma, alpha activity is not noticeable until the sugar level falls to approximately 35 mg. per cent in the venous blood (Lennox, Gibbs and Gibbs). If it drops to 18 mg. per cent, the frequency of the waves is 2 to 4 per second. Animal experiments (Moruzzi et al.) show a complete cessation of electrical activity after the blood sugar reaches a critical level of about 20 mg. per cent. Termination of hypoglycemia reverses the changes brought on by insulin. Himwich et al. believe that the clinical symptoms, the EEG manifestations, and the changes in brain metabolism occur simultaneously. Similar findings are reported by Hoagland et al., who state that the alpha activity is proportionate to the rate of the carbohydrate metabolism of the brain. There is no doubt that, in a general way, brain metabolism, clinical signs, and brain wave patterns are correlated, but one is not the absolute mirror of the other. Occasionally, we have observed signs of slow wave patterns in patients under insulin who did not display clinically impressive signs of hypoglycemia. The electroencephalogram cannot be used at present as a reliable index of the degree of hypoglycemia. This was confirmed in studies by Weinland and Weinland. In hypoglycemic convulsions Gibbs and Murray found spike seizure discharges of high voltage indistinguishable from those in epilepsy.

Lemere tried to employ the electroencephalogram as a basis for the selection of patients for treatment but the findings were not confirmed by Grey Walter. The value of the electroencephalogram in the diagnosis of schizophrenia is still a controversial matter. It is true that abnormal findings are not uncommon, but none of them can be considered as specific for the illness. It is difficult, therefore, to interpret changes which supposedly occur in the wave pattern after insulin treatment. McNeil et al. have been unable to demonstrate lasting brain damage after insulin treatment. Hoagland, et al., in interpreting the effects of insulin shock treatment on the electric brain waves of schizophrenics, pay special attention to the delta waves. As a measure, they devised the delta index. In about 88 per cent of the cases, a diminution of the delta index was seen as the patient improved. Transient relapses and remissions of the patients were correlated with an increase or decrease in the delta index. In several patients the delta index changed prior to any other objective change in the symptoms. These authors believe that this index is an interesting physiologic measure of the trend of an individual's psychosis. In 8 out of 10 schizophrenics studied, Knott et al. found an increased alpha index following insulin treatment which was particularly evident in the frontal area. There were no uniform, notable deviations in slow activity.

Neuropathology of Hypoglycemia

Many investigations on experimental hypoglycemia in animals were reported before and after the introduction of insulin treatment for schizophrenia. The first publication on the effect of large doses of insulin on the central nervous system was made by Stief and Tokay who demonstrated that high doses of insulin lead to irreversible changes. Weil et al. showed that doses up to 70 units produce no damage but that more than 200 units injected over a period of two months severely damage the cerebral neurons. Accornero found diffuse, severe alterations only in animals who died in coma; for the most part reversible and only few irreversible cell changes and areas of rarifications in most layers were encountered in animals which did not die in coma. Little or no irreversible damage after therapeutic doses of insulin was found by Schmid. Neumann et al. saw no changes not found in control animals. There is some evidence (Finley and Brenner) that only after several hours of hypoglycemic coma do neuropathologic changes become irreversible. Winkleman and Moore, who experimented with very large doses of insulin leading to death, found severe damage to the nerve cells in practically all areas of the nervous system including the spinal cord and the cells of the posterior root ganglia; Schereschewsky et al. observed alterations in the sympathetic ganglia of the solar plexus. In hypoglycemic dogs who died under convulsions, Schaltenbrand found changes particularly in the Ammon's horn. In a monograph, Lorentzen presents an extensive experimental study on rabbits treated with insulin. He uses Einarson's gallocyamin-chromalum method which gives a quantitative measure for the nucleic acid content of the nerve cells and thus, registers the structural activity changes of the cells. It was shown that repeated insulin shocks induce an increasing chromophoby of the nerve cells. Some cells, especially in the fifth layer, pass through irreversible cellular atrophy, developing into cell shadows. After cessation of the treatment, in most areas the chromophoby will be replaced by the normal activity picture, with chromoneutrality as the central point. However, a certain number of cells degenerate into cell shadows and disappear permanently.

The first investigation disclosing irreparable damage in human brains of patients dying in hypoglycemic coma was made by Bodechtel, and of those dying in insulin treatment for schizophrenia by Kobler. It may be objected that patients who die in prolonged coma usually develop a pulmonary infection which in itself could be responsible for some of the neuropathologic changes; however, the material studied by Ferraro and Jervis offers sufficient conclusive uniformity. According to them, the morphologic alterations were of both a vascular and cellular character. The nerve cell changes ranged from chromatolysis and shrinkage to severe colliquation and formation of cell shadows; homogenizing alterations and Spielmeyer's *ischemic nerve changes* were frequently encountered. The majority of the cells were altered and the architecture of the cortex markedly changed. Areas of loss of nerve cells were irregularly distributed and appeared in all cortical layers. The glia reaction varied. Vascular changes, such as endothelial proliferation of small vessels and capillaries with swelling of the endothelial cells, were considered as contributory to the ischemic changes. Ferraro believes that some of the pathologic changes are similar to those encountered in other conditions accompanied by vasospasms, such as epilepsy, eclampsia, arteriosclerosis, and so on.

A study based on 6 fatal cases of hypoglycemia was reported by Lawrence et al. In every case there was widespread degeneration and necrosis of nerve cells with corresponding microglial and macrogial proliferation. The predominating types of degeneration were homogenizing and severe nerve cell changes. The cerebral cortex, caudate nucleus, and putamen were most affected. In 2 cases, widespread glial fibrosis of the cerebral and cerebellar white matter was a striking feature. In another group of 6 cases, studied by Jansen and Waaler, small perivascular hemorrhages were found in nearly all the brains. On the other hand, the changes demonstrated in the nerve cells were comparatively slight, and in some of the brains there were no changes at all. The conclusion was that changes after insulin treatment are due to circulatory disturbances, and that no permanent changes occur. The possibility that the histological changes in insulin fatalities are caused by convulsions was denied by Rauch because of their minimal intensity in electric shock convulsions. The suggestion that severe histologic lesions occur only after hypoglycemic convulsions was refuted by Weil et al. These authors, Meyer, and many others consider intracellular anoxia as the main cause of the nechosis; while others, among them Wohlwill, hold alkalosis and other metabolic disturbances responsible. Hassin compares his findings with those described in patients dying from barbiturates and other poisoning and holds that neither vascular changes nor anoxemia are likely to be of pathogenic importance. Schmid considers the findings as an immediate result of the excessive output of adrenaline in response to insulin.

Massive hemorrhages and softenings in the brain were reported in the literature on hypoglycemia prior to the introduction of insulin treatment. A fresh hemorrhagic infarct involving the parieto-occipital lobes was found by Zeitlofer et al. in a young woman of 22, who died in coma. Schmid described changes in the adrenals and hypophysis and hypertrophic changes in the insular apparatus of the pancreas. Nicolajev found small foci of necrosis in the liver and discusses the possibility that they are responsible for the changes in the glia. Few reports on pathology outside the central nervous system are available. Brain changes are undoubtedly the most important pathology in hypoglycemic treatment; but the question remains unsettled whether chemical or circulatory changes or both are pathogenic factors.

Prognosis

Since the introduction of insulin treatment, a number of authors have studied the results of the treatment and have tried to formulate prognostic principles. The evaluation of the basic prognostic factors apparently remains the same as before the shock treatment era. Although most of the prognostic signs are present before treatment, some appear during the treatment and will be discussed separately. Most prognostic factors for the response to treatment outlined in this chapter are equally valid for insulin and convulsive therapy. The entire question of prognosis in schizophrenia was reviewed by Zubin et al.

Opinions differ on the importance of heredity in relation to the outcome of a schizophrenic psychosis. With regard to age, it is the general consensus that schizophrenic patients below the age of 15 do not respond well and spontaneous and shock treatment recovery rates are low. In the older age groups, observations are conflicting. Freudenberg considers that age has no decisive influence on the outcome. Chase and Silverman believe that onset of illness after 40 is unfavorable. Cheney and Clowe think that the best prognosis may be made for a person below 30 years of age. Ross and Malzberg found that patients over 25 responded better than those below that age. Concerning the importance of sex, Cheney and Clowe, as well as the New York State Insulin Commission, found better results in male patients; Chase and Silverman saw no difference between male and female patients; and von Braunmühl observed only negligible differences. It is interesting that the spontaneous remission rate was found to be higher in females than in males (Blair).

The most important factors in evaluating prognosis are acute onset of the psychosis and duration of illness prior to treatment. The best results are obtained with patients who are ill not longer than one year (Müller, Cheney and Clowe, and Dukor, Ross and Malzberg, Freudenberg, and many others). After two years, recovery and improvement figures sink rapidly. After five years' duration, only a small percentage of schizophrenic patients recover. The only exceptions are those patients in whom symptom-free periods have occurred during the illness. Improvement is achieved in chronic patients, but it is usually temporary and the quality of the improvement is none too impressive. This is not to say that no chronic schizophrenic is amenable to treatment; it simply indicates that the cures are exceptions which test the above stated rule.

The usefulness of this prognostic factor is somewhat reduced by the fact that it is not easy to fix reliably the duration of psychoses in many patients. Insidious development is not uncommon, and a schizoid, prepsychotic personality sometimes merges imperceptibly into a psychosis. In our experience careful anamnestic and personality studies have revealed that many patients have been sick for a longer period of time than is recognized by their relatives or physicians.

Previous attacks are usually considered a favorable prognostic sign if the patient made a good adjustment during the remission and if he is treated soon after the occurrence of the new attack (Küppers, Müller, Chase and Silverman, Harris). However, the clinical impression is that even though the majority of patients respond to treatment within each new attack, this response becomes progressively less complete. There is more and more "scar formation" in the sense of increasing personality changes, particularly emotional flattening and other residues.

The type of schizophrenia is of considerable importance for the prognosis. Most statistics demonstrate the efficacy of insulin treatment in the paranoid and catatonic forms; hebephrenic and simple types are much less amenable to treatment (Müller, Chase and Silverman). Insulin treatment has changed the prognostic outlook for paranoid schizophrenics, this form having previously shown no great tendency to spontaneous recovery. Küppers agrees with Müller that the paranoid form of schizophrenia responds well to insulin, but he has found a rather high relapse rate in follow-up studies.

The excited catatonic patient with massive hallucinations and delusions responds well, the stuporous catatonic less well. In the stuporous catatonic cases, the combination treatment of insulin with electroshock or metrazol is superior to insulin employed alone. It has been pointed out by many authors (Langfeldt, Hirschman, Lewis) that the best results are seen not in cases of typical schizophrenia in the sense of Kraepelin's dementia praecox, but in atypical schizophrenia or, as Langfeldt terms them, the "schizophrenoid psychoses." In this latter group he includes cases which on admission suggest schizophrenia but later are found to be composed of mixed manic-depressive or reactive, paranoid, hysterical, and schizophrenic features. Many of these patients show symptoms of an exogenous psychosis or there is present much reactive psychogenic material. Meduna recently expressed the opinion that only schizophreniform syndromes which are exogenous, and which he describes under the term "oneirophrenia," have a favorable treatment prognosis while the cases of true schizophrenia remain uninfluenced.

The response to shock treatment is relatively poor in some schizophrenic groups in which the personality remains well preserved. One group of schizophrenics, where usually no deterioration takes place, is represented by the late paranoids. Response to shock therapy here, however, is quite unsatisfactory. The same is true for those schizophrenics who show primarily a neurotic syndrome, though in a schizophrenic setting. They were described by Hoch and Polatin as pseudoneurotic form of schizophrenia; they show little tendency to deteriorate but at the same time do not respond well to shock therapy.

Manic-depressive features in a schizophrenic psychosis are considered by many as favorable prognostic signs, as are pyknic body build and sociable, extroverted makeup. Müller, Plattner and Fröhlicher emphasize, however, that the presence of manic-depressive symptoms in their insulin-treated cases definitely indicate a poor prognosis, in contrast to their cases with spontaneous remission where manic-depressive symptoms were of favorable import. It should be pointed out that insulin is not very effective in the manic-depressive psychoses and it is therefore a matter of question why it should be more effective in the schizophrenias with manic-depressive coloring.

The prognosis is especially good in patients with definite precipitating factors, or, as Kronfeld and Sternberg pointed out, in schizophrenic psychoses of a reactive nature where the mental disturbance is an acute response to an emotional or physical stress situation. The favorable outcome of those acute cases with much psychogenic material is in sharp contrast to the therapeutic response in the "pseudoneurotic" form of schizophrenia.

The presence of hallucinations is not an unfavorable sign. Delusions are of little significance from a quantitative point of view, but of considerable significance from a qualitative angle (Blair). Bizarre, dereistic elaborations, somatic and hypochondriacal delusions, point to a more unfavorable outcome. Menzies believes that it is important to know whether the patient has obtained satisfaction in his unreal world or is still fighting against it. He believes that paranoid patients respond better than the others because they are dissatisfied with the world of fantasy they have invented. Prolonged existence of negativism, command automatism, catatonic posturing, stereotypes, and grimacing are not favorable signs. Regression to an infantile level does not mitigate against a favorable prognosis if the affective contact remains fairly good and an intellectual regression does not occur simultaneously. Marked incoherence and other speech disturbances, emotional and intellectual deterioration are of serious import, particularly if they manifest themselves in connection with a clear sensorium and are not associated with a confusional state.

The constitutional makeup is considered by many to be of some importance. Dinther and Jansen, Freudenberg, Cheney and Clowe and many others found the pyknic or athletic body type prognostically more favorable than the asthenic and dysplastic type. Among personality make-ups extroverts and cyclothymics have a better outcome under treatment than those with a schizoid-autistic personality structure. Unfavorable are shiftlessness and psychopathic features.

Polonio and Slater have used a point system in a prognostic study in insulin treatment. They assigned two points to duration of illness of less than one year, and one point each to a good premorbid personality and the presence of precipitating factors. Eighty-four per cent of patients who scored four points, had good results. This is valid in all treatment procedures applicable in schizophrenia.

In the section "Psychological Investigations," we mentioned the studies of workers who used the Rorschach method and various sorting tests for prognostic purposes. It was generally found that patients who showed only emotional impairment had a good prognosis, whereas those who displayed intellectual deterioration experienced an unfavorable outcome.

An important prognostic aid appears to be the application of sodium amytal; 2 to 7½ grains of sodium amytal is injected intravenously. Harris et al., Gottlieb and Hope, Hoch and others found that if, on injection of sodium amytal, schizophrenic patients responded favorably by a lessening of their negativism, becoming more normal in speech, ideation, and behavior, they were apt to respond well to shock treatment; while those who remained untouched by the drug generally showed an unfavorable outcome.

Hoch et al. used the psychogalvanic reflex to investigate the responses of 40 schizophrenic patients tested before and after they received insulin treatment. In general, along with the clinical improvement of the patient, the abnormal characteristics of the psychogalvanic reflex often seen in untreated schizophrenic patients diminished or disappeared. In some instances, the psychogalvanic reflex continued to be abnormal even though the clinical condition of the patient appeared much improved. These patients usually relapsed. Similar observations were made by Solomon, Darrow and Blaurock.

A prognostic test of four convulsive treatments was recommended by von Braunmühl before a long and costly course of insulin treatment is started. Patients who failed to respond to four convulsions with clinical improvement have, according to him, a poor prognostic outlook even with the most intensive insulin treatment. In our experience, although there have been some exceptions to this rule, the test is extremely valuable in all prognostication of schizophrenics. Temporary removal of symptoms after a few convulsive treatments proves that such symptoms are still reversible.

The various prognostic criteria should be evaluated before treatment is applied. However, as there are many exceptions to the above-mentioned prognostic rules, every patient should be treated as soon as possible regardless of the outlook. As yet we have no absolute prognotic signs and, therefore, we should not exclude patients from treatment because the outlook is unfavorable. Some patients have shown surprisingly good results in spite of unfavorable prognosis, while others with good prognosis have failed to improve.

Attempts to draw prognostic conclusions from clinical observations made during the treatment remained inconclusive. A link between improvement and insulin sensitivity or insulin resistance was assumed by some but denied by others. Various metabolic and sympathetic regulative mechanisms could also not be related to prognosis. Gain of weight during the treatment seems to be a favorable prognostic sign; but it should be remembered that also deteriorated schizophrenics may gain weight steadily.

Results of Insulin Coma Treatment

The number of publications on the results of insulin coma treatment is enormous. A great many of them, however, are based on very small numbers of patients. Others have limited value because their material is not broken down on the basis of duration of illness. Since the effectiveness of all shock treatments is essentially limited to patients with relatively short duration of illness, papers which do not separate acute and chronic cases may present either too favorable results because the acute cases prevail or too discouraging results because chiefly chronic cases were treated.

Statistics from large groups of hospitals are also frequently inconclusive as they collect dissimilar material from institutions which may differ widely regarding diagnostic principles, type of patients admitted, intensity of treatment, and evaluation. But in spite of these various possibilities of error, sufficient statistical material is available to draw some conclusions which seem reasonably safe.

The first statistical report on insulin treatment in schizophrenia was made by Dussik and Sakel, who even then recognized the necessity of distinguishing between acute and chronic cases. They reported 88 per cent remissions among the group of patients ill less than six months; in 70 per cent the remission was considered complete ("full remission"). Shortly afterwards the Yugoslavian workers, Berglas and Susic, obtained 70 per cent remissions in acute cases. In schizophrenics of long standing they made the interesting distinction between alert and dull schizophrenics and found that in the former group 27.7 per cent and in the latter only 4.3 per cent experienced remissions. The first negative report came from Wilna (Borysowiz et al.) with the statement that results with insulin treatment did not exceed the rate of spontaneous remissions. However, study of their paper shows that no deep coma was used, the duration of the individual hypoglycemic state was kept brief, and the number of shocks was limited to fifteen. Thus the first dissenting voices were obviously due to inadequate intensity of treatment as were many later reports of failures.

Müller, in a 1937 survey, pointed out that the first reports on insulin treatment showed 70-80 per cent remissions in cases of less than six months' duration. Hospitals reporting without distinguishing between acute and chronic cases claimed between 40-50 per cent remissions for such mixed material. These figures for acute cases and for mixed material became more or less standard figures provided that insulin, convulsive, or combined treatment were adequately applied.

The most extensive material on insulin treatment was gathered by the Department of Mental Hygiene of New York from its various State Hospitals. Ross, together with the statistician, Malzberg, and other co-workers, reported this material in various papers. The New York figures (Ross) for insulin-treated schizophrenics of less than six months' duration show 29.2 per cent recovered and 30.2 per cent "much improved" cases. Since the differentiation between recovered and much improved will vary from hospital to hospital and from one examiner to the other, it became customary to consider these two groups together under the common heading of "remission." In European studies the terms, "full remission" for recovered and "social remission" for much improved cases, are employed. Adding up the figures for the two groups in the New York statistic, 59.4 per cent remissions were obtained. In cases of seven to twelve months' duration the remission rate is still as high as 51.3 per cent. A definite drop occurs in the next group of cases of one to two years' duration of illness; only 37.9 per cent remissions are reported. The figures for the remission rate of cases of several years' duration cannot be evaluated as no distinction is made between chronic patients who had been ill continuously for several years and those more favorable cases that had had previous episodes but with long symptom-free periods. Of all the subjects treated with insulin, 65.4 per cent showed some degree of improvement (recovered plus much improved plus improved) as compared with only 22.1 per cent in an untreated control group, making a ratio of nearly 3:1 in the New York group. It is only 2:1 or slightly less in most other reports on insulin treatment. This unusually favorable ratio in the New York report is due to the low figure for spontaneous remissions with which the treated groups were compared.

Another report of comparable institutional material in Switzerland was made by Müller. Here, the remission rate (social and full remissions together) reached 59.1 per cent in cases up to six months' duration. Müller found that by limiting the statistics to hospitals applying intense treatment, viz., cases with at least sixty treatment days, the figure went up to 65.3 per cent. Still the rates of 52.1 per cent and 61.3 per cent in the more adequately treated group were obtained in cases of between six months' and one year's duration of illness, but only 27.3 per cent and 31.6 per cent respectively in cases of one to two years' duration. Beyond two years of illness the remission rate dropped to 11.3 per cent or, after elimination of inadequately treated cases, 14.1 per cent. This report demonstrates equally well that the peak for the curative effect in insulin treatment is one year's duration of illness. The percentage of cases which benefited at least to some degree was 66.7 per cent in the total Swiss material, taking acute and chronic cases together. It was 66 per cent in similar German statistics (Küppers). The ratio between these figures and those for untreated groups in the same countries was usually 2:1.

Comparison between treated and untreated subjects from the same hospital is the most desirable proof of the efficacy of the treatment, but few reports are available which fulfill this condition. Bond and Rivers reported on such comparable groups from the Pennsylvania Hospital in Philadelphia, which they had been able to follow for many years. One of the interesting features of their work is the striking difference in the remission rate between cases treated from 1936-1938, when tentative, comparatively mild, treatment was given by various physicians of the hospital, and cases treated later when deeper and longer comas were applied and treatment was left in the hands of one experienced physician. The more important figures are those from the second series showing the optimal results to be obtained with the method when its potentialities were fully utilized. In cases of less than one year's duration the remission rate on Bond and Rivers' early insulin group was 46 per cent, in the more adequately treated group 79 per cent. The remission rate in the same hospital prior to shock treatment varied between 10 per cent and 20 per cent. Bond, whose experience has spanned both the preshock and the shock area, also feels that the quality of remissions in insulin-treated patients is of a much higher standard than in those not so treated. The follow-up of their treated group revealed the following: the remission rate for the total number treated by them in the Pennsylvania Hospital was 55 per cent at the end of treatment, 42 per cent after one year, 36 per cent after two years, 31 per cent after three years. The long range remission rate was therefore still twice as high as that of the control cases.

On the same material West et al. showed later that 63 per cent of the original patients in remission had relapsed, but that 50 per cent of the relapsed group improved again with a second course of treatment. In a hospital with very similar material Cheney and Clow obtained only 48 per cent improvements at the end of treatment, and 36 per cent six months to two years later. These percentages resemble those given by Bond and Rivers for their less intensively treated group. The same is probably true for the skeptical conclusions drawn from Rennie's material in which even the number of insulin treatments averaged only 36, and the figure of Gottlieb and Huston, who gave only 30 treatments, is lower than reported by most workers. If Boling et al. found results with light comas very similar to those they obtained with deep coma, this is contrary to the general experience; however, they, too, found that patients with longer duration of illness fared better under deep than under light comas. Other negative reports were published by Notkin et al., Gralnick, and recently Gottlieb and Huston. These authors, in a new study, matched three groups of schizophrenics treated with brief psychotherapy, insulin and ECT without finding any significant difference in clinical status after one to four years. Also Appel et al. found no difference in a five-years' follow-up between patients subjected to insulin and to hospitalization without specific therapy. Ackner et al. came to equally negative conclusions, when they compared patients who had been obviously treated with an inadequate number of comas, with another group given only barbiturate sleep.

The limitations of the purely statistical approach from large groups of hospitals is demonstrated by differences among three such reports. The Temporary Commission on State Hospital Problems in New York on 1128 schizophrenics treated with insulin compared with the same number of untreated patients led to results and conclusions that were obviously beyond what can be expected from the treatment. The opposite extreme is represented by figures reported by Penrose and Marr who found treated patients only slightly superior to untreated patients. Again more favorable were the figures published by the State of New Jersey which most closely approached figures from individual workers with a discharge rate of 39.3 per cent before insulin treatment, but 61.9 per cent after the introduction of shock treatments. Finiefs, on the basis of 1000 cases, stressed the more rapid and frequent improvements and the strikingly better quality of the improvements. Other satisfactory results were obtained by Fitzgerald, Kwalwasser and Robinson, and Freudenberg. It may be mentioned here that in the Soviet Union insulin treatment is being used extensively, and that it is given preference over ECT. It is often combined with sleep treatment and other therapeutic modalities.

It is undoubtedly true that relapses are frequent and that the long-range prognosis is not satisfactory. Kolle and Rückdeschel who reported disappointing figures after 10 to 17 years, rightly acknowledge the significance of immediate results and years of well-being before the relapse. The same point was made by Hinko and Lipschutz. In a first survey on relapses Horwitz et al. found only 8.4 per cent early relapses, but 25 per cent after a year in their own material. Most statistics regarding early relapses range between these two figures. Müller found 6.5 per cent relapses in acute cases, and 13 per cent in those ill for more than one year when treatment was started. Patients who improved only slightly have a much higher relapse rate than those in full remission. Müller, Küppers, Runge, Chapuis and Georgi agree that the stability of full remissions is very satisfactory. Haddenbrook demonstrated that treated remissions are far more stable than spontaneous remissions. He compared his 30 per cent relapse rate of shock treated patients after three years with Kraepelin's relapse rate of 54.2 per cent after the same three year period for spontaneous remissions which after five years even rose to 78 per cent. If M. Bleuler saw insulin remissions only in schizophrenics with an episodic course, Müller rightly points out that Bleuler based his skeptical attitude on a material of patients with an average duration of more than four years, when remissions are known to be rare in shock treatments.

Studies comparing not only untreated and treated cases but comparing insulin treatment and ECT are rare. A study by Leiberman et al. from the Bethlehem Royal and Maudsley Hospitals comparing a group treated in 1934 and 1935, and a second group treated from 1948-1950 shows that the latter group treated with shock treatments did definitely better. There was also some evidence that insulin coma was superior to ECT. Feuerlein rightly pointed out that most patients submitted to insulin, had already failed under ECT, or were treated with combined insulin-convulsive therapy. In his much quoted paper entitled "The Insulin Myth" Bourne denies that insulin results are greatly superior to those obtainable with electro-convulsive therapy.

In recent years several large-scale statistics have been published compiling material from various studies on untreated as well as treated schizophrenics. L. Alexander, and Appel et al. found approximately 29 per cent, and Staudt and Zubin a somewhat higher figure of significant clinical improvement under purely custodial treatment. Alexander's series of more than 9000 insulin-treated patients showed 61.3 per cent significant clinical improvement or 2.1 times greater than the untreated group. The two other studies also found a higher favorable outcome in treated than in untreated cases, but noticed a levelling off of the improvements over the years.

Much criticism has been expressed regarding inadequate statistical procedure, neglect of the psychological effect of the insulin procedure on the patient, and particularly of the lack of untreated controls (David). We clinicians are very much aware of these shortcomings, but to withhold treatment from one group of patients would be unjustifiable. In our opinion sufficient evidence is available for the value of active therapy as compared to the pre-shock era, and clinical experience cannot be entirely meaningless.

The introduction of pharmacotherapy with neuroleptic drugs in schizophrenia makes it particularly important to establish as clearly as possible what optimal results had been obtainable with previously available treatments. This question can be best answered by results obtained, when insulin coma and convulsive therapy were combined as was actually done by most experts.

A follow-up of such material treated by Georgi with combined treatment, has been published by Chapuis and, later, by Chapuis and Georgi. The average number of treatments was seventy to eighty days of hypoglycemia and ten to twenty convulsions. The rate for full and social remissions in acute cases of less than six months' duration was 81.5 per cent. When improvements were added to the remissions, 94.6 per cent of these patients benefited to some extent from the treatment. During an observation period of five years, 70 per cent of the remissions remained stable. After an observation period up to seven years in some cases, this figure was still more than 50 per cent. It was found that during the last two years the number of relapses increased only among the social remissions; no further relapses occurred among the full remissions. In fact, 70 per cent of the full remissions remained stable for three to seven years. Chapuis, comparing the original results obtained with straight insulin and those of later years with combined treatment, found the combination superior in catatonics but not in paranoids.

An elaborate evaluation of combined insulin-convulsive treatment was published by von Braunmühl based on five years' experience during which combined insulin and convulsive therapy was mainly, though not exclusively used. Treatment and follow-up were in the hands of the same physician so that this report on 563 institutionalized cases has great uniformity. Schizophrenics of less than six months' duration showed 56.3 per cent remissions, of which 33.8 per cent came to a full remission, with normal affectivity and other finer features being fully restored; 22.5 per cent showed a good remission with only slightly impaired affectivity. A further group (20.3 per cent) of good "defect remissions" capable of work brought the percentage of "social cures" to 76.6 per cent. The rates remained almost as good for the period of six months to one year (50.5 per cent cures and 62.8 per cent "social cures"). These latter figures are particularly convincing since short psychotic episodes of perhaps symptomatic type are already automatically eliminated in this group of patients who have been psychotic not less than six months. After one year's duration of illness there is a distinct decrease in effectiveness. In cases of one to two years' duration, figures drop to 25.8 per cent cures with 15.5 per cent additional good defect remissions. Cases of more than two years' duration give no more than 4.9 per cent remissions of any type, while older cases with previous remissions again show in the new attack of their illness rather favorable results with 35.3 per cent cures and an additional 23.5 per cent good defect remissions, or a total of 58.8 per cent social cures. Further features of interest in this study are the results with the various subtypes in cases up to one year's duration:

Catatonic excitements	66.3 per cent cures
Paranoids	57.7 " " "
Catatonic stupors	55.5 " " "
Hebephrenics	26.0 " " "

There was no difference in the rates for male and female patients.

Relapses in the whole material during the five years' period occurred in cases of:

less than 6 months' duration of illness in 9.6 per cent of the cured and 32.0 per cent of the improved;
6 months' to 1 year's duration in 22.8 per cent of the cured and 8.7 per cent of the improved;
more than 1 year's duration in 28.3 per cent of the cured and 12.8 per cent of the improved.

The distribution of relapses again demonstrates the importance of early treatment. It should be added that the majority of relapses occurred within the first year after treatment; many of these cases were successfully retreated. This is probably the most elaborate study on insulin treatment and should be a yardstick for our therapeutic efforts with any of the treatments available for schizophrenia today.

One of the few reports on insulin results that was published after the introduction of modern pharmacotherapy is by Alexander and Bindelglas from the Rockland State Hospital. Aside from a 50 per cent discharge rate, the authors mention 22 patients who did not respond to reserpine or chlorpromazine, and of this group 12 still responded to insulin therapy, although they had been started on this method rather late. The authors warn against delaying insulin too long in patients with only symptomatic improvement under drugs. There are a few comparative studies (Boardman et al.; Patton and Garneau) between chlorpromazine and insulin in a group of previously untreated schizophrenic patients which come to the conclusion that the two methods are equally effective. Such studies ignore the fact that insulin and convulsive therapy are measured in terms of what has been achieved at termination of treatment while neuroleptic drugs are mostly continued indefinitely, and are, therefore, measured in terms of their results during rather than after their application.

Insulin coma treatment remains a treatment applicable only in schizophrenia. Some attempts in other mental disorders have been made, thus Borgarello has reported improvement in depressions, Engelman et al. in manic patients. However, most workers who have used insulin in the affective disorders have combined it with convulsive therapy since Küppers pointed out that insulin alone is unsatisfactory in depressions. J. H. Taylor has recommended the use of insulin in the paranoid type of involutional psychosis, adding electric shock if no improvement occurs after twenty insulin treatments; in involutional melancholia he uses both methods simultaneously. Fariello has used insulin treatment in general paresis. Dussik has successfully treated the paranoid syndromes seen in general paretics after a course of malaria treatment; this was not confirmed by Müller. Some workers have mentioned favorable results in other organic psychoses.

Statistical evaluation comparing a representative group of insulin-treated schizophrenics with a matched group of patients treated with ECT or with neuroleptic drugs, can hardly be expected at this point. However, the experience of those who are still actively engaged in insulin coma treatment in various parts of the world, and of those of us who accumulated a wealth of clinical observations with all the various treatments, suggests strongly that insulin even more than ECT achieves remissions in schizophrenics that are not obtainable with presently available drugs. This conclusion based on many individual cases, is not meant to distract from the enormous value of pharmacotherapy in the management of schizophrenics in whom a lasting remission is not obtainable. Many hospitals discontinued insulin treatment prematurely before any longterm results with the neuroleptic drugs were available. Since the technical difficulties and dangers of insulin coma treatment have been diminished, this method should be retained as an important tool in the treatment of schizophrenia.

CHAPTER V

Psychosurgery

Introduction

Psychosurgery went through important changes during the last fifteen years. The introduction of new drugs considerably reduced the number of operations, eliminating most chronic schizophrenics who, already before, had been recognized as giving the least favorable results, and who greatly benefited from the neuroleptic drugs. The resurgence of psychosurgery is due to a better selection of patients and to more restricted operations which avoid undesirable personality changes. If properly applied, psychosurgery is a valuable therapeutic method which gives most gratifying results in patients who had been unresponsive to all other treatments and who usually are more appreciative than any other group. Favorable results can be better predicted and are more lasting than in most other treatments available in psychiatry. The renewed interest in this field was illustrated by an Editorial in *Lancet* in 1964 stating that these "operations have been among the most striking developments of our medical times."

Systematic work in this field started when Moniz conceived the idea of frontal lobe surgery on mental patients. Historically, the discovery of psychosurgery goes back to the Swiss psychiatrist Burckhardt, who, on December 29, 1888, performed the first brain operation on a psychotic patient. His report, published in 1890, shows that he clearly saw many of the problems which determine present-day developments in the field. When he performed the first operation Burckhardt's aim was to change a very assaultive patient into a quiet, harmless individual. His original concept was that sensory stimuli of abnormal quality and intensity reaching the motor area caused the patient's impulsiveness. He therefore cut the connections between motor and sensory area in the parietal lobe. A definite improvement was obtained after the first operation on the right side, but only after a total of four operations, including the left hemisphere, did the patient become perfectly quiet and cooperative. It is fascinating to find in the detailed case report such familiar features of lobotomized patients as the occasional outbursts of temper which were always short-lived, and the postoperative persistence of hallucinations in which the patient lost all interest.

In a second case, Burckhardt interrupted fibers between central area and frontal lobe. This patient, who also lost his aggressiveness entirely, actually represents the first case of *frontal lobe* surgery for mental disorders (1889). In 3 more cases an attempt was made to give relief from auditory hallucinations by means of temporal cortical excision. Burckhardt, rightly encouraged by his results in cases with obviously hopeless prognosis, recommended continuation of selective cortical excisions in view of the lack of any other available treatment for such conditions. However, these attempts were abandoned and taken up again only after several decades by Egas Moniz in Lisbon, Portugal, who was apparently unaware of Burckhardt's work.

Moniz based his procedure on physiological and clinical observations of frontal lobe function. He first experimented by injecting alcohol into the frontal lobes. The first operation was carried out by Moniz and Lima in 1935. In his monograph published in 1936, Moniz reported on 20 cases and developed the theory that the operation was designed to interrupt the formation of persistently faulty cellular synapses which lead to abnormal mental processes. The only European country where this work was taken up with some enthusiasm was Italy (Rizzatti).

Full credit for rescuing Moniz's work from probably the same fate as Burckhardt's earlier attempts goes to W. Freeman, who together with J. Watts performed the first such operation in the United States on September 14, 1936. Their efforts met with strong opposition and found few followers until favorable reports from England led to a greater acceptance of the method.

Anatomy, Physiology and Pathology of the Frontal Lobes

The anatomy of the frontal lobes and their connections will be discussed only so far as they relate to psychosurgery. The gross anatomy in its surgical implications was best described by Freeman in his various writings. Fiber connections of the frontal lobes were studied mainly by A. Meyer and his coworkers, who were able to base their report (given at the International Congress Psychiatry in Paris in 1950) on the histological study of 122 brains from patients after prefrontal lobotomy.

The frontal lobe reaches posteriorly and inferiorly to the rolandic and sylvian fissures. The "prefrontal' area is that part of the frontal lobe which lies anterior to the motor area. The term "prefrontal" was uncommon prior to its use by Moniz; it was debated by some and Menge tried to introduce the term "frontopolar lobotomy."

Descriptive anatomy distinguishes between a superior, medial and inferior frontal gyrus, the latter being subdivided into an opercular, a triangular and an orbital part. On the medial surface of the brain, the cingulate gyrus lies between frontal gyri and corpus callosum, and on the base of the brain we find the gyrus rectus. At the base, the frontal lobe extends to the olfactory trigone and the anterior edge of the insula.

According to Freeman and Watts, burr holes at the lower end of the coronal suture allow an instrument to be passed through the frontal lobe just anterior to the frontal horn of the lateral ventricle. They use as principal landmark the sphenoidal ridge, which can be easily reached with the leucotome.

The cytoarchitecture of the frontal cortex permits division into a granular and an agranular portion. In describing cytoarchitectural areas, Brodmann's classification will be used. Our main concern here is the prefrontal cortex, represented by areas 8 to 12, 45, 46, and 47. It is mostly granular, except for areas 8 and part of 9, which form a transitional zone to the agranular posterior part of the orbital surface. Macroscopic identification of the areas is difficult because of the unsatisfactory landmarks on the skull and on the cortex. It is also interesting that Beck et al. showed great variations of these areas between the two hemispheres, even in the same person.

The afferent fibers at the prefrontal region arise in their majority in the dorsomedial nucleus of the thalamus. Many different authors studying retrograde degeneration in the dorsomedial nucleus, with its magnocellular and parvocellular portion, have contributed to our knowledge of the thalamofrontal projections. McLardy presented a diagram of thalamic projection at the frontal lobe, based on 54 hemispheres with different lobotomy lesions; this confirmed the findings of Walker that the medial portion of the dorsomedial nucleus of the thalamus projects to the orbital region and the lateral portion to the convexity of the frontal lobe. Hassler demonstrated that the nucleus consists of a number of cellular units each of which projects to a different part of the frontal cortex. He also showed that the connections between frontal lobe and thalamus run both ways. This work of Hassler and Jung and others indicates that the relationship between cerebral cortex and thalamus is a very intimate one. Due to the representation of every area of the cerebral cortex in the thalamic nuclei and due to the double track circuit to and from the thalamus, no irritation of the cerebral cortex can take place without also irritating the thalamus. Therefore, the cortical gray and the subcortical gray might mutually influence each other. Clark showed that there is also an intimate two-way relationship between the frontal lobes and the hypothalamus. There is some difference on details but there is essential agreement that the most important frontal connections come from the dorsomedial nucleus of the thalamus. There are, however, also projections from other nuclei of the thalamus to the frontal lobes; e.g., from the anterior nucleus to the cingulate gyrus.

The efferent connections of the frontal lobe are much smaller. No retrograde degeneration after isolation of the prefrontal region has been found as yet, with the one exception of the anterior cingular area. There is much controversy with regard to the efferent fiber connections of the frontal lobe, which were studied extensively by Mettler in animals and by Meyer et al. in the brains of lobotomized patients. Also the intracortical short and long association systems are not yet well understood, and studies on psychosurgical materials have contributed little to our knowledge of these connections.

Clinicoanatomical correlations are the main point of interest in any discussion of psychosurgery. Earlier attempts to localize function in the frontal lobe, based on clinicopathological observations (Kleist and many others), were reviewed extensively by Freeman and Watts in the first edition of their monograph. Such observations of brain injury, tumors and other lesions were rarely limited to the prefrontal region. Therefore, their value for localization of function was necessarily limited. The data derived from psychosurgery have certainly contributed more to the understanding of the physiology of the frontal lobe than any previous work. This is true although neither prefrontal lobotomy as a blind operation nor even the open procedures permit an accurate appraisal of the actual cut made by the surgeon. The material collected by A. Meyer and his group has led to important insight into the clinicoanatomical relations. One of their conclusions was that cases with cuts totally or partially behind the granular cortex (so-called posterior cuts) present such undesirable symptoms as restlessness, vasomotor and trophic lesions of the skin, persistent incontinence of urine, nutritional deficiencies and respiratory failure. The patients often die from the late effects of the operation and, as a whole, have a much shorter survival time than those with exclusively prefrontal cuts. It is assumed these patients die due to impairment of their vegetative regulation. This is an assumption; the details of such a "vegetative" death are unknown. Furtado found a high late mortality rate in Moniz and Lima's first cases.

In Meyer's material, bilateral lesions of the granular frontal cortex cause characteristic personality changes, but there was no evidence of rigid localization of mental functions in selected areas of the frontal cortex. There was some slight positive correlation between the involvement of the orbital cortex and degree of personality changes, but these findings were overshadowed by the *quantitative* relationship between the degree of the personality change and the extent of prefrontal area isolated or ablated. Hoch as well as Kalinowsky emphasized that the operation is essentially a quantitative therapy. A few psychiatrists (Dax and his co-workers) saw some evidence in favor of specific functions in different areas, but most clinical experience with the various surgical methods supports the concept of a primarily quantitative relationship between personality changes and operation. McLardy and Meyer point out also that, among cases of equal prognostic potentialities, clinical improvement varies directly with the amount of prefrontal cortex isolated from its white matter. Their finding that the central segment is of prime importance is in agreement with the foregoing statement because the frontothalamic fibers collect in this region. The anatomical correlates of postoperative personality changes are roughly the same as those of clinical improvement, although it may be that isolation of the orbital cortex increases the personality changes, while the anterior cingular region (area 24) appears to play a small part in determining personality changes. As their work went on, Meyer's group began to regard the frontal lobe more and more as a functional entity, and a study based on 102 brains confirms that clinical improvement is related to the number of fibers severed rather than to any given location.

Pathological findings in brains of patients who have died early after prefrontal lobotomy has not shown anything unexpected. Freeman and Watts found that two weeks after operation, proliferation of blood vessels with increase of astrocytes and connective tissue results in the formation of a scar. Frequently, the head of the caudate nucleus is involved, and a cyst communicating with the ventricle has occasionally been found. The most common statement in all pathological reports on lobotomy material involves the variety of operative lesions, which was particularly stressed by Stengel and Carse. They stated that the actual anatomical findings after prefrontal lobotomy had little relation to what the surgeon, following Freeman and Watt's technique, did "or rather thought he had done." Some pathological studies as well as pneumoencephalographies (Donovan et al.) demonstrated cortical atrophy. A microscopic study by Yokoi led to interesting findings of gliosis in the pathways severed by the operation. The gliosis extended with the length of time after the operation.

It is not possible within the scope of this book to give a complete review of all the available clinical material and experimental findings referring to the effect of frontal lobe and other brain lesions on mental behavior. Much experimental work has been done without direct relation to clinical work in psychosurgery and actually preceded it. Ever since Fritsch and Hitzig associated the frontal lobe with mental behavior, physiologists have been interested in this problem. Ferrier had described the loss of active interest in their suroundings in monkeys whose frontal lobes had been extirpated; Bianchi noticed that unilateral destruction of the frontal lobe led to only negligible changes, while removal of this area on both sides was followed by definite changes in behavior. Such well documented cases as the one reported by Brickner showed that bilateral frontal lobe lesions cause more definite changes than unilateral ones. However, it should be noted that unilateral frontal lobectomy also leads to outspoken mental changes, as shown by Feuchtwanger, Goldstein, Kleist, and others. A thorough study of the type of personality changes which can be observed after unilateral frontal lobectomy was presented by Rylander and was later supplemented by the same author with studies on patients after prefrontal lobotomy.

Animal experimentation, on which Moniz' discovery was actually based, was done by Jacobsen, who demonstrated in his monkeys that even bilateral frontal lobe lesions interfered little with intelligence. However, the animals showed very pronounced emotional changes. Such monkeys, contrary to normal experimental animals, were "quite impervious to any frustrating effect of errors." They failed to show any pleasure when they succeeded with experimental tasks, and no displeasure in case of failure. The analogy between these observations and the experience in psychosurgery is obvious. More recent animal experiments were stimulated by special problems connected with clinical work in psychosurgery. Thus, Freudenberg et al. observed the effect of partial leucotomy on monkeys of the Rhesus macaque type. The greatest contributions to the physiology of the frontal lobes have undoubtedly been made by work on lobotomized patients rather than by animal experimentation. The physiological and psychological observations obtained on patients who have undergone frontal lobotomy and similar brain operations will be presented in later sections.

Various Techniques in Psychosurgery

The psychiatrist should be acquainted with the different surgical procedures used in psychosurgery. He must be able to discuss with the neurosurgeon the proper indications for and especially the extent of the cut to be performed. A great number of methods have been used contributing considerably to our knowledge in this field. Some were only technical modifications, others differ in their clinical effect. In their survey on the various neurosurgical procedures Falconer and Schurr emphasized the need for good team work between psychiatrist and neurosurgeon.

Moniz and Lima's Original Method (Prefrontal Leucotomy)

This technique will be described briefly not only because of its historical interest but because it is apparently still being used in some countries as a smaller operation. Burr holes are made 3 cm. lateral to the midline and 3 cm. in front of the auricular line. While originally alcohol was used for the destruction of brain tissue, later on a leucotome was inserted. This is first done in the anteromedial direction and several spherical incisions are made. Then the leucotome is removed and reintroduced in an anterolateral direction, where again spherical cuts are made. The original instrument used by Moniz and Lima had a wire loop which protruded when pressed upon. With this instrument the scores were cut in various depths of the white matter in both hemispheres.

Standard Lobotomy by Freeman and Watts

The standard operation is a "blind" procedure performed through small lateral burr holes. The white matter in both frontal lobes is sectioned in the plane of the coronal suture directly down to the sphenoidal ridge. The operation is performed under local anesthesia where this is possible; in disturbed patients general anesthesia is usually applied. The coronal suture which crosses the midline 13 cm. from the glabella, is outlined on the skull. Its lower end lies at a point 6 cm. superior to the zygoma and 3 cm. posterior to the lateral rim of the orbit. An incision 5 cm. long is made over the lower end of the coronal suture following the plane of the suture. When the suture line is visible on the skull, a burr hole 1.5 cm. in diameter is made through its lower end, and the hole slightly enlarged with a rongeur. The same is done on the other side and a cannula inserted through a cortical incision in the left frontal lobe aiming at the opposite burr hole. Then the sphenoidal ridge, as the second landmark, is located by inserting the cannula towards the base of the skull at an angle of about 40 degrees with the sagittal plane; it usually strikes the sphenoidal ridge at a depth of 4 to 5 cm. In this plane the standard operation is performed by introducing the leucotome and making sweeping movements of 30 to 40 degrees with a radius of 4.5 cm. The incisions are then deepened toward the midline and orbital cortex by radial stab incisions. The same is done on the other hemisphere. The location of the incisions is verified by the injection of 0.5 cc. lipiodol.

A more radical operation was used when patients had been sick for a long time, or had failed under a standard lobotomy. In this operation the cuts were performed posterior to the sphenoidal ridge. Freeman and Watts also described a minimal operation in the plane of their standard operation but omitting the incision into the upper quadrant. This "lower quadrant lobotomy" is one of many partial operations described in the next chapter.

Modified Lobotomies

Partial operations have been performed in order to arrive at a therapeutic effect with minimal damage. Unilateral prefrontal lobectomy was recommended in 1936 by Ody in Switzerland, who had a fair result in a schizophrenic patient. Since then unilateral lobotomies have been tried repeatedly for psychiatric conditions, but, as a whole, with limited success. The unilateral operation is often sufficient to relieve intractable pain (Scarff). Other partial operations are the bimedial operation (Greenblatt et al.), where only the two medial halves of the frontal lobe are cut; sections of the orbital areas only (Hofstetter et al., Reitman); and any other variety of partial cuts of the white matter of the frontal lobes (Carrillo), some of which will be discussed presently.

The only selective operation considered as having different effects is the isolation of the orbital lobes by Reitman. His triad of symptoms indicative of orbital lesions was extroversion, increased motor activity and euphoria. The best results, therefore, were obtained in patients with introversion, blockage, emotional dulling and depersonalization. Such symptoms as aggressiveness or any state of excitement are not markedly influenced by this operation (Egan). The majority of workers in the field saw only a quantitative difference between partial and complete lobotomies. During the last years the orbitomedial regions of the frontal lobes are considered perhaps the most important areas for the removal of emotional symptoms (Busch et al. in Denmark, Hirose in Japan, Le Beau in France and others).

Bimedial lobotomy by Greenblatt and Solomon is the best documented partial lobotomy in this country. It developed from the open operation by Poppen. The aversion of neurosurgeons against blind operations first led Lyerle in 1947, to operate with an osteoplastic flap. Our own material, without any fatality, seems to confirm the safety of this approach. The largest material of open operations was reported by Poppen who first paid special attention to the fibers in the inferior or orbital parts of the frontal lobes. The largest material operated by him, consisted of bimedial leucotomies, and the excellent results of these partial lobotomies were well documented in various publications by Greenblatt and his group.

In England, McKissock used both, the open and blind approach, in his rostral leucotomy, which largely corresponds to what is now known in the U. S. as the widely used pre-coronal lobotomy. His original blind rostral leucotomy is made just in front of the coronal suture. In a later modification the burr holes are made 5 or 6 cm. anterior to the coronal suture and 2 cm. lateral to the midline. The needle is passed to strike the orbital plate between its middle and anterior third, and is then angulated laterally 2 cm. at its tip. This "rostral leucotomy G." based on Grantham's work, concentrates on the inferior medial quadrants. Pippard prefers McKissock's original blind rostral leucotomy as superior and showing less intellectual damage than the "rostral leucotomy G." In a comparison with the standard operation Pippard showed that if a rostral leucotomy fails standard leucotomy offers no additional advantages.

In addition to surgical cuts chemical lobotomies have been tried. Aside from Moniz who used alcohol, Woringer injected 0.5 per cent uroselectane as necrotizing solution, and Mandl a 6 per cent phenol solution. Meyers et al. injected procaine. Attempts were made injecting first small amounts of chemicals, and if no clinical results were obtained, destroying further fibers with additional injections. Scherer and Winne injected procaine as a prognostic test for lobotomy.

Electrocoagulation as a means to destroy the ventromedial quadrant of both frontal lobes was introduced by Grantham in 1951. He first used it for the relief of intractable pain and later in psychiatric patients. This method is said to avoid two undesirable side-effects, the personality changes and convulsive seizures which might occur after other methods of lobotomy. The tips of the electrodes are passed to a point about 2 cm. of thc floor of the skull and their position checked by x-ray. Current is then applied to produce cylindric lesions 2 cm. long and 1.5 to 2 cm. in diameter. There was one fatality among the first 132 patients.

Favorable reports on patients operated upon with this technique were given by McIntyre et al. Ayd, in a more recent paper, published several years after introduction of the neuroleptic drugs, stresses the immediate results and the saving of expensive medication as factors which make this operation preferable to drug therapy in many instances.

Ultrasonic waves producing local necroses are used by Lindstrom and by Fry. Lindstrom et al. claim that such sonic treatment produces a functional alteration of prefrontal white matter without anatomical changes. The possibility of optic nerve damage which occurred in two cases in the beginning, is now considered to be eliminated. There is no chance of injuring vessels or to damage cortical tissue because the beam of high frequency sound will limit its effects in the white substance.

A stereotaxic "progressive leucotomy" is recommended by Crow et al., who insert many thin gold needles leaving them for several months and studying the effects of electric stimulation. When the most effective sites are found, they are electrocoagulated. Le Beau and Dondey test the effective sites by injecting a two-way cannula and cooling by evaporating liquid butane in stages, achieving first a reversible, and by cooling further, a destructive effect. According to Freeman, stereotaxic operations were also performed by Honda, as well as Sano in Japan. Turner severs fibers in the roof of the temporal horn, then, if relapses occur, he extends the incisions stereotaxically down through the hippocampus and the underlying formations. Noting in 1965 an increasing number of requests from psychiatrists for operations, this neurosurgeon now prefers for depressions and tension states a lower quadrant section which, for obsessional neuroses, is extended upwards, thus modifying the operation with the type of illness.

Cortical Operations

LOBECTOMY AND GYRECTOMY: While lobotomy concentrates on the interruption of the frontal pathways in the white matter, cortical operations were also attempted. Peyton et al. excised the frontal areas in an operation which they called "prefrontal lobectomy."

Limited cortical excisions were first promoted by Penfield et al. in the hope of sparing parts of the frontal cortex and thereby diminishing the sacrifices in the field of personality. Penfield carried out bilateral symmetrical removal of cortex in varying patterns, and called this operation "bilateral frontal gyrectomy." The ablations of cortex were carried out along fissure lines. All ablations were performed anterior to the coronal suture. Bilateral ablations of cortex in a superior mid-frontal zone produced confusion, incontinence, automatic movements and apathy, which disappeared slowly; this syndrome remained absent in more anterior ablations. The authors consider gyrectomy as a difficult, long and somewhat dangerous procedure. Their psychiatric evaluation has led to the conclusion that it is of no greater value than lobotomy and does not merit continuance.

TOPECTOMY: In 1948 a group of workers from various fields of science, the Columbia-Greystone Associates, reported on selected partial ablations of frontal cortex. The purpose of the study, which was conceived by the neuroanatomist, F. Mettler, was the evaluation of such selective ablations in human psychotic subjects. The operation, performed by J. Lawrence Pool, consisted of symmetrical excision of various areas of the frontal cortex, and was called "topectomy." The best results from this first Columbia-Greystone Project (which was followed by other investigations by the same group of workers) were obtained with the removal of Brodmann's areas 9, 10, and 46. The full effect of topectomy was not obtained unless the rostral part of area 9 and the caudal part of area 10 were included. Later, Pool as well as Hoch found that no one specified area of the frontal lobe governs the therapeutic results, and that the amount of brain substance removed was a decisive factor in the therapeutic outcome. Topectomies were also performed by the French neurosurgeon Le Beau and some others. It has now been mostly abandoned because the operation is technically difficult, and followed by a high rate of postoperative epilepsy.

CINGULECTOMY: This is another method of cortical extirpation recommended by Le Beau, and also independently by Whitty et al. It is a very complicated operation which makes it necessary to open up the great longitudinal fissure down to the corpus callosum. The anterior part of the cingulate gyrus on either side is then removed by subpial suction. It seems to produce a minimum of personality defects, and is supposed to be most valuable in obsessions, tensions and anxiety. Falconer and Schurr feel that this operation is relatively ineffective. On the other hand, Livingston finds a low surgical risk, high anatomical accuracy and good results with bilateral cingulate cortex isolation in the treatment of psychoses and neuroses. More recently, Cassidy et al. reported on a simpler closed cingulotomy with electrocoagulation. Cingulectomy is preferred by Lewin in obsessional neuroses, while he prefers orbital leucotomy in depressions.

CORTICAL UNDERCUTTING: An operation which seems to have found followers in many countries was introduced by Scoville under the name of "selective cortical undercutting." His technique makes it possible to detach certain areas of the frontal cortex by making a line of cleavage to the relatively avascular junction of gray and white matter by means of a suction tip and spatula, thus interrupting the long association fibers of the overlying cortex.

The following advantages over cortical ablations are given by Scoville. The undercutting can be accomplished through a 1½ or 2 inch trephine bone button in one hour's time as compared to three or four hours for cortical ablations through a bilateral cranioplastic flap. It requires only a 2 or 3 cm. straight cortical incision to accomplish the undercutting of an area 6 cm. by 4 cm. or larger, leaving no raw, exposed surface, and does not interfere with the blood supply to adjacent areas. It should lessen the incidence of epilepsy and no large vessels have to be interrupted. Cortical undercutting has been performed in three different areas: the anterior medio-lateral surface of the frontal lobes (Brodmann's areas 9 and 10), the orbital surface, and the medial surface of the brain cingulate gyrus.

The most interesting conclusion of Scoville's work was that almost identical therapeutic results were obtained with undercutting of these different areas, but he later felt that anterior (superior) undercutting is not only less effective but also most liable to produce undesirable personality changes. The medial operation is technically complicated. The best results with the least side-effects were obtained with orbital undercutting as it was performed by Tow and Lewin and other English workers.

Another technique of "Restricted Orbital Undercutting" was described in England by Knight. An extensive follow-up study of his material was undertaken by Sykes and Treadgold in 1964. Perhaps the deathrate for this operation of 1.5 per cent and convulsions in 16% were higher than expected, but behavior changes were found in only 5% of the cases.

In Japan, Hirose has done outstanding work with orbito-ventromedial undercutting. The cut with this supraorbital approach involves the gyrus orbitalis medialis, gyrus rectus, and the small inferior part of the medial surface which contains the gyrus supraorbitalis and maybe a small part of the gyrus cinguli. This operation differs from Scoville's undercutting in that the cuts made by Hirose are much more restricted and produce less confusional states and other side-effects. The area of operation also differs from Knight's stereotactic operation of the orbitomedial quadrants. Both obtained the same favorable results, and both have selected their material very carefully.

In elderly patients with depressions who are more and more considered excellent candidates for psychosurgery, Knight noticed a greater mortality if the subjects were weak and frail. In this group he, therefore, recommends a "stereotactic tractotomy" of the substantia inomminata below the head of the caudate nucleus. Such stereotactic operations avoid infarction or hemorrhage in the region of the striatum, thus eliminating the after-effects of such an involvement seen in other operations. He implants seeds of radioactive yttrium Y.90, which only produces a symptomatic effect up to 3 mm. from the seed's surface. Under x-ray control rows of radioactive seeds were implanted in the substantia innominata. The lesions are approximately 2 cm. long, 1 cm. wide and ½ cm. in vertical extent bilaterally. These small lesions prove harmless and fully beneficial. In 130 cases no mortality and no persistent post-traumatic epilepsy occurred. Some patients were in their eighties, and the results compared well with open psychosurgical interventions.

Thalamotomy

Interruption of frontothalamic connections is usually considered the purpose of all psychosurgical procedures. This can be performed on the cortical level, in the white matter connecting frontal cortex and thalamus, and finally on the thalamus itself. Such "thalamotomy" was first conceived by Spiegel and performed by Wycis. In order to overcome the variability of the skull, they used as a roentgenographic landmark the pineal gland, or, if this were not calcified, the suprapineal recess, demonstrated by means of pneumoencephalography. The stereotaxic techniques of Horsley and Clark, used for a long time in animal experiments, were applied in this operation. The instrument used by Spiegel and Wycis, which they call stereoencephalotome, can be fitted to each individual skull and permits precise localization of areas within the skull. Lesions in the dorsomedial nucleus of the thalamus are made by electrolysis, using direct current, or by electrocoagulation. Lesions were also made in the hypothalamus ("hypothalamotomy"). The advantage of this method is said to be the absence of undesirable personality changes and also of postoperative convulsions. The results in the hands of the originators of the method were favorable. No clinical reports from other workers are available, except from Baudouin and Puech, who perform thalamotomies from a temporal trephine opening. Recently Spiegel et al. reported success with thalamotomy in lobotomy failures.

Transorbital Lobotomy

A route different from the operations described so far was used by Fiamberti. In 1937, he proposed the transorbital approach to the frontal lobes, which had been previously used for ventriculography in Italy. Freeman must be credited with the wider application of this technique, which, contrary to all other procedures, can be performed by the psychiatrist himself. The method is simple and the recovery period short. On Freeman's suggestion, anesthesia was given by means of several electrically induced convulsions, a technique for which the psychiatrist is better equipped than for other methods of general anesthesia. Another reason for Freeman's preference for this anesthetic is his assumption that the convulsions disorganize cortical patterns underlying the psychosis and that the operative cuts prevent these patterns from reforming. The patient is given two electric shock treatments, which permit operation on one side. He then receives a third electric shock treatment, or, if he becomes restless, even a fourth before the second side is done.

The technique of transorbital lobotomy is as follows: The upper eye lid is lifted away from the eye ball, and the point of a leucotome introduced into the conjunctival sac until it rests in the vault of the orbit. This is usually 3 cm.

from the midline. The shaft of the instrument is aimed parallel to the bony ridge of the nose and the base of the instrument driven with a hammer through the orbital plate. At a depth of 5 cm. from the margin of the upper eye lid, i.e., 3 cm. within the frontal lobe, the handle is moved as far laterally as the orbit will permit. This movement severs the basal portion of the thalamofrontal fibers. Returned to the midline, the instrument is then driven until a 7 cm. mark is reached and the handle is moved 20 degrees medially and 30 degrees laterally in order to sever the superior portion of the thalamofrontal radiation, which is supposed to be that part underlying areas 9 and 10 of Brodmann. To these two cuts Freeman later added a "deep frontal cut." The deep frontal cut is performed when the handle of the instrument is in the lateral position at the 7 cm. mark. At this moment the handle is strongly elevated until the shaft lies as nearly parallel as possible to the orbital plate. From this position the handle is then returned to the parasagittal plane and withdrawn. The operation is always performed on both sides.

Sometimes it is difficult to withdraw the instrument when the bone is very thick. Therefore, Moore replaced Freeman's "ice-pick-like" instrument with a "transorbitoma" whose shaft is elliptical in cross section and has a gentle increase in caliber from the point of the hilt, thus preventing the instrument from running through the orbital plate too fast when struck with a mallet, and also allowing easy removal. The instrument also has an extension arm which permits one to visualize the movements of the instrument on the surface of the skull.

Postoperative care is minimal. The operative area is considered sterile, yet sulfadiazine, 1.0 Gm. every four hours for four doses, is usually given. Edema and ecchymosis of varying degree develop and small compresses are therefore applied to the eye lids prophylactically if the patient is cooperative. Vomiting occurs in a fair percentage of cases, but inertia, incontinence, and other postoperative symptoms as seen after standard lobotomy are usually not observed.

Complications are undoubtedly rarer than in other procedures. This is particularly true for convulsions. The lesser degree of personality changes will be discussed later. Operative deaths are less frequent; Freeman reported 3 per cent mortality in the standard lobotomy, as compared to 1 per cent with the transorbital approach.

In the hands of Freeman as well as Moore, the technique of transorbital lobotomy has shown results which come close to, and, in a report by Freeman, even surpass the results of standard lobotomy. In the second edition of their book, Watts disagrees with Freeman. Our own limited experience with transorbital lobotomies was unsatisfactory, but maybe our cuts were less extensive than those by workers who report good results (Freeman, Moore, Jones, Shanklin, and Freyhan). Different consistency of the brain and the possibility that the entire brain is moved by the instrument rather than cut, were mentioned by Edwards as factors that make it difficult to judge the extent of the lesion. Stender reported injections of the patient's own blood into the brain by the transorbital cut.

Parietal, Temporal and Occipital Lobotomies

Evidence from experience with psychosurgery weighs heavily against specific function of certain areas in the frontal lobes. The further question arises of how far destruction of other cortical areas and their pathways leads to changes similar to those of frontal lobe operations.

Parietal lobotomies were performed by Yahn et al. They operated on the parietal lobe in order to interrupt the pathways running from the frontal to the occipital lobe (fasciculus longitudinalis superior) in a place where section of the frontothalamic fibers could be avoided. The results, although not entirely negative, were unsatisfactory, but it is difficult to draw conclusions from their material because most of their cases also had failed under a previous prefrontal leucotomy.

Temporal lobotomy was practiced by Obrador. He based his attempts on the animal experiments by Klüver and Bucy, who had shown that bilateral removal produced profound changes in emotional behavior. Obrador penetrated 4-5 cm. through a temporary burr hole in order to reach the uncus and beginning of the hippocampus, and to attack the "circuit of emotions" described by Papez. The operation gave favorable results in cases that had not benefited from a preceding prefrontal lobotomy. A patient in whom the symptoms reappeared after a few days was benefited by subsequent prefrontal lobotomy. A patient under our own observation had vivid auditory hallucinations as the only symptom; a bilateral temporal lobotomy did not make the voices disappear, but a subsequent topectomy of the frontal lobe also failed to improve the patient's condition.

Operations on the temporal lobe, particularly anterior temporal lobectomies were performed for psychomotor epilepsy. Falconer and Schurr gave a survey on this work by Hill et al., and some others. They showed that the aggressive outbursts mostly respond to this operation, while paranoid. depressive and other symptoms remain unchanged.

An interesting experiment was made by Freeman and Williams who operated on the amygdaloid nuclei for the removal of auditory hallucinations; but it seems that this approach was not continued.

Torkildsen performed occipital lobotomy on a blind deteriorated patient who had destroyed his eyes following orders from his "voices." There was no improvement, the patient's hallucinations continuing, and a subsequent prefrontal lobotomy also failed to bring about any change.

The material presented from these operations outside of the frontal lobe is too meager to answer the question of how far such operations can be effective. The effect on some individual cases with gun shot wounds through these areas seemed to favor the idea that the changes observed after prefrontal lobotomy are not specific for the frontal lobe. However, even if the evidence presented in psychosurgery in other than frontal areas were more convincing, the frontal lobes—as neurologically "mute" areas—still would be the site of choice for this form of therapy.

Complications

The most frequent complications are operative hemorrhages. They may occur during the operation, when they can usually be easily taken care of if the operation is performed under direct vision. In blind operations they are treated by enlargement of the trephine opening.

Neurological focal signs must always be regarded as complications. It has been mentioned that these signs may be due to cuts placed too far posteriorly, involving the motor area or the basal ganglia. But if they occur only some time after the operation they are usually due to hemorrhage, or, less frequently, to an infection. Sjoekvist et al. demonstrated such hemorrhages by displacement of the injected lipiodol. Occasionally hemorrhage also occurs in less extensive operations, such as transorbital lobotomy. We saw such hemorrhage in a transorbital case which later came to autopsy due to pulmonary embolism. In a second case which later was explored surgically, the hemorrhage could be diagnosed from hemiparetic symptoms developing shortly after the procedure. Infection after lobotomy may consist of infection of the wound itself, or of brain abscess or meningitis. Infections are well controlled with antibiotics. In some cases, meningism was observed a few days after the operation but cleared up spontaneously. Some workers have been impressed by the frequency of edema of the legs and bullae and other trophic disturbances in lobotomized patients.

Convulsive seizures are the most frequent complications after psychosurgery. They mostly occur a few months or even years after the operation and are usually few in number. Many patients have but one convulsion, or perhaps two to three, within a few days, and never again show this symptom even if they are not placed under anticonvulsive medication. They are never very numerous in any patient. They cannot be predicted because it has been shown that patients with a preoperative abnormal EEG are not predisposed to seizures. An incidence of 3.3 per cent was reported in the series of 1000 leucotomies reported by the English Board of Controls. It appears that this figure is unusually low, and that the reported occurrence of seizures is higher in most individual follow-ups. Dax noticed that the larger the cortical damage, the more frequent the attacks. He also found that convulsions are favored by damage to the upper parts of the frontal lobes. Topectomy, which produces a larger cortical scar, leads to a higher incidence of seizures. Dilantin is used routinely after the operation to prevent the occurrence of seizures (1½ grains, three times a day for about a year).

Fatalities are extremely rare after open operations, more frequent with closed procedures. Freeman and Watts reported a mortality rate of 3 per cent. In transorbital lobotomies, Freeman had a death rate of only 1 per cent, Edwards more than 2 per cent. The English Board of Controls had reported 3 per cent operative and another 3 per cent postoperative deaths in closed prefrontal lobotomies. Later Maclay reported from the same hospital group a death rate of only 2 per cent. Many of these complications occurred in large mental institutions. In our own material operated on in specialized neurosurgical setups by Scarff, Pool, Ransohoff, no fatalities have occurred.

Postoperative Course

The immediate postoperative course is mainly a surgical problem. It depends on the type of operation performed. After a standard lobotomy the patient is usually deeply confused. Patients after less extensive operations, are sometimes surprisingly well-oriented, and patients after transorbital lobotomies often show hardly any disorientation. After standard lobotomies, patients persistently deny that they have been operated on and give the most far-fetched explanations for their head bandage. The temperature after lobotomy is moderately elevated. The patient's inertia is often very pronounced and may prevent him from moving at all; this, and the often shallow respiration, may result in pulmonary atelectasis.

Some patients are temporarily incontinent for urine. It is a rare occurrence in patients with well preserved personality and after smaller operations. There is no evidence that incontinence depends on any lesion of a bladder center in the frontal lobe. It is felt by some that the incontinence is part of a general psychological behavior. Rinkel et al. examined incontinent lobotomized patients cystometrically and found a hypertonic spastic bladder which they explained as being due to the surgical liberation of the autonomic nervous system from supranuclear inhibitory centers. In Partridge's careful follow-up studies the frequency of occasional urinary incontinence was 9 per cent after six months, 4.6 per cent after twelve months, and 3.2 per cent after two years. The smaller operations done nowadays eliminated incontinence as a problem except for the first postoperative days.

Various papers deal with the nursing requirements after lobotomy (Behnken and Merrill, Carse).

Physiological Changes

Physiological changes after lobotomy and other psychosurgical methods are unimpressive, and the return to a hemeostatic equilibrium is surprising. This was particularly well demonstrated after topectomy in the Columbia-Greystone Project; all physiological changes were studied closely, and where changes did occur they were rather transitory.

Body weight shows the most striking changes in patients after psychosurgical interventions. The changes are not so clearly related to the clinical improvement as they are in shock therapy. Some patients improve without gaining weight; others gain much weight without improving. Lobotomized patients often eat ravenously, a phenomenon which is not limited to the immediate postoperative period but can still be observed after years. This occurs not only in patients who are deteriorated and without any concern for their appearance but even in some with negligible personality changes who are displeased with their gain of weight. Partridge found increase of weight in 90 per cent of his cases. In two-thirds of these patients the excessive gain began to disappear after a while and their weight leveled off (although usually remaining above the premorbid normal) before the first postoperative year was over.

Sleep is known to be disturbed in the great majority of those mental patients who are candidates for lobotomy. It is, therefore, remarkable that it was restored to normal in 90 per cent of the cases, according to Partridge.

Menstruation, which is also often disturbed in psychotics, became regular in 15 out of 19 lobotomized women, in which it had been irregular or absent prior to the operation.

The relationship of frontal lobe surgery to the autonomic nervous system in man found special attention on the part of Rinkel et al. Studies of the peripheral sympathetic nervous system with intravenous injection of epinephrine hydrochloride, and of the parasympathetic system with stimulation of the carotid sinus reflex in lobotomized patients showed an overreaction of the autonomic nervous system to direct stimulation, but the autonomic equilibrium was re-established after some time. Epinephrine also lowered the skin temperature in lobotomized patients more than in controls (Fairman et al.).

Electroencephalographic studies after lobotomy are available in a fair number. The scarcity of changes was demonstrated in the first study made by Davis. Immediate postoperative electroencephalograms show high-voltage, slow waves in both frontal leads, hyperactivity to hyperventilation, and in some cases one to three months later short sequences of 6 per sec. activity of moderate amplitude. In most cases, the abnormal pattern disappeared within one to three months. Other workers (Greville and Last, Stevens and Mosovich) found that in the majority of cases electroencephalographic changes persist for a considerable length of time. According to Levin et al., slow activity is diffuse during the drowsy postoperative state, but when somnolence disappears the slow activity becomes concentrated frontally and may persist for years. In topectomies, Zingarelli also demonstrated slowing, but in some cases the EEG did not show any abnormalities at all. In transorbital lobotomy, usually no electroencephalographic changes are found. The interesting problem of how far postoperative convulsions can be predicted from the electroencephalogram has been answered by most authors in the negative. There is no evidence that those patients who show an abnormal EEG for a longer period of time after the operation will develop seizures later on. Adams et al. found progressive electroencephalographical changes in the sense of frontal asynchrony and slow activity which became constant only after three years; they assume that this was due to delayed degeneration of commissural fibers linking nuclei of the left and right thalamus.

Neurological focal signs are conspicuously absent after prefontal lobotomy as well as after partial ablations of the frontal cortex. Where they occur, they are temporary and probably caused by such complicating factors as hemorrhage, inadvertent extension of the cut beyond the proposed area or edema. Slight hemiparesis or paresis, pathological reflexes (mostly on one side), aphasia and various syndromes referable to the basal ganglia (masked facies, plateau speech) may be present for a short time.

In the topectomy material studied by the Columbia-Greystone workers, special attention was paid to neurological changes. The most striking finding was the absence of certain symptoms as, for instance, aphasia after bilateral removal of Broca's area.

Sensory function is most strikingly changed in the field of pain perception. However, there is no actual loss of sensory perception in any particular area of distribution of sensory pathways. What is impaired is a more complicated and not yet fully understood mental process of attachment or detachment which modifies the primary sensory perception into a secondary awareness of caring or not caring (Hoch). It is this change in the patient's reaction to his pain which suggested to Freeman and Watts the use of prefrontal lobotomy in cases of intractable pain. It has been found that the less extensive operations are often sufficient ("minimal operation" of Freeman and Watts; "unilateral lobotomy" of Scarff). It may be mentioned that in lobotomized patients the perception of applied pain, for example in the usual sensitivity test to a needle, is not only preserved but the reaction of the patient to painful stimuli is even accentuated. This latter mechanism parallels the exaggerated reactivity of lobotomized patients to all types of stimuli, which has been tested in various ways.

Psychological Changes

The much feared personality changes which were a frequent side-effect of the larger standard lobotomies, are no longer noticeable in the type of patient selected today for the newly devised smaller operations. The fear of personality changes is still the main reason for the reluctance on the part of many psychiatrists to recommend psychosurgery. All those working in this field and seeing the remarkable clinical results, regret this attitude by physicians who never had any contact with actual cases.

The previous practical importance of frontal lobe personality changes and their great theoretical interest suggests their intensive discussion in this book. It was surprising that even in patients with obvious personality changes psychological tests did not reveal any impairment in the performance of lobotomized patients. It soon became obvious that our available psychological tests are not fitted to measure the types of changes offered by these patients, and that careful clinical observations—including the patient's behavior in all possible life situations—is necessary for a full appraisal of his personality changes. In the following discussion, psychological test findings will be dealt with only briefly; more space will be given to conclusions gained from interviews with the patient and with those who have lived with him. It has been recognized, now, that many personality changes attributed to the operation were due to the schizophrenic process. They are almost absent after the newer limited operations in the type of non-deteriorated cases that are now considered the best candidates for psychosurgery.

Psychological tests for psychosurgical patients were first used by Hunt in Freeman and Watts' material. Psychometric testing of the patient's intellectual abilities revealed no obvious decrease in intelligence. Performance was slow and inaccurate during the first weeks after the operation, but this impairment was largely regained after a few months. Often responses were better than before, which is easily explained by the relief from psychotic or neurotic symptoms which had interfered with the performance of these tests before the operation. These original findings by Hunt, obtained with a battery of 15 tests, were confirmed by a great number of other psychologists The only change observed was some difference in the patient's behavior during the test. It is understandable, therefore, that such performance tests as the Rorschach, although failing to show changes in quantitative records, showed qualitatively fewer neurotic trends, less concern over performance, less self-criticism and other changes of behavior. According to Grassi, a graphic Rorschach (which differs from the verbal Rorschach in that it requests the individual to sketch the impressions he just described) revealed impairment of abstract organization and inability to shift from a concrete to an abstract approach. This impairment, also shown in the Grassi block substitution test, disappeared almost entirely within the first year.

Freudenberg and Robertson found a significant loss on the Kohs' block test, the Bender Gestalt test, and on the "Paired Association" test. Lobotomized patients gained considerably less than a control group on sorting tests. A test that shows some changes after the operation is the Maze test (Porteus and Peters). Rylander as well as Petrie was able to find a reduction of the I.Q. with the usual psychometric testing. Landis, Zubin, et al. tested topectomized patients. Most of the changes disappeared about four months after the operation. The number of transient changes was greatest in selected ablations of the frontal cortex near the motor area, and decreased as one moved forward from agranular to granular cortex.

The first attempt to adjust psychological concepts to the clinically observed behavior changes was Halstead's introduction of his concept of "biological intelligence." In a special category or grouping test, the subject is required to grasp or comprehend essential similarities or differences in test figures presented in a multiple choice situation by means of a special production apparatus. However, it was seen again that the test devised by Halstead showed very little impairment. Goldstein stated that only those capacities are impaired which require the abstract attitude, while those which can be performed in a concrete way are intact. The Greystone-Columbia investigators found no impairment of the abstract attitude after topectomy.

Personality tests devised specifically for the changes after psychosurgery were introduced by Robinson. She worked on Freeman and Watts' material and based her tests on man's "sense of his own self-continuity." Such self-continuity, the duration of one's essential identity through changing experiences, is basic to all personality development. A high degree of self-continuity leads to tensions and, in some circumstances, to mental symptoms. Her hypothesis is that psychosurgery alters the structure of the self in reducing self-continuity. In the Robinson-Freeman Self-regarding Span Test, the patient is directed to talk about a certain subject, and later about himself, as long as he can. In the Robinson-Freeman Sensibility Questionnaire, the patient is asked such questions as whether he worries about the future, whether he feels hurt easily, what embarrasses him, and so on. Lobotomized patients are not able to speak about themselves for the same length of time as are emotionally upset patients prior to the lobotomy. It is obvious that such tests come closer to the simple psychiatric interview technique than to an objective psychological test.

A most extensive psychological study was published by Tow on the previously used frontal leucotomy in the plane of the coronal suture. His patients who were tested before and after the operation, showed reduction of intelligence, vocabulary, flexibility and especially abstraction ability among other findings. Qualitative changes include lack of perseverance, irritability, inability of the patient to fix more than one concept in his mind at the same time. Indecisiveness and rigidity of attitude were seen particularly in the "sorting test," when, having discovered one principal of sorting, the patient was unable to pass on from this to a new one. Where the patient has to conform to a certain pattern the performance approximated more nearly the preoperative performance than in a completely unstructured situation such as the writing of an autobiography. The author concludes that there is an impairment of the powers of abstraction and of synthesis; of perception of relations and differences; of the ability to deal with complex situations, planning and thinking out of the next action and its consequences; and of appreciation of one's own mistakes.

Personality changes, although rare today, will still be described in some detail because of their clinical interest. They are more noticeable when the patient is observed in his daily life, in his contacts with his family, on the job, and in his spare time. Rylander was the first to describe these changes, when he wrote of patients who had undergone unilateral frontal lobectomy that their behavior is most embarrassing to the relatives, who are the best judges of these changes. The relatives of one of Stroem-Olsen's patients made the classic statement: "For him the operation did miracles, if we only did not have to live with him."

Many contrasting traits enter into the patient's postoperative personality. It will be shown later, on the basis of some instances, how the operation in different individuals can lead to entirely different reactions to certain problems or situations. This explains why listings of postoperative changes contain so many different and apparently contradictory features. The observations of Greenblatt et al. on the material of the Boston Psychopathic Hospital show the above-mentioned especially clearly. Hoch found that the most conspicuous damage from the operation was a certain inertia or apathy. The patient shows little sustained effort especially concerning intellectual performance, or drive to creative achievement. Sublimated tendencies are impaired; there is very little anticipatory goal-setting present, and no foresight. A "don't care" attitude, day to day living in happy equanimity is seen. Depth of emotional experience is reduced. Social sentiments are also often impaired.

The most rewarding effort to understand what is changed in these patients was made by Partridge. His study to which frequent reference is made, is based on 300 cases, all of whom were personally seen by the author before and after operation regardless of time and distance. Partridge summarized the postoperative personality in the following way: "The trends are towards a lowered postoperative drive. On the affective side, this is paralleled by a reduction in the intensity of emotional experiences. The net effect is to make the patient on the whole less responsive. This is chiefly noticeable in such more rather than less subtle ways as diminished appreciation and sense of obligation and considerateness. The patient is thus slightly more primitive, less critical of himself, of things, and of other people. The reduction in self-criticism leads to an increase of confidence and to a loss of self-consciousness, and therefore to an increased extraversion. The tendency of the extraversion is toward the comfortable and the pleasurable, with an avoidance of difficulty and effort. The patients tend intellectually to be more empty, with restricted interests and simpler satisfactions."

All postoperative personality changes are more noticeable at home than in the presence of strangers, for whom the patient keeps up an appearance. In patients in whom schizophrenic deterioration can be ruled out, these postoperative changes are often hardly noticeable even with larger operations.

It is now in order to discuss the patient's behavior in various given situations. Much emphasis has been placed on his ability to seek employment or to hold a job. Our own experience has convinced us that employment as a measure of the patient's condition is not too revealing. Many of our patients who have shown rather poor results are employed in some family enterprise or by friends who, for various motives, are willing to put up with their shortcomings. They are often late for work or do not show up at all on days when they do not feel like working. In spite of this, we agree with Freeman and Watts that the fair number of patients who make an occupational adjustment after severe mental illness plus a mutilating brain operation is a proof for the efficacy of the operation.

Such typical postoperative symptoms as lack of inhibition may lead to rather contrasting changes. A patient who had been prevented by his neurotic inhibitions from expressing his feelings may postoperatively become quite outspoken; another neurotic patient, with a very aggressive personality, driven by his ambitions, may become much more pleasant and contented than he had ever been before. The complicated interplay between the patient's prepsychotic personality, the mental abnormality for which he is operated on, and the surgical interference with frontal lobe function explains why only very thorough evaluation of the various factors can make it possible to predict whether, for instance, an alcoholic after lobotomy will drink less or, on the contrary, drink in an even more uninhibited way. If he drank because of some tension, he will probably stop drinking because he feels no need for it any more. If he drank for other reasons, the loss of restraint might make him drink with less inhibition. The interplay between the "lower drive, the lessened restraint and the simpler mentation" (Partridge) acts in rather different ways on the personality of operated patients.

A few aspects which led to some special investigations may be discussed briefly. Frank noticed the disappearance of dreams as well as day dreams after lobotomies. The same was seen by Piehler, who found that the absence of dreams is not permanent, but that when they return their intensity had faded, and that the mood derived from the dream, which usually persists after the awakening, is less differentiated than in normals. The patient's lack of emotional response and of fantasy life, his failure to reproduce memories, and the lesser affective charge of dream-producing unconscious conflicts may be responsible for this phenomenon.

The effect of psychosurgery on sexual activity seems to be less of a problem than would be expected after an operation that removes inhibitions. It appears that the sexual urge is reduced in many patients, and therefore complaints of unrestrained sexual behavior are rare. Patients who have had neurotic difficulties in their sexual relations often find better sexual adjustment and gratification than ever before. The unexpectedly rare occurrence of indecency led Rüsken to the conclusion that sex behavior, including inhibitions and taboos, is so deep-rooted that it is not easily influenced by such personality changes as caused by lobotomy. There is no evidence that latent homosexuality, which is supposed to be frequent in schizophrenics, becomes overt after psychosurgery. Freeman observed some patients whose sexual activity increased shortly after the operation but subsided to normal levels within a few months. Some of Piehler's patients reported that fantasies leading to masturbation had become less pronounced, and that masturbation therefore could be more easily suppressed.

Some authors have paid special attention to the patient's creative ability. Reitman describes what he calls a "creative spell." This occurs quite unexpectedly shortly after the operation in some patients who had never been artistically inclined. This phenomenon dies out quickly after a few weeks or months, when the patients show the lack of creative artistry which in an early report was described by Freeman and Watts as one of the main features of the postoperative state, and which was again studied by Dax, Ashby, and Bassett. No loss has been found in copying, but original artist's work was impossible even for those who had such abilities before the operation. Two of Dax's patients complained that they had lost the "vividness" of their concepts or could not put things down, although they could see them.

Some reports suggest that the attitude toward religion suffers as a result of lobotomy. Others describe patients who became more interested in religion after lobotomy. In many instances the attitude toward religion remains unaffected. It can be assumed that, like all feelings, the religious feeling also becomes somewhat shallower, and Rüsken stressed the quite unproblematic attitude of these patients regarding "Weltanschauung" and religion. It is probable that a negative attitude toward religion will appear only in patients who had such a negative attitude before the operation but were hiding it. In others a more positive attitude which had been kept inside, will be displayed more freely. This example, like many others, shows that the operation may affect the same personality feature in entirely different ways. As a whole, in many respects lobotomy acts as a "revealer rather than as an originator" (Stengel and Carse).

More recently tests were used to measure the improvement obtainable with psychosurgery. What Kral and Elidge describe as the operated patient's "emotional equilibrium on the basis of which he can function more satisfactorily," Levinson and Meyer's psychological testings define as lower scores on neuroticism and increase in extraversion. A different approach was taken by Kelly et al., based on increase in the forearm blood flow in chronic anxiety states. In patients after modified leucotomy they found a highly significant fall in forearm blood flow together with a fall in heart rate, blood pressure, as well as anxiety self-rating based on various rating scales.

Rehabilitation; Psychotherapy

Rehabilitation of the lobotomized patient seemed to be an obvious and promising task, and much discussion has been devoted to it ever since the beginning of work with psychosurgical methods. However, the opinion of different workers about the most likely methods of rehabilitation have varied considerably. It appeared to be a sound hypothesis that the time after lobotomy would offer good opportunities to build up the patient's personality along new lines, but Greenblatt pointed out the great difficulty in the selection of programs for the patient's rehabilitation.

Freeman recommends early discharge of the patient to his family. Few are in favor of such early discharge, and it is our belief that there is no necessity to discourage the family by the unpleasantness of the immediate postoperative state, which can hardly be a good basis for the re-establishment of finer human relations. It is understandable, therefore, that most workers prefer a longer rehabilitation period in the hospital as we do.

Some detailed programs have been worked out in private hospitals (Burlingame). Among the Boston Group, Hyde et al. have clearly demonstrated that certain patients improve under a program which includes careful planning of their activities and rectifying their deficiencies, but that others improve more readily when they are left alone without any pushing, persuasion, education or stimulation of aspiration. Time is a more important factor than anything we can offer these patients. Nevertheless, every effort should be made to help them in their readjustment, applying all modern methods of social psychiatry.

Lobotomized patients present problems so different from any other type of patient that special wards for them had been advised for the rehabilitation and, if feasible, vocational re-training of these patients in simple tasks. Here occupational therapy certainly has a very important task (Kalinowsky). The occupational therapist will learn better to deal with the special problems of these patients when he concentrates on work with them in special shops set up for them. They must be prodded more than the average psychiatric patient, and suggestions must be stronger even if the patient flares up occasionally.

Rehabilitation in the home is facilitated if the patient is discharged from a special ward or followed by the same social worker familiar with the quite specific problems of the family group. Much more attention should be given to the training of social workers along these lines because in the resocialization of these patients they can accomplish more than in many other groups of patients. Knowledge of the patient and his relatives before the operation enables the social worker during the postoperative stay in the hospital to prepare the family for the acceptance of the patient and his shortcomings, and later to straighten out difficulties when they arise after the patient has returned home. This can be best accomplished, if one and the same social worker follows the patient through all these stages.

The role of formal psychotherapy in the rehabilitation of the psychosurgical patient has been discussed but little. This is partly explained by lack of interest in and antagonism against psychosurgical procedures on the part of most psychotherapeutically interested psychiatrists. It has to be admitted, however, that psychotherapy in the true sense of the word has only limited possibilities for these patients, who may be quite suggestible but with whom a real transference relationship is difficult. Working with them in psychotherapy of any kind is a frustrating experience. Directive psychotherapy is hampered by the rapidity with which they forget any advice or admonition given them, and deep psychotherapy requires an emotional attitude which these patients lack. It was an early theoretical objection against lobotomy made by Roemer that the patient would feel no more urge to work out his problems in psychotherapy. This seems to be true in some way but few attempts have been made to work with these patients in any systematic manner. Hoch has pointed out that patients who undergo psychosurgery in general show unchanged dynamics after operation; but even though the basic structure is apparently unchanged, marked alterations are seen in the patient's behavior. This was shown by Cattell, who found that a certain suggestibility and the patient's dependence on the therapist are increased, with a more childlike quality. Dynamically, however, the patient is less malleable and is rather indifferent and inelastic in respect to interpretation. It is a challenging question as to how far there is still a need to change such a patient after the anxiety which was caused by his problems has been relieved in spite of the persistence of the problems.

Indications and Results

Psychosurgical procedures reduce anxiety and the emotional impact of delusions and other symptoms shown by many different psychiatric patients. This explains why psychosurgergy can be indicated in a great variety of psychiatric disorders. As a matter of fact, there are few chonic conditions in psychiatry, where brain surgery has not been tried. It is only lately that stricter indications have been agreed upon. The original experience was mostly obtained in schizophrenia which is no longer the primary indication for psychosurgery. This is partly due to the introduction of neuroleptic drugs, but also to the realization that deteriorated schizophrenics are poor candidates for frontal lobe surgery. The English surgeon McKissock, more recently, noticed the striking change in the type of clinical case referred for psychosurgery, and remarks "It seems evident that psychiatrists have now a fairly clear concept of the type of symptomatology or syndrome likely to be beneficially affected by the operation. This has been reflected in a marked diminution in the numebr of deteriorated schizophrenics offered for surgery, although a number of dangerous or disturbed patients are still referred and can often be adequately sedated by a standard prefrontal operation. There has been a corresponding increase in number of patients suffering from the symptoms of anxiety, tension, agitation and depression who have failed to respond to all the other accepted forms of treatment. It is in this group as well as in the obsessional states that limited leucotomies seem to produce eminently satisfactory, even if not perfect results." This statement, published in 1959 after several years of modern psychopharmacology reflects very well our own appraisal of the problem. After these general remarks indications and results in various psychiatric disorders will be discussed separately, and reference be made to some of the older concepts and their changes during recent years.

Schizophrenia

During the first years of experimentation with prefrontal lobotomy it was natural that the most hopeless cases were selected for this new procedure. As time went on, many experienced workers in the field realized that deterioration cannot be stopped by lobotomy, and that it is of ominous prognostic significance for the outcome of an operation. It soon became obvious that the least deteriorated patients offered the best prognosis and the least side-effects. The introduction of neuroleptic drugs changed the picture even more radically. It was found that chronic disturbed schizophrenics were also the best candidates for pharmacotherapy. Some statements claimed that psychosurgery was a thing of the past. However, the usefulness of neuroleptic drugs has limitations. There are patients with unsatisfactory response, and there are others who do respond but refuse medication after discharge from the hospital. There are furthermore those who need such large amounts of the drugs that the side-effects make them uncomfortable or unable to lead a normal life. Therefore, psychosurgery continues to have a place in the treatment of schizophrenia in selected cases.

No patient should be considered for surgical procedures who has not been tried adequately on all other types of therapy. This was strongly emphasized by such an experienced authority on shock treatments as M. Müller in whose extensively treated schizophrenics still two-thirds could be listed as "improved" after the operation. Today it must be requested that pharmacotherapy has also been given an ample trial, especially in the chronic schizophrenics, where neuroleptics are the treatment of choice.

No steadfast rule can be established regarding the question of how early to operate. Adequate shock treatment can be applied well before one year of illness has elapsed. It is often difficult for the consultant who must decide on the indication for psychosurgery to judge whether the patient had adequate treatment. Too often patients have several series of 4 or 5 electric shocks, relapse each time, and are then considered as shock treatment failures. Such treatment must be regarded as inadequate, and we usually recommend an intensive course of ECT or combined insulin-electric shock in patients where we doubt the adequacy of the previous therapy. If no remission can be obtained, pharmacotherapy under proper supervision in the hospital followed by pharmacotherapy at home should be tried, and only if this fails should psychosurgery be considered.

The prognosis of psychosurgery in an individual schizophrenic depends on many factors. First to be mentioned is the prepsychotic personality, and this applies to the schizophrenic as well as to any other psychiatric patient subjected to psychosurgery. Schizophrenics, more often than other patients, have an inadequate personality to begin with. Even where the onset of the psychosis can be clearly determined (which is, of course, not always the case), the patient has frequently shown shortcomings and character traits detrimental to his postoperative prognosis. Patients who did not make a good working adjustment even before they became sick, and who were also unable to make a positive emotional or sexual adjustment, can hardly be expected to do so, even though their most disturbing symptoms are improved by lobotomy. A thorough evaluation of the patient's prepsychotic personality may avoid disappointments. Odegaard, however, warns that overemphasis on the importance of the prepsychotic personality can be deceiving. He believes that what is known as the permanent personality of the patient is often a superficial mask which serves as a cover for deeper layers of the mind which may emerge only postoperatively.

The most significant prognostic factor of unfavorable nature is the degree of deterioration. Psychosurgery does not improve emotional or intellectual deterioration. The personality changes caused by frontal lobe surgery are in some respects similar to the original mental changes of the schizophrenic patient, and it is often difficult to differentiate them. It is now generally realized that many of the personality changes in lobotomized patients had been wrongly attributed to the frontal lobe surgery, but that they are actually signs of schizophrenic deterioration.

In an individual case it is often difficult to determine how far the patient is deteriorated and how far the clinical picture is still reversible. A catatonic who has no contact with his surroundings may be either deteriorated or only blocked. In the latter case, the condition is still reversible. Various means are available to determine whether a chronic patient may still improve. A simple way is the "prognostic electric shock test" (Kalinowsky), which is based on the experience that even patients without lasting benefit from a full course of shock therapy are still apt to show a transitory improvement after 3 or 4 convulsions. Such positive response demonstrates that the patient's condition is still reversible. A negative response makes the reversibility of the psychotic syndrome questionable. Hoch and his co-workers have demonstrated the value of pharmacodynamic tests for the prognosis of psychosurgery.

The prognostic significance of the various schizophrenic symptoms for the outcome of psychosurgical methods has been studied intensively. Certain groups of symptoms are favorably influenced, while others are not influenced at all. Rees states that patients who exhibit any of the following symptoms to a marked degree, will benefit most from the operation: anxiety, groundless fears about the future, suicidal tendencies, self-mutilation, states of tension, destructiveness and attacks of uncontrollable violence. In the first edition of their book, Freeman and Watts give a list of symptoms and the frequency with which they are relieved by prefrontal lobotomy. This list is headed by introversion, preoccupation, and nervous tension. More informative is their primary prognostic criterion; namely, the degree of emotional tension in proportion to which success can be anticipated. This working hypothesis has proved most useful in the selection of cases for prefrontal lobotomy, although it should not be the only yardstick.

Certain symptoms which present an important indication for surgery may persist after the operation, though in an innocuous form. According to Stengel, hallucinations were unchanged in 117 out of 154 cases, reduced in 8, and eliminated in only 29. Delusions were unchanged in 116 patients out of 160, reduced in 22, eliminated in 22. When they reappear, they usually do not regain their earlier importance to the patient. He loses interest in them progressively, and after several years they may disappear for good; the importance of this observation on the dynamics of delusions and hallucinations is obvious. While Müller noticed that they hardly ever disappear, Freeman and Watts found disappearance of hallucinations in 18 out of 19 cases in their first listing of symptom responses. In our own experience, delusions and hallucinations often have not disappeared even in patients with favorable outcome.

Anxiety, frequent in schizophrenia as in many other psychiatric conditions, is more susceptible to psychosurgery than any other symptom. Where it is a dominating symptom, as in the pseudoneurotic form of schizophrenia (which will be discussed later), it makes for a particularly favorable prognosis. The same is true for obsessions, compulsions, tension, ruminations, physical symptoms, hypochondriacal preoccupations and other neurotic symptoms as they may occur in any schizophrenic.

Some symptoms which, as a whole, are considered to be of ominous prognostic significance in schizophrenia may disappear. This was seen with unexpected frequency in mannerisms and stereotypies. We observed that even giggling frequently disappeared, although the final outcome in most of these cases was poor because such symptoms as giggling, stereotypies, and mannerisms often appear only in far progressed and deteriorated cases. Müller felt that mannerisms and stereotypies can disappear as long as they are not yet automatisms, void of all emotional charge. Depression, usually of good prognosis with shock therapy, does not respond with the same reliability to psychosurgery. Depressive mood may persist postoperatively and even lead to suicidal attempts. In a group of patients in whom deep depersonalization was the primary symptom, Shorvon saw remarkable improvement in all cases. Freeman and Watts' listing of individual symptoms also notes depersonalization as one of the more favorable ones.

The most ominous prognostic signs for spontaneous as well as shock remissions are known to be long duration of illness and insidious onset of the psychosis. They are of lesser prognostic value in psychosurgery. Late paranoid schizophrenics usually develop their symptoms quite insidiously, and yet, contrary to their poor response to shock therapy, they do well under psychosurgery. The same is true for pseudoneurotic schizophrenics. In both these groups, also, the duration of illness is not necessarily of ominous significance; while in those types of schizophrenia which tend to deteriorate, the longer duration of sickness makes for an increasingly poor outcome.

In Partridge's opinion the chances for recovery are diminished after more than five years of illness. It also appears that delusions have a greater tendency to persist after lobotomy if they have previously become constant and firmly fixed. The less there are variations and fluctuations of the disease, the poorer the prognosis after psychosurgery, or, for that matter, after any other means of treatment. This is an important point against any set time limit. Extensive experience in diagnosis and prognostic evaluation is more necessary in the decision regarding the best time for psychosurgery than in any other part of psychiatric work.

Results. The difficulty of listing results statistically has been encountered in all types of psychiatric treatments. In psychosurgery, a statistical evaluation is even more uncertain because not the disorder in toto but certain symptom constellations are influenced. The terms "recovered," "much improved," "improved," and "unimproved" are difficult to apply to a treatment that reduces the intensity of certain symptoms, modifies the expression of others and, to make things even more complicated, can add new symptoms. Freeman and Watts list their results in two different ways: once according to occupational status, grouping the patients as "employed," "keeping house," "being inactive at home" and "remaining in an institution." This classification depends too much on the attitude of the family and the insistence of the psychiatrist on pushing patients into some kind of employment. The other grouping used by Freeman and Watts is the differentiation between "good," "fair," and "poor" results. This, of course, is quite subjective, and the literature on psychosurgery shows how many different definitions are given for these terms. Some statistics are based on the discharge rate from the hospital. This has been criticized because of the entirely different policies as to discharges and because of the different types of material in various hospitals.

Results should be listed from as many aspects as possible. A very informative attempt was made by Ström-Olsen, and Tow, who tabulated the social results separately in two groups: an institutional group operated on only for "nursing improvement," and a second ambulatory group operated on for "complete social rehabilitation." They furthermore classified the results in individual patients under different headings, such as "illness" (assessment of symptoms only), "status" (social adaptation at home or in the hospital), "work," "pleasure" (capacity for enjoyment), "bad features" (objectionable behavior trends). A fairly practical way of listing results is the use of a series of numbers, from 1 for excellent, to 5, meaning most unfavorable outcome, as it was done at the Brain Research Project of the New York State Psychiatric Institute. The shortcomings of the usual means of evaluating results led Sands and Malamud to the recommendation of a rating scale analysis for individual symptoms. Each patient is rated in terms of his own premorbid personality, then the quantity and direction of well-defined manifestations of his disease process can be studied. Such a rating scale approach was also used by Rothschild and Kaye in lobotomy material.

In spite of many difficulties the conclusions drawn from various statistics show a certain uniformity. In mixed schizophrenic material, most statistics from the time prior to the introduction of neuroleptic drugs show one-third of the patients as much improved and usefully employed, a second third as improved, mostly at home or as working patients in an institution; and another third unimproved. Clinically oriented psychiatrists will find that individual cases of their own experience and detailed reports as given in the monographs by Freeman and Watts, the Boston Group (Greenblatt et al.) and particularly by Partridge, contribute more to our knowledge than large statistics.

Subdividing schizophrenia into various subtypes some conclusions can be made. In chronic catatonic excitement the aggressive behavior and the often dangerous response to delusions and hallucinations can be reduced. "Periodic psychoses" have been studied by Jones and McCowan, who saw the periodicity disappear in a number of catatonics. They assume that cutting the connections between hypothalamus and cortex is responsible for interruption of periodicity. There are reports, however, that the patients suffering from periodic psychosis continue to show exacerbations after surgery, although they are less severe. Catatonic stupors show a much poorer result which is all the more regrettable as also available neuroplegic drugs have the least to offer in these cases. Reitman recommended an orbital cut as a means of increasing their initiative.

Paranoid schizophrenics are promising candidates. This is particularly true for the late paranoids, patients who develop delusions at the age of 40 years or more, and the group described by Kraepelin as paraphrenia. Their personality is usually well preserved, and their prepsychotic personality has often been good, particularly as to their work record. Some of these are among the best results in our lobotomy material.

Simple schizophrenics and hebephrenics who respond poorly to shock therapy as well as drugs have the same poor response to psychosurgery. The primary schizophrenic symptoms such as emotional flattening and disturbance of thinking, dominate the picture and there are few or no symptoms readily influenced by psychosurgery.

The pseudoneurotic form of schizophrenia (Hoch and Polatin) is represented by neurotic symptoms of various kinds. Patients are dominated by diffuse anxiety, and show obsessions, phobias and a great variety of neurotic symptoms. These are associated with many mechanisms of schizophrenia not seen in true neurotics. The symptoms are more bizarre, the patient shows a deeper withdrawal from reality, and in sodium amytal interviews more florid schizophrenic symptoms can often be elicited. Intensive psychotherapy is indicated but often unsuccessful. Shock treatments have little to offer in this group, also results of psychopharmacology are disappointing in many instances. Psychosurgery relieves the dominant symptom of pain-anxiety and, therefore, radically reduces the patient's suffering. The less extensive operations are sufficient in most cases, and therefore personality changes can be avoided. This group of patients represents the most gratifying chapter in work with psychosurgery, as reported by Hoch and his co-workers, and later by many others.

The outcome in any lobotomized patient can be determined only after a year and sometimes later. The modification of symptoms on the one hand, and the temporary postoperative symptoms on the other hand, complicate the situation. An equilibrium between the various resulting and often contradictory features after the operation is frequently reached only after a considerable length of time. Contrary to other types of treatment in psychiatry, the outcome tends to improve as time goes on, and steady improvement is often observed over a period of several years.

Although individual case reports and experience on small, well studied groups are more informative than large statistics, some of these larger reports should be discussed. The "Report of the English Board of Control on Prefrontal Leucotomy in 1000 Cases," which appeared in 1947 contains data obtained at a time when psychiatrists were still quite reluctant to submit patients to the operation. Therefore, an unusually large number of chronic, deteriorated patients must be included in this survey. The discharge rate for schizophrenics was 23 per cent, not including patients who had been discharged but later relapsed. In a chronic schizophrenic material with an average duration of illness of 7.4 years, Oltman, et al. reported in another collective study that 37.4 per cent were able to leave the hospital, and a total of 56.7 per cent exhibited significant improvement. In material from one single hospital, Worthing et al. reported 29 per cent returned home, and a favorable behavior response in two-thirds, including those chronic patients who remained in the hospital. This material was reviewed with favorable conclusions in a follow-up by Barahal. Some studies with entirely negative results like the one from England by Robins are difficult to explain considering the very favorable overall picture of the more than 10,000 patients leucotomized in England and Wales which were reviewed again in 1961 by Tooth and Newton for the British Ministry of Health. An interesting observation of severely chronic schizophrenic twins of whom only one was operated, showed that the lobotomized twin did considerably better than his co-twin (Weatherly and Deabler). Figures for patients made worse by the operation are surprisingly low even in older material from the time, when deteriorated patients were operated with larger cuts. Today they are definitely absent in the experience of workers limiting surgery to selected cases and performing smaller operations.

Affective Disorders

The use of antidepressive drugs and the almost specific effect of electric shock treatment in the affective disorders limits the number of patients in whom psychosurgery is indicated for depressions. In some statistics, manic-depressive cases are more numerous, but the question arises as to how far the diagnosis was correct. The differentiation between manic-depressive psychosis and schizophrenia is, at times, not easy. A more liberal selection of affective disorders for psychosurgery is advocated by Freeman. While relief from anxiety is almost constant, the depressive mood, in whatever setting it occurs, may easily continue—although often with diminished depth.

A larger material of manic-depressive patients was studied by Stengel and Carse, who noticed an immediate effect on most depressive or manic conditions. They observed, however, that in some cases the manic-depressive episodes continued, although they became less severe, so that patients who previously had had to be hospitalized each time could now be kept at home. This report did not bear out Jones and McCowan's observation that the periodicity of both manic-depressive and schizophrenic episodes disappears after lobotomy. Partridge noticed persistence of a depressive mood, and sometimes a swinging into manic states after the operation even in patients who had not been manic before. Like Carse and Stengel, he noticed much better results in manic-depressives without manic episodes, compared to those who had had manic attacks. An attempt on Partridge's part to break up the depressed group into more endogenous and more reactive depressions led to the conclusion that in depressions on an endogenous basis the results are far less satisfactory than in those where the illness was considered mainly reactive.

Both relapses and failure of the operation to interrupt the depressive phase led Lopez Ibor to a rather negative attitude toward lobotomy for such affective disorders. The poor response of depressions was illustrated by M. Müller in two cases of suicide in depressed patients after lobotomy. One of these had never made a suicidal attempt in nine previous years of illness, which suggests postoperative loss of inhibition and increased impulsiveness as explanation for this incident. The only suicide after psychosurgery observed by us, occurred in a writer who had been operated very successfully for an intractable neurosis but every few years suffered from a depression which responded well to ECT. When he felt such a depression coming on, which had not yet been noticeable to the family, he committed suicide.

More recent reports seem to indicate that certain depressions may respond very well to psychosurgery. Some follow-ups in England show convincingly what some of us have seen in individual cases, namely that patients with chronic depressions may be excellent candidates for psychosurgery. This concerns mainly those chronic depressions of the older group in whom somatic delusions, hypochondriacal symptoms or other atypical features accompany a depression, patients in whom ECT has only a temporary unconvincing effect. A detailed study of 105 cases of depression treated with prefrontal leucotomy was presented by Elithorn with excellent results. Equally good results in depressions were reported by Sykes and Treadgold after orbital undercutting. They found the best outcome in endogenous depressions, while Sargant obtained better results in exogenous depressions. Also McKissock reported that two-thirds of his depressions left the hospital after the operation compared to only one-third of his schizophrenics. According to Myerson and Myerson, Greenblatt et al., and the just mentioned English workers, older patients of the involutional psychosis group respond equally well. Involutional psychosis of the so-called mixed or paranoid type give similar results as nondeteriorated schizophrenics.

Old age does not preclude favorable results. Thorpe published an evaluation of prefrontal leucotomies in 50 patients over 65 years of age, mostly suffering from affective disorders. All but 2 showed appreciable improvement. In 35 a complete remission with disappearance of all symptoms was obtained. Five to nine years later 32 were still alive and 25 fully recovered. The author concludes that after lower quadrant leucotomy two-thirds can be expected to recover. There is little danger of postoperative mental deterioration, and patients are "able to live the remainder of their lives with added years of equanimity." Scoville in a recent follow-up on orbital undercutting found better results in depressed older patients than in the younger age group. Pippard also singles out persistent depressive states in older patients, especially those with obsessive personality, as particularly good prospects.

The most recent British report (1968) by Post et al. demonstrates convincingly the favorable prognosis which a depressive element in the patient's symptomatology has on the outcome of bimedial leucotomies. In their material elderly depressed patients did best. Most interesting is that by separating obsessive states with and without depression, it appeared that those with some depressive admixture were the ones who showed satisfactory results.

Psychoneuroses

The best results of psychosurgery are obtained in severe intractable psychoneuroses. If psychosurgery in these often seriously handicapped patients is not more widely used, it is due to the fear of personality changes in these highly intelligent patients. However, since psychoneurotic patients do not show emotional or intellectual deterioration due to their illness, personality changes failed to occur even with larger operations. Since the introduction of modified lobotomies the most brilliant results are obtained in these patients who usually had been unsuccessfully treated for many years.

The first to recognize the potentialities of prefrontal lobotomy in psychoneuroses were Freeman and Watts, who were able to report excellent results in neurotics classified as obsessive-compulsive and obsessive-ruminative tension states, as well as in tension states without particular differentiation. It appears that those neurotics in whom anxiety is the essential symptom can be influenced favorably by relieving the anxiety quantitatively, while not affecting the basic neurosis. There is no evidence that the underlying psychodynamics of the individual case are a determining factor in the final outcome, which is favorable in the vast majority of cases. It is a highly responsible task for the psychiatrist to balance the severeness of the patient's neurotic suffering against possible side-effects. Fortunately these are minimal in psychoneurotics where less extensive operations are sufficient.

Obsessive-compulsive neurosis, as the most chronic and psychotherapeutically least responsive group, presents the most important indication. Such patients, often unable to live a normal life for years and decades, and frequently confined to their homes, tortured constantly by their compulsions and obsessive fears, obtain relief from their suffering with adequate psyschosurgery. Partridge showed that obsessive-compulsive ruminations yield more readily to operation than does ritualistic behavior. The longer the duration of an obsessive-compulsive neurosis, the more the rituals are entrenched in the patient's behavior; and the more automatically and without variation rituals are perpetuated, the greater the possibility that postoperatively some rituals persist, though with less anxiety, and no longer disabling the patient. According to Post et al., obsessive states responded best, when some element of depression was present.

To mention a few statistics: The English Board of Controls reported 17 recovered and 6 improved out of 29 obsessives, with equally good results in "other" neurotics. In 1949, Freeman and Watts listed 121 "obsessive and psychoneuroses," of which 57 per cent showed good, 28 per cent fair and 11 per cent poor results; 4 per cent had died at the time of this follow-up. Results were almost the same in the group of anxiety neuroses. Most cases listed as psychosomatic disorders also seemed to have benefited. In 23 thoroughly studied cases of Partridge, 11 could be considered as very good results in every respect, 9 showed substantial and 2 additional cases moderate but still distinct gains. Only one was unimproved. Various surveys showed similarly good results including series of transorbital lobotomies reported by Freeman as well as Moore.

Hoch reported on 21 patients, most of whom had been diagnosed and treated for a long time as severe psychoneurotics but who subsequently were determined as actually belonging in the "pseudoneurotic" schizophrenic group. These patients underwent topectomy; 4 per cent recovered, 10 per cent were much improved, 48 per cent improved, 24 per cent slightly improved, and only 14 per cent remained unimproved. The improvement in these patients has sometimes been very impressive because they lose practically all their incapacitating symptoms and are able to work and live without anxiety and tension. In most of them, personality impairments after the operation have not been present or have been minimal. A good lobotomy result in a unique case of chronic battle neurosis was described by Sargant and Stewart.

Intensive psychotherapy and pharmacotherapy must be tried prior to brain surgery in all types of neuroses. In patients who have failed under such methods optimal results with minimal side-effects can be obtained by means of the less extensive psychosurgical procedures. This has been proven in all reports including those that appeared after the introduction of neuroleptic drugs (Slocum et al., Tucker). There are some successful operations reported in patients suffering from psychosomatic disorders such as hypertension, ulcerative colitis and others, but the case material is too small to judge the efficacy of psychosurgery in these cases. Tucker indicates that one group of neuroses with poor results are those with hysterical reactions. The overall picture in neuroses and anxiety, tension, obsessions and compulsions is extremely gratifying in our own recent material.

Hypochondriasis

One of the best indications for psychosurgery is severe hypochondriasis. This disease entity, often diagnosed as involutional psychosis but probably more closely related to the schizophrenic group, is represented by patients who, usually between the age of 50 and 60, begin to develop and be progressively dominated by hypochondriacal ideas. Their complaints become increasingly bizarre. One of the typical features is a resentful attitude toward the relatives if they question the somatic complaints or do not show enough sympathy. Thus, these patients make life miserable for themselves and for those around them and sooner or later, become complete invalids. Prefrontal lobotomy strikingly relieves their self-preoccupation. It was this type of patient in whom Freeman first realized the possibility of neutralizing the patient's worry over his pain, an observation which led to the recommendation of lobotomy for intractable pain.

Hypochrondriacal trends as a symptom in many other psychiatric conditions both psychotic and neurotic, are also relieved by frontal lobe surgery. Where hypochondriasis is the main symptom, a favorable outcome results in practically all cases. The lack of deterioration which is one of the characteristics of these patients, even when their somatic delusions become more and more fantastic, is another factor in their favor. The only prognostically unfavorable feature may be an unpleasant premorbid personality, with resentfulness and aggressiveness which can interfere with the patient's postoperative adjustment.

Drug Addiction; Alcoholism; Psychopathic Personality

Operations on patients with intractable pain demonstrated that they were afterward able to give up an addiction to morphine or other drugs without difficulty. It was a natural thought, therefore, to operate on patients where the addiction rather than the pain was the leading symptom. Some of the cases reported under this heading have obviously been schizophrenic; some apparently belonged to the group of psychopathic personality.

Withdrawal symptoms are usually not noticed in addicts after successful psychosurgery, although Freeman gave examples of patients who, a few days after the drug had been discontinued, developed rapid pulse and respiration, sweating, and restlessness. In our own material of pain cases, such withdrawal symptoms have not been seen. They were not seen either by LeBeau and Gaches, who concluded from their absence that all withdrawal symptoms are caused by the patient's anxiety, and that anxiety is actually the cause of most drug addictions. It is for this reason that they consider topectomy or other psychosurgical measures as the best treatment.

Lobotomy for drug addiction as well as alcoholism has not yet been studied sufficiently to arrive at a definite appraisal of its value. The outcome depends largely on the patient's underlying disease which led to alcoholism or drug addiction. Even more important is his attitude toward alcohol or drugs. A thorough study of the dynamics in each individual case should help to predict the final result. Some carefully observed cases reported by Partridge, demonstrated very well how those who take drugs or alcohol not only without any remorse whenever they feel any physical or emotional discomfort, but with a feeling of justification will not benefit from the operation. On the other hand, those who fight their addiction, but are subject to unbearable distress which they try to overcome with the drug, have a better prognosis. If drugs are used for self-regulation of anxiety and tension, the prognosis for the operation is much better than if no tension or anxiety symptoms are present. Because the operation usually reduces or eliminates anxiety and tension symptoms, the alcohol or drug abuse is also eliminated. In some cases reported by Greenblatt et al. the lobotomy performed for some other psychiatric condition led to alcohol abuse, because the operation obviously "facilitated the change from self-consciousness, inhibitions and social anxiety to overconfidence, lack of restraint, hedonic indulgence and alcohol addiction."

Lobotomized patients diagnosed as psychopathic personality have been reported here and there, but psychopathic personality is defined in so many different terms in the literature of various countries that only cases described in some detail can be considered in a discussion of this indication for psychosurgery. The aggressive and destructive behavior of asocial psychopaths has been an occasional reason to perform the operation. Its application to criminals found undue attention in the daily press. A survey of the literature shows that actual experience is still negligible. It should be realized that the patient's criminal trends will remain the same and may easily be exhibited with less restraint after the operation than before. Also sexual deviations may be exhibited with less restraint after the operation. An often mentioned but inconclusive case is that of a sexual psychopath, originally reported as improved, who was later described again by Friedlander and Banay as a "psychosis following lobotomy." Thorough study of the dynamics of a sexual deviate may lead to a rare recommendation of psychosurgery with the intent to relieve anxiety, if this, or abnormal tension, seem to be responsible for the abnormal behavior. We had a patient whose abnormal sexual behavior (nymphomania) was eliminated because tension and anxiety were markedly reduced by the operation. Cases reported by Partridge under the heading of psychopathic personality show the difficulty of defining this disease group. He describes inadequate psychopaths with an overwhelming sense of insecurity and also with hysterical paralysis, screaming attacks and hypochondriacal ideas. Such patients found relief and learned to live with themselves. Patients classified as schizoid psychopaths by this author could equally well have been listed as schizophrenics. Several isolated cases and a study by Whalen et al. dedicated specifically to the effect of psychosurgery on psychopathic personalities led to serious doubts regarding this indication except in very carefully selected cases.

Mental Deficiency

Mental defectives have frequently been operated on because of their aggressive behavior. The results in these cases are, of coures, limited to an improvement in the patient's management. It has been pointed out that the degree of mental deficiency is not unfavorably influenced, and that in some cases the removal of aggressive and disturbed behavior makes it even possible to start with some training which had been impossible prior to the operation. Such cases, operated on at an early age by the French authors Klein and Tardieu, led to the claim that psychosurgery has an important place in child psychiatry. Of two larger reports from English institutions for mental defectives, one by Mackay quotes extremely satisfactory cases, while another by Engler comes to rather unsatisfactory conclusions. In Engler's report, both an unusually high fatality rate and the incidence of postoperative convulsions made this indication for lobotomy more than questionable. Very few patients improved; many more showed deterioration of their conduct. Engler arrives at the conclusion that only defectives with a relatively higher degree of intelligence as well as a higher standard of personality are promising candidates for lobotomy. In the United States, Angus reported on two children who could not be kept in a highgrade training school because of their behavior, but who were returned to the school after the operation and made a good adjustment. A feebleminded patient reported by Greenblatt et al. could be diagnosed as Propfschizophrenia. This patient, who had been completely withdrawn, became a wage earner after lobotomy. It appears that neither flat rejection of mental defectives nor indiscriminate operating is the answer, but rather a careful selection of each individual case on its own merits.

Epilepsy

Epilepsy is often accompanied by aggressive behavior, irritability, moodiness, and a great number of other psychiatric symptoms. In some of these cases an organic brain condition may be responsible for both the convulsions and the mental symptoms. In others, "idiopathic" epilepsy seems to be the proper diagnosis. Numerous authors have mentioned institutionalized epileptics in whom the operation removed aggressive behavior and other disturbing symptoms. Post-lobotomy seizures do not appear to be more frequent in patients who have already suffered from epilepsy. Baretto et al. even operated on epileptics with some success not only for the psychiatric symptoms but also for their convulsions. These workers based their attempts on the idea that epilepsy is the result of lack of balance between the two hemispheres, and that lobotomy can correct the predominance of the one hemisphere. Whatever the justification of this reasoning, they were able to show that almost one-third of their material had fewer seizures after the operation, and that only in 1 per cent was an increase noticed. The absence of a greater occurrence of post-lobotomy convulsions in epileptics, seen also by other authors, suggests that the etiology of post-traumatic epilepsy after a brain operation is different from that of idiopathic epileptic fits. Therefore, convulsions as such do not represent a valid objection to psychosurgery as a therapeutic procedure for the psychiatric complications of epilepsy. More experience, however, must be accumulated before the indications in this group of patients can be properly judged.

Various Indications

Cachexia as a symptom in various diseases was seen to respond well by Lopez Ibor. He mentioned good results not only in cases associated with depression but also in some other conditions; an example was a patient with Alzheimer's disease who regained excellent physical health in spite of continued intellectual impairment. In patients with cachexia less extensive operations seem to be sufficient. The syndrome of anorexia nervosa has also been mentioned occasionally as a possible indication for psychosurgery. Improvement of such psychosomatic conditions as ulcerative colitis and neurodermatitis is sometimes seen. Special attention was paid to this problem by Sargant who included asthma in the list of psychosomatic disorders responding well to modified leucotomy. After the operation the attacks may still occur, but the diminished tension makes them shorter, and finally lets them die out. The recent French literature contains two very convincing reports on psychosurgery by electrocoagulation of two conditions with psychosomatic connotations. Cattan et al. reported on twelve cases of ulcerative colitis with excellent results; most of the patients had already been considered for ileostomy or colostomy. In most cases one cerebral electrocoagulation was sufficient, in others a second coagulation through the previous trephine opening was performed. The same group of workers (Fumusau et al.) reported on electrocoagulation for intractible gastric and duodenal ulcers. In four out of five cases excellent results were obtained; intestinal surgery had been impossible because of various physical contraindications.

Organic brain diseases, other than those mentioned in previous chapters, may also present rare indications for surgery. Schwartz reported a case of Parkinson's disease with depression where the depression was lifted. Postencephalitic patients with behavior disorders, obsessional traits, and aggressiveness as described after the epidemic of 1918, were successfully operated on by Rizzatti, and similar favorable results were reported by Holland et al.

Psychosurgery in children was originally performed by Freeman and Watts apparently with poor results. Holland et al. reported on 12 disturbed children and adolescents. They observed relief of hostility in all but one; seven of the patients were in school or at work. Surgery was recommended only if the prognosis was poor and the behavior problem so severe that nothing short of permanent institutional care was foreseeable. More patients suffered from chronic childhood schizophrenia, some were postencephalitic cases.

Multiple Lobotomies

It could be expected that the need for reoperation would become more frequent with the introduction of smaller operations. The type of case in whom this problem comes up, is usually one who greatly improved after the operation, but after weeks, months or even years relapses, manifesting identical symptoms as those for which the operation had been originally performed. In such cases it must be assumed that the original cut had been insufficient. Freeman has just reported on a follow-up of 414 patients who had been reoperated on once or twice. In our own material we are forced with increasing frequency to ask the surgeon for reoperation because of our efforts to keep the first operative cut at a minimum in order to avoid personality changes. Fortunately, we did not see personality changes in the subsequent operations either.

In reoperations many neurosurgeons now concentrate on the basal portions of the frontal lobes, particularly the orbito-medial quadrants. The importance of the dorso-medial nucleus of the thalamus has been questioned by many recently. Freeman, lately, failed to find retrograde degeneration in this nucleus in transorbital lobotomies even if they had been successful. In the original standard lobotomies, retrograde degeneration in this nucleus was a typical neuropathological finding. Freeman now also questions the belief that the extent of the lesion decides on the success of the operation because results can be obtained with minimal lesions in the orbito-medial quadrants. As long as these questions are not answered and the most desirable location of the cut is not determined, the need for reoperation in patients with reoccurrence of symptoms will be unavoidable. Sufficient evidence is available that such secondary operations can lead to a more permanent result. Interesting in this connection is a patient of Sargant's in whom a fourth "open" operation showed that in three previous "closed" ones the important lower medial quadrant had not been reached.

In many instances of a relapse or of the persistence of some symptoms it will be indicated to apply other treatments rather than to reoperate. Sargant has repeatedly emphasized the possibility to use other psychiatric treatments after a partially successful leucotomy. This applies, for instance, to those patients whom we have mentioned already, and on whom Birley commented, where depressive episodes occur after lobotomies. They respond to antidepressant drugs or ECT and are no candidates for reoperation. However, more frequent are those in whom reoccurrence of the original symptoms requires a second psychosurgical procedure.

General Remarks

In view of the excellent results of psychosurgery in well selected cases it is to be regretted that this entire therapeutic approach has come under such heavy criticism from the most diverse quarters. Objections came from such different sides as organically oriented psychiatrists concerned with psychological changes after brain injuries, and from some psychoanalysts opposed to any type of somatic treatment. Interesting enough, several psychodynamically oriented psychiatrists recently emphasized the value of brain operations in selected cases, among others Brody, Cattell, Kubie (quoted by Slocum et al.). Psychosurgery became a political issue when Soviet Health Authorities prohibited the operation by an official decree in 1950, although it should be mentioned that apparently disappointment in results has been the true reason for this radical decision. Legal issues were discussed in the Stanford Law Review. It also became a religious issue according to some statements in the literature, but actually no verdict against the operation has ever been passed, and according to a discussion by Father Gerald Kelly, lobotomy and similar operations are justified when indicated as the proper treatment in mental illness, and when the expected advantages will outweigh the possible evils. The sweeping statement was most unjustified that these operations are no longer necessary after neuroleptic drugs had been introduced. Actually psychosurgery has very definite indications. It is fair to say that psychosurgery is not the treatment of choice in any particular disease entity. Each case, whatever the diagnosis, must be decided on its own merits. The more treatment procedures are available in psychiatry the less need will there be for such drastic methods as a brain operation. At present, there are still many chronic psychiatric patients in whom no other treatment has brought sufficient relief. In these cases psychosurgery must be given serious consideration, and will yield many satisfactory results unobtainable with other methods.

CHAPTER VI

Various Pharmacological and Other Methods

The preceding chapters dealt with those somatic treatments which are more or less widely used in psychiatry today. This leaves a number of important areas of somatic psychiatric therapy to be discussed. They include some pharmacological methods which preceded the new era of psychopharmacotherapy. Others, such as the use of lithium salts, were known in general medicine long ago, but their value in psychiatric disorders is just being recognized. Some of these drugs probably deserve a firm place in the general chapter on pharmacotherapy. Others have a limited range of application, or are used only in certain countries; others were of interest at one time or another and, although they are now rarely applied, continue to be of theoretical interest. We feel that even those more or less discarded methods are still important from the point of view of research, and, therefore, should not be omitted from a book on all somatic treatment attempts in psychiatry. Some approaches, such as endocrinological therapy, are old but may have some promise for the future. The following chapter includes a great variety of pharmacological and other physical methods. It also contains special sections on various pharmacological means to assist in the overall treatment of special groups of patients such as alcoholics and drug addicts. Attempts to bring some order into these miscellaneous subjects were abandoned as artificial and unrewarding. Their entirety represents an attempt to give a full account of all types of therapeutic efforts made, including those which are only somatic adjuncts to psychotherapeutic methods which by themselves are not the subject of this book.

Continuous Sleep Treatment

Prolonged sleep as a treatment for mental symptoms is rather old. However, the systematic use of "continuous sleep treatment" was introduced by Klaesi in 1922. His method of keeping the patient in a barbiturate narcosis for a considerable time can be considered as the first systematic procedure of organic treatment in the endogenous psychoses. Duration and depth of the narcosis seem to determine the effectiveness of the treatment, although opinion to the contrary has been expressed. In acute anxiety states, as seen particularly during the war, it was used as a form of first aid (Sargant and Slater). A review of the literature was presented by Clapp and Loomis.

The drug originally recommended for continuous sleep treatment was somnifen. A high percentage of complications suggested its replacement or combination with other drugs. Various mixtures of barbiturates, chloral hydrate, and paraldehyde were recommended, the best known being Cloetta's mixture, which is usually applied rectally. Somnifen, given orally, has been used by Walsh. Great technical skill is required to avoid complications, particularly of a cardiovascular and renal nature. The patient is kept in a sleep-like state for ten or more days. The narcosis is reduced temporarily to permit feeding and excretion of stool and urine. At the end of the narcosis the medication should be reduced slowly in order to avoid the convulsions which may follow the sudden withdrawal of most drugs used for this treatment. Another withdrawal symptom is presented by delirium-like psychotic reactions. It is interesting that Heldt, who reported on prolonged sodium amytal narcosis, sees an important part of the treatment in this delirium which usually sets in two or three days after cessation of administration of the drug if this has been stopped abruptly. His results were favorable in a great variety of psychiatric disorders.

The best results were reported in the manic-depressive psychoses. Manic excitements responded better than depressions. In depression the agitated type benefited more than the retarded patient. In schizophrenia patients in catatonic excitement reacted better than patients in catatonic stupor.

Klaesi stressed the psychological aspect, believing that after the treatment the patient is weakened and looks for help. This simplifies the psychotherapy which should immediately follow the awakening of the patient. Others stressed the organic side of the treatment. Since the introduction of shock therapy it is used very little except in the Soviet Union. It seems, though, that lately Soviet psychiatrists draw a clear line between Klaesi's original method of rather deep barbiturate narcosis which they consider dangerous, and their own method of inducing sleep, partly with hypnotics, partly with conditioning. They claim results similar to those obtained with insulin treatment with which it is often combined alternating the two methods in various ways. According to Ivanov-Smolenski, schizophrenics with florid symptomatology respond better to insulin, those with bland symptomatology do well under sleep therapy. In the United States neither form of sleep therapy is being used much, while in some European countries sleep treatment has a firm place as a hospital procedure in patients with various psychiatric disorders. This is particularly true for well-staffed private hospitals with sufficient personnel to care for patients under this treatment.

The more symptomatic sedative effect of the method is today largely replaced by the neuroleptic drugs. It is interesting that in Switzerland chlorpromazine and reserpine have been frequently used in darkened rooms keeping the patient in a sleep-like state for several days in a way similar to the previously used method of Klaesi. A combination of prolonged sleep therapy with barbiturates and phenothiazines has also been recommended. Ey and Faure use mixtures of long and short acting barbiturates potentiated with chlorpromazine resulting in 16 to 20 hours of sleep per day. Recently Sargant et al. were able to enhance the combined effect of iproniazid and other antidepressants plus ECT by simultaneous light continuous narcosis with chlorpromazine and barbiturates in otherwise untractable chronic tension states.

Narcotherapy

Sodium amytal, introduced by Blackwenn, was seen by Lindemann to alter mental states in relatively small doses when injected slowly intravenously. Sodium amytal, sodium pentothal, and other barbiturates such as the German Evipan sedate the patient and, at the same time, produce a lack of inhibition, and in some individuals also a psychomotor discharge. These drugs injected intravenously, were seen to remove such symptoms as mutism and refusal of food in catatonics. Their usefulness became more important in overcoming resistance and inducing the patient to communicate his ideas and experiences. Horsley introduced the term narcoanalysis. Other terms like narcosuggestion, narcocatharsis, narcohypnosis, narcosynthesis, or the combining term, narcotherapy, are used for the application of these drugs when used in connection with psychotherapy.

Three to 7½ grains of amytal are injected slowly until the patient is in a state of relaxation. The needle is left in place during the treatment so that an additional amount of the drug can be injected. The method is relatively harmless, but acutely ill patients and those with liver or kidney disease and severe hypertension should not be so treated. In many patients, delusions and hallucinations can be elicited which formerly were not disclosed. Moreover, focal psychodynamic points in the psychoses and neuroses are easily found, because tensions, anxieties, and preoccupations are eliminated from the clinical picture and the patient is able to verbalize where formerly he was too dominated by his symptoms to do so.

Sodium amytal and the similar pentothal were extensively used by Horsley, Grinker and Spiegel, Hoch, Sargant and Slater in war neuroses and are also used in civilian neuroses. Our experience shows that of these, conversion hysterias, anxiety states, and some psychosomatic disorders, like stomach ulcers, colitis, and postconcussional syndrome, respond favorably. More deeply structuralized neuroses, like anxiety hysterias and obsessive-compulsive states, respond only temporarily to this treatment. Sodium amytal is used today chiefly as a form of short psychotherapy where we try to eliminate the neuroses in just a few sessions. It is not an instrument to be used in connection with extensive psychotherapy or prolonged analysis. There are two methods of using the treatment which are usually combined. The first method is the so-called narcosuggestive treatment where the patient, after receiving sodium amytal, is brought to a hypnosis-like state in which he receives suggestions concerning his neurotic symptomatology. The other method is the so-called narcoanalysis in which the patient under the influence of amytal associates freely and discharges emotional material. Many workers use the narcosuggestive and narcocathartic procedures simultaneously.

In narcosuggestive or narcocathartic procedures it is undesirable to make the patient somnolent and unresponsive. Slurred speech and nystagmus are useful signs to determine the depth of the seminarcotic state. A deeper narcotic state is only used by Brickner et al. who developed a technique in which intensive psychotherapeutic work is done while the patient is actually under narcosis but presumed to absorb some of the material presented to him during this state.

It is a rare complication of narcotherapy that in well-integrated but psychotic patients an acute syndrome is released under the influence of intravenous sodium amytal. This may occur in the treatment of cases with latent schizophrenia. As far as narcotherapy of frank psychotics is concerned, the sodium amytal technique is of very little therapeutic value. It is possible, for an hour or so, to influence a depression or catatonic state and restore the patient to normalcy; but such an improvement never lasts and the patient relapses shortly into his previous state. A combination of narcotherapy and insulin shock treatment was introduced by Levy and Perry and mentioned in the chapter on insulin shock therapy. Under the term "narcostimulation" La Verne and, recently, the Indian psychiatrists Neki and Kishore use a combination of barbiturate narcosis and non-convulsive doses of metrazol or leptazol in the treatment of depression and other psychiatric conditions.

Acetylcholine

In 1937, Fiamberti recommended intravenous injections of the drug acetylcholine as a less drastic method of applying "shock therapy." He pointed out that the only common feature of insulin and convulsive therapy is the provocation of violent vascular modifications, and concluded that the curative effect should be seen in a "vascular storm."

The most striking effect is cardiac arrest for thirty to fifty seconds. The patient turns extremely pale shortly after the injection and becomes unconscious. There are twitchings of the face and extremities and usually an extensive spasm but never clonic movements reminiscent of the clonic phase of an epileptic seizure. A case described by Cohen et al. underwent a dramatic remission after a dangerous episode in which he was considered probably dead, and which was followed by a comatose condition of one hour's duration. There are favorable reports, especially in Italy, where Fasanaro in a comparative study obtained results superior to those with insulin and convulsive therapy, particularly in chronic cases. Fiamberti, whose technique we could observe as quite simple and not very unpleasant to the patient, had no fatalities. He gives acetylcholine bromide in doses up to 600 mgm., and limits the method to schizophrenics, where he, and Fabbri reported good results.

Contrary to this, Lopez Ibor used acetylcholine chloride up to 200 mgm. in anxiety neuroses. Reactions are limited to some respiratory difficulty, coughing and slow pulse. Several intravenous injections a week up to a total of 40 are given. On the basis of their own experience Sargant and Slater consider this method worthy of trial in various neuroses and tension states.

The use of acetylcholine has never become widespread. Some controlled studies have been reported. Pare gave 110 outpatients mostly suffering from depressive reactions or a mild obsessive compulsive state, 200 mg. acetylcholine at weekly intervals for 30 weeks. Controls received intravenous calcium gluconate which gives sensations similar to those produced by acetylcholine. Although over 50 per cent of the patients improved there was no significant difference between those receiving acetylcholine and those on calcium gluconate. However, Maria et al. confirmed the value of acetylcholine even after the introduction of chlorpromazine, and they also combined the two drugs. Hawkins and Tibbetts were unable to demonstrate any superiority in acetylcholine treated neurotics as compared to a group given a placebo.

Carbon Dioxide

Carbon dioxide for psychiatric conditions had first been tried by Loevenhart et al., who, in 1926, reported on such treatment in psychotics. It was successful in some catatonic patients as far as disappearance of catatonic stupor was concerned, but this effect was only of very short duration; lasting improvements could not be obtained. After some attempts by others (Hinsie et al.) it was given up as unsuccessful in psychotics. Attempts in psychoneurotics had not been made until 1947, when Meduna first published a report on carbon dioxide therapy in psychoneurotics.

The technique consists in inhalation of a mixture of 30 per cent CO_2 and 70 per cent O_2. Originally Meduna had experimented with 20 per cent CO_2 but found that the introductory phase, during which the patient may suffer from dyspnea and a choked feeling, was unduly prolonged. He also tried a slow increase of the CO_2 content of the inhaled gas but found it less comfortable for the patient. At the first treatment, 20 to 25 respirations are given. After 8 to 16 respirations the patient usually loses consciousness. At this time, psychomotor excitement of various forms may be seen. Later, the lower extremities and, to a lesser degree, the upper extremities are slightly flexed, and the hands show carpal spasms, reminding one of tetanic signs in hyperventilation. We have seen many other manifestations of strio-pallidar type, when we have increased the number of respirations to 50 or even 100. At this point the pupils may become rigid, and a decerebrate rigidity-like state may develop. Meduna, however, usually did not give such a large number of respirations. He determined the number by the therapeutic response of the patient and increased only if the patient did not show any improvement after a few treatments. In his experience only 3 or 4 out of a hundred patients stopped the treatment because of the anxiety experienced during the initial phase. The number of treatments necessary to achieve clinical results varied from 20 to 150.

According to Meduna, the treatment is ineffective in obsessive-compulsive neuroses and cases of hypochondriasis. Good results are obtained in patients with conversion symptoms, anxiety neuroses, personality maladjustment, and emotional instability. Of 100 psychoneurotic patients with personality maladjustment, 68 were considered cured. Most of them were chronic cases, and a group with particularly good results was represented by stutterers. The contraindications are severe hypertension, active pulmonary tuberculosis, cardiovascular disease, severe emphysema, acute allergic respiratory reactions or respiratory or cardiovascular sensitivity to CO_2. Moriarty does not regard pregnancy as a contraindication.

The treatment is explained by the theory that psychoneurosis is due to an abnormally low threshold of stimulation with respect to normal stimuli, or by a relatively low threshold of stimulation with respect to stimuli of exceptional strength. In either case, treatment is intended to raise the threshold of stimulation to the normal level of resistance to noxious stimuli from within or from without. This postulate seems to be fulfilled by repeated administration of carbon dioxide.

A number of other investigators presented reports which are arriving at cures and improvements ranging from 50 to 80 per cent. A second monograph on the treatment was edited by Meduna in 1958 with clinical trials on various types of patients and some interesting physiological and psychological investigations. LaVerne introduced a rapid coma technique as compared to Meduna's slow coma technique. He uses higher concentrations, usually 70 per cent CO_2 in O_2 mixtures for one to seven consecutive breaths. This reduces the excitement to seconds and carries the patient quickly into unconsciousness. It is superior to the standard technique in anxiety states, obsessive-compulsive disorders, phobias, psychosomatic and conversion hysteria. In a comparative study Peck found superiority over psychotherapy in anxiety and phobic reactions. One of us (L.B.K.) gave up to 100 respirations in one treatment leading to rather deep unconsciousness. Improvements were seen, but they were not lasting. Some patients, however, become quite dependent on the treatment as also seen by Kindwall.

Wilcox uses the patient's reactions under CO_2 "as reports back from the patient's conscious mind to the therapist." He uses them in both non-coma and coma doses of CO_2 as indication of psychotherapeutic progress and sees the aim of such a method of "psychopenetration" in producing a symptom-free person with very mild reaction to CO_2 sleep. A CO_2 abreaction technique was used by Milligan. He avoids unconsciousness and prefers it to narcoanalysis using intravenous barbiturates, and to abreaction with inhalation of nitrous oxide and ether.

There have been a number of conflicting reports about the efficacy of the treatment, even in conditions where benefit was claimed by Meduna. Thus, Arthurs et al. found that objective measurements of stuttering frequency and rating of stuttering severity failed to reveal any improvement in 14 patients given 30 to 70 administrations each, although there was some decrease in speech anxiety. They attempted to eliminate any close relationship between doctor and patient, and question whether this accounts for the discrepancy between their results and those of Meduna.

Hawkings and Tibbetts in a controlled clinical trial concluded that the treatment has no specific therapeutic effect in neuroses. They believe that the regular attendance for treatment in itself may be a beneficial factor. Similar conclusions were reached by Hargrove and his co-workers, who found psychotherapy alone to be much more effective than a combination of CO_2 and psychotherapy which produced added problems of transference and resistance to impede recovery. Moriarty, however, after a four year experience with 7500 treatments given to 290 patients, concluded that it was of benefit in anxiety tension and phobic states, as well as in migraine and spastic colitis. It was of little value in the psychoses or in firmly established obsessive-compulsive neuroses. Shorvon found it effective in depersonalization states. Although still in 1962 Uhler reported favorably on it in anxiety states with somatic symptoms and in personality conflicts, we believe that it is rarely used today.

Nitrogen Inhalation Treatment; Nitrous Oxide

One theory on the effective agent in insulin and convulsive therapy holds that the common factor is a diminished cerebral metabolism. It was logical, therefore, for attempts to be made to subject mental patients to short periods of anoxia. Trials in producing artificial anoxemia for the treatment of mental illness were made by Alexander and Himwich with the inhalation of nitrogen. The patient goes through the same changes as with insulin except that the duration of the various stages of disintegration of brain function is limited to seconds rather than hours. Determination of the arterial blood oxygen concentration gives about 20 per cent, i.e., half the concentration reached at the end of a convulsion in metrazol therapy. Nitrogen, administered by an anesthetist, is permitted to flow at a rate of 6 liters per minute for six minutes.

A comparative study with nitrogen inhalation treatment was made by Sillman and Terrence; they administered the treatment five times a week, the average number of treatments being forty. The results, which were compared with those of insulin and metrazol treatment in the same hospital, were entirely unsatisfactory. Büssow et al. noted changes of mood which they consider as an unspecific reaction.

Nitrous oxide (N_2O) inhalation has also been used for hypoxemia by Alexander and Himwich who later replaced it with nitrogen. In the preshock era Zador, in 1928, experimented with nitrous oxide in normal individuals and in psychotics. In the psychotics he noticed clinical changes which suggested some therapeutic value. Work with nitrous oxide was later taken up by Lehmann and Bos who noticed the difference between the effects of nitrous oxide and nitrogen inhalation. Nitrous oxide produces euphoria in the induction phase ("laughing gas"). They prefer it to other inhalation treatments because it gives no feeling of suffocation or other physical discomfort. Although a facilitation of mental processes was seen, this is followed by sedation. In manic excitements, daily administration of nitrous oxide has controlled and terminated the attack in some cases. Nitrous oxide is also useful for narcoanalysis.

Ether; Trichlorethylene

Ether has been used in psychiatry from time to time for therapeutic purposes. The same is true for alcohol. Ether found more systematic application for two different purposes. One is the technique of abreaction, for which it was recommended by Sargant and Slater. Here it is actually an adjunct to psychotherapy. It supposedly depresses the highest psychic centers, thus producing disinhibition and excitation to a greater extent than sodium amytal does. According to Shorvon and Slater, it is preferable to barbiturates because the patient is less apt to fall asleep and therefore better able to retain the material discussed.

While in these abreaction procedures ether is inhaled, Ferraro recommended the use of ether applied by the drip method as a possible cure for affective disorders. A solution of ether, 2.5 to 5 per cent in glucose and saline is administered by slow phleboclysis. The amount of solution given is generally from 750 to 1000 cc., and the flow regulated from 25 to 100 or even 180 drops per minute. This lasts two to three hours and 10 to 30 daily applications are given.

Trichlorethylene was used by Rees et al. as a therapeutic aid in psychotherapy. Compared to other inhalation methods, it has the advantage of a faster effect and abscence of nausea. It is also considered by Rees et al. as superior to nitrous oxide, which is too transient for prolonged psychotherapy, and to intravenous barbiturates, where the sedative effect may prevent resumption of normal activity for hours. Like nitrous oxide, ether and other gases, trichlorethylene is recommended for eclectic use in psychotherapy, including narcoanalysis, narcosynthesis, abreaction, relaxation procedures and reinforcement of reassurance.

Lithium

Lithium salts enjoyed a vogue in the nineteenth century for the treatment of gout and a variety of other disorders, but they fell into disuse because of the alarming reports of their toxicity and their replacement by safer and more effective therapeutic agents. Their use in psychiatric conditions was first suggested by Cade in Australia in 1949, who developed the idea of using lithium in the treatment of psychotic excitement from the experimental observation that lithium carbonate produced a short period of lethargy and unresponsiveness to stimuli in guinea pigs who, however, remained fully conscious.

Cade reported favorable response in manics with no hypnotic effect and since this first study there have been a number of others which emphasized the efficacy of lithium salts in manic states. Schou and his co-workers in Denmark treated a series of manic patients alternately with lithium and a placebo. They made a cautious assessment at the end of the trial, bearing in mind the tendency of mania to remit spontaneously, and out of their 38 patients they found that 14 had responded to such an extent that in their opinion it was highly improbable that changes during treatment were due to spontaneous variation. Rice, in a trial with a mixed group of patients found that it had a special sedative action on manics, and where schizophrenics were improved, it was the affective element which was influenced.

There is a general consensus that the drug is of benefit in manic conditions. Noack and Trautner found that the best response was in the acute case and they do not consider it of value in chronics. Schou, in a review of the literature, points out that a total of 80 per cent cures and improvements have been reported in manics. Schou, in a similar trial to the one described for manic patients, obtained no benefit with lithium in endogenous depression. Andreani, however, reported improvement in 10 out of 24 depressed patients, but since the trial was uncontrolled, spontaneous improvement cannot be excluded. Glesinger regards severe depression, particularly associated with agitation, as a contra-indication and depression has been reported as a side-effect from the drug. However, recently the value of lithium for prophylactic use in both manic and depressive episodes has been recognized.

Lithium is usually used as lithium carbonate in 300 mg. capsules. Other salts used are lithium citrate, lithium acetate, and according to a Soviet report by Mosketi et al., lithium iodate.

The therapeutic dose in an acute attack should be 600 mg. three times a day, although slow daily increase might be advisable to avoid side-effects. The maintenance or prophylactic dose should be 300 mg. three times a day. The serum lithium concentration is an indicator of the lithium effect. It should not be lower than 0.6 m-equiv./l. and not higher than 1.6 m-equiv./l. The therapeutic dose of 600 mg., three times a day, should not be given ordinarily for more than a week, and—if necessary, after a few ECT's for severe manic excitement—be replaced by the prophylactic dose of 300 mg. three times a day. Rice advises a rest day once weekly in order to allow for complete elimination of the drug and reduce the incidence of toxic symptoms. Lithium replaces sodium in the body and as a protection against accumulation, with its attendant risk of toxicity, Roberts advises administration of additional salt in the diet. Lithium should not be given to patients on a salt-free diet, or when strongly indicated, only in sufficiently small dosage to be handled by the kidneys under these circumstances (Schou).

Studies show that 50 per cent is excreted in the urine 6-7 hours after ingestion, but the remainder is excreted only slowly over a period of 10 days. Noack and Trautner found that manic patients appeared to retain considerably higher amounts at the beginning of treatment, and that excretion of lithium reflects the clinical state in that the patients tend to retain more as long as mania lasts and to excrete more as the condition begins to abate. Lithium clearance is slower with increasing age. In any one patient the renal lithium clearance is remarkably constant.

The toxic effects described are abdominal pain with anorexia, nausea, vomiting or diarrhoea, drowsiness, ataxia, giddiness, tinnitus, blurred vision, thirst, polyuria with dilute urine, and a fine tremor commencing in the hands. These symptoms occur at a serum level of 2mEq/l. As the level rises to 3-4mEq/l there is the development of confusion, nystagmus, epileptic fits, hypo- or hyperreflexia, fasciculations of the muscles and a recurrence of diarrhoea and vomiting, followed by the onset of coma. The first fatality reported in psychiatric practice by Roberts, was of the development, on the eighth day of treatment, of epileptic fits leading to status epilepticus and death from circulatory failure, in a 57 year old female being treated for psychotic excitement. Glesinger reported a death from encephalopathy and advocated the use of cylotropin (40 per cent hexamethylenetetramine, 16 per cent sodium salicylate and 1 per cent caffeine) in doses of 10-22 cc. intravenously or intramuscularly daily for this complication.

In a more recent study Schou distinguishes between side-effects which are inconvenient rather than dangerous, and true lithium poisoning. The borderline of 2 m-equiv/l between the two is not absolute. Side-effects may be seen when serum lithium peak values remain below 1 m-equiv/l. In 8 cases of lithium poisoning observed in Denmark, in 15 years, it was primarily the central nervous system that was effected. Consciousness was severely impaired, and in some patients coma developed. Attacks of hyperextension of arms and legs were seen, and 2 patients had epileptic seizures. On the other hand, kidney function and electrocardiogram were affected only moderately and reversibly. Plasma sodium and potassium concentrations did not change significantly. Three of the patients died from pulmonary complications. No antidote is known. Treatment with sodium chloride and potassium chloride was ineffective. Treatment of severe lithium intoxication must be symptomatic and of the same type that is used in other cases of narcotic poisoning.

In some cases the EKG shows a flattening of the T wave or sometimes an inversion. Visual and tactile hallucinations may occur and abnormalities of the EEG, increase of voltage and the appearance of frequencies of 3-4 cps have been reported.

Animal experimentation indicates that the main toxic effect of the drug is on the kidney tubules in the form of a water-losing nephritis unaffected by large doses of the antidiuretic hormone (Radomski et al.). These changes are completely reversible in the early stages, but if lithium administration continues after the initial urinary symptoms appear the animals develop degenerative changes in the kidney tubules, with oliguria or anuria and azotemia.

Contraindications are renal disease or any illness affecting kidney function, decompensated heart disease, Addison's Disease because of the disturbance of sodium metabolism and any other condition in which sodium balance is interfered with. Noack does not regard a stable condition of cardiac disease, arteriosclerosis or hypertension as necessarily preventing treatment with lithium. In view of the EEG abnormalities reported, care should be taken in patients with a history of epilepsy. In pregnant women the problem of possible teratogenic effect was examined. Contrary to findings in certain lower organisms, no untoward results had been seen in babies whose mothers were on continuous lithium medication. Yet one should try to avoid giving lithium during the first three months of pregnancy.

Careful clinical and laboratory control is necessary. Before treatment is started determination of creatinine or blood urea nitrogen, sedimentation rate, blood pressure, electrocardiogram, and analysis of the urine for protein and formed elements must be available. The serum lithium concentration should be used to monitor treatment. If it is too low, either the patients are not taking their tablets, or the dosage is inadequate. The flame photometric serum lithium determination is a rapid and accurate test. Weekly determinations are advised during therapeutic lithium doses, but no strict rules can be given for how often serum lithium concentration should be determined during maintenance therapy.

The opinion of those who have used the drug is that, provided there is careful clinical observation lithium is a safe therapeutic agent. French workers have reported on the successful use of both chlorpromazine and ECT with it (Teulié et al.). The period during which improvement is noted is slightly longer with lithium than with ECT, but there is the advantage of a lack of the confusion which may result from the frequent treatments required to control manics with ECT, as well as the fact that relapse is common in ECT.

The prophylactic value of lithium salts has been established convincingly by Schou. This is certainly true for the manic phase, and there seems to be increasing evidence that it applies also to subsequent depressive phases. The prevention of manic states is of paramount importance because once a manic phase sets in, patients are usually unwilling to undergo any treatment. Prophylactic treatment can be started at any time during a manic or depressive episode. In severe cases, where the patient must be hospitalized because of manic excitement, ECT may have to be initiated, but in such cases as well as in depressions prophylactic medication with lithium salts can be started simultaneously.

The practical significance of prophylactic treatment is evidenced by the difficulty to treat patients who have both manic and depressive episodes by means of other available drugs. In such cases antidepressants easily elicit manic phases, and neuroleptics given in a manic phase are apt to lead to a depression. So far prophylactic ECT is the best treatment, but the simpler application of lithium salts, in our experience, has replaced ECT in some patients who had been treated for years with other means. This includes a 75 year old man in whom previous attempts to replace monthly ECT's given over 20 years, with maintenance drug therapy had failed to prevent the mostly manic episodes.

The usefulness of lithium in depressions claimed by some and questioned by others, was studied most recently by Fieve et al. in careful investigations. They found hardly any therapeutic effect in acute endogenous depressions, while the prophylactic use of lithium did decrease the depth of the depression, but did not change the frequency of their occurrence.

Lithium salts are of particular value in patients where the cycles of manic and depressive mood swings follow each other so rapidly that no therapeutic or prophylactic treatment has any chance of becoming effective before the next phase occurs. An unpublished observation by Jenner reported by Schou of a successfully treated patient with a 48-hour cycle is most convincing. While the effect of lithium salts in other psychotic patients remained unconvincing, the conclusion is justified that in manic depressives this treatment is of great practical and perhaps of equally great theoretical significance.

Histamine Therapy

Marshal and Tarwater, on the assumption that psychoses are allergic responses and hence capable of nonspecific desensitization treated patients with histamine phosphate and peptone solution. Hill publised a monograph on combined treatment with histamine and insulin. He as well as Robb et al. expected favorable results from the alteration in capillary permeability and cerebral blood flow, secondary effects of a vascular shock and a general "shock to the bodily economy." Intramuscular injections of a 1:1000 solution of histamine were used, with the dosage slowly increased to a maximum of 7 mg. Various vasomotor symptoms and general discomfort, headache, and palpitations were observed, lasting for thirty to sixty minutes. A drop in blood pressure was always noticed.

Histamine treatment in psychiatric disorders was again recommended by Sackler et al. on the basis of a somewhat different idea. These authors, looking for a common denominator in ECT and insulin, made the observation that a vasodilating agent was apparently liberated by the passage of an electric current through living tissues, and that there was an increase in gastric hydrochloric acid during ECT, which increase might in part be attributable to the effect of a histamine-like agent released by this procedure. Histamine was given intramuscularly, starting with 3 mg. of histamine base in 6 to 9 cc. of saline, divided into two doses, the second of which was given after an interval of 45 minutes. The total number of treatments ranged from 9 to 70. The authors treated schizophrenics, manic-depressives and involutionals, and seemed to obtain as good results with histamine as with ECT. In a second paper, Sackler et al. found that histamine-refractory patients, when receiving ECT after the histamine, showed results superior to those obtained in patients who had ECT alone. Shortly after the original publications reports from different hospitals were presented. Hoch, adding up these results, arrived at a recovery rate, for instance, for manic depressives, of 30 per cent which is considerably less than that obtained with ECT. A study by Hoffa and Parsons in schizophrenics was too small to permit conclusions.

Malononitrile; Succinylnitrile

In 1947, on the basis of theoretical concepts of Casperson, Hydén and Hartelius reported on attempts at increasing the nucleo-protein content of ganglion cells by intravenous injection of malononitrile. After quantitative studies made by microspectrographical methods of the nucleo-protein content of the nerve cells of rabbits, they made similar determinations on human brain tissue of mental patients who underwent frontal lobotomy. They found that the amount of nucleo-protein in certain ganglion cells of psychotics was significantly less than in normal persons.

Malononitrile was administered in doses of 3 to 6 mg. per kilogram of body weight at 2 to 4 day intervals. An hour after the injection of 5 per cent malononitrile, sodium thiosulfate was given which counteracts toxic symptoms such as nausea. The clinical results reported by the originators of the method were that in endogenous depressions the drug first accentuated psychomotor retardation and depression but later produced psychomotor spontaneity and euphoria. In schizophrenics, initial accentuation of catatonic symptoms was later followed by improved contact and mental release.

A study by MacKinnon et al. could not confirm the favorable results reported by the originators of the method. Neither improvements nor other alterations in the mental picture were seen. Hartelius, in a later article, tried to explain these negative results by the fact that sodium thiosulfate was administered too early and before the malononitrile could have achieved results. The period during which malononitrile takes effect should be one hour. In material treated since the publication of the first paper, Hartelius again reported favorably. Each patient was given an average of 1,250 mg.; the average individual dose was 2.4 mg. per kilogram of body weight; the average number of treatments was 8.

Delay et al. experimented with succinylnitrile, a chemical substance closely related to malononitrile. The results were not encouraging.

The therapeutic attempts with malononitrile found new significance through work by Cameron based on the malononitrile nitrate studies by Hydén and Hartelius, Cameron tried to influence memory disturbances in senile psychoses with ribonucleic acid, and later with Cylert described in the next chapter.

Chemical Treatment of Senile Psychoses

Ribonucleic Acid

In 1956 D. E. Cameron started to use nucleic acids in aged patients. These attempts were based on work by Hydén. He and Hartelius had shown that malononitrile, or probably its reaction product malononitrile dimer, stimulated the large nerve cells of the central nervous system to an increased production of nucleic acid in protein substances. This malononitrile produce speeds up synthesis of ribonucleic acid (RNA). It was found that rats subjected to a learning experiment, showed an increased amount of RNA in nerve cells. Cameron started with the use of deoxyribonucleic acid (DNA) given intravenously in association with intrathecal hyaluronidase, the latter being added to improve the blood-brain barrier permeability. The work was continued with the use of RNA because of its apparent closer relationship to protein synthesis. It could be shown that RNA favorably affects memory deficits in the aged. The result was marked most in the arteriosclerotic, next in the presenile (Alzheimer's and Pick's diseases) and least in the senile psychoses. Intravenous administration gives more marked results than oral administration. One prefers RNA 10 per cent buffer solution, the basic material being obtained from yeast. The injections were usually given three times per week. It must be realized that the clinical improvement which is more visible in moderate than in severe cases of memory impairment, does not necessarily prove the validity of the theory on which the treatment is based. It is interesting that Kral, in a personal communication, confirmed the favorable clinical impression but also noticed improvements in depressions without organic memory impairment. A few studies by other investigators, some with negative results, have appeared since.

Magnesium Pemoline (Cylert)

This is a substance which stimulates the RNA synthesis in the brain and has been demonstrated to improve memory in healthy individuals. Talland et al.

using it in chronic Korsakoff patients, found some general improvement but no evidence of a reliable effect on memory disorders. Using a placebo and metamphetamine as controls and giving Cylert in a single dose of 50 mg., also over a period of three weeks in doses of 25 and 50 mg., they conclude that some improvement may be due to the general stimulatory properties of the drug rather than to its specific impact on learning and remembering. More favorable results were obtained by Freyhan et al. who gave magnesium pemoline, 75 mg. daily, for three weeks to patients with organic brain syndrome. They also used a placebo and dextroamphetamine with amobarbital, each patient serving as his own control, one group starting with the amphetamine, the other with the magnesium pemoline. The Wechsler Memory Quotient increased significantly on both active compounds. There was, however, a significant difference in favor of magnesium pemoline over the amphetamine compound. Clinical evaluation of psychostimulant effects revealed more effective results with the amphetamine compound. Thus, while magnesium pemoline is the weaker psychostimulant, its effect on memory improvement was superior.

Nicotinic Acid and Nicotinamide in Schizophrenia

On the basis of a biochemical theory regarding faulty adrenochrome metabolism in schizophrenics Hoffer and Osmond, 15 years ago, started to treat schizophrenic patients with massive doses of nicotinic acid, penicillamine and ascorbic acid. In 1966, they were able to report very successful treatment of acute and chronic schizophrenics. It consisted of daily oral doses of 1 to 2 grams of nicotinamide adenine dinucleotide (NAD), also known as dephosph-pyridine-nucleotide (DNP). In a recent long-term follow-up Hoffer concluded that the majority of acute patients receiving nicotinic acid or nicotinamide responded much better to the overall treatment, when these vitamins were included, than did a comparison control group. Also chronic schizophrenics as a group did better, although the majority of these patients did not benefit. His conclusions were based on readmission rates and also on the fact that no suicide occurred in any treated patient. This therapeutic approach found very wide publicity, and corroboration by other workers was hoped for. The first control study was done with a very elaborate methodology but a small number of patients by Kline et al. together with a group from the American College of Neuropsychopharmacology. Ten patients were treated with the material, and ten matched patients received placebo. No convincing improvement was seen in either group, aside from some placebo effect which occurred in both groups.

Equally negative results were reported in some acute cases by Kline himself outside this study. Hoffer and Osmond objected to the way the substance had been administered. It should be given in enteric-coated capsules to avoid the presence of free nicotinic acid, while actually the NAD should arrive intact in the blood. Other authors (Gallant et al.) used both enteric-coated and other material at 4 grams a day, and found little improvement with either method, and certainly no improvement in chronic deteriorated schizophrenics as had been claimed by the originators of the method. A survey on the chemical implications of this treatment was made by Neumann who clinically saw an activation of psychotic symptoms but no improvement. He quotes some more favorable results by Chinaglia. Although some of the results obtained by the originators even in extremely chronic schizophrenics were quite amazing and justify further serious control investigations, the presently available knowledge of cases so treated, does not seem to prove the efficacy of this new pharmacological approach.

Atropine and Scopolamine Treatment

Based on therapeutic results in chronic cases of encephalitis, Hoch used atropine in other mental patients, particularly catatonic schizophrenics in the early 1930's. He used doses up to 20 mg., but results remained entirely negative which proved to him that catatonia was not an extrapyramidal symptom.

Repeated toxic doses of atropine sulfate by intramuscular injection were applied to mental patients by Forrer. The patients were treated three to six times per week with 32 to 200 mgms per treatment. The first reaction to the injection is a drying of the mouth and mucous membranes, the skin becomes warm and dry, while an evanescent rash may appear over the face, neck and upper parts of the body. Brief acceleration of the pulse and respiration, with a slight rise of B.P. are followed by a return to normal levels. This is followed by restlessness, excitement, confusion, giddiness, muscular incoordination and speech disturbance with disorientation and visual hallucinations. Then the patient passes into coma from which there is spontaneous awakening.

Forrer and his co-workers regard the main indication for this treatment to be anxiety and agitation, regardless of diagnostic category. They therefore advocate its use in the neuroses including obsessional neurosis with anxiety, and in the psychoses apart from depression in which it is ineffective.

The most serious complication is hyperthermia (treated with ice-packs); it is unclear whether this is of central or peripheral origin. Hyperthermia was the cause of death in the one fatality in 10,000 treatments. Contraindications to the treatment are glaucoma, impairment of cardiac function, marked malnutrition since there is weight loss with the treatment, and severe liver disease as atropine is detoxified in the liver. The drying of mucous membranes may lead to an activation of an old sinusitis or otitis media. At present there is no antidote to atropine, but according to Forrer there is a wide margin of safety.

The improvement reported in a percentage of cases of diversified diagnostic categories—mania, schizophrenia, neurosis—is difficult to explain on theoretical grounds, apart from Forrer's general postulate that it permits reintegration of the shattered ego. In this connection the recent work of Ackner et al. claims equal efficacy of coma with insulin and barbiturates, and the question of whether it is the coma rather than the coma-producing agent which is of therapeutic benefit in schizophrenia, is of interest. The coma rather than the drug atropine may explain the results.

Stimulated by Forrer's work with atropine Goldner experimented with scopolamine. Since l-isomers of the belladonna alkaloids are biologically much more effective than the d-form, and since scopolamine is the l-isomer of hyoscine, scopolamine was given intramuscularly in doses of 5 to 30 mg. initially, increased in subsequent treatments by 5 or 10 mg. to a maximum of 100 mg. (5 cc. of the usual solution). In a few minutes this leads to a sleeplike state with some involuntary movements which later lead to extensor rigidity and opisthotonus. The patient develops hyperthermia. After 4 to 6 hours he arouses with symptoms of a delirium. Physostigmine salicylate appears to be a specific antagonist for use in scopolamine therapy. Results are described as "favorable in selected cases of schizophrenic and manic reactions."

Hormone Therapy

In a recent monograph, M. Bleuler made a complete survey of endocrinological treatments in mental disease. Of only historical interest are attempts like castration in schizophrenics, epileptics, and hysterical psychopaths. The same is true for thyroidectomy in schizophrenics and manic-depressives, implantation of various endocrine glands, and irradiation of the hypophysis.

The hypothesis that adreno-cortical activities have some etiological importance in schizophrenia led to an attempt to treat chronic schizophrenics with bilateral adrenalectomy. Apter gave a clinical follow-up six years after the operation of four such patients, and came to the conclusion that this operation does not influence the clinical course. Similar attempts were made by Allen and Brostel. Elmadjian et al. observed two adrenalectomized schizophrenic patients in whom the adrenals were removed for other reasons than the psychosis. They made the interesting observation that, although the operation did not change the thought disorders and other schizophrenic symptoms, these disappeared every time the patient lapsed into an adrenal crisis. In Cushing's disease adrenalectomy can remove schizophreniform reactions (Hickman et al.). Attempts to use ACTH or cortisone in the treatment of schizophrenia were made by Cohn et al. with good results, while Glaser and Hoch, and many others did not see convincing benefits from such treatment.

In general it must be admitted that even if certain endocrine symptoms can be changed, the mental symptoms usually remain uninfluenced. One of the exceptions is hypothyroidism as cause of cretinism in children, where endocrine treatment is known to be effective. In the major psychoses endocrinological therapy has not yet found a definite place. It has to be seen to what extent M. Reiss' attempts to investigate psychotics from all endocrinological angles, will lead to more definite indications for hormone therapy in psychiatric disorders.

Treatment with hormones had its widest application as replacement therapy in involutional psychoses. Results were poor. Convulsive therapy became the treatment of choice. Yet, the wish to use etiologically better founded methods explains why attempts to combine shock treatments with hormones are still made. This has been done not only in involutional cases but also in post-partum psychoses. Successful combination of insulin treatment and progesterone was reported by Billig and Bradley. These authors injected progesterone twice monthly, mostly on the twelfth and fourteenth days following the first day of the preceding menstruation. This was found to be of benefit in the alleviation of psychotic symptoms which were activated during the post-puerperal and premenstrual period. Testosterone was given successfully in depressions by

Altschule and Tillotson, who used it as a substance with strong anabolic effects rather than as a specific sex hormone. M. Bleuler and Züblin gave large doses of the hormone of the other sex to depressives but obtained rather unreliable results; some patients became euphoric, while others showed an aggravation of their depression. The euphorizing effect of cortisone-like substances in combination with ascorbic acid was used by Cranswick and Hall in various types of psychoses. Their favorable results in depressions were confirmed by Büssow, who found a similar unspecific effect with the male and female sex hormones. In endogenous depressions Büssow and Ottlik obtained results with extracts from the entire hypophysis followed by injections of ascorbic acid.

Hormones can be used effectively in the premenstrual tension syndrome which is characterized by a mixture of physical and mental symptoms—anxiety, tension, depression and irritability, with feelings of abdominal discomfort, painful swollen breasts and an increase in body weight—occurring in the latter half of the menstrual cycle. The evidence suggests that these symptoms are produced by water retention due to an abnormal elevation of the oestradiol/progesterone ratio (Greene and Dalton). Treatment has been directed to the production of dehydration by means of diuretics. Progesterone has been used to compensate for any imbalance of the oestrogens. It is given orally as ethisterone 5 mg. b.i.d. for twelve days before the onset of menstruation, increasing to 10 mg. b.i.d. if necessary. Alternatively, androgens which are also oestrogen antagonists may be given in the form of methyl testosterone 10 mg. daily, for the same period of time. This is reported to be as effective as ethisterone, but has the disadvantage of possible virilizing side effects. L. Rees reports that with the use of ethisterone there has been relief of both psychological and physical symptoms.

Attempts to Influence Metabolism

Metabolic changes in mental diseases found in various investigations have been the basis for therapeutic attempts. Their advantage over most other procedures is seen in the fact that they have a rationale. Yet, actual effectiveness has remained limited. Gjessing found abnormalities in the nitrogen metabolism in cases of schizophrenia with periodic course. His procedure of following the metabolic changes of catatonics through various phases was unique, but the actual therapeutic gain was small. His recommendation was a combination of thyroid extract in increasing doses up to 0.45 Gm., together with dietary measures. Later Danziger et al. successfully treated periodic catatonia by raising the basal metabolic rate with thyroid without regard to the nitrogen balance.

Based on observation of acidity in the blood and spinal fluid following shock treatment, Steinfeld believed that the acidosis is an important factor in the therapeutic mechanism of shock therapy. In accordance with similar ideas of Delay, he first used acidifying drugs, and later produced acidosis by dietary measures. He claims results with shock therapy in such dieting patients where it had failed without the acidifying diet. He feels that a ketoneproducing diet together with acidifying drugs may be sufficient to achieve results without shock therapy, but no clinical reports are available.

Georgi and his co-workers, studying manic-depressives and involutional depressions, noticed a disturbance in cholesterol metabolism and advised intramuscular injection of adrenal cortex preparations. An attempt to influence the course of a schizophrenic psychosis through support to the liver was made by Piaget. It had been demonstrated by several investigators and confirmed by Georgi that the hippuric acid synthesis of the liver is impaired during acute exacerbations of schizophrenia. Piaget, therefore, tried to support the liver by a diet poor in fat, rich in carbohydrates and proteins, and by administration of methionine, choline, inositol, enzymes and glucose. In almost all schizophrenics, the improvement of the liver function was accompanied by a distinct improvement of the mental condition.

In connection with these attempts to change the metabolism, it may be mentioned that the hypothesis of an endotoxic origin of catatonic episodes led Kielholz to the advocation of blood transfusions in such patients. After withdrawal of 500 to 800 cc. of blood, an infusion of the same amount was given together with 100 to 200 cc. of glucose solution on five subsequent days. Further work to study metabolic changes and possibly to determine an endotoxic etiology of mental disease might one day lead to more specific therapeutic recommendations. More recent work by Heath in the USA, Arnold in Austria and others who isolated certain chemical substances in schizophrenia, did not yet lead to practical results.

Treatment of Alcoholism (Emetics, Antabuse, etc.)

Even though alcoholism like drug addiction is a psychological problem, drugs are a helpful adjunct in the effort to keep the alcoholic away from alcohol for various lengths of time.

1. *Conditioning with emetics* is a combination of psychological and somatic approaches. This method, originally used in Russia, consists of administration of emetine or apomorphine followed by the intake of alcohol. The association with nausea makes the alcohol distasteful to the patient. After some time the conditioning wears off, and the procedure must be repeated at certain intervals. For technical details we are referring to the work of Voegtlin. It appears that the unpleasant features of this method prevented it from wider use which it undoubtedly deserves. Recently, more reports, mostly favorable, appear. According to Williams, the proper degree of aversion is reached when even the sight or smell of alcohol produce nausea. Desrulles and Fellion first subject their patients to a detoxication treatment with strychnine followed by dietary and supportive measures. Sargant and Slater gave amphetamine, 10 mgm. two and a half hours before the injection with emetine which is followed by injections with pilocarpine and ephedrine.

The treatment should never be given to those in poor physical health, especially patients with renal or cardio-vascular diseases, hepatic cirrhosis or any condition that might be exacerbated by vomiting, such as esophageal varices, peptic ulcer or hernia. Active psychosis has been named as a contraindication but Thompson and Bielinski reported improvements in a number of cases of psychoses treated with emetine aversion therapy. The majority of these reactions were due to alcoholism or associated deficiency states, but some of these psychoses had started prior to the excessive drinking.

The effect of the conditioning should be reinforced by antabuse. Social treatment is equally important, and use can be made of such valuable agencies at AA (Alcoholics Anonymous), where the alcoholic will meet others with the same problem.

Other authors who used emetics successfully, expressed different theoretical concepts. Dent administers apomorphine to the point of vomiting but considers this therapeutic effect as not due to the subsequent aversion which is only temporary but to the drug-induced reduction of anxiety and tension. He also tried it orally in out-patients. Since conditioning in animals can only be achieved if the stimulus produces an experience that is meaningful to them, Franks believes that any stimulus in alcoholics, in order to be successful, must involve the whole configuration of feelings associated with drinking alcohol. He, therefore, suggests that conditioning should also attempt to produce the pleasure and feeling of well-being associated with alcohol with the help of something innocuous. Therefore, the patient should be taught to use sweets and other harmless substitutes for the relief of anxiety. In other words, it is not sufficient to produce an association of nausea with alcohol which is inevitably of short duration. The conditioning can only be lasting when alcohol is replaced by a harmless substitute from which the patient derives similar satisfaction as from alcohol.

2. *Antabuse* (*tetraethylthiuramdisulfide*) or *Disulfiram* was introduced in Denmark by Hald et al., who noticed that persons ingesting this substance during experiments showed discomfort after consumption of alcohol. In the first large survey on their clinical experience, Jacobsen and Martensen-Larsen reported favorable results which were later confirmed by most other workers. Antabuse as such does not produce any symptoms in the vast majority of cases. However, when a person under antabuse medication takes alcohol the following symptoms appear: General flushing after five or ten minutes, with an unpleasant subjective feeling of heat in the face, vasodilatation elsewhere, pronounced reddening of the sclerae, increased pulse rate and a slowly progressing fall in blood pressure. After thirty to sixty minutes, nausea sets in, the flushing disappears, and the patient becomes pale; still later, vomiting may occur if the patient has consumed a larger amount of alcohol. Even if there is no vomiting, the general discomfort is pronounced for several hours and reminds the patient of an unduly severe hangover. These symptoms are explained by formation of acetaldehyde in the blood when antabuse and alcohol are combined.

The effect of antabuse is to inhibit the enzyme responsible for the breakdown of acetaldehyde during alcohol metabolism. Thus acetaldehyde is released and brings about the characteristic symptomatology. At least part of this syndrome is a histamine reaction and in cases where it is necessary to terminate the symptoms abruptly, anti-histamines may be given intravenously. The reaction can be inhibited by the intravenous injection of 1 Gm. of ascorbic acid.

The application which we prefer is as follows: The patient, who must be free from alcohol, is given doses of 1 to 2 Gm. of antabuse for three days. On the third or fourth day a test dose of alcohol is given. Originally the patient was advised to take the amount of alcohol he usually needed to feel an effect. In this way doses of 3 to 4 ounces of whiskey were consumed by the patient during the test. In view of some rather severe toxic reactions with such amounts, the general tendency is to limit the dose to 1 or 2 ounces, which is sufficient to give the patient considerable discomfort without the threatening symptoms. He is then kept on one tablet of 0.5 Gm. antabuse daily, which is enough to produce a strong reaction with alcohol. Even it he omits the drug one or several days, the blood level of antabuse is still high enough to give a reaction with alcohol.

R. Fox on the basis of a very extensive experience, does not consider the antabuse test a necessary preliminary to maintenance medication of antabuse. It is true that the test is unpleasant, but it is our experience that patients who are not given the test, often consider it a bluff when they are simply told about the discomfort they would experience from alcohol, while under antabuse. If they do drink in spite of the warning, the toxic reaction might be much more dangerous than when a test dose is given under medical supervision, and countermeasures are available. Fox also feels that it is sufficient to maintain patients on smaller daily doses of 0.25 gram (half a tablet).

The toxic symptoms can be rather severe. The most threatening manifestation during a test is the fall in blood pressure, particularly of the diastolic pressure, which in some instances cannot even be read. If the patient's condition becomes threatening or if he loses consciousness, ephedrine intravenously and other methods to counteract shock must be applied. An early fatality occurred in a patient who received antabuse in the middle of a heavy drinking spell. An occasional threatening collapse was seen not infrequently when too much alcohol had been given in the test. Bowman et al. noticed electrocardiographical changes in two patients, and a myocardial infarction in another patient who drank while under antabuse. Markham and Hoff took EKG's during tests. There were no critical clinical reactions but definite changes appeared in the EKG in 91 per cent of the cases attributed to the toxic effect on the myocardium of the metabolites of the reaction. The changes were reversible but the authors indicated that it is wise to withhold antabuse (disulfiram) if there is any suspicion of cardiac abnormality. The dangers even in the physically healthy are emphasized by McCabe and Wilson who found evidence of severe cardiac embarrassment in the EKG during the alcohol-antabuse reaction in 35 per cent of patients in the fourth and fifth decade of life in whom the previous work-up had not revealed any cardiac abnormality.

Other complications are psychotic reactions which Bowman et al. consider as being results of alcohol withdrawal but which others suspect to be a toxic effect of the antabuse. Bennett et al. interpret it as antabuse action in patients with some liver dysfunction or previous brain damage or both. Hayman and Wilkins reported six cases of polyneuropathy due to disulfiram. Møller-Madsen points out the danger of chloroform and trilene for anesthesia in patients receiving antabuse since both contain small amounts of alcohol. A high oxygen percentage in the anesthetic and in intravenous drip containing ascorbic acid in glucose is recommended for such cases.

No absolute contraindications have been described by Jacobsen and Martinsen-Larsen but Barrera listed myocardial failure and coronary disease as contraindications, and recommends caution in patients with enlarged thyroid, cirrhosis of the liver, nephritis, diabetes, pregnancy and epilepsy. In our opinion, the initial administration of antabuse and the alcohol test should be undertaken in a hospital.

The shortcoming of antabuse is that it depends on the patient's cooperation. However, in those who are anxious to give up their drinking it is a great help when these patients are momentarily tempted to drink. The relapse rate is high but antabuse medication can be started again, and sometimes the relapse has a good psychological effect on the patient who had thought that he could handle his urge for alcohol without the drug.

3. *A citrated calcium carbimide (C.C.C.)* was the result of reports of the cardiovascular effects of antabuse which led to a search for a drug with similar properties but without its toxicity. In 1956 Ferguson reported on a drug called C.C.C.–citrated calcium carbimide–composed of two parts by weight of citric acid added to one part of highly purified calcium carbimide (cyanimide) and incorporated in a slow release tablet containing 50 mg. of the carbimide. Its action in inhibiting acetaldehyde metabolism is the same as that of antabuse, but it is absorbed much more rapidly and its effect lasts for only about 24 hours. A single dose of 50 mg. will sensitize an individual to alcohol. Smith et al. confirmed the lack of disturbing cardiovascular symptoms during C.C.C.-alcohol reactions.

4. *Metronidazole (Flagyl):* This drug had been used since 1959 for trichomonas vaginitis and urethritis, when J. A. Taylor described in 1964 as a side observation that patients under this drug lost their taste for alcohol. Slowly they even develop an aversion to alcohol, but only mild to moderate antabuse-like reactions. The drug also improves the hypermetabolic state of delirium tremens. The dose recommended is metronidazole 250 mg. one to three times a day. Headache, asthmatic symptoms and bad taste were side-effects, sometimes leading to discontinuation of the drug by patients. Lehmann et al. in a favorable report on the drug also mentions its usefulness for alcohol withdrawal with doses of 1000 mg. four times a day in patients with various alcohol psychoses. Sogliani prefers the drug to antabuse in cardiac patients, because side-effects are less severe. It seems to be a useful new addition to the treatment of alcoholism, is similar to antabuse, has less violent reactions to alcohol, and is apparently better accepted by the patient. Most reports are favorable (Bonfiglio and Donadio, Semer et al., Goodwin).

5. *Chlormethiazol (Distraneurin):* Chlormethiazol is uniquely effective in the treatment of delirium tremens. In this condition the neuroleptic drugs are more and more recognized as being contraindicated because of their circulatory effects. Chlormethiazol was found to be the best compound for therapeutic use, after Thiazol had been studied in France as one of the two components of Vitamin B_1 (Thiamine).

Aside from an anticonvulsant action, chlormethiazol has a strong sedative and hypnotic effect. In Sweden, Osterman et al. tried it first, and Giacobini and Salum gave a survey on 159 cases of delirium tremens treated without a fatality. An increasing number of French, Swedish and German publications agree on the superiority of this drug compared to previous methods in delirium tremens. The German preparation with the trade name Distraneurin is available in tablets of 0.5 g., and also in 0.8 per cent solution. Oral medication with an initial dose of 1 to 1½ g., usually leads to a sleep-like state which is maintained with additional doses. Gastager et al. did not succeed with oral usage and, like many others, prefer intravenous infusions. The delirious manifestations usually clear up after 24 to 48 hours. Electroencephalographic studies by Amber and Bergener seem to prove that the effect is obtained through stimulation of subcortical areas which are assumed to be the points where alcohol has its main effect in the CNS. The usefulness of the drug in pre-delirious states underscores its preventive value. It is also indicated in other organic brain disorders with psychomotor restlessness, e.g., in senile conditions.

6. *Other attempts* should be briefly mentioned. Insulin in subcoma doses has been used since the 1920's, but is of limited value except for improving the general condition of the alcoholic. It also reduces withdrawal symptoms from alcohol and the tension which often leads to drinking. Today chlorpromazine and other neuroleptic drugs are used for this purpose. The occasional use of convulsive therapy for the psychiatric conditions underlying alcoholism in certain cases has been mentioned in the chapters on these treatments. ACTH and cortisone have also been recommended. Hormonal therapy was developed by J. J. Smith for alcoholism, and adrenocorticotropic hormone was administered.

A wider use of these hormones has been made in delirium tremens. Here, also large doses of vitamins were recommended. Richter reported that thyroid extract greatly increased the craving for sugar in rats. After he indicated similar craving for alcohol the thyroid extract also induced the rats' craving for alcohol, and he suggests similar attempts in man.

Lysergic acid diethylamide (LSD) has been used in a group of 20 recalcitrant alcoholics by R. Fox in a hospital setting in doses of 200 micrograms. A follow-up showed a rather high number of lasting improvements. Even though the author does not exclude a placebo effect or the total hospital regime as responsible for the improvements, she feels that this indication of LSD should be further investigated.

In spite of the psychological basis in most cases of alcoholism, the poor psychotherapeutic results make it necessary to try the various somatic treatments which are often extremely useful even in serious cases of alcoholism.

The Treatment of Drug Addiction

Pharmacotherapy and other somatic treatments have been used in three different ways in the management of addiction to opiates, to alleviate the withdrawal symptoms, to replace opiates with less harmful drugs, and to use the antagonistic action of certain chemicals to opiates.

Withdrawal symptoms in drug addiction had been alleviated with insulin hypoglycemia and also with a few ECT's as has been discussed in the chapters on these treatments. After the introduction of chlorpromazine this drug alone as well as in combination with insulin and barbiturates has been recommended. Fraser and Isbell could demonstrate the failure of neuroleptic drugs in the treatment of abstinence from opiates.

Methadone is not only being used for quite some time in morphine and heroin addiction as a substitute for the opiate during the period of withdrawal, but more recently it is recommended to replace the harmful opiates as a less harmful drug for an indefinite period of time. Its usefulness for gradual withdrawal of opiates is based on the effect that its withdrawal produces fewer symptoms than the withdrawal of opiates. Therefore, the usual procedure is to give 1 mg. of methadone to replace 4 mgs. of morphine, 1 mg. of dilaudid, 2 mg. of heroin, 20-30 mg. of demerol or 20-30 mgs. of codeine. In most cases 10-20 mg. of methadone, twice daily by the oral route is sufficient. In heavy opiate intake higher doses of methadone might be necessary. After 2 or 3 days the methadone can be reduced at approximately two day intervals to 50, 30, 10 and 5 per cent of the amount which just prevents the appearance of abstinence symptoms. No such scheme of withdrawal is required with cocaine and marihuana.

The high relapse rate in the withdrawal of opiates led to the idea of keeping patients under medical control on a lasting regime with methadone. Dole and Nyswander experimented with the use of methadone in ambulatory treatment of addicts. Such a regimen helps maintain a therapeutic relationship and enhances efforts at rehabilitation. The use of drugs with an antagonistic action to morphine and other opiates is the more recent way of pharmacological treatment of addicts. Cyclazocine, a benzo-morphane derivate is, like nalorphine an analgesic and has a fairly long lasting antagonistic action to morphine. The usual procedure is to detoxify the patient with methadone within 4 to 7 days, and then to give cyclazocine, starting with 0.2 mg. per day, and increase 0.2 mg. every day. The desired dose reached within 15 days is 4 mg. given in a single dose each morning. After this dose has been reached, it is demonstrated to the patient that self-administration of 50 mg. i.v. heroin fails to have the usual euphoric and general systemic effects. The effect of one dose of cyclazocine usually lasts for 20 to 24 hours. Side-effects are increased libido, constipation and some general nervousness. It is interesting to note that cyclazocine has also an antidepressant effect. On withdrawal from cyclazocine some withdrawal symptoms such as irritability, depression and paranoid ideation can be described.

The search for better antinarcotics without side-effects and without withdrawal symptoms led to experimentation with another antagonist, naloxone (n-allyl-noroxymorphone) recommended by Blumberg et al. and Jasinski et al. Fink et al. found that 200 mg. of naloxone orally blocks the euphoric effect of heroin and that the side-effects obtained with cyclazocine are absent. They also demonstrated that in EEG recordings the desynchronization and increased theta and beta frequencies seen with other antinarcotics like nalorpine and cyclazocine are missing.

Barbiturate withdrawal may be followed by epileptic fits and examination of the EEG during this period shows progressive slowing with paroxysmal bursts of high voltage. There is danger of convulsions up to the seventh day, and gradual withdrawal should avoid tremor and muscle twitchings which show that the dosage is being cut too rapidly (Isbell and White). Dilantin should be given at the same time. The other withdrawal symptoms of barbiturate intoxication are delirium-like states which can be well controlled with chlorpromazine. Since chlorpromazine is epileptogenic these patients should also receive anticonvulsive medication. The same treatment is advised for withdrawal syndromes of the same nature which were recently observed in meprobamate addiction and also after abuse of chlordiazepoxide (Librium).

Psychopharmacotherapy with Anti-epileptic Drugs

It is beyond the scope of this book to discuss the diagnostic problems of the various psychiatric disorders in connection with epilepsy. It can be debated to what extent behavior problems in children, certain cases of aggressive psychopaths, and some other syndromes are actually related to epilepsy even though electroencephalographic findings suggest such causality. Seizure discharges from the temporal lobes have been found with particular frequency in psychotic syndromes labeled as psychomotor epilepsy. In many of these conditions anticonvulsive therapy is of limited success.

Dilantin sodium (sodium diphenylhydantoinate), introduced by Merritt and Putnam as an anticonvulsant, was soon recognized as also having a striking effect on psychic equivalents. This led Kalinowsky and Putnam to attempts to treat various nonepileptic psychotics with dilantin. Symptomatic improvements were seen in a large number of patients. No specific effect in any particular type of mental illness was observed, and no cures were obtained. Disturbed patients showed the best response. In the schizophrenic group catatonic excitements improved greatly but patients in catatonic stupor remained uninfluenced. Hallucinations disappeared in only one patient, and even in this case they returned four days after dilantin had been discontinued. In the manic-depressive group manic excitements showed by far the best results. In a majority of patients the excitement subsided; twice patients changed from a manic attack into a depression. The purely symptomatic action of dilantin was demonstrated by the fact that discontinuation of the drug usually led to relapse after the same four or five days required for the anticonvulsive effect of dilantin to wear off. It is also in accord with experience in epilepsy that dilantin influences mental symptoms only when given in doses close to the toxic level (four to five capsules of 1½ grains daily). Freyhan obtained similar results.

The above mentioned clinical results and some attempts by later investigators have not been correlated to electroencephalographic findings. A different approach to the problem was undertaken in children with behavior problems. An unusually high percentage of abnormal electroencephalographic patterns suggested to some authors a connection of these disorders with epilepsy. Walter and Kirkpatrick used dilantin in behavior problem children with abnormal electroencephalographic findings. All the children showed a definite clinical improvement.

Twenty-five years after the original use in non-epileptics the self-observation of a prominent layman led to a study of its use in neuroses. Turner used 0.1 gm. daily in a variety of patients with findings of dependency, irritability, anxiety, obsessive-compulsive and other neurotic symptoms. His conclusion was that "Dilantin is an effective agent in the relief of symptoms in a variety of neurotic disturbances. It is particularly effective in relief of neurotic depression, tension and irritability, especially in persons with obsessive or passive-dependent personalities."

Chemically somewhat related to dilantin is phenurone (phanacetylurea). This drug is of special value for psychic equivalents or psychomotor epilepsy, while it is inferior to dilantin in grand mal seizures of epilepsy. Gibbs et al. noticed remarkable improvements in psychomotor seizure under average doses of 2.5 Gm. (up to 5 Gm.) of phenurone but they also saw aggravation of psychiatric manifestations in some cases. A toxic psychosis in a patient simultaneously showing evidence of acute liver damage was described by de Jongh. Other complications like severe skin conditions and blood dyscrasias are further evidence of the great toxicity of the drug which for this reason is not widely used in spite of its apparent superiority in psychomotor epilepsy over dilantin.

Mysoline (ethylphenylhecahydropyrimidine dione) is a newer anticonvulsant which is also said to have an effect on the psychiatric manifestations of epilepsy. It can be given up to 1.5 Gm. daily and seems to be less toxic than phenurone.

Fever Therapy

The various methods of inducing fever as treatment for mental illness represent the first successful organic therapeutic approach in psychiatry, but their usefulness largely remained limited to specific infections of the nervous system. Wagner-Jauregg's starting point was the frequently reported spontaneous improvement of psychoses during infectious diseases, but he had already noticed that such observations applied chiefly to cases of general paresis. The technique of inoculation with malaria, which turned out to be the best controllable infection for the treatment of mental patients, has been dealt with extensively in monographs by Gerstmann and by Dattner. Results remained disappointing in the nonsyphilitic psychoses (Hinsie). Physical methods of fever therapy are described in the book by Neymann on Artificial Fever. The introduction of penicillin treatment for general paresis has demonstrated even more convincingly that it is the infectious agent which is treated in general paresis. Many, though not all, workers feel that penicillin alone is equally effective as malaria. Kierland and O'Leary treated successfully neurosyphilitic patients with oral aureomycin (60 Gm. given in 2 to 4 Gm. daily doses).

Fever treatment in other psychoses was tried with unspecific provocation of fever by means of sulfur in oil. The Danish psychiatrist, Schroeder-Knud, used it first in 1924 in general paresis with the idea of supplementing or replacing malaria treatment with a simpler method, and later in nonsyphilitic psychoses. Sulfur in oil was used mainly as sulfosin 1 per cent. The injection is given at night; the temperature rise occurs six to eight hours later. One to three series of eight to ten injections each were recommended.

A study of the treatment of dementia praecox with malaria, other infectious diseases, nonspecific organic substances, as well as sulfur was made by the French authors Claude et al. They reported a recovery rate of 10 per cent and improvements in 30 per cent of the cases treated. Buscaino, who considers schizophrenia a toxic condition, produces fever by means of vaccines. In Germany pyrifer and other preparations consisting of various bacilli were used. Fuster reported on chronic schizophrenics who failed under insulin or convulsive therapy but responded to a combination of fever therapy and electric shock, the so-called pyretoelectric convulsive therapy. However, fever treatment in schizophrenia has only been used by few psychiatrists.

Refrigeration Therapy: Hypothermia

Reports on the use of refrigeration ("frozen sleep") in the treatment of malignant diseases led to similar attempts in schizophrenia. Talbott and Tillotson induced hypothermia in psychotics by placing the patient between a pair of blankets through which a refrigerant was circulating at a temperature of 32° or less. The body temperature was reduced below 85°, and a minimum temperature of 74.6° was observed in one patient. Although some patients showed clinical changes, the result was unsatisfactory. One of the ten patients treated died from cardiovascular failure during treatment. After some equally unsatisfactory reports interest was revived when chlorpromazine was introduced as "hibernation therapy" by French authors. The hypothermia claimed for "hibernation" with chlorpromazine and similar drugs was minimal. Combining refrigeration and drug-induced hypothermia, Fisher and Greiner described a case of acute catatonic stupor with a pyrexia of 107°. They used ice packs to bring down the patient's temperature to 80°, at which temperature she was allowed to remain for 36 hours. Together with this, they administered intravenous chlorpromazine, 75 mgm, as well as fluids and antibiotics. After cessation of refrigeration the temperature returned spontaneously to a normal level after a brief rebound rise to 101°. The mental condition showed a gradual return to a level which permitted discharge six weeks later. The authors suggest that wider use should be made of hypothermia in the treatment of disturbed and physically poor-risk patients.

Photoshock

Cossa and Gastaut noticed that intermittent photic stimulation lowers the threshold to metrazol convulsions, and they recommend this combination under the name of photoshock. They used visual stimuli with a rhythm of 15 flashes per second applied with a stroboscope. Gastaut claims that this also reduces anxiety after the treatment. Photoshock without convulsion was described by Flanigan et al. who combined photic and chemical stimulation in the following way: They gave a standard dose of 1 cc. of 5 per cent hexazoletriazol intravenously and followed this 5 to 15 seconds later by photic stimulation which they repeated in regular intervals. The patient usually shows myoclonic movements. Such stroboscopically induced dysrhythmia of the electroencephalographic pattern, together with the action of an analeptic drug acting supposedly on the diencephalon, seems to achieve results similar to ECT, but the authors admit that further investigations are required to support this conclusion. Photoshock with convulsions is being considered superior to ECT without photostimulation by Ulett because it is said to produce a more gradual onset of seizures, less confusion, and good clinical results, particularly in depressions. A combination of photic, sonic and tactile stimuli was recommended in various psychiatric disorders by Lovett et al. as "Bombardment therapy."

Cerebral Pneumotherapy

Cerebral pneumotherapy was introduced by Delay et al. It was used with lumbar or suboccipital gas injection or ventriculogram. The method was found accidentally in a patient in whom a pneumoencephalogram had been performed for neurological reasons, and in whom amelioration of mental symptoms could be observed. In a series of patients so treated, temporary as well as lasting improvements were seen. Temporary changes were particularly striking in manic states which cleared up for a period of up to four weeks, but then reappeared. Also in schizophrenic excitement states a temporary relief was noted. Lasting changes are most frequent in melancholia, where the episode may clear up entirely (Deshaies and Le Pourbiet). Also aggressive oligophrenics respond well. Most clinicians saw only temporary results. Borel combines it with insulin, fever therapy and ECT. He replaces the entire spinal fluid with air. Abely uses oxygen and injects a larger amount than he withdrew spinal fluid in order to facilitate the ascension of the oxygen. He also uses ozone. The originators of "pneumoshock" as it is also called, explained the results with an effect on the regulating centers of the diencephalo-hypophyseal area. There is no evidence that this theoretically interesting treatment is still used anywhere.

Other Therapeutic Attempts

A number of pharmacotherapeutical attempts of the past did not fulfill the hope of their originators. They will be mentioned only briefly. Methylguanidine, a substance found in the urine of burned individuals, was seen to improve schizophrenia. Lactic acid has been used in depressions because its content in the blood is raised after convulsive therapy. Prostigmine has been tried in involutional psychoses to counteract aberrations in vegetative tonus. Cannabis-like drugs such as synhexyl were used in depressions because of their euphorizing effect. Attempts with tuberculin as well as gold salts were made in France based on concepts that certain psychoses are related to tuberculosis.

Glutamic acid, said to increase mental and physical alertness in mental defectives, has also been tried in schizophrenia but has found no wider use. Tetraethyl ammonium chloride was recommended in anxiety states because it counteracts acetylcholine.

Cameron treated persistent anxiety states with adrenaline in an effort to desensitize the adrenal sympathetic nervous system which remains overactive in anxiety states even after removal of the precipitating conflict. The signficance of the adrenals also figured in Rockwell's recommendation of dibenamine hydrochloride which is an effective adrenergic blocking agent.

Theories of reduced blood circulation in the brain led to the administration of various cerebral vasodilators such as folliculine with caffeine (Baruk and Racine), amylnitrate, stellate ganglion block by means of procaine (Karnosh and Gardner). A "vascular therapy" has been tried in Germany with such drugs as euphyllin, hydrergin, theophyllin, nicotinic acid (von Baeyer and Tellenbach quoted by Hippius and Jantz) in mild depressions particularly of older age. In senile and arteriosclerotic psychoses metrazol was used unsuccessfully by Gross and Finn, and intravenous iodide by Wilson and Hohmann, but abandoned because of two fatalities. In a variety of conditions Straube tried aminophenazone by intravenous injections of 2 to 5 cc.

Oral hypoglycemic agents have already been mentioned in the chapter on Insulin Coma Treatment. Frost used the euphorizing and anti-hallucinogenic effect on the hypoglycemic drug carbutamide alone as a therapeutic approach to schizophrenia. He thought of schizophrenia being a toxic-infectious encephalopathy which could be favorably affected by the bacteriostatic action of sulphonamides like carbutamide. Gouldman et al. did not confirm his favorable impression.

A method introduced in Russia is the use of "antireticulocytotoxic serum" (Bogomoletz). Outside of the Soviet Union similar sera are available in France and Italy. These attempts are based on the significance of the mesenchyma for all healing processes in the human organism. The serum is prepared by immunization of rabbits with human mesenchymal tissue, in particular spleen and bone marrow. This is supposed to stimulate the restorative and productive functions of connective tissues whose dysfunction is supposed to be characteristic of the schizophrenic process. Some cases showed marked improvement under this treatment alone, but apparently it is considered mainly as a good basis for the application of other forms of treatment. Ewalt and Bruce made similar attempts without seeing significant clinical changes.

It may be mentioned here that another method tried in the Soviet Union under the name of "colloidoclastic shock treatment" consists in the intravenous administration of 5 to 20 cc. of incompatible blood. The dose is increased with each injection, and the patient is supposed to have a strong vasomotor and autonomic reaction lasting 5 to 25 minutes, followed by a febrile reaction varying in intensity and duration. The statistics in early cases of schizophrenia compared favorably with insulin treatment.

Introduction of ions of magnesium into the brain with his method of transcerebral "dielectrolysis" was recommended by Bourgignon in various mental conditions, especially in depressions, but it also brought temporary improvement in a case of dementia praecox. While calcium ions are effective in neuralgias and other neurological conditions, they are ineffective in depressions, where dielectrolysis with magnesium is the most promising method, and, according to Bourgignon, sometimes superior to shock therapy.

A therapeutic attempt of great theoretical interest was made by Cerletti: It was based on his conclusion that the convulsive seizure releases all nervous, humoral, biochemical, endocrine reactions regulated by the diencephalic-neurovegetative systems which are organized phylogenetically for the defense of the organism. Cerletti formulated the theory that repeated electrically induced convulsions form a substance in the brain, and he called this substance "acroagonine." His idea was to produce this substance in animals by means of repeated electric shock treatments. A suspension of cerebral material of such animals was prepared in phenotic water and injected intramuscularly into various psychiatric patients. In many cases there was a marked improvement in affect and in their anxiety. Transient benefit in psychotics was seen by Kornmüller who used extracts from the brains of electroshocked rabbits. If these extracts were injected into other animals the electroencephalogram showed characteristics similar to those seen after ECT. A similar idea was the basis for Doussinet and Thévenot's report on intravenous injection of 10 to 15 cc. of serum from electric shock-treated patients into others. Cerletti also made experiments to show that these "acroagonines" increased the resistance of animals against certain infections. The therapeutic value of this method in mental disorders has not been established but it is an interesting attempt to reproduce the beneficial effect of electric shock in an indirect way. If it turns out to be unsuccessful, it should not discourage similar attempts which, some future day, may enable us to reproduce the cerebral changes occurring in convulsive therapy with less complicated and better understood methods.

CHAPTER VII

Theoretical Remarks

Psychiatry differs from other fields of medicine in a deplorable lack of facts on which all psychiatrists can agree. There is no generally accepted etiology of most mental diseases, and the entire foundation of the specialty of psychiatry is based on theories believed by some, and opposed by others. It is, therefore, not surprising that attempts to explain treatment procedures vary with the theoretical approach of the observer. This in itself leads to differences in explaining the mode of action of treatments. The matter is complicated by the fact that all psychiatric treatments were found empirically, and only later theories were developed to explain their action. Many theories were offered for one individual method, and efforts to find a common denominator for several treatments with similar effects have also been made. None of these attempts was satisfactory. The following chapter tries to list the theories presented in the literature, and to scrutinize their validity.

Pharmacotherapy

While in the field of the later discussed shock treatments physiological and psychological theories were primarily based on the individual belief of those who developed them, pharmacotherapy seemed to offer a more scientific basis of theoretical considerations. It must not be overlooked, however, that no theoretical concepts led to the introduction of any of the new drugs into psychiatry. Even the hope that they would contribute to a better understanding of the pathophysiological manifestations underlying psychiatric disorders, was not yet fulfilled. The same hope had been expressed when shock treatments were introduced. Thus far, all forms of therapy were equally disappointing in this respect. In pharmacotherapy the interest of the basic sciences was greater than in previous somatic treatments, and it was justified to expect that this chemical approach would lead to better knowledge of the biochemical basis of psychopathological manifestations and their changes under the influence of known chemicals. Actually, the various theories presented for the action of the empirically found neuroleptics are still quite speculative. Some clearly defined theories on certain antidepressant drugs turned out to be inapplicable to other drugs with the same clinical effect. The following theoretical considerations are presented mainly as a starting point for further efforts.

The main basis for theory formation in pharmacotherapy is animal experimentation and observations in humans. Most pharmacological properties have already been described in the chapters on the various drugs or groups of drugs. It soon became apparent, and is today the generally accepted view that the side-effects of psychotropic drugs in humans have the greatest significance for an understanding of their mode of action. It can even be expected that clinical-pharmacological longitudinal studies of these side-effects will be more revealing regarding their therapeutic mechanism than animal experimentation. There is already a consensus that extrapyramidal motor side-effects are an indicator of the neuroleptic action of the drug. These characteristic side-effects of neuroleptic drugs permit the conclusion that neuroleptics exert their main effect on the brain stem. Consequently it is assumed that this effect on the brain stem is probably also the basis of their therapeutic action. This opinion is supported by a great many older clinical psychiatric observations which demonstrate that all noxious agents with effect on the brain stem lead to a triad of extrapyramidal motor, vegetative, and psychopathological effects. In the case of the brain stem effects of neuroleptics it can be stated that the psychopathological manifestations of the drugs are used therapeutically, while their extrapyramidal and their vegetative effects are considered to be side-effects because both these sets of physical symptoms are unwanted from a practical standpoint. If, however, one looks at these physical symptoms from a theoretical standpoint, they should not be taken merely as side-effects but as an integral part of the total action of these most beneficial psychotropic drugs. Their action in the brain stem is not limited solely to the extrapyramidal motor nuclei but affects the thalamus, the hypothalamus, and the reticular formation as well.

Theoretical considerations regarding the antidepressants originally centered around the possible connection between monoamine oxidase inhibition and antidepressive effect. Later, when the tricyclic antidepressants were introduced, it became more and more apparent that it is probably not justified to try to explain the therapeutic antidepressive action with a single biochemically or pharmacologically identifiable effect. One has to assume a correlation of the antidepressive action with a pattern of various pharmacological properties. Thus, effective antidepressants have such different characteristics as anticholinergic action, tetrabenazine or reserpine reversal, and noradrenaline-potentiating effect.

The action of the various new drugs have also been explained in psychoanalytical terms. Sarwer-Foner edited a volume with numerous contributions on "The Dynamics of Psychiatric Drug Therapy." A contribution by Ostow infers that neuroleptics and antidepressants primarily affect a function which

Freud hypothesized "psychic energy," which is ultimately derived at from instinctual impetus. Ostow stipulates that the phenothiazines decrease the amount of psychic energy available to the ego, while iproniazid increases it.

There are many psychoanalysts who reject pharmacotherapeutic support to patients under psychotherapy for theoretical reasons. It is difficult to see why, for instance, a patient should not be given relief by means of drugs because it has been claimed that this may diminish his efforts to work out his problems with the psychotherapist. A more valid objection to the use of the new drugs is that such symptoms as feeling of depersonalization might be produced by certain drugs, and, like other side-effects, interfere with the patient's cooperation in psychotherapy. These are considerations in which the theoretical concepts of the individual psychiatrist influence his attitude regarding the use of drugs. True contributions to the understanding of drug action have not been made by psychodynamic interpretations. Unlike the literature on the so-called shock treatments, publications on psychotropic drugs have never seriously questioned their purely organic effect.

Most interesting attempts have been made frequently since the beginning of the psychopharmacotherapeutic era in 1952 to draw conclusions from the effect of the new drugs on the pathophysiology of the psychoses which are treated with these drugs. It can be expected that in the future psychotropic drugs, aside from their enormous practical importance for therapy, will also play a decisive role in basic science research related to psychiatry. This can be expected, although the various working hypotheses presented so far concerning the pathophysiology of schizophrenia in connection with psychopharmacology did not withstand critical testing. Examples are the serotonin theory and the adrenochrome theory. At present, the emphasis of pathophysiological research has shifted to the field of endogenous depressions. Extensive studies have been made in this area of research concentrating on the biogenic amines, mineral and water metabolism, and plasma cortisol concentration. They received a new impetus recently from the most promising therapy of manic-depressive psychoses with lithium salts. The tremendous potential of biological research in connection with the various new drugs is realized by an increasing number of psychiatrists.

Insulin and Convulsive Treatments

In the area of shock treatments, many theories have been presented, many of them without actual foundation in facts. Some overlap, and some express the same idea in different terms. This made it possible for Gordon to collect the surprising number of fifty different theories. We still agree with Nolan D. C. Lewis that "at the present time there is no theory as to the nature of the shock treatments sufficiently comprehensible to be taken very seriously."

The therapeutic action is explained by some authors on an organic basis, others believe that shock treatments effect essentially a psychogenic cure. The so-called somatic theories will be discussed first. The first explanation was advanced by Sakel concerning insulin treatment. The theory of insulin action was obviously evolved during or after the introduction of the treatment as an afterthought. Sakel himself realized that his theory was not too convincingly elaborated. He once wrote: "The mistakes in theory should not be counted against the treatment itself, which seems to be accomplishing more than the theory behind it."

Sakel believed that in schizophrenia the nerve cell develops an exaggerated activity, becomes oversensitive to the normal stimuli of the outside world and elaborates these stimuli excessively. "To restore normal conditions again," he writes, "one has to either limit the supply of excitant material, or else diminish combustion in the cell by muffling it." He conceives the action of insulin as being due to neutralization of the excitant, which he believes to be a hormone, and to the vagotonic muffling of the cell. He further assumes that in schizophrenics, the phylogenetically youngest intracellular connections are injured, and the more ancient nerve pathways are activated. As the disease progresses, these normally obliterated pathways dominate the scene. The stronger the harmful influence of the disease, more and more deeply seated pathways are involved successively until phylogenetically ancient pathway patterns are reached which prove to be resistant to the toxic influences. Sakel also assumes a short-circuiting of the pathways between the nerve cells. Insulin shock treatment, according to him, reverses all these processes by blockading the cell through influence on the vegetative centers so that the injured or confused pathways are not exposed to further stimuli. By means of this artificial rest, the normal pathways recuperate and attain their former prominence. In schizophrenia, vegetative subcortical centers are assumed to be the site of the primary disturbance, of which the abnormal psychotic symptoms are secondary manifestations.

It is apparent that this hypothesis of Sakel's is far too vague and speculative to offer convincing evidence on the action of insulin shock. It leaves completely unresolved the questions as to how and where this overaction of the nervous system originates in schizophrenia, and, furthermore, what kind of physical-chemical process is responsible for the "blockade" of the cell or the short-circuiting of the pathways. Nor does this theory elucidate the etiology of schizophrenia which is a necessary shortcoming of all theories on treatments of this disease.

A similar theory centering on cell destruction was evolved by Arnold. He assumes that insulin leads to an acute disorganization of carbohydrate metabolism of the ganglion cell which first interferes with cell function and ends in cell destruction. This effect of insulin is limited to those ganglion cells which for genetic reasons are predisposed to a disturbance in carbohydrate metabolism.

Meduna's introduction of the metrazol treatment was based on premises which proved to be incorrect, but, as so often happens in science, an erroneous working hypothesis yielded an effective therapeutic weapon. We owe to it not only the pharmacological convulsive therapy but also the electric convulsive therapy for which no new theories have been developed by their inventors. Meduna's theoretical basis for the introduction of the convulsive treatment was the assumption that epilepsy and schizophrenia are antagonistic to each other.

He found, in his clinical studies, that these two disorders very rarely occurred together. Moreover, his biochemical investigations supported this theory as determinations of uric acid, creatinine, nitrogen content, and blood sugar suggested that schizophrenics and epileptics had a different biochemistry. In addition, he made clinical observations which emphasized the beneficial effects of spontaneously occurring epileptic convulsions in schizophrenic patients.

Meduna's assumption that schizophrenia and epilepsy are antagonistic to each other has been refuted by a number of authors. The biochemistry of both disorders is so complicated and still so obscure, that no theory of similarity or antagonism regarding these two diseases can be formulated at the present time. In strong contrast to von Meduna's original concept of a biological antagonism between the two diseases, attempts have been made to establish a positive relationship between schizophrenia and epilepsy on the basis of electroencephalographic findings. This, however, was disproved by Hoch, who demonstrated in a genetic, electroencephalographic, and clinical study that the two disorders are neither related nor opposed to each other. The observation by Meduna that spontaneous epileptic attacks in schizophrenia influence favorably the clinical symptomatology is probably more valid. However, contrary to clinical evidence brought forward by other workers, Esser, on the basis of 10,000 patients surveyed in the literature, arrives at the conclusion that epileptic convulsions are not infrequent in catatonia and in many cases are not followed by improvement. But the main argument against von Meduna's theory is the fact that convulsive treatment is most effective in the manic-depressive psychoses. The great therapeutic value of convulsive therapy in the affective disorders was recognized, but not until several years after the theoretical foundation for the treatment of schizophrenia with convulsions had been developed. A theory of a biological antagonism, therefore, would have to be extended to cover the affective psychoses as well.

After Sakel and Meduna had given the first theoretical explanations for the treatments devised by them, other authors advised theories which were partly elaborations of previous ones; again, others suggested some new mechanisms that might be responsible for the improvement, with more and more emphasis on the common denominators in view of similarities in the effectiveness of insulin and convulsive therapies. Georgi believes that alteration of the nerve cell membrane is responsible for the success of these therapies. Evidence of this membrane alteration is found in a reduction in the amount of sugar in the cell, which is produced slowly in the hypoglycemic coma and quickly with metrazol and electric shock. Demole and Freudenberg expressed similar ideas. Von Angyal believes that hypoglycemia affects the metabolism in the brain cells due to reduction of the sugar content followed by compensation and an increased metabolism stimulating the cells that are in a state of malfunction or degeneration. Similarly, Küppers thinks that metabolic exhaustion in the nerve cells due to insulin provokes a counteraction and finally restores the cells to normal functioning. An unknown toxic substance is assumed by Danziger to accumulate in the body. This substance might depress the rate of heat production by inhibiting one of the respiratory enzymes. Shock therapy is assumed to remove the postulated toxic material. This idea is similar to the assumption that in epilepsy the convulsion eliminates toxic substances, and insulin, by way of sweating, does the same. Cerletti formulated the theory that convulsions bring the organism to a state which is close to death, thereby arousing a reaction of extreme biologic defense in producing a substance he calls agonine, which exerts the therapeutic effect. Pappalardo explains the effect of shock as well as of fever therapies as means of modifying the defense mechanism of the organism via the reticuloendothelial system. Ewald believes that all shock treatments have a marked influence on the diencephalon whose regulatory mechanisms are intensely stimulated under any kind of shock treatment. He speaks of a "massage of the diencephalic centers" and states that changes in the vegetative regulation, expressing themselves, among other symptoms, by increased weight, are the important therapeutic factors. His theory follows logically his ideas on the origin of schizophrenia which he localized essentially in the diencephalon. In a paper on electric shock therapy, Ewald and Haddenbrock lists various observations to support this theory.

A similar concept is Delay's and Mallet's, that the shock treatments exert a sedative effect on hyperthymias (manic states) and a stimulating effect on hypothymias (depressive states). The action of the treatment is explained as excitation of the diencephalon in the hyperthymias and as depression of the diencephalon in the hypothymias. Thus, it is postulated that the vegetative centers in the brain are influenced. Delmas-Marsalet's theory of dissolution and reconstruction of the mechanism of ECT is in many respects related. Delay and also Delmas-Marsalet expounded their theories in monographs on the subject.

Attempts were made to determine whether cerebral oxidation was the common denominator for the action of all shock treatments. High insulin doses prevent the utilization of carbohydrates by the central nervous system and indirectly reduce the oxidation of the brain, as demonstrated in human beings by Damashek and Myerson, and in animals by Himwich et al. Oxygen consumption of the brain drops during insulin treatment and the basal metabolism of the nervous system is reduced by about 60 per cent. The reduction in the metabolism of the brain is actually even greater if we consider that during hypoglycemia the circulation time of the blood in the brain is reduced by about 25 per cent. Serejski is of the opinion that it is not so much the reduction of oxygen as the inability to utilize oxygen that is important in this metabolic alteration. He finds relatively high oxygen content in the veins of the brain during insulin treatment. In convulsive treatments anoxemia due to a general cyanosis was quite apparent before anesthesia techniques were used. Also, cerebral anoxemia is assumed to be present, at least temporarily, caused by the vasoconstriction during convulsions. In electrically induced convulsions, Wortis et al. found interference with oxygen uptake. Due to the anoxia, a reduction in brain metabolism ensues, to be supplanted by a compensatory hyperactivity after the convulsion. In the light of experience with ECT under anesthesia during which the patient is not anoxic but rather oversaturated with oxygen, it is difficult to maintain the theory of anoxia as an important factor in this treatment.

Gellhorn believes that the sympathetic adrenal system dominates the vagoinsulin system in the normal person. In schizophrenia, however, clinical evidence exists pointing to a deficient sympathetic reactivity. The therapeutic effect of shock treatments in schizophrenia is due to the stimulation of the sympathetic adrenal system. This leads to a shift in the balance existing between the centers of the sympathetic adrenal and vagoinsulin systems. Prolonged excitation of the sympathetic centers by the shock treatments restores the disturbed autonomic balance and exerts far reaching effects on the cortex itself. According to Gellhorn, the fact that inhibited conditioned reflexes can be restored by subjecting the animal to insulin coma or to convulsions supports this interpretation. In insulin coma treatment and prolonged narcosis, the hypothalamic stimulation is a release phenomenon, the cortical control being abolished; in convulsive treatment, direct excitation of the hypothalamus takes place. Ivanov-Smolenski also believes that the common therapeutic factor in shock treatments is the production of cortical decompression or inhibition coupled with subcortical release and vegetative mobilization. Abely et al. hold that the effect of ECT is determined by a short sympathetic stimulation followed by prolonged parasympathetic excitation with stimulation of the anterior hypothalamus and the acidophile cells of the hypophysis. We repeatedly expressed the view that ECT exerts its influence on the diencephalon. This view based on clinical observations regarding sleep, weight, and menstrual changes, was supported by M. Roth in electroencephalographical studies which also suggested the primary effect of ECT on the diencephalon.

There is no doubt that changes in the vegetative nervous system can be demonstrated experimentally and clinically during and following shock treatment. It is also apparent that vegetative regulations are changed, as evidenced by improvement in sleep, appetite, weight, digestion, and circulation. It is still uncertain, however, whether or not these changes are concomitant manifestations occurring with mental improvement rather than the basis of mental improvement. It has not been demonstrated conclusively that an alteration in vegetative regulations is the actual cause of schizophrenia; therefore, biochemical changes during successful treatment are not necessarily the cause of mental improvement. Moreover, these theories do not take into consideration the differences which exist between manic-depressive psychoses and schizophrenia and some other mental conditions in which shock treatments are generally effective in varying degrees.

Of particular interest is the response to treatment of organic psychoses. The removal of psychotic syndromes in general paresis, of postinfectious psychoses and even psychotic syndromes in cases of pernicious anemia, led Fernandes and Polonio to the conclusion that the shock therapies and leucotomy have no bearing on the etiological causes of the psychoses. According to their concepts, psychotic symptoms arise from deviations of biopsychological functions caused by the noxious factors which, once in existence, may persist for a longer or shorter time. This may lead to the conclusion that we treat only symptoms or groups of symptoms, if we want to extend Bonhoeffer's concept of symptomatic psychoses to the symptoms of schizophrenia or manic-depressive psychosis, assuming that schizophrenia is a toxic disease acting secondarily on the brain.

On the basis of histopathological examinations, Stief formulated the theory that hypoglycemic coma and convulsive therapy produce spasms in the brain capillaries which eliminate diseased nerve cells, thereby bringing about the desired therapeutic results. That the vascular origin of cellular changes is disputed was discussed in the chapters on neuropathology. A more important objection to this theory is that there is no histopathological evidence that in schizophrenia diseased cortical cells are responsible for the mental pathology. Stief's theory fits in with the theories of the efficacy of frontal lobotomy. In the light of these concepts, shock treatment is considered a milder form of surgical procedure. While shock treatments may temporarily impair the function of cortical cells, in frontal lobotomy pathways are permanently cut between the cortical and subcortical centers. Both procedures supposedly lead to a reduction in cortical stimulation. LaValette assumes that the organic reaction in convulsive therapy produces a personality change on which the patient can reconstruct his personality.

Coma has also been credited as being the common therapeutic factor, whether caused by hypoglycemia or by convulsive therapy. Not only is coma brought about in hypoglycemia but the patient is in an equally comatose condition during and shortly after a convulsion as indicated by the term "electrocoma treatment" (Fettermann). Coma as the common denominator was suggested not only by those who consider therapeutically effective the pathophysiologic changes occurring in the brain during coma, but also by some who incline to psychologic explanations.

In this connection it is tempting to speculate on the old theory of the detoxifying effect of epileptic convulsions. Recent work that psychoses are caused by certain chemical substances in the brain, would fit into this concept that a treatment like ECT which removes so completely many psychotic syndromes, works through elimination of such disease-producing substances. A theory of this kind would be supported by the observation of Arneson and Ourso that in bromide intoxication an electrically induced convulsion not only removes the psychotic symptoms but also reduces the bromide level in the spinal fluid faster than, e.g., hemodialysis. If this can be demonstrated for a known psychosis-producing substance like bromide, it might be equally true for still unknown substances producing the so-called functional psychoses. This would be in line with findings of increased membrane permeability following ECT, and the redistribution of electrolytes and fluid from intracellular to extracellular spaces which Brown et al. demonstrated in depressions responding to ECT, and, by the way, in those responding to imipramine.

A new approach to the effective mechanism in ECT was presented by Cohen et al. Animal experimentation suggests that REM-sleep deprivation can be alleviated by ECT and, since sleep disturbances accompany depressions in most cases, the effect on REM-sleep deprivation might be the critical factor in the successful course of treatment. Green and Stajduhar were quoted as seeing special importance in the normalization of a disturbed sleep-dream-cycle.

One of the few available experimental studies on clarifications of some of the main problems in ECT was published in a monograph by Ottosson. His questions concern the assumption of most clinicians that the convulsion rather than the electric current is responsible for a therapeutic effect, and, secondly, whether the memory impairment is a consequence of the seizure or a direct effect of the current as had been assumed by those who claimed diminished memory impairment with certain modifications of current. Ottosson uses the anticonvulsive effect of lidocaine, a local anesthetic which abolishes electrically induced seizures and grand mal attacks in epileptics. He applied ECT to three groups, all of them receiving barbiturate and succinylcholine. The first two groups were given supraliminal and liminal electric stimuli, and it is shown that the electroencephalographic pattern is the same, characterized by an electric silence followed by delta waves. The lidocaine-modified seizures of the third group had hardly any electric silence and no delta activity. The clinical improvement is impaired, when lidocaine is given, and the conclusion can be drawn that the depression-relieving effect must be due to seizure activity and not to the current as such. The memory impairment, however, is only slightly less in ECT with lidocaine which permits the conclusion that a great part of the memory disturbance is accounted for by effects of the current other than the seizure. This most informative study on the action of ECT was later supplemented by the fact that unilateral ECT produces less memory impairment in spite of a generalized seizure, but that in our clinical experience it is therapeutically less effective. The relationship between memory impairment and therapeutic effect remains unproven.

Soon after the first organic theories of the action of insulin coma and convulsive therapy appeared, other psychiatrists expressed a psychogenic point of view. These workers believe that the somatic part of the treatment is only incidental and that prolonged sleep, insulin, or convulsive therapies only prepare the soil for intensive psychotherapy. Maier was one of the first to advance the idea that the more intimate contact with physician and nurses produced by shock treatments exerts a marked psychotherapeutic effect on the patient. Somewhat similar views have been expressed by Schatner and O'Neill, who reason that with the patient helpless and dependent, the physician becomes a mother surrogate, the patient establishes a better transference and therefore becomes more psychotherapeutically approachable. This is true of insulin treatment, which requires a great deal of attention, but is less applicable to electric shock treatment, where the patient is returned to the general ward soon after the treatment or returns home soon after an office treatment. Furthermore, in many private institutions with large medical staffs, considerable attention was paid to the individual patient before the shock era; yet the results were not comparable to those with shock treatment. If rendering the patient helpless or unconscious were sufficient to produce recovery, many other forms of treatment, such as fever treatment, anesthesias, continuous sleep would be as effective as the shock treatments but such is not the case.

Another group of authors emphasizes the psychotherapeutic value of the psychic "shock." They assume that the treatments actually produce a shock in the patient. However, it is quite evident that the so-called shock treatments usually do not produce any mental shock. Also on the physical level "shock" treatments present no phenomena similar to surgical shock which is a different and fairly well defined pathological condition. Some of these theories were evolved only because the patient was visualized as undergoing some form of mental shock. The patient is usually amnesic during insulin or convulsive treatment and is unable to report on his experiences or impressions during the state of unconsciousness. This naturally does not mean that there are no experiences in that condition, but since it is impossible to obtain any facts on these perceptions, it is pure assumption to say that the experience is that of mental shock. Jelliffe, and others believe that the patients undergo the experience of impending death followed by the feeling of rebirth, and the impetus of these sensations is so great that it breaks the autism of the patient and eliminates the regression and narcissism. We mentioned previously that these experiences of impending death are rather uncommon in insulin-treated patients and in those treated with electric convulsive therapy. Furthermore, there is the question of why it is that all the medieval tortures inflicted on the insane failed to produce impressive therapeutic results, especially when they were inflicted on a conscious person in whom the so-called emotional shock or death threat must have been much more intense. Millett and Mosse found that in patients treated by electric shock the treatment is desired because it is felt to be fitting punishment acceptable from the hands of a trusted and kind doctor-father who really wishes to do no injury but to temper retribution with mercy. Ideas of battering down the patient's defense mechanism, are based more on the impressions of somebody who saw the treatment before muscle relaxation was used or envisages it as a painful "electric shock." The patient himself is often afraid of the first "electric shock" for the same reason but is relieved that the experience has not been unpleasant. He may develop an unexplained fear during later treatments. But the fear *of* the treatment should always be differentiated from the fear *produced by* the treatment. Furthermore, many patients who display fear in connection with shock treatments do not improve, while many who display no fear do improve. In electric shock treatment it is a common experience that psychoneurotics express more fear of the treatment than any other group of patients and yet they show the poorest results.

Schilder tried to combine psychogenic and organic theories, stating that the victory over the death threat expressed in the epileptic fit and lingering in the perceptual and aphasic difficulty enables the individual to start life and normal relations with human beings all over again. The hypomanic elation which often follows the epileptic fit is the joy of rebirth; the previous fixations of libido lying in a more personal layer of experience are removed by recovery from a catacylsmic catastrophe in the depth of the organism. "But," Schilder emphasizes, although "the result of the treatment are psychologically understood, it does not mean that metrazol treatment acts as a psychologic agent in the common sense. Its effects are deeper than the effects of what is called psychic influence. This is an organic treatment reflected in psychologic attitudes. Just as in insulin treatment, the organic processes of regeneration are put in action, metrazol convulsions seem to bring with themselves a reconstruction which also serves the more labile organic structures which serve emotions and which are damaged by the process of schizophrenia. The forces liberated by metrazol and insulin treatment come from layers which are generally not accessible to the processes which are usually called psychic." Flescher feels that the therapeutic process of ECT implies a specific and dynamic pathogenous element which cannot be referred to a higher psychic level such as fear or need of help. He himself tries to understand ECT through the function of epileptic attacks, in which, according to him, considerable amounts of destructive energies are discharged.

Psychoanalytic theories of shock treatment have been formulated by Jelliffe, Glueck, Bychowski, and others. Glueck believes that the shock treatment facilitates emotional catharsis and is a highly condensed recapitulation of the process by means of which the fate of the egodystonic impulses is determined —the process which takes place normally in cases of ontogenetic development and artificially in the course of psychoanalytic therapy. Bychowski believes that in the psychoses the pathologic ego dominates the healthy one which experiences a rebirth and fortification through insulin; between these two a battle rages until the shock reduces the pathologic ego. The cathartic abreaction then permits psychoanalytic approach and influence. Frosch and Impastato maintain that the various clinical changes seen during and following convulsive therapy reflect the degree to which the ego defenses succeed in controlling the emergence of previously repressed libidinous and aggressive impulses consequent to the drastic physical assault of the convulsion and the attendant disorders of memory defect and altered body image.

There have been some who assert that the amnesia produced in convulsive shock treatment is a therapeutic factor. For instance, the theory of Brain and Strauss postulates the presence of faulty electrical patterns in the brain, which are altered by the treatment, the resulting amnesia allowing time for the brain to become accustomed to simplified patterns. It should be pointed out, however, that amnesia does not occur regularly in shock treated patients. It is not often present in the insulin-treated patients, and it is usually temporary. The loss of familiarity which plays a certain role in the psychological literature on ECT (Zubin, Janis) has the same weak point as the amnesia theory, namely, that often the organic symptoms are either not present or clear up in a short time after the treatment, and yet, in many cases the recovery persists. The temporary blotting out of symptoms does not affect the ultimate outcome of therapy.

A neurophysiologic-adaptive theory was presented by Fink et al. who stated that in ECT an induced change in brain function precedes the milieu in which behavioral changes can occur depending on the characterologic disposition of the subject. As indices of cerebral function they measured the degree of induced delta activity in the EEG, and changes in orientation and awareness of illness after intravenous injection of amobarbital sodium. In the amobarbital test the patient is asked a standard set of questions, and changes in orientation, denial of illness, confabulation and reduplication are considered as indicative of altered brain function. It was found that patients with high denial scores are those who improve best under ECT. These findings were considered to support the hypothesis advanced by Weinstein and Kahn that the mechanism of therapeutic action of electrically induced convulsions lies in the creation of altered brain function in which the patient might express his problems in a new symbolic fashion, particularly in the form of denial. Other theories also tend to combine physiological and psychological mechanisms. In an analogy to similar insulin theories, Benda using Selye's general adaptation syndrome, considers the convulsion as a severe stress to which the body adapts and thereby mobilizes general defences. Ploog applies ideas about psychic counter regulation to ECT. L. Alexander tried to come to a better understanding of the mode of action by means of a study of the distinctive operations of the ego.

In connection with psychogenic theories of shock treatment, it is necessary to discuss again the question of psychotherapy in conjunction with these treatments. The theoretical implication of this question is whether the somatic treatments are treatments in their own right, or whether they are only part of the over-all psychological treatment of the patient, or, as is still claimed by many, an adjunct to psychotherapy. This question is still sometimes heatedly discussed for ECT. Actually, no study is available that proves the necessity of psychotherapy by comparing the results in patients who received psychotherapy during or after ECT with those who did not. A synthesis of psychotherapy and all somatic treatments was assumed by Barahona Fernandez because during somatic therapy of the actual sickness the patient simultaneously undergoes some kind of psychotherapy to reestablish his place in the world. In practice, results in large hospitals, unable to provide any form of psychotherapy during shock treatments, were apparently not worse and indeed sometimes even better than those in hospitals providing intensive psychotherapy.

Mention should be made here of some comparative studies which try to determine the therapeutically effective factor by comparing groups of patients treated with ECT and anesthesia without ECT. N. Q. Brill et al. came to the conclusion that neither the electricity nor the motor convulsion are responsible for improvements; and Heath et al. saw no therapeutic effect at all in any of the groups they treated with ECT or simulated ECT or no treatment. These studies were made in chronic schizophrenics. Therefore, if they meant to prove that a convulsion is not more effective than anesthesia without a convulsion, this confirms only the known fact that ECT has little to offer in chronic schizophrenia. It does not contradict the clinical experience of a predictable effect of ECT in other psychiatric disorders. In a paper on hypnosis Stratas describes patients with a disconnected electrode on their head, who were told they were going to have ECT. These patients supposedly recovered as well as patients who had real ECT. If this is to prove that such hypnotic suggestions cure depressions, all clinical experience before and after the discovery of convulsive therapy stands against such assumption.

An attempt was made by Knight to designate the organic forms of treatment and especially shock therapy as "strong arm method" in contrast to the "gentle" form of treatment, meaning psychotherapy or psychoanalysis. Hoch took exception to this differentiation of therapy. Shock treatments, lobotomy, and other procedures were not devised to intimidate patients, to purge patients, or to force them to desist from expressing symptoms. The treatments were introduced as the basis of certain theoretical conceptions and, more important, of empirical observations. Some of the theoretical concepts which were offered as a basis of these treatments turned out to be invalid. The same, however, can be said for many psychoanalytic concepts.

Empirically, the organic treatments produced results. The evaluation of these results is naturally open to discussion, and no final determination of their value has as yet been made. Even so, we know approximately what they are able to accomplish. The organic treatments rapidly accumulated considerable statistical material which could be analyzed and criticized. By comparison, the psychotherapeutic approaches have practically no statistics or the number of patients evaluated and reported is very small. Therefore, it is more difficult to appraise the efficacy of these treatments; this is especially true for psychoanalytical treatment in the psychoses. The indiscriminate use of the somatic treatments, particularly of electric shock therapy, must be deplored. However, indiscriminate use of psychotherapy also occurs. For instance, we do not think that treatment with analysis or other psychotherapy is justified in a markedly depressed patient who is not able to establish a good transference with the therapist, and becomes agitated due to a procedure that he is unable to follow and which brings up traumatic material which, in his state of agitation and agony he is unable to digest. These patients often become worse under such treatment but usually very quickly recover with electroshock treatments.

In all theoretical considerations of shock therapy there is a great tendency to single out certain observational factors, such as memory impairment or confusion, unconsciousness, and so on, and to try to explain all the actions of the treatments by one or the other of these changes seen. We are in full agreement with Von Baeyer that the shock treatments are not etiological treatments because the basic personality organization, the matrix on which the psychosis grows, is not touched. The recurrence of manic-depressive psychosis or the frequent relapses in shock-treated schizophrenics indicates that even though symptoms of the disorder can sometimes be fully removed, some of the underlying basic factors are not eliminated. With such special drugs as mescaline, pervitin, etc., it is possible to reactivate the psychosis, which also would indicate that a complete elimination of the etiological mechanisms is not achieved. However, lack of etiological basis should not be assumed as an argument against any form of treatment. Many valuable methods in other fields of medicine are proof that it would be entirely unjustified to reject methods because they are purely symptomatic in nature.

Psychosurgery

Theories which try to explain *frontal lobotomy and other psychosurgical procedures* are fewer in number than those brought forward for the shock treatments, and have a better foundation in clinical observation, although it must be repeated that none is entirely satisfactory. The hypothesis of Egaz

Moniz, who introduced frontal lobotomy, has been mentioned already. It is in certain ways too general to be useful, and some of his specific statements concerning mental illness as being caused by faulty fiber connections are not generally accepted.

Freeman and Watts demonstrated that the therapeutic results were obtained by section of the thalomofrontal radiation followed by a degeneration of the dorsal medial nucleus of the thalamus which, in turn, produces a bleaching of the affect. They assume that the dorsal medial nucleus of the thalamus is the physical substrate of emotion. Their explanation that the so-called functional psychoses are produced by worry, which is reduced by the operation because the self-involvement of the patient is reduced, is too simple an explanation for the origin of the functional psychoses, even though a nucleus of truth may be in it. Their belief that without the frontal lobes, which have a tendency to overelaborate on anxiety and worry, no functional psychoses could develop, is open to question: elimination of the frontal lobe functions in many patients does not improve the psychosis, and relapses after frontal lobotomy may occur which would not be the case if existence of frontal lobe function were the sole prerequisite for a functional psychosis. It is probable that the origin of the functional psychoses goes beyond the function of the frontal lobe and involves other than the cortical areas of the brain as well.

Partridge, in his monograph on prefrontal leucotomy, clearly states that the modus operandi of leucotomy is not solved. He believes that the most important change after lobotomy is in the thalamus. He considers the thalamus an organ which integrates perceptions, emotions, and patterns of behavior, and believes it is also linked with the hypothalamus, through which autonomic influences are exerted. Partridge feels the schizophrenic disturbances are due to an impairment of this integrating function, which is seemingly favorably altered after operation. This actually does not solve the complicated question of improvements and personality damage seen after psychosurgery but does focus attention on a part of the brain which is probably implicated in mental sickness. Halstead, Hebb, and lately Landis have offered hypotheses based on their psychological investigations. Their description of the alterations which take place after frontal lobe surgery illuminates some aspects of the impairment of function in the frontal lobes without, however, offering a comprehensive understanding of all the alterations of function which are seen. They do not illuminate the etiology of the disorders involved, and do not actually explain the modus operandi of the surgical procedures.

Studies made on different brain-operated patients indicate that a very intimate relationship exists between the cerebral cortex and thalamus, and that a two-way circuit exists between the cortical gray matter and the subcortical gray matter, which mutually influence each other. Therefore, personality alterations can be achieved by ablating cortex, operating on the thalamus, or by cutting connections between thalamus and cortex. Today the connections between frontal lobe and thalamus are especially emphasized. However, it is necessary to recall that the long association fibers connecting the cortical areas of different lobes are also of great importance. We believe that these twofold connections within the cortical areas, and between cortex and thalamus explain why after frontal lobotomy the alterations of psychic functioning are not more severe. The basic intellectual and emotional functioning of the individual remains intact after frontal lobotomy even though the more subtle cognitive and conative performances are altered. If the basic functions of the person were concentrated in the frontal lobes alone, we could expect personality function after frontal lobotomy to show very serious alterations which actually are not even seen after frontal lobectomy. The changes are much less marked than prior theories of the function of the frontal lobe have indicated. Most likely, when parts of the frontal lobe are separated from other parts of the brain, the other cortical areas are able to take over. We believe that the basic intellectual and emotional life of the individual which is necessary for his personality functioning is not localized in the frontal lobe alone, but is distributed over the whole cortex, with the thalamus also having some function in it. This, of course, does not contradict the observation that the highest symbolic functions, such as creativeness, planning and the fusion of emotional and intellectual performances, depend on normal functioning by the frontal lobes. We do not believe that psychosurgery alters the basic structure of the neurosis or psychosis. Most patients who have undergone psychosurgery show in general unchanged dynamics. The retention of the basic psychodynamic structure is clearly seen in schizophrenic patients, and, it is possible with drugs like mescaline to reactivate the original psychosis even some time after the operation. The symptoms which reappear are usually not as intense but are the same in quality. Therefore, we believe that psychosurgery points to an important problem in psychiatric therapy. Most of our treatments, especially the psychotherapeutic ones, mainly consider the qualitative approach to the different disorders. By analyzing the psychodynamic factors in a case we try to find out what conflicts in what constellations produce the emotional disorder. Thus we may overlook the fact that many of these conflicts can be present in a person without emotional disease becoming apparent with the patient being obsessed by his fears or dominated by his hallucinations and delusions. Only these dominating symptoms are eliminated or reduced by psychosurgery. An analogy exists in patients who suffer from intractable pain, where the pain is not eliminated but the patient's response to the perception of the pain experience is altered by lobotomy. We think that in psychosurgery we are dealing with a quantitative treatment which leaves many of the underlying disease processes unimpaired; the patient, however, does not perceive his difficulties any more, is no longer disorganized by them, and is thereby enabled to function. The same quantitative approach is applicable to the therapeutic effect of the neuroleptic drugs which may not always remove certain symptoms completely but reduce them sufficiently to allow the patient to live with them.

Final Remarks

The discussion of the theoretical aspects of the various somatic treatments has shown that most of them are poorly understood, or even entirely obscure in their mode of action. The expectation that the newer somatic treatments would throw some light on the etiology of the mental disorders for which they are applied, has not yet been fulfilled. A great deal of research will still be necessary to explain the mode of action of the treatments hitherto available, and thus help us at some future day to arrive at better understood means of treating psychotic disorders. At present, we can say only that we are treating empirically disorders whose etiology is unknown, with methods whose action is also shrouded in mystery.

Bibliography

Abbott, P., Blake, A., and Vincze, L.: Treatment of mentally retarded with thioridazine. Dis. Nerv. Syst. *26*:583, 1965.

Abdul Hameed, J. M., and Haley, T. L.: Psycho-sedative properties of three indolylethyl-piperazine derivatives. Brit. J. Pharmacol. *26*: 186, 1966.

Abel, H. H., Brock, N., and Lenke, D.: Zur Pharmakologie und Toxikologie des Neurolepticums 3-Chlor-10-(γ-[N′-β′-(1″-methyl-2″-oxo-imidazolidyl-3″)-aethyl-N-piperazinyl]-propyl)-phenothiazin-dihydrochlorid. II. Mitteilung: Subakute und chronische Toxizität an Ratten und Hunden. Arzneim.-Forsch. *17*:323, 1967.

Abély, P., Borenstein, P., and Puech, J.: La pneumothérapie cérébrale par l'oxygéne pur. Sem. Hôp. Paris *27*:1145, 1951.

——, Loine, B., and Assailly, A.: Une hypothèse sur le mode d'action de l'électrochoc. Ann. méd. psychol. *106*:453, 1948.

——, Vanecloo, M., and Chaneac, H.: La pneumothérapie cérébrale par l'ozone. Ann. méd. psychol. *109*:588, 1951.

Abraham, H. C., Kanter, V. B., Rosen, I., and Standen, J. L.: A controlled clinical trial of imipramine (Tofranil) with out-patients. Brit. J. Psychiat. *109*: 286, 1963.

Abramov, A. A., and Kopeliovic, B. I.: Roentgenoskopie beim Electroschock. Nevropat. i. psikhiat. *18*: 60, 1949.

Abrams, A. L.: Imipramine in enuresis. Amer. J. Psychiat. *120*: 177, 1963.

Abrams, R.: Daily administration of unilateral ECT. Amer. J. Psychiat. *124*:384, 1967.

——, and De Vito, R. A.: Clinical efficacy of unilateral ECT. Dis. Nerv. Syst. *30*: 262, 1969.

Abramson, H. A.: The use of LSD in Psychotherapy. Transactions of a Conference on d-Lysergic Acid Diethylamide (LSD-25). New York: Josiah Macy Jr. Foundation, 1960.

Abse, D. W., Dahlstrom, W. G., and Tolley, A. G.: Evaluation of tranquilizing drugs in the management of acute mental disturbance. Am. J. Psychiat. *116*:973, 1960.

Accornero, F.: Paralisi radiale durante lo shock insulinico. Atti del convegno sulla terapia moderna della schizofrenia. Milano: 1937.

——: Experimental histopathological researches on insulin shock. Am. J. Psychiat. *94* (Supp.):130, 1938.

——: Comportamento del polso, della respirazione, della pressione arteriale e della temperature durante l'elettroshock. Riv. sper. di freniat. *64*:459, 1940.

——, and Anderson, M.: L'elettroshock nella psichiatria infantile. Lavoro Neuropsichiatr. *3*:231, 1948.

——, and Guerra, A.: Contributo alla interpretazione die disturbi motori transitori susseguenti a terapie da shock (elettroshock e insulinico). Giorn. Psichiat. e Neuropatol. *3*:1, 1958.

Ackner, B. H., and Oldham, A. J.: Insulin treatment of schizophrenia. Lancet *1*:504, 1962.

Adams, C. L., Gibbs, E. L., and Gibbs, E. A.: Asynchronism of electrical activity of frontal lobes during sleep; a late sequel of frontal lobotomy. Arch. Neurol. & Psychiat. *77*:237, 1957.

Adamson, W. C.: Chlorpromazine and Mental Health. Philadelphia: Lea and Feibiger, 1955.

Adlin, E. V., Sher, E. B. and Berk, N. G.: Fatal reactions following the ingestion o meprobamate. A.M.A. Arch. Int. Med. *102*:484, 1958.

Aidin, R.: Chlorpromazine jaundice. Brit. Med. (letter) *1*:342, 1958.

Ainslie, J. D., Jones, M. B., and Stiefel, J. R.: Practical drug evaluation method. Imipramine in depressed outpatients. Arch. Gen. Psychiat. *12*:368, 1965.

Aird, R. B.: Clinical correlates of electroshock therapy. A.M.A. Arch. Neurol. & Psychiat. *79*:633, 1958.

Aivazian, G. H.: Thioridazine in treatment of mental disorders. J. Tennessee M. A. *52*:446, 1959.

——, and Reese, H. C.: Clinical evaluation of promazine therapy for schizophrenia. Dis. Nerv. Syst. *20*:472, 1959.

——: Clinical evaluation of diazepam. Dis. Nerv. Syst. *25*:491, 1964.

de Ajuriaguerra, J. ed.: Monoamines et système nerveux central. (Symp. Bel-Air, Genève, Septembre 1961). Genève, Georg et Cie. S.A.; and Paris, Masson et Cie, 1962.

Akimoto, H., Honda, Y., and Takahashi, Y.: Pharmacotherapy in narcolepsy. Dis. Nerv. Syst. *21*:704, 1960.

Alexander, F. A. D., and Himwich, H. E.: Nitrogen inhalation therapy for schizophrenia. Am. J. Psychiat. *96*:643, 1939.

Alexander, L.: Nonconvulsive electric stimulation therapy. Am. J. Psychiat. *107*:241, 1950.

——: Treatment of Mental Disorder. Philadelphia: W. B. Saunders Co., 1953.

——: Therapeutic process in electroshock and the new drug therapies. Psychopathological considerations. J.A.M.A. *162*:966, 1956.

——: Chemotherapy of depression—use of meprobamate combined with benactyzine. J.A.M.A. *166*:1019, 1958.

——, and Löwenbach, H.: Experimental studies on electroshock treatment. 1. The intracerebral vascular reaction as an indicator of the path of the current and the threshold of early changes within the brain tissue. J. Neuropath. & Exper. Neurol. *2*:139, 1944.

Alexander, S. P., and Bindelglas, P. M.: Insulin coma therapy in patients resistant to chemotherapy. Dis. Nerv. Syst. *17*:220, 1956.

——, and Neander, J. F.: The use of hyaluronidase with insulin in insulin coma therapy. Psychiat. Quart. *30*:89, 1956.

Allen, A. G., and Black, A. V.: Near-fatal case of intoxication with meprobamate, treated with electro-stimulation and levarterenol. Ohio State Med. J. *52*:1303, 1953.

Allen, C., and Broster, L. R.: A further case of paranoid psychosis successfully treated by adrenalectomy. Brit. M. J. *1*:696, 1945.

Allen, V. S.: Trifluoperazine in the treatment of drug-resistant Schizophrenics. J. Clin. & Exper. Psychopath. *20*:247, 1959.

Almansi, R., and Impastato, D. J.: Electrically induced convulsions in the treatment of mental diseases. New York State J. Med. *40*:1315, 1940.

Alpers, B. J., and Hughes, J.: Changes in the brain after electrically induced convulsions in cats. Arch. Neurol. & Psychiat. *47*:385, 1942.

——, and ——: The brain changes in electrically induced convulsions in the human. J. Neuropath. & Exper. Neurol. *1*:173, 1942.

Alsen, M., and Frey, T. S.: Om behandling av alkoholpsykoser med Truxal. Svenska Läk.-Tidn. *56*:3344, 1959.

Alsen, M., and Johanson, E.: Experience with chlorpromazine therapy amongst a male psychiatric clientele. Nord. psykiat. Medlemsbl., *10*:207, 1956.

Altschule, M. D.: Physiologic observations in mental disease. Bull. New England Med. Center *11*:229, 1949.

——: Further observations on vagal influences on the heart during electroshock therapy for mental disease. Am. Heart J. *39*:88, 1950.

——: Adrenal apoplexy following electronarcosis therapy. New England J. Med. *253*:191, 1955.

——, Ascoli, J., and Tillotson, K. J.: Extracellular fluid and plasma volumes in depressed patients given electric shock therapy. Arch. Neurol. & Psychiat. *62*:618, 1949.

——, Cline, J. E., and Tillotson, K. J.: Fall in plasma protein level associated with rapid gain in weight during course of electroshock therapy. Arch. Neurol. & Psychiat. *59*:476, 1948.

——, Cram, J. E., and Tillotson, K. J.: Hemoconcentration after electrically induced convulsions in man. Arch. Neurol. & Psychiat. *59*:29, 1948.

——, Parkhurst, B. H., and Tillotson, K. J.: Decreases in blood eosinophilic leucocytes after electrically induced convulsions in man. J. Clin. Endocrinol. *9*:440, 1949.

——, Sulzbach, W. M., and Tillotson, K. J.: Significance of change in the electrocardiogram after electrically induced convulsions in man. Arch. Neurol. & Psychiat. *58*:716, 1947.

——, and ——: Effects of electrically induced convulsions upon respiration in man. Am. J. Psychiat. *103*:680, 1947.

——, and Tillotson, K. J.: The use of testosterone in the treatment of depressions. New England J. Med. *239*:1036, 1948.

——, and ——: Effects of electroconvulsive therapy on water metabolism in psychotic patients. Am. J. Psychiat. *105*:829, 1949.

Altschuler, M.: Massive doses of trifluoperazine in the treatment of compulsive rituals. Amer. J. Psychiat. *119*:367, 1962.

Ambrozi, L., und Birkmayer, W.: Zur Therapie der senilen Depression mit Protriptyline. Klin. Med. *22*:115, 1967.

Amler, G., and Bergener, M.: Elektroencephalographische Veränderungen bei der Behandlung des Delirium tremens mit Chlormethiazol und ihre Interpretation. Arzneimittel-Forschung. *15*:837, 1965.

Andermann, K.: Electroencephalographic evidence of personality changes produced by ataraxic drugs in mentally disturbed patients. Med. J. Austr. *2*:1, 1957.

Andersen, H., and Sarauw, E.: Tofranil treatment of endogenous depressions. Acta psychiat. et neur. scandinav. *34*:387, 1959.

Andreani, G., Caselli, G., and Martelli, G.: Rilievi clinici ed elettroencefalografici durante il trattamento con sali di litio in malati psichiatrici. G. Psiachiat. Neuropat. *86*:273, 1958.

Angst, J.: A clinical analysis of the effects of Tofranil in depression. Longitudinal and follow-up studies. Treatment of blood-relations. Psychopharmacologia. *2*:381, 1961.

——: Insidon als Antidepressivum. Vergleich mit Tofranil: Katamnesen. Nervenarzt. *34*:76, 1963.

——: Vergleich der antidepressiven Eigenschaften von Amitriptylin und Imipramin.

Psychopharmacologia *4*:389, 1963.
——: Intoxikationen mit Psychopharmaka. Ther. Umschau *22*:178, 1965.
——, Brandenberger, H. and Herrmann, B.: Suicid mit Opipramol (Insidon ®). Psychopharmacologia *11*: 174, 1967.
——, and Kind, H.: Poliklinische und klinische Erfahrungen mit einem Dibenzodiazepinderivat bei depressiven Zustandsbildern. Schweiz. med. Wschr. *94*:759, 1964.
——, and Pöldinger, W.: Vergleichende klinische Erfahrungen mit Protriptylin bei depressiven Verstimmungszuständen verschiedener Genese. Arzneim.-Forsch. *16*:893, 1966.
Angus, L. R.: Prefrontal lobotomy as a method of therapy in a special school. Am. J. Ment. Deficiency *53*:470, 1949.
Angyal, L. von: Über die motorischen und tonischen Ercheinungen des Insulinschocks. Ztschr. f. d. ges Neurol. u. Psychiat. *157*:35, 1937.
——, and Gyarfas, K.: Über die Cardiazolkrampfbehandlung der Schizophrenie. Arch. f. Psychiat. *106*:1, 1936.
——, and Juba, A.: Über Erfahrungen mit Elektroschock Behandlung. Arch. f. Psychiat. *116*:553, 1943.
Anton-Stephens, D.: Preliminary observations on the psychiatric uses of chlorpromazine (Largactil). J. Ment. Sc. *100*:543, 1954.
Appel, K. E., Myers, J. M., and Schoflen, A. E.: Prognosis in psychiatry. Results of psychiatric treatment A.M.A. Arch. Neurol and Psychiat. *70*:459, 1953.
Applebaum, A.: An ophthalmoscopic study of patients under treatment with thioridazine. Arch. Ophthal. *69*:578, 1963.
Apter, N. S.: Bilateral adrenalectomy in chronic schizophrenic patients: *6* years after. Am. J. Psychiat. *115*:55, 1958.
Archer, J. D.: Effects of chlorpromazine on maze performance of albino rats. Fed. Proc. *13*:332, 1954.
Archer, S., Wylie, D. W., Harris, L. S., Lewis, T. R., Schulenberg, J. W., Bell, M. R., Kullnig, R. K., and Arnold, A.: 1-(Indolyalkyl)-4-arylpiperazines: A new class of tranquilizers. J. Amer. Chem. Soc. *84*: 1306, 1962.
Arduini, A., and Arduini, M. G.: Effects of drugs and metabolic alterations on brain stem arousal mechanisms. J. Pharmacol. & Exper. Therap. *110*:76, 1954.
Arenillas, L.: Amitriptyline and body weight. Lancet *1*:432, 1964.
Arieti, S.: Histopathologic changes in experimental metrazol convulsions in monkeys. Am. J. Psychiat. *98*:70, 1941.
Arneson, G. A., and Butler, T.: Cardiac arrest and electroshock therapy. Amer. J. Psychiat. *117*:1020, 1961.
——, and Ourso, R.: Bromide intoxication and electroshock therapy. Amer. J. Psychiat. *121*:1115, 1965.
Arnold, O. H.: Results and efficacy of insulin shock therapy. *In* M. Rinkel: Insulin Treatment in Psychiatry. New York: Philosophical Library, 1959.
——, and Böck-Greissau, W.: Elektroschock und Muskelrelaxantien. Wien. Ztschr. f. Nervenheilk. u. d. Grenzgeb. *4*:326, 1951.
——: Klinische Erfahrungen mit dem Neuroleptikum Truxal. Wien. med. Wschr. *109*: 892, 1959.
——: Combined electroshock—Tofranil therapy of melancholia. Wien. med. Wschr. *110*:250, 1960.
——, and Deisenhammer, E.: Erste Erfahrungen mit dem Intensivneuroleptikum N 746. Wien med Wschr. *112*:558, 1962.
——, and Foitl, G.: Die Behandlung der endogenen Depression mit Amitriptyline. Wien. med. Wschr. *111*:272, 1961.
——, and Kryspin-Exner, K.: Klinische Erfahrungen mit dem Antidepressivum Protriptyline (MK 240). Wien. med. Wschr. *114*:883, 1964.
Arthurs, R. G. S., Cappon, D., Douglass, E., and Quarrington, B.: CO_2 therapy with stutterers. Dis. Nerv. Syst. *15*:123, 1954.
Aschieri, G.: Contributo clinico alla chimoterapia delle sindromi depressive con considerazoini nosografiche. Minerva Med. *50*:3043, 1959.
Ashby, W. R.: The effects of convulsive therapy on the excretion of cortins and ketosteroids. J. Ment. Sc. *95*:275, 1949.
——, and Bassett, M.: The effect of leucotomy and creative ability. J. Ment. Sc. *95*:418, 1949.
Atkin, I.: The psychology of shock therapies and of leucotomy. J. Clin. Psychopathol. *7*:731, 1946.
Atkinson, R., and Rubin, R. T.: Electroconvulsive treatment and severe cardiovascular disease. Amer. J. Psychiat. *121*:249, 1964.
Atkinson, R. M., and Ditman, K. S.: Tranylcypromine: A review. Clin. Pharmacol. *6*:631, 1965.
Aubertin, E., Martin-Dupont, C., and Tavernier, J.: Tentative de suicide par la Chlorpromazine et al Phénobarbital. Sém. Hôp., Paris. *30*:2307, 1954.
Avenarius, R., Fischer, H. and Meyer, J.-E.: Zur Behandlung der symptomarmen Schizophrenie mit sehr hohen Dosen Reserpin und Orphenadrin. Psychiat. Neurol. *142*:13, 1961.
Avery, L. W., and Campbell, L. K. Shock therapy as an aid to the withdrawal of morphine in addiction. Dis. Nerv. Syst. *2*:333, 1941.
Ayaslioglu, Y., and Lange, M.: Psychische Veraenderungen bei einem Enzephalitiskranken. Schw. Arch. Neurol. Neurochir. Psychiat. *98*:297, 1966.
Ayd, F. J., Jr.: Chlorpromazine therapy for anxiety associated with electroshock therapy. Confinia neurol. *16*:168, 1956.
——: Fatal hyperpyrexia during chlorpromazine therapy. J. Clin. & Exper. Psychopath. *17*:189, 1956.
——: The dermatologic and systemic manifestations of chlorpromazine hypersensitivity. J. Nerv. & Ment. Dis. *124*:84, 1956.
——: A Clinical evaluation of methylphenidylactate hydrochloride (ritalin). J. Clin. Exp. Psychopath. *18*:342, 1957.
——: A clinical report on benactyzine hy-

drochloride. New Eng. J. Med. *257*:669, 1957.
——: The treatment of anxiety, agitation and excitement in the aged. A preliminary report on Trilafon. J. Am. Geriat. Soc. *5*:92, 1957.
——: Treatment of ambulatory and hospitalized psychiatric patients with perphenazine. Dis. Nerv. System. *18*:394, 1957.
——: Value of the Grantham lobotomy. South. Med. J. *50*:939, 1957.
——: Prolonged administration of chlorpromazine (Thorazine) hydrochloride. J.A.M.A. *169*:1296, 1959.
——: Prolonged use of reserpine in schizophrenia. In N. S. Kline, ed.: Psychopharmacology Frontiers. Boston: Little, Brown & Co., 1959.
——: Amitriptyline (Elavil) therapy for depressive reactions. Psychosomatics *1*:320, 1960.
——: A critique of antidepressants. Dis. Nerv. Syst. *22*:(suppl.)32, 1961.
——: Recognizing the depressed patient. With essentials of management and treatment. New York, Grune & Stratton, 1961.
——: Prolonged perphenazine therapy and thyroid function. Amer. J. Psychiat. *120*:592, 1963.
——: Perphenazine: A reappraisal after eight years. Dis. Nerv. Syst. *25*:311, 1964.
——: Amitriptyline: Reappraisal after six years experience. Dis. Nerv. Syst. *26*:719, 1965.
——: A clinical evaluation of pargyline hydrochloride (Eutonyl) in the management of mental depression. Internat. J. Neuropsychiat. *1*:233, 1965.
Ayres, C. M.: The relative value of various somatic therapies in schizophrenia. J. Neuropsychiat. *1*:154, 1960.
Azima, H.: Imipramine (Tofranil): a new drug for the depressed. Canad. M. A. J. *80*:535, 1959.
——, and Durost, H.: Effects of promazine in mental syndromes. Canad. M. A. J. *76*:442, 1957.
——, ——, Arthurs, D., and Silver, A.: The effect of RO-5-0831/1 (Marplan) in depressive states. Am. J. Psychiat. *116*:453, 1959.
——, ——, and Cahn, C.: Vesprin and mepazine: two new phrenotropic substances. Am. J. Psychiat. *114*:747, 1958.
——, Silver, A., and Arthurs, D.: The effects of G-33040 in depressive states: A multiblind study. Amer. J. Psychiat. *119*:465, 1962.
——, ——, and ——: Effects of G-33040 (Ensidon) and G-35020 (Pertofrane) on depressive states. A comparative multiblind study. Canad. Med. Ass. J. *87*:1224, 1962.
——, and Wittkower, E. D.: Anaclitic therapy employing drugs. Psychoanalyt. Quart. *26*:190, 1957.
Bacon, R. L., and Rosvold, H. E.: Effects of electric convulsion shock on pregnancy in rats. Proc. Soc. Exper. Biol. Med. *69*:287, 1948.
Baeyer, W. von: Vergleichende Psychopathologie der Schocktherapien und der praefrontalen Lobotomie. Fortschr. d. Neurol. u. Psychiat. *17*:95, 1949.
——: Die moderne psychiatrische Schockbehandlung. Stuttgart: Georg Thieme, 1951.
——: The clinical and psychopathological mode of action of somatic therapies. Compr. Psychiat. *5*:146, 1964.
Bagchi, B. K., Howell, R. W., and Schmale, H. T.: Electroencephalographic and clinical effects of electrically induced convulsions in treatment of mental disorders. Am. J. Psychiat. *102*:49, 1945.
Bair, H. U., and Herold, W.: Efficacy of chlorpromazine in hyperactive mentally retarded children. Arch. Neurol. & Psychiat. *74*:363, 1955.
Baird, E. E.: The effect of insulin on the blood picture. J. Nerv. & Ment. Dis. *105*:85, 1947.
Baker, A. A.: Observations on the effect of Largactil in psychiatric illness. J. Ment. Sc. *101*:175, 1955.
——, and Thorpe, J. G.: Assessing a new phenothiazine. J. Ment. Sc. *104*:855, 1958.
Baker, J. P.: A controlled trial of ethylcrotonylurea J. Ment. Sc. *105*:853, 1959.
Balduzzi, E.: In tema di terapia dell'anoressia mentale: considerazioni a proposito dell'insorgenza di reazioni bulimiche dopo elettroshock. Note e Riv. Psichiat. *47*:64, 1955.
Balestrieri, A.: Su di un nuovo farmaco ad azione negli stati depressivi (Tofranil-G 22355). Giorn. Psichiat. e neuropatol. *1*:1, 1959.
Ban, T. A., Ferguson, K., and Lehmann, H. E.: The effect of clopenthixol on chronic psychiatric patients. Amer. J. Psychiat. *119*:984, 1963.
Bankhead, A. J., Torrens, J. K., and Harris, T. H.: The anticipation and prevention of cardiac complications in electroconvulsive therapy. Am. J. Psychiat. *106*:911, 1950.
Barahal, H. S.: 1000 prefrontal lobotomies—a five-to-ten-year follow-up study. Psychiat. Quart. *32*:653, 1958.
Barahona Fernandes, H. J.: Hirnanatomie and -physiologie. Psychische Funktionsänderungen nach der präfrontalen Leukotomie. Nevernarzt *23*:101, 1952.
——: Synthese psychotherapeutischer und somatischer Behandlungsverfahren in der Schizophrenie. Arch. Psychiat. Nervenkra. *197*:52, 1958.
Barbour, J. P., jr.,: Maintenance therapy of chronic psychotics with perphenazine. Amer. J. Psychiat. *120*:176, 1963.
Barek, A., Burgermeister, J. J., Rey-Bellet, J., Tissot, R. et de Ajuriaguerra, J.: Niamid parentéral à hautes doses dans les syndromes dépressifs. (Essais de corrélations cliniques et biologiques). Psychiat. Neurol. (Basel) *149*:257, 1964.
Barison, F.: Rilievi di psicopatologia sul risveglio dal coma insulinico. Atti del convegno sulla terapia moderna della schizofrenia. Milano: 1937.

Barker, J. C., and Baker, A. A.: Deaths associated with electroplexy. J. Ment. Sci. *105*:339, 1959.
——, Jan, I. A., and Enoch, M. D.: A controlled trial of mebanazine ('Actomol') in depression. Brit. J. Psychiat. *111*:1095, 1965.
Barker, Ph., and Fraser, I. A.: A controlled trial of haloperidol in children. Brit. J. Psychiat. *114*:855, 1968.
Barnard, R. D., and Barnard, J. F.: An effect of meprobamate withdrawal in rats. Lancet *2*:47, 1957.
Barnes, R. J., Kong, S. M., and Wu, R. W. Y.: Electrocardiographic changes in amitriptyline poisoning. Brit. Med. J. *3*:222, 1968.
Baron, A.: Doppelblindversuch mit einem Dibenzodiazepin-Derivat bei geriatrischen Patienten. Med. Welt *18*:388, 1967.
Barrera, S. E., Lewis, N. D. C., Pacella, B. L., Kalinowsky, L. B.: Brain changes associated with electrically induced seizures. Tr. Am. Neurol. A. *31*:1942.
——, Osinski, W. A., and Davidoff, E.: The use of antabuse (tetraethylthiuramidisulphide) in chronic alcoholics. Am. J. Psychiat. *107*:9, 1950.
Barretto, A. C.: Psicocirurgia: técnica, acidentes, em 418 doentes operados. Neurobiologia *12*:168, 1949.
——, Velasco, O. P., Bairao, I. S., Da Costa, E. M., and Bernardinelli, E.: Lobotomy in epilepsy. Lisbon: Psychosurgery, 1949.
Barron, A., Rudy, L. H., and Smith, J. A.: Clinical evaluation of a secondary amine, nortriptyline. Amer. J. Psychiat. *121*:268, 1964.
Barron, S. P., and Sullivan, T. M.: The use of the cardiac pacemaker in an ECT-Induced cardiac arrest. Amer. J. Psychiat. *124*:395, 1967.
Barsa, J. A.: The dual action of the tranquilizers. Am. J. Psychiat. *114*:74, 1957.
——: Use of chlorpromazine combined with prochlorperazine. Am. J. Psychiat. *114*: 1112, 1958.
——, and Kline, N. S.: Combined reserpine-chlorpromazine therapy in disturbed psychotics. Am. J. Psychiat. *111*:780, 1955.
——, and ——: Treatment of 200 disturbed psychotics with reserpine. J.A.M.A. *158*: 110-113, 1955.
——, and ——: Comparative study of reserpine, chlorpromazine and combined therapy. A.M.A. Arch. Neurol. & Psychiat. *76*:90-97, 1956.
——, and ——: Use of meprobamate in the treatment of psychotic patients. Am. J. Psychiat. *112*:1023, 1956.
——, and Saunders, J. C.: Deanol (Deaner) in the treatment of schizophrenia. Am. J. Psychiat. *116*:255, 1959.
——, and ——: Thioridazine (Mellaril) in the treatment of chronic schizophrenics. Am. J. Psychiat. *116*:1028, 1960.
——, and ——: Trifluoperazine combined with chlorpromazine. Am. J. Psychiat. *116*:925, 1960.
——, ——, and Kline, N. S.: Trifluoperazine in the treatment of chronic schizophrenia. Am. J. Psychiat. *115*:812, 1959.
——, and ——: Amitriptyline (Elavil), a new antidepressant. Amer. J. Psychiat. *117*: 739, 1961.
——, and ——: Chlorprothixene in the treatment of psychotic patients. Amer. J. Psychiat. *119*:468, 1962.
——, and ——: A double blind study of a new chlorprothixene preparation. Amer. J. Psychiat. *121*:493, 1964.
——, and ——: A comparative study of tranylcypromine and pargyline. Psychopharmacologia *6*:295, 1964.
Barten, H. H.: Toxic psychosis with transient dysmnestic syndrome following withdrawal from Valium. Amer. J. Psychiat. *121*:1210, 1965.
Bartholomew, A. A.: An evaluation of tranylcypromine ("Parnate") in the treatment of depression. Med. J. Australia *49/1*:655, 1962.
Bartholomew, L. G., and Cain, J. C.: Abdominal pain following use of chlorpromazine. J.A.M.A. *163*:733, 1957.
——, ——, Frazier, S. H., Petersen, M. C., Foulk, W. T., Soule, E. H., Fleischer, G. A., and Owen, C. A., Jr.: Effect of chlorpromazine on the liver. Gastroenterology 1096, 1958.
Barucci, M.: Contributo alla conoscenza ed all' interpretazione della sindrome extrapiramidale di reserpina. Riv. Patol. Nerv. Ment. *78*:483, 1957.
Baruk, H.: La catatonie experimentale par la Chlorpromazine. La posologie et la methode d' administration la plus efficace en thérapeutique psychiatrique. L'Encéphale *45*:474, 1956.
——, Launay, J. and Roberti, A.: Action therapeutique du 7044RP dans les Névroses Obsessionelles, les Nérvoses Digestives et les États de Cénestopathies. Ann. med.-psychol. *116*:149, 1958.
——, and Racine, M.: Essai de traitement circulatoire de la démence précoce ancienne par la folliculine et al caféine. Ann. méd.-psychol. *104*:169, 1946.
Bassa, D. M., and Vora, H. D.: Evaluation of efficacy of imipramine in depressive disorders: A double-blind study. Amer. J. Psychiat. *121*:1116, 1965.
Basset, J., Jude, J.-P., Delcroix, A., Vouin, Ph. et Mahon, P.: Utilisation du Benpéridol en mileu psychiatrique hospitalier. Ann. méd.-psychol. *125/1*:568, 1967.
Batt, J. C., and Dally, P.: Abreaktion durch Anwendung von Nebenhirnrindenhormonderivaten. Medizinische *19*:802, 1958.
——, Kay, W. W., Reiss, M., and Sands, D. E.: The endocrine concomitants of schizophrenia. J. Ment. Sc. *103*:240, 1957.
Battegay, R.: Vergleichende Bewertung antidepressiv wirksamer Psychopharmaka, unter besonderer Berücksichtigung von Pertofran (Desmethylimipramin). Nervenarzt *34*:371, 1963.
——: Entziehungserscheinungen nach abruptem Absetzen von Neuroleptica als Kriterien zu ihrer Differenzierung. Nervenarzt *37*:552, 1966.
Batterman, R. C., Grossman, A. J., Leifer,

P., and Mouratoff, C. J.: Clinical evaluation of day time sedatives. Postgrad. Med. *26*:502, 1959.

Baudouin, A., et Puech, P.: Premiers essais d'intervention directe sur le thalamus (injections, électrocoagulation). Rev. neurol. *81*:78, 1949.

Bauer, A.: Klinische Erfahrungen mit Thioridazin (Melleril-Sandoz) anhand von 202 Fällen, zugleich ein Beitrag zur Problematik der Behandlung endogener Depressionen. Nervenarzt *33*:321, 1962.

——: Verlaufsanalyse der durch zentral anticholinergisch wirkende Substanzen erzeugten Psychosen an Hand von 70 Fällen. Arzneim.-Forsch. *16*:233, 1966.

Bauer, H. G., Seegers, W., Krawzoff, M., and McGavack, T.: A clinical evaluation of ectylurea (Nostyn). New York State J. Med. *58*:520, 1958.

Baumer, L., and Baumgartl, J.: Klinische Erfahrungen mit Bischolin-succinat-dijodid bei der Elektroschocktherapie. Nervenarzt *24*:66, 1953.

Bayles, S., Busse, E. W., and Ebaugh, F. G.: Square waves (BST) versus sine waves in electroconvulsive therapy. Am. J. Psychiat. *107*:34, 1950.

Beard, B. H., and Harris, T. H.: A near fatality from curare preceding electroshock therapy. Dis. Nerv. Syst. *7*:276, 1946.

Beaudouin, H. Joyeut, J., and Quercy, D.: Le traitement par l'électro-choc et les petites doses d'insuline dans 18 cas de schizophrénie. Ann. Méd.-psychol. *106*: 636, 1948.

Beck, E., McLardy, T., and Meyer, A.: Anatomical comments on psychosurgical procedures. Dig. Neurol. & Psychiat. *17*:570, 1949.

Beckenstein, N.: Results of metrazol therapy in schizophrenia. Psychiatric Quart. *13*: 106, 1939.

Bedson, H. S.: Coma due to meprobamate intoxication. Lancet *1*:288, 1959.

Beek, M. in der, and Schmidt, G.: Empfindungssensationen und Angst in der Schocktherapie. Nervenarzt *18*:384, 1948.

Behnken, P. B., and Merrill, E. G.: Nursing care following prefrontal lobotomy. Am. J. Nursing *49*:431, 1949.

Beiglböck, W., and Dussik, T.: The physiology of the hypoglycemic shock in the treatment of schizophrenia. Am. J. Psychiat. *94* (Supp.):50, 1938.

Bein, H. J., Gross, F., Tripod, J., and Meier, R.: Experimentelle Untersuchungen über "Serpasil" (Reserpin). Schweiz. Med. Wchnschr. *83*:1007, 1953.

Belin, J., and Griffiths, B.: Un "Equilibrant," le T.P. 21 ou Melleril. Lyon méd. *91*:911, 1959.

Bell, E., and Karnosh, L. J.: Tetra-ethyl ammonium chloride as an adjunct in treatment of psychovisceral manifestations of ansiety. J. Nerv. & Ment. Dis. *108*:367, 1948.

Bell, J. L., Tauber, H., Santy, A., and Pulito, F.: Treatment of depressive states in office practice. Dis. Nerv. Syst. *20*:263, 1959.

Bellet, S. Kershbaum, A., and Furst, W.: The electrocardiogram during electric shock treatment of mental disorders. Am. J. M. Sc. *20*:201, 1941.

——, Freed, H., and Dyer, W. W.: The electrocardiogram during insulin shock treatment of schizophrenia and other psychoses. Am. J. M. Sc. *198*:533, 1939.

Benaim, S.: Use of hydroxydione in psychiatry. Brit. Med. J. *2*:801, 1959.

Bender, L.: Twelve year follow-up study on metrazol treated children and adolescent schizophrenics. Presented at 116th meet. of N. Y. Soc. for Clin. Psychiat., 1950.

——, and Cottington, F.: Use of amphetamine sulfate (benzedrine) in child psychiatry. Am. J. Psychiat. *99*:116, 1942.

Benedek, L.: Insulinschockwirkung auf die Wahrnehmung. Berlin: 1935.

Bengzon, A., Hippius, H., and Kanig, K.: Some changes in the serum during treatment with psychotropic drugs. J. Nerv. Ment. Dis. *143*:389, 1966.

Bennett, A. E.: Preventing traumatic complications in convulsive shock therapy by curare. J.A.M.A. *141*:322, 1940.

Bennett, A. E.: Misconceptions concerning hazards of curarization with electroshock. Dis. Nerv. Syst. *9*:219, 1948.

——, McKeever, L. G., and Turk, R. E.: Psychotic reactions during tetraethylthiuramdisulfide (Antabuse) therapy. J.A.M.A. *145*:483, 1951.

——, and Wilbur, C. B.: Convulsion shock therapy in involutional states after complete failure with previous estrogenic treatment. Am. J. M. Sc. *208*:170, 1944.

Bennett, I. F.: Hormonal and other blood changes occurring during insulin hypoglycemia treatment. *In* M. Rinkel: Insulin Treatment in Psychiatry. New York: Philosophical Library, 1959.

——, Cohen, D., and Starer, E.: Isoniazid in treatment of the chronic schizophrenic patient. A.M.A. Arch. Neurol. & Psychiat. *71*:54, 1954.

——, Letonoff, T. V., Winick, W., and Dohan, F. C.: Relationship of blood glucose to changes in "insulin sensitivity" during insulin shock therapy, A.M.A. Arch. Neurol. & Psychiat. *78*:221, 1957.

——: The constellation of depression: Its treatment with nortriptyline. II. Clinical evaluation of nortriptyline. J. Nerv. Ment. Dis. *135*:59, 1962.

——: Is there a superior antidepressant? *In* S. Garattini, and M. N. G. Dukes, Eds.: Antidepressant Drugs. Amsterdam, Excerpta Med. Found., Internat. Congr. Ser. *122*:375, 1967.

Bensoussan, M. P., and Villiaumey, E. M.: Note sur les premiers résultats de l'utilisation d'un nouveau médicament dépressolytique: le chlorhydrate de pipradol. Ann. méd-psychol. *114*:438, 1956.

Bente, D., Denber, H. C. B., Hartung, M.-L., and Ranneberg, K. M.: Extrapyramidalmotorische und elektroenzephalographische Reaktivität unter neuroleptischer Medikation. Ergebnisse einer vergleichenden Buta-

perazin-Studie bei einer amerikanischen und einer deutschen Patientengruppe. Pharmakopsychiatrie *1*:27, 1968.
——, Engelmeier, M.-P., Heinrich, K., Hippius, H. and Schmitt, W.: Methodenkritischer Beitrag zur klinischen Wirksamkeitsprüfung von Psychopharmaka. *In* P. B. Bradley, F. Flügel, P. H. Hoch, Eds.: Neuro-Psychopharmacology, vol. *3*:63, (CINP, München 1962). Amsterdam, Elsevier, 1964.
——, ——, ——, ——, and ——: Zur klinischen Wirkungsanalyse antidepressiver Pharmaka: Ergebnisse mit Amitriptylin. Arzneim.-Forsch. *14*:490, 1964.
——, ——, ——, ——, and ——: Zum Wirkungsbild eines Antidepressivums aus der Dibenzodiazepin-Reihe-Wander 91/HF 1927 (Noveril). *In* D. Bente, and P. B. Bradley, Eds.: Neuro-Psychopharmacology, Vol. *4*:431, (CINP, Birmingham 1964). Amsterdam, Elsevier, 1965.
——, ——, ——, ——, and ——: Klinische Untersuchungen über eine neue Gruppe tricyclischer Neuroleptika. (Substanzen mit 7-gliedrigen heterocyclischen Zentralringen). *In* H. Brill, J. O. Cole, P. Deniker, H. Hippius, and P. B. Bradley, Eds.: Neuro-Psychopharmacology, Vol. *V*:977, (CINP Congr. Washington 1966). Amsterdam, Excerpta Med. Found. Internat. Congr. Ser. No. 129, 1967.
——, ——, ——, ——, and ——: Klinisch-statistische Untersuchungen über die thymoleptischen Therapie- und Begleiteffekte des Melitracen (Trausabun ®). *In* H. Brill, J. O. Cole, P. Deniker, H. Hippius, and P. B. Bradley, Eds.: Neuro-Psychopharmacology, vol. *5*:1135, (CINP, Washington 1966). Amsterdam, Excerpta Med. Found., Internat. Congr. Ser. No. 129, 1967.
——, ——, ——, ——, and ——: Dimensionsanalytische Untersuchungen zur Symptomatologie medikamentös behandelter Depressionen. Arzneim.-Forsch. (in press).
——, Flegel, H., Katscher, H. and Pfeiffer, W.: Das klinische Wirkungsbild des Floropipamid. Ergebnisse mehrjähriger klinischer Untersuchungen. Arzneim-. Forsch. *16*:312, 1966.
——, Hippius, H., Pöldinger, W. and Stach, K.: Chemische Konstitution und klinische Wirkung von antidepressiven Pharmaka. Arzneim.-Forsch. *14*:486, 1964.
——, and Itil, T.: A comparison of the action of various phenothiazine compounds on the human EEG. *In* P. B. Bradley, P. Deniker, C. Radouco-Thomas, Eds.: Neuro-Psychopharmacology, vol. *1*: 496, (CINP Congr. Rom 1958). Amsterdam, Elsevier, 1959.
——, and ——: Clinico-electroencephalographic investigations. *In* N. Kline, Ed.: Psychopharmacology Frontiers. London, Churchill, 1959.
Bercel, N. A.: Clinical trial of thioridazine in private practice. Amer. Pract. Digest Treatm. *12*:44, 1961.
Berenstein, S., and Levi, R.: Verhütung von Zwischenfällen bei Insulinkuren durch Adenosintriphosphorsäure (Atriphos). Schweiz. Med. Wchnschr. *1948*: 1200, 1948.
Berg, S., and Robbins, E. S.: A pharmacological report on PM-1090. J. Neuropsychiat. *1*:32, 1959.
Berger, F. M.: The Pharmacological Properties of 2-methyl-2-n-propyl-1, 3-propanediol dicarbamate (Miltown), a new interneuronal blocking agent. J. Pharm. & Exper. Ther. *104*:468, 1952.
Berger, F. M., and Ludwig, B. J.: Meprobamate and related compounds. *In* M. Gordon, Ed.: Psychopharmacological Agents, Vol. I: 103, Medicinal Chemistry; A Series of Monographs, Vol. 4. New York, Academic Press, 1964.
Berger, M.: The use of cerium oxalate to reduce incidence of emesis in deep insulin therapy. Am. J. Psychiat. *106*:865, 1950.
Berkwitz, N. J.: Faradic shock treatment of the "functional" psychoses. J. Lancet *59*: 351 1939.
Bernath, A. K.: Modification of anxiety subsequent to insulin-induced mild hypoglycemia. *In* M. Rinkel: Insulin Treatment in Psychiatry. New York: Philosophical Library, 1959.
Bernstein, S.: Serial observation on the physiological and psychological changes in patients reacting with a depression to reserpine. J. Mt. Sinai Hosp. *24*:89, 1957.
Bernthsen, A.: Zur Kenntnis des Methylenblau und verwandter Farbstoffe. Berichte der Dtsch. Chem. Ges. *16*:2896, 1883. No. 511.
Berson, S. A., and Yalow, R. S.: Insulin antagonism, insulin antibodies and insulin resistance. Am. J. Med. *25*:155, 1958.
Bersot, M.: Autoobservation de l'électrochoc. Ann. med.-psychol. *101*:488, 1943.
Berzewski, H., and Hippius, H.: Das klinische Wirkungsbild des Neurolepticums 3-Chlor-10-(γ-[N′-β′-(1″-methyl-2″-oxo-imidazolidyl-3″)-aethyl-N-piperazinyl]-propyl)-phenothiazin-dihydrochlorid (Chlorimpi-phenin). Arzneim.-Forsch. *17*:329, 1967.
Besson, F.: Chloropromazine et voies biliares. Schweiz. med. Wchnschr. *86*:1020, 1956.
Betts, T. A., Kalra, P. L., Cooper, R., and Jeavons, P. M.: Epileptic fits as a probable side-effect of amitriptyline. Lancet *1*:390, 1968.
Bhaskaran, K., and Nand, D. S.: Clinical trial with a (2-piperidyl) benzhydrol hydrochloride (Meratran) and methylphenidylate (Ritalin) in chronic apathetic schizophrenics. Ind. J. Med. Sc. *13*:117, 1959.
——, Subrahmanyan, P., and Satya Nand, D.: Fatal bone-marrow aplasia complicating prochlorperazine therapy. Amer. J. Psychiat. *119*:373, 1962.
Biagi, R. W., and Bapat, B. N.: Intrahepatic obstructive jaundice from amitriptyline. Brit. J. Pscyhiat. *113*:1113, 1967.
Bianchi, J. A., and Chiarello, C. J.: Shock therapy in the involutional and manic-depressive psychoses. Psychiatric Quart. *18*:118, 1944.
——, and ——: Comparative results of

electric shock and metrazol convulsive treatment in dementia praecox. Psychiatric Quart. *21*:304, 1947.
Bianchi, L.: The mechanism of the brain and the function of the frontal lobes. Edinburgh: Livingstone, 1922.
Bidder, T. G.: Localized-convulsion electroconvulsive treatment. Anesthesiology *23*: 266, 1962.
Biddy, R. L., and Smith, K: Shock treatment. *In* E. A. Spiegel, Ed.: Progress in Neurology and Psychiatry. New York, Grune & Stratton, 1966.
Biel, J. H., Horita, A., and Drukker, A. E.: Monoamine oxidase inhibitors. (Hydrazines). *In* M. Gordon, Ed.: Psychopharmacological Agents, Vol. I: 359, Medicinal Chemistry; A Series of Monographs, Vol. 4. New York, Academic Press, 1964.
Bielfeld, K.: Über die Anwendung eines neuen Phenothiazin-derivates in der Geburtshilfe, insbesondere unter der Geburt. Zbl. Gynäk. *82*:1205, 1960.
Billet, J., Pagés, P. LaFon, R., and Billet, M. and B.: Les accidents et incidents de la cure de Sakel. Ann. méd.-psychol. *109*:23, 1951.
Billig, O., and Bradley, J. D.: Combined shock and corpus luteum hormone therapy. Am. J. Psychiat. *102*:783, 1946.
Bindelglas, P. M., Dee, G. H., and Enos, F. A.: Medical and psychosocial factors in enuretic children treated with imipramine hydrochloride. Amer. J. Psychiat. *124*:1107, 1968.
Bini, L.: Ulteriori ricerche biochimiche sul coma insulinico. Atti del convegno sulla terapia moderna della schizofrenia. Milano: 1937.
——: Experimental researches on epileptic attacks induced by the electric current. Am. J. Psychiat. *94* (Supp.):172, 1938.
——: Ricerche sperimentali sulla fisiopatologia degli apparati cardiovascolare e respiratorio nell'elettroshock. Riv. sper. de freniat. *64*:4, 1941.
——, and Bazzi, T.: L'elettroshockterapia col metodo dell'annihilimento nelle forme gravi di psiconeurosi. Rassegna di neuropsichiat. *1*:59, 1947.
——, and Puddu, V.: Ricerche sperimentali sulla fisiopatologia degli apparati cardiovasculare e respiratorii nell'elettroshock. Riv. sper. di freniat. *64*:653, 1940.
Binzley, R. F., and Anderson, J. L.: Prolonged coma in insulin treatment of dementia praecox. Psychiatric Quart. *12*: 477, 1938.
Bird, E. G., Goss, J. D., and Denber, H. C. B.: Chlorpromazine in the treatment of mental illness. Am. J. Psychiat. *111*: 930, 1955.
Birkmayer, W.: Beobachtungen über Augenbewegungen im Cardiazolkrampf. Arch. f. Psychiat. *109*:542, 1939.
——, and Danielczyk, W.: Die Behandlung von Depressionen mit Tofranil. Klin. Med. *14*:337, 1959.
Birley, J. L. T.: Modified frontal leucotomy: A review of 106 cases. Brit. J. Psychiat. *110*:211, 1964.
Bischoff, G.: Insulinkur und Leberfunktion. Psychiat.-neurol. Wchnschr. *40*:142, 1948.
Bishop, M. P., and Gallant, D. M.: Behavioral toxicity associated with benzquinamide (Quantril) therapy in schizophrenic patients. Amer. J. Psychiat. *120*: 180, 1963.
Bjørn, S., and Rasmussen, C.: Sordinol ® (Clopenthixol) in the treatment of schizophrenics. Acta psychiat. scand. *39*:427, 1963.
Blachly, P. H., and Gowing, D.: Multiple monitored electroconvulsive treatment. Compr. Psychiat. *7*:100, 1966.
Blachly, P. H., and Semler, H. J.: Electroconvulsive therapy of three patients with aortic valve prostheses. Amer. J. Psychiat. *124*:137, 1967.
Blackwell, B., and Marley, E.: Hypertensive interactions between MAOI and foodstuffs. *In* H. Brill, J. O. Cole, P. Deniker, H. Hippius, and P. B. Bradley, Eds.: Neuro-Psychopharmacology, Vol. *V*:578, (CINP, Washington 1966). Amsterdam, Excerpta Med. Found. Internat. Congr. Ser. No. 129, 1967.
——, ——, Price, J., and Taylor, D.: Hypertensive interactions between monoamine oxidase inhibitors and foodstuffs. Brit. J. Psychiat. *113*:349, 1967.
Blair, D.: Prognosis in schizophrenia. J. Ment. Sc. *86*:378, 1940.
——, and Brady, D. M.: Recent advances in the treatment of schizophrenia: group training and the tranquillisers. J. Ment. Sc. *104*:625, 1958.
Bleuler, M.: Das Wesen der Schizophrenieremission nach Schockbehandlung. Ztschr. f. Neurol. *173*:553, 1941.
——: Endokrinologische Psychiatrie. Stuttgart: Georg Thieme, 1954.
——, and Stoll, W. A.: Clinical use of reserpine in psychiatry: comparison with chlorpromazine. Ann. New York Acad. Sc. *61*:167, 1955.
Blignault, A. P.: Electric coma treatment of mental disorder; a preliminary report. South African Med. J. *28*:409, 1954.
Bliss, E. L., Migeon, C. J., Nelson, D. H., Samuels, L. T., and Branch, C. H. H.: Influence of E.C.T. and insulin coma on level of adrenocortical steroids in peripheral circulation. A.M.A. Arch. Neurol. & Psychiat. *72*:352, 1954.
Bloomfield, S., Simard-Savoie, S., Bernier, J., and Tetreault, L.: Comparative analgesic activity of levomepromazine and morphine in patients with chronic pain. Canad. Med. Ass. J. *90*:1156, 1964.
Blumberg, H., Dayton, H. B., and Wolf, P. S.: Narcotic antagonist activity of Naloxone. Fed. Proc. *24*:676, 1965.
Board of Control (England and Wales): Results in 1000 leucotomies. London: H. M. Stationery Office, 1947.
Boardman, R. H.: Fatal case of toxic hepatitis implicating chlorpromazine. Brit. Med. J. *2*:579, 1954.
——, Lomas, J., and Markowe, W.: Insulin and chlorpromazine in schizophrenia. Lancet *2*:487, 1956.

Bobon, J., Bobon, D. P., Breulet, M., Colinet, M., Devroye, A., Korn, M., and Pinchard, A.: Un traitement d'urgence de l'agitation: le droperidol (R 4749). Acta neural. psychiat. belg. *68*:103, 1968.

——, Collard, J., Delree, Ch., and Gernay, J. M.: Le Spiropéridol. Acta neurol. psychiat. belg. *63*:991, 1963.

——, ——, and Demaret, A.: Un nouveau neuroleptique à effet hypnogène différé: le Dipipérone (R 3345), butyrophénone carbamidée. Acta neurol psychiat. belg. *61*:611, 1961.

——, ——, and ——: L'imipramine à doses faibles en gériatrie mentale. Acta neurol. psychiat. belg. *62*:559, 1962.

——, ——, and Pinchard, A.: Un neuroleptique à effets hypnique et akinétique prépondérants: le benzpéridol (R 4584), 8° butyrophénone. Acta neurol. psychiat. belg. *62*:566, 1962.

——, Gernay, J. M., Collard, J., Goffioul, F., and Breulet, M.: Mauvais caractère et Neuleptil. A propos d'une expérience clinique belgoluxembourgeoise (1963-1964). Acta neurol. psychiat. belg. *68*:154, 1968.

Bockner, S.: Controlled clinical trial of methylpentynol (Oblivon). J. Ment. Sc. *103*:218, 1957.

Bockoven, J. S. Greenblatt, M., and Solomon, H. C.: Treatment results in the major psychoses. New England J. Med. *244*:357, 1951.

Bodechtel, G.: Der hypoglykämische Schock und seine Wirkung auf das Zentralnervensystem. Deutches Arch. f. klin. Med. *175*: 188, 1933.

Boissier, J. R., Simon, P., and Lwoff, J. M.: Etude pharmacologique d'un neuroleptique à action prolongée: l'énanthate de fluphénazine. Med. Pharmacol. exp. *14*:435, 1966.

Boling, L., Ryan, W., and Greenblatt, M.: Insulin treatment of psychotic patients: Comparative results with deep- and light-coma treatment. Am. J. Psychiat. *113*: 1009, 1957.

Bolles, M. M., Rosen, G. P., and Landis, C.: Psychological performance tests as prognostic agents for the efficacy of insulin therapy in schizophrenia. Psychiatric Quart. *12*:733, 1938.

Bonafede, V. I.: Chlorpromazine (Thorazine) treatment of disturbed epileptic patients. Arch. Neurol. & Psychiat. *77*: 243, 1957.

Bond, E. D.: Continued follow-up results in shock therapy and in control cases. Am. J. Psychiat. *97*:1024, 1941.

——, and Rivers, T. D.: Further follow-up results in insulin-shock therapy. Am. J. Psychiat. *99*:201, 1942.

——, and ——: Insulin shock therapy after seven years. Am. J. Psychiat. *101*:62, 1944.

——, and Shurley, J. T. Insulin therapy and its future. Am. J. Psychiat. *103*:338, 1946.

Bonello, F. J.: Chlorpromazine in general practice. Internat. rec. Med. *169*:197, 1956.

Bonfiglio, G., and Donadio, G.: Risultati della sperimentazione clinica di un nuovo farmaco (metronidazolo) nella cura dell' alcolismo. Cronico. Lav. Neuropsichiat. *38*:135, 1966.

Bonhoeffer, K.: Die symptomatischen Psychosen im Gefolge von akuten Infektionen und inneren Erkrankungen. Leipzig: F. Deuticke, 1910.

Borel, M. J.: Traitement de la schizophrénie par la soustraction massive de liquide céphalo-rachidien suivi d'injection d'air combinée à I'insuline et al pyréthotherapie. Ann. méd.-psychol. *107*: 51, 1949.

Borenstein, P., Gekiere, F., Cujo, Ph., and Thouvenot, M.: Evaluation des effets thérapeutiques d'un neuroleptique par la confrontation des données cliniques et paracliniques. A propos d'une expérience de deux ans de la thioridazine. Psychiat. Neurol. (Basel) *153*:1, 1967.

Borgarello, G.: L'insulinoterapia nello stato depressivo, prevalentemente involutivo. Atti del convegno sulla terapia moderna della schizofrenia. Milano: 1937.

Borup Svendsen, B., Faurbye, A., and Kristjansen, P.: Comparison of the effect of thioridazine and chlorpromazine on chronic schizophrenic psychosis using double blind technique. Psychopharmacologia *2*:446, 1961.

Borysowicz, J., Paradowski, J., Rose, J., Witek, S., and Zalewski, W.: Insulin treatment of schizophrenia. Rocznik Psychjatrycny *28*:26, 1936.

Bos, C., and Lehmann, H. E.: Studies on psychiatric patients undergoing nitrous oxide treatments. J. Ment. Sc. *94*:509, 1950.

Bourgignon, M. G.: Résultats de la diélectrolyse en psychiatrie. Ann. méd. psychol. *106*:469, 1948.

Bourne, H.: The insulin myth. Lancet *2*:964, 1953.

Bowers, M. K., and Berkowitz, B.: Clinical observations on the effects of electroconvulsive therapy in the hypnotic state. J. Nerv. & Ment. Dis. *118*:355, 1953.

Bowes, H. A.: The ataractic drugs: the present position of chloropromazine, Frenquel, Pacatal and reserpine in psychiatric practice. Am. J. Psychiat. *113*:530, 1956.

Bowman, K. M., Miller, E. R., Dailey, M. E., Simon, A., Frankel, B., and Lowe, G. W.: Thyroid function in mental disease measured with radioactive iodine I^{188}. Am. J. Psychiat. *106*:561, 1950.

——, and Simon, A.: Studies in electronarcosis therapy. Am. J. Psychiat. *105*:15, 1948.

——, ——, Hone, C. H., MacKlin, E. A., Crook, G. H., Burbridge, N., and Hanson, K.: A clinical evaluation of tetraethylthiuramdisulphide (Antabuse) in the treatment of problem drinkers. Am. J. Psychiat. *107*:832, 1951.

Boyd, D. A., Jr., and Brown, D. W.: Electric convulsive therapy in mental disorders associated with childbearing. J. Missouri M. A. *45*:573, 1948.

Brachman, P. S., McCreary, T. W., and Florence, R.: Agranulocytosis induced by

trimeprazine. New England J. Med. *260*: 378, 1959.
Bradley, P. B.: Phenothiazine derivatives: *In* W. S. Root and F. G. Hofmann, Eds.: Physiological Pharmacology. A comprehensive treatise, Vol. I: The Nervous System—Part A: Central Nervous System Drugs, p. 417. New York, Academic Press, 1963.
——, and Fink, M.: Anticholinergic drugs. Amsterdam, Elvesier, 1968.
Brandner, M.: Methoden zur Beurteilung antidepressiv wirksamer Substanzen mit spezieller Berücksichtigung von Mono-Chlor-Imipramin G 34 586. Schweiz. Arch. Neurol. Neurochir. Psychiat. *93*:137, 1964.
Bratfos, O., and Haug, J. O.: Electroconvulsive therapy and antidepressant drugs in manic-depressive disease. Acta Psychiat. Scand. *41*:588, 1965.
von Brauchitsch, H.: Endokrinologische Aspekte des Wirkungsmechanismus neuroplegischer Medikamente. Psychopharmacologia *2*:1, 1961.
Braun, M., and Parker, M.: The use of glucagon in the termination of therapeutic insulin coma. Am. J. Psychiat. *115*:814, 1959.
Braunmühl, A. von: Das Azoman bei der Krampfbehandlung der Schizophrenie. Psychiat.-Neurol. Wchnschr. *40*:515, 1938.
——: Die Insulinschockbehandlung der Schizophrenie (unter Berücksichtigung des Kardiazolkrampfes). Berlin: J. Springer, 1938.
——: Fünf Jahre Schock- und Krampfbehandlung in Eglfing-Haar. Arch. f. Psychiat. *114*:410, 1942.
——: Insulinshock und Heilkrampf in der Psychiatrie. Stuttgart: Wissenschaftliche Verlagsgesellschaft, 1947.
——: Ein neues Gerät für die Heilkrampfbehandlung mittels elektrischen Stromes. Fortschr. d. Neurol. u. Psychiat. *19*:325, 1951.
Brazier, M. A. B.: The effects of drugs on the electroencephalogram of man. Clin. Pharmacol. Ther. *5*:102, 1964.
Breitner, C.: Localized electric stimulation of the diencephalon in the treatment of mental disorders. Dis. Nerv. Syst. Suppl. *18*:14, 1957.
Brick, H., Doub, Jr., W. H., and Perdue, W. C.: A comparison of the effects of amitriptyline and protriptyline on anxiety and depressive states in female prisoners. Internat. J. Neuropsychiat. *1*:325, 1965.
Brickner, R. M.: The intellectual functions of the frontal lobes; a study based upon observation of a man after partial bilateral frontal lobotomy. New York: Macmillan, 1936.
——, Porter, R. T., et al.: Direct reorientation of behavior patterns in deep narcosis. Arch. Neurol. & Psychiat. *64*:165, 1950.
Brill, H., and Binzley, R. F.: Involuntary eye movements as a criterion of depth in insulin coma. Am. J. Psychiat. *96*:177, 1939.
——, and Kalinowsky, L. B.: Asphyxial episodes and their prevention in electric and other convulsive therapies. Psychiatric Quart. *16*:351, 1942.
——, and Patton, R. E.: Analysis of 1955-1956 population fall in New York State mental hospitals in first year of large-scale use of tranquillizing drugs. Am. J. Psychiat. *114*:509, 1957.
——, and ——: Analysis of 1955-56 population fall in New York State mental hospitals in first year of large-scale use of tranquilizing drugs. Amer. J. Psychiat. *114*:509, 1957.
——, and ——: Clinical-statistical analysis of population changes in New York State mental hospitals since introduction of psychotropic drugs. Amer. J. Psychiat. *119*:20, 1962.
Brill, J. M.: Treatment of the acute alcoholic with injectable thioridazine. Amer. J. Psychiat. *120*:496, 1964.
Brill, N. Q., Crumpton, E., Eiduson, S., Grayson, H. M., Hellmann, L. I., and Richards, R. A.: Relative effectiveness of various components of electroconvulsive therapy: experimental study. A.M.A. Arch. Neurol. & Psychiat. *81*:627, 1959.
Brodie, B. B.: Interaction of psychotropic drugs with physiological and biochemical mechanisms in brain. Modern Medicine *4*:453, 1959.
Brody, E. B.: Superego, introjected mother, and energy discharge in schizophrenia: contribution from the study of anterior lobotomy. J. Am. Psychoanal. A. *6*:481, 1958.
Brody, I. A.: Shock after administration of prochlorperazine in patient with pheochromocytoma. Report of a case with spontaneous tumor destruction. J.A.M.A. *169*:1749, 1959.
Brody, M. B.: Prolonged memory defects following electrotherapy. J. Ment. Sc. *380*:777, 1944.
——: Leucotomy as an instrument of research. Proc. Roy. Soc. Med. *40*:149, 1947.
——, and Moore, B. E.: Prefrontal lobotomy; a review of recent literature. Connecticut M. J. *10*:409, 1946.
Broggi, F. S.: Modified electrotherapy versus anti-depressant drugs. J. Maine M. A. *53*:219, 1962.
Brooke, G.: Imipramine. Lancet *7102*:568, 1959.
Brooks, C.: The use of reserpine (Serpasil) in mentally ill epileptics. Dis. Nerv. Syst. *18*:275, 1957.
Brooks, G. W.: Experience with the use of chlorpromazine and reserpine in pyschiatry. New England J. Med. *254*:1119, 1956.
——: Withdrawal from neuroleptic drugs. Am. J. Psychiat. *115*:931, 1959.
Broussolle, P., and Dubor, P.: Preliminary appraisal of the clinical effects of a new neuroleptic. Bordeaux, Cong. Alien. Neurol., 1956.
——, Perrin, J., Maurel, H., Lambert, P., Achaintre, A., Balvet, P., Beaujard, M., Revol, L., Requet, A., and Berthier, C.: La Prochlorperazine en psychiatrie: expérience tirée de 240 cures. Presse méd. *65*:1628, 1957.

——, and Rosier, Y.: Evolution des symptômes neurologiques dus aux neuroleptiques. (Bilan de 344 cures). Ann. méd.-psychol. *117/I*:140, 1959.
——, ——, and Pauget: Carbamate de methylpentimol. J. Med. Lyon. *41*:123, 1960.
Browne, M. W., Kreeger, L. C., and Kazamias, N. G.: A clinical trial of amitriptyline in depressive patients. Brit. J. Psychiat. *109*: 692, 1963.
Brown, D. G., Hullin, R. P., and Roberts, J. M.: Fluid distribution and the response of depression to E.C.T. and Imipramine. Brit. J. Psychiat. *109*:395, 1963.
von Brücke, F. Th., and Hornykiewicz, O.: Pharmakologie der Psychopharmaka. Berlin—Heidelberg—New York, Springer, 1966.
Bruno, A., and Allegranza, A.: The effect of haloperidol on the urinary excretion of dopamine, homovanillic and vanilmandelic acids in schizophrenics. Psychopharmacologia *8*:60, 1965.
Bruyn, G. W.: Thiopropazate dihydrochloride (Dartal) in the treatment of Huntington's chorea. Psychiat. Neurol. Neurochir. *65*: 430, 1962.
Bucci, L., and Saunders, J. C.: Methotrimeprazine for control of the acutely disturbed. Amer. J. Psychiat. *120*:905, 1964.
Bucher, H. W., and Stucki, P.: Kardiale Komplikationen bei einer Vergiftung mit Desipramine (Pertofran). Schweiz. med. Wschr. *97*:519, 1967.
Bückmann, L.: Beriberisymptome bei der Hypoglykämietherapie der Schizophrenie. Nervenarzt, *10*:412, 1937.
Bulley, K. G., and Greene, B. L.: Incidence of pulmonary tuberculosis in schizophrenic patients following metrazol convulsive therapy. Am. J. M. Sc. *201*:504, 1941.
Burch, B. H., Hughes, C. L., Bishop, C. D., Droske, L. Z., and Gericke, O. L.: Lung abscess in the mentally ill as an indication of electric shock treatment. Dis. Chest *36*:52, 1959.
Burchard, J. M.: Pharmakopsychiatrische Untersuchungen über die Wirkungsweise der Opiumalkaloide bei endogenen Psychosen. Nervenarzt *29*:103, 1958.
Burckhardt, G.: Über Rindenexcisionen, als Beitrag zur operativen Therapie der Psychosen. Allg. Ztschr. f. Psychiat. *74*:463, 1890.
Burian, H. M., and Fletcher, M. C.: Visual functions in patients with retinal pigmentary degeneration following the use of NP 207. Arch. Ophthal. *60*:612, 1958.
Burk, H. W., and Menolascino, F. J.: Haloperidol in emotionally disturbed mentally retarded individuals. Amer. J. Psychiat. *124*:1589, 1968.
Burke, J. C., High, J. P., Leffan, R. J., and Ravaris, C. L.: Depot action of fluphenazine (Prolixin) enanthate in oil. Fed. Proc. *21*:339, 1962.
Burlingame, C. C.: Rehabilitation after leucotomy. Proc. Roy. Soc. Med. *42*:31, 1949.
Burns, B. H.: Preliminary evaluation of a new anti-depressant, trimipramine, by a sequential method. Brit. J. Psychiat. *111*: 1155, 1965.
Busch, E., Halmsted, O., Lund, O., Nevin, J. and Thelle, P.: Orbitomedial undercutting in mental disease. Danish Med. Bull. *2*:10, 1955.
Burshstein, M. L.: On the problem of artificially enhancing the convulsive tendency in schizophrenics. Nevropat. i psikhiat. *16*:50, 1947.
Buscaino, V. M.: L'iperpiretoterapia della schizofrenia. Progressi di Terapia, 1951.
Busch, E., Halmsted, O., Lund, O., Nevin, J., and Thelle, P.: Orbitomedial frontal undercutting in metal diseases. Danish Med. Bull. *2*:10, 1955.
Büssow, H.: Cortisonartig wirkende Substanzen bei endogenen Depressionen. Nervenarzt *22*:401, 1951.
——, Dunker, E., and Albrecht, H.: Über die Wirkung von Stickstoffatmung auf Zustandsbild und Verlauf endogener Depressionen. Nervenarzt *18*:229, 1947.
——, and Lindner, W.: Inverse Doriden-Wirkung im Verlauf einer Reserpin-Behandlung von Depressionen. Dtsch. med. Wschr. *83*:500, 1958.
Buxbaum, G.: Fünf Jahre einfache und kombinierte Insulinshocktherapie an der Landes-Heil- und Pflegeanstalt Göttingen mit katamnestischen Ergebungen. Ztschr. f. Neurol. 177, 1944.
Bychowski, G.: Psychoanalyse im hypoglykämischen Zustand. Internat. Ztschr. f. Psychoanal. *23*:540, 1937.
Cade, J. F. J.: Lithium salts in treatment of psychotic excitement. M. J. Australia *2*:349, 1949.
Cahn, C. H.: Complications during reserpine therapy. Am. J. Psychiat. *112*:64, 1955.
——, and Lehmann, H. E.: Perphenazine: Observations on the clinical effects of a new tranquillizing agent in psychotic conditions. Canad. Psychiat. Ass. J. *2*:104, 1957.
Cahn, L. A.: The influence of clopenthixol (Sordinol®) on the libido of the male. Psychiat. Neurol. Neurochir. *68*:67, 1965.
Calwell, W. P. K., Jacobsen, M., and Skarbeck, A.: A comparative study of oxypertine and trifluoperazine in chronic schizophrenia. A new application of the Wing rating scale. Brit. J. Psychiat. *110*:520, 1964.
Cameron, D. E.: Adrenalin administration in persistent anxiety states. Am. J. M. Sc. *21*:281, 1945.
——: The use of nucleic acid in aged patients with memory impairment. Amer. J. Psychiat. *114*:943, 1958.
——, Kral, V. A., Solyom, L., Sved, S., Wainrib, B., Beaulieu, C., and Enesco, H.: RNA and memory. *In*: Galio, J. (Ed.): Macromolecules and Behavior New York, Appleton Century Crofts, 1966.
——, Lohrenz, J. G., and Handcock, K. A.: The depatterning treatment of schizophrenia. Compr. Psychiat. *3*:65, 1962.
——, and Pande, S. K.: Treatment of the

chronic paranoid schizophrenic patient. Canad. M. A. J. *78*:92, 1958.
——, Sved, S., Solyom, L., Wainrib, B., and Barik, H.: Effects of ribonucleic acid on memory defect in the aged. Amer. J. Psychiat. *120*:320, 1963.
Campan, L., and Parant, R.: Hibernation pour un coma prolongé grave compliquant une cure de Sakel. Anesth. *10*:99, 1953.
Campanella, G., and Guida, A.: α-Ethylcrotonylurea: a new drug of "tranquillising" action Minerva Med. *49*:890, 1958.
Campbell, J. D.: Manic-depressive disease in children. J.A.M.A. *158*:154, 1955.
Cannicott, S. M.: Unilateral electro-convulsive therapy. Postgrad. Med. J. *38*:451, 1962.
——: The technique of unilateral electroconvulsive therapy. Amer. J. Psychiat. *120*:477, 1963.
——, and Waggoner, R. W.: Unilateral and bilateral electroconvulsive therapy. Arch. Gen. Psychiat. *16*:229, *1*967.
Caplan, G.: Treatment of epilepsy by electrically induced convulsions, Brit. M. J., April 14, 1945, p. 511.
Cares, R. M., Asrican, E., Fenichel, M., Sack, P., and Severino, J.: Therapeutic and true effects of chlorpromazine among 3014 hospitalized cases Am. J. Psychiat. *114*: 318, 1957.
Carey, B., Weber, M., and Smith, J. A.: Methyl-phenidylacetate hydrochloride (Ritalin) in the treatment of chronic schizophrenic patients. Am. J. Psychiat. *113*:546, 1956.
Carney, M. W. P., Roth, M., and Garside, R. F.: The diagnosis of depressive syndromes and the prediction of E.C.T. response. Brit. J. Psychiat. *111*:659, 1965.
Carrillo, R.: Leucotomia selectiva. Lisbon: Psychosurgery, 1949.
Carse, J.: The nursing requirements for prefrontal leucotomy. Nursing Times *40*:165, 1944.
——, and Slater, E.: Lymphocytosis after electric convulsion. J. Neurol., Neurosurg. & Psychiat. *9*:1, 1946.
Carter, Ch. H.: Nortriptyline HCl as a tranquilizer for disturbed mentally retarded patients: A controlled study. Amer. J. Med. Sci. *251*:465, 1966.
Carter, J. T.: Types of personal life memories forgotten following electro-convulsive therapy. Am. Psychologist *8*:330, 1953.
Casey, J. F., Lasky, J. J., Klett, C. J., and Hollister, L. E.: Treatment of schizophrenic reactions with phenothiazine derivatives. A comparative study of chlorpromazine, triflupromazine, mepazine, prochlorperazine, perphenazine, and phenobarbital. Amer. J. Psychiat. *117*:97, 1960.
Cash, P. T., and Hoekstra, C. S.: Preliminary curarization in electric convulsive shock therapy. Psychiatric Quart. *17*:20, 1943.
Cassidy, W. L., Ballantine, H. T., Jr., and Flanagan, N. B.: Frontal cingulotomy for affective disorders. Recent Advances in Biological Psychiatry. Vol. 8. New York, Plenum Press, 1966.
Cattan, R., Carasso, R., Frumusan, P., Nataf, P., Soupault, R., and Bucaille, M.: Indications et résultats des interventions pré-frontales dans les recto-colites ulcérohémorragiques. Sem. hôp. Par. *33*:507, 1957.
Cattell, J. P.: A psychodynamic study of topectomy patients. Am. J. Psychiat. *107*: 373, 1950.
——: Psychopharmacological agents: a selective survey. Am. J. Psychiat. *116*:352, 1959.
——, and Malitz, S.: Revised survey of selected psychopharmacological agents. Am. J. Psychiat. *117*:449, 1960.
Cavka, V.: Über die Augensymptome bei Kranken, welche mit der Cardiazol- und Insulinschocktherapie behandelt waren. Arch. f. Psychiat. *109*:721, 1939.
Cazzullo, C. L.: Rapporti fra i risultati delle indagini sperimentali e delle esperienze cliniche in psicofarmacologia. Minerva Medica *54*:3155, 1963.
Centini, D., and Bandettini di Poggio: Ricerche biochimiche in schizofrenia durante l'ettroshock, Rassegna di studi psichiat. *28*:875, 1939.
Cerletti, U.: L'Elettroshock. Riv. sper. di freniat. *64*:209, 1942.
——: L'electrochoc. Congrés Internat. de Psychiat. *4*:1, 1950.
——: Old and new information about electroshock. Am. J. Psychiat. *107*:87, 1950.
——, and Bini, L.: L'Elettroshock. Arch. gen. di neurol., psichiat., e psicoanal. *19*:266, 1938.
——: Le alterazioni istopatologiche del sistema nervoso nell'elettroshock. Riv. sper. di freniat. *64*:2, 1940.
Cernáček, J.: Die therapeutische Anwendung des Electroschocks ausserhalb des Gebietes der sogenannten grossen Psychosen. Wien. med. Wchnschr. *30/31*:433, 1943.
Cesaroec, Z., and Nilsson, L.: The effect of electroshock and imipramine treatment on figural fluctuations in a group of psychiatric patients. Acta Psychiat. Scand. *41*:131, 1965.
Challas, G., and Brauer, W.: Tourette's disease: Relief of symptoms with R 1625. Amer. J. Psychiat. *120*:283, 1963.
Challiol, V.: Electric shock therapy of schizophrenia; action of phenobarbital on convulsive crises. Riv. sper, di freniat. *64*:635, 1940.
Chanoit, P., Deshaies, G., Mignot, H., Rouquette, Sivadon, P. et de Verbizier, J.:
Etude thérapeutique d'un nouveau neuroleptique: La propériciazine. Presse méd. *71*:339, 1963.
Chantraine, J., and Pairoux, R.: Contribution clinique à l'étude du chlorprothixène. Acta neurol. psychiat. belg. *60*:846, 1960.
Chapel, J. L., Brown, N., and Jenkins, R. L.: Tourette's disease: Symptomatic relief with haloperidol. Amer. J. Psychiat. *121*:608, 1964.
Chapman, W. P., Rose, A. S., and Solomon, H. C.: A follow-up study of motor withdrawal reaction to heat discomfort in pa-

tients before and after frontal lobotomy. Am. J. Psychiat. *107*:221, 1950.
Chapius, R.: Cinq ans d'insulino-et convulsive-therapie chez 210 malades mentaux. Schweiz. Arch. f. Neurol. u. Psychiat. *51*:26, 1953; *52*:1, 1943.
——, and Georgi, F.: Traitements de choc dans les dépressions et les schizophrénies Schweiz. Arch. f. Neurol. u. Psychiat. *15*:66, 1945.
Charatan, F. B. E.: An Evaluation of chlorpromazine (Largactil) in psychiatry. J. Ment. Sc. *100*:882, 1954.
——, and Bartlett, N. G.: The effect of chlorpromazine (Largactil) on glucose tolerance. J. Ment. Sc. *101*:351, 1955.
Charpentier, P., Gailliot, P., Jacob, R., Guadechon, J., and Buisson, P.: Récherches sur les dimethylaminopropyl-n-phenothiazines substituées. Compt. rend. *235*-59, 1952.
Chase, L. S., and Silverman, S.: Prognostic criteria in schizophrenia. Am. J. Psychiat. *98*:360, 1941.
Chatrian, G. E., and Petersen, M. C.: The convulsive patterns provoked by Indoklon, Metrazol and electroshock. Clin. Neurophysiol. *12*:715, 1960.
Cheney, C. O., and Clow, H. E.: Prognostic factors in insulin shock therapy. Am J. Psychiat. *97*:1029, 1941.
——, Hamilton, D. M., and Heaver, W. L.: Metrazol as an adjunct to the treatment of mental disorders. Psychiatric Quart. *15*:205, 1941.
Chesrow, E. J., Kaplitz, Sh. E., Breme, J. T., Sabatini, R., Vetra, H., and Marquardt, G. H.: Nortriptyline for the treatment of anxiety and depression in chronically ill and geriatric patients. J. Amer. Geriatr. Soc. *12*:271, 1964.
Childers, R. T.: Two cases of urinary retention in females on amitriptyline. Amer. J. Psychiat. *120*:912, 1964.
Cieslak, G.: Komplikationen der Reserpinbehandlung. Nervenarzt *31*:102, 1960.
Clapp, J. S., and Loomis, E. A.: Continuous sleep treatment. Am. J. Psychiat. *106*:821, 1950.
Clark, W. E. Le Gros: The connections of the frontal lobes of the brain. Lancet *1*:353, 1948.
Claude, H., Coste, F., and Dublineau, J.: Etude comparée des pyretothérapies parasitaires, bactériennes, organiques et chimiques dens le traitement de la démence précoce. I. Congrès Français de Thérapeutique. Paris: 1933.
——, Ey, H., and Dublineau, J.: Pyretothérapie souffrée et chrysothérapie associées dans le traitement de certaines démences précoces. I Congrès Français de Thérapeutique. Paris: 1933.
——, and Rubénovitch, P.: Thérapeutiques biologiques des affections mentales. Paris: Masson et Cie., 1940.
Cleckley, H., and Templeton, C. M.: Prolonged coma in insulin therapy of the psychoses. Am. J. Psychiat. *97*:844, 1941.
Cleghorn, R. A., Graham, B. F., Saffran, M., and Cameron, D. E.: A study of the effect of the pituitary ACTH in depressed patients. Canad. M. A. J. *63*:329, 1950.
Clement, A. J.: Atropine premedication for electric convulsion therapy. Brit. M. J. *1*: 228, 1962.
Close, H. P.: The use of electroshock therapy in treating psychiatric patients with associated pulmonary tuberculosis. Am. J. Psychiat. *106*:352, 1949.
Clute, K. F., and Fitzgerald, G. W.: Anuria following electroshock therapy. Canad. M. A. J. *59*:426, 1948.
Coffin, S.: Curare-modified E.C.T. Brit. M. J. *4614*:1050, 1949.
Cohen, H., and Freireich, A. Z.: Trilafon in the treatment of chronically psychotic hospitalized patients. Am. J. Psychiat. *115*:452, 1958.
Cohen, H. B., Duncan, R. F., and Dement, W. C.: Sleep: The effect of electroconvulsive shock in cats deprived of REM sleep. Science *156*:1647, 1967.
Cohen, I. M.: Complications of chlorpromazine therapy. Am. J. Psychiat. *113*:115, 1956.
——, and Archer, J. D.: Liver function and hepatic complications in patients receiving chlorpromazine. J.A.M.A. *159*:99, 1955.
Cohen, S.: Clinical experiences with pipradol and a pipradol-reserpine combination. Int. Rec. Med. *169*:751, 1956.
——, Leonard, C. V., Farberow, N. L., and Shneidman, E. S.: Tranquilizers and suicide in the schizophrenic patient. Arch. Gen. Psychiat. *11*:312, 1964.
Cohn, J. B., Karnosh, L. J., and Stecher, R. M.: Clinical trials with cortisone in the treatment of chronic schizophrenia. Dis. Nerv. Syst. *12*:291, 1951.
Cohn, R.: Electroencephalographic study of prefrontal lobotomy. Arch. Neurol. & Psychiat. *53*:283, 1945.
Coirault, R., Girard, V., Jarret, R. et Rouif, J.: Nouvelle conception thérapeutique en psychiatrie: le chimiochoc sans perte de conscience avec le 7843 R. P. (Premières données). Ann. méd.-psychol. *117/I*: 160, 1959.
——, ——, ——, and ——: Le chimio-choc au 7843 R.P. [Di-méthyl-sulfamido-3-(N-méthyl-pipérazinil-propyl)-10-phénothiazine]. Ann. méd-psychol. *117/II*:45, 1959.
Cole, C. E., Patterson, R. M., Craig, J. B., Thomas, W. E. Ristine, L. P., Stahly, M., and Pasamanick, B.: A controlled study of the efficacy of iproniazid in treatment of depression. A.M.A. Arch. Gen. Psychiat. *1*:513, 1959.
Cole, J. O.: Drug therapy. *In* Progress in Neurol. & Psychiat., E. A. Spiegel, ed. New York: Grune & Stratton, 1959.
Collard, J., et Lecoq, R.: Benpéridol et placebo: Une étude "double blind" chez les névroses en traitement ambulatoire. Acta neurol. psychiat. belg. *64*:353, 1964.
Collard, J. F., and Maggs, R.: Clinical trial of acepromazine maleate in chronic schizophrenia. Brit. Med. J. *1*:1452, 1958.
Columbia-Graystone Association: Selective

partial ablation of the frontal cortex. Edited by F. A. Mettler. New York: Paul B. Hoeber, 1949.
Condrau, G.: Klinische Erfahrungen an Geisteskranken mit Lysergsäurediäthylamid. Acta psychiat. et neurol. *24*:9, 1949.
Connecticut Lobotomy Committee: Moore, B. E., Friedman, S., Simon, B., and Fariner, J.: A cooperative clinical study of lobotomy. The frontal lobes. A. Research Nerv. & Ment. Dis. Proc. *27*:769, 1948.
Connell, M. M., Poley, B. J., and McFarlane, J. R.: Chorioretinopathy associated with thioridazine therapy. Arch. Ophthal. *71*: 816, 1964.
Connell, P. H.: Amphetamine psychosis. London: Chapman & Hall, 1958.
Consbruch, U., and Faust, C.: Vergleichende Längsschnittbetrachtung der Serumeiweiss-verhältnisse bei exogenen traumatischen Psychosen und bei endogenen Psychosen unter der Behandlung mit Reserpin, Iminodibenzylderivat und Phenothiazinen. Arch. f. Psychiat. u. Z. Neur. *197*:279, 1958.
Conway, H., and Osmond, H.: Lung abscess following electro-convulsive therapy: description of a case. J. Ment. Sc. *94*:953, 1948.
Cook, L. C.: Convulsion therapy. Recent progress in psychiatry. Ed. by G. W. T. H. Fleming. London: 1944.
——, and Sands, D. E.: Spinal injuries in convulsive therapy. Am. J. M. Sc. *87*:230 1941.
——, and Walter, W. G.: The electroencephalogram in convulsion induced by cardiazol. J. Neurol. & Psychiat. *1*:180, 1938.
Cooper, A. J.: The action of mebanazine, a mono amine oxidase inhibitor antidepressant drug in diabetes—Part II. Internat. J. Neuropsychiat. *2*:342, 1966.
——, and Keddie, K. M. G.: Hypotensive collapse and hypoglycaemia after mebanazine—a monoamine-oxidase inhibitor. Lancet *1*:1133, 1964.
Cooperberg, A. A., and Eidlow, S.: Hemolytic anaemia, jaundice and diabetes mellitus following chlorpromazine therapy. Canad. M. A. J. *75*:674, 1956.
Corbella, T., and Piredda, F.: Una nuova applicazione dell'elettroshockterapia: Il trattamento della malattia ulcerosa gastroduodenale. Minerva Med. *40*:896, 1949.
Cordoba, E. F., and Lopez Ibor, J.: La monoclorimipramina en enfermos psiquiatricos resistentes a otros tratamientos. Act. Luso Espagn. Neurol. Psiquiat. *26*:91, 1967.
Cordoba, J., Francis, J. M., Pigem, J. H., Gurcia, J., and Polach, J.: El electroshock en las neurosis vasomotrices troficas. Medicina Clinica *7*:53, 1946.
Cornu, F.: Psychopharmakotherapie. *In* H. W. Gruhle, R. Jung, W. Mayer-Gross, and M. Müller (Eds.): Psychiatrie der Gegenwart Forschung und Praxis, Bd. I/2: Grundlagen und Methoden der Klinischen Psychiatrie, pp. 495. Berlin-Göttingen-Heidelberg, Springer, 1963.
Corsellis, J. A. N., and Meyer, A.: Histological changes in the brain after uncomplicated electro-convulsant treatment. J. Ment. Sc. *100*:375, 1954.
Cossa, P., Bougeant, H., and Lombard, A.: La cure de Sakel dans les états schizophréniques. Ann. méd.-psychol. *106*:23, 1948.
——, and Gastaut, H.: Une nouvelle technique de chocs convulsants en psychiatrie. Ann. méd.-psychol. *107*:184, 1949.
Costa, E., and Himwich, H. E.: Brain serotonin metabolism in insulin hypoglycemia. Present. at Internat. Biochemic. Congress, Vienna, 1958.
——, and Rinaldi, F.: Biochemical and electroencephalographic changes in the brain of rabbits injected with 5-hydroxytryptophan (influence of chlorpromazine premedication). Am. J. Physiol. *194*:214, 1958.
Cottington, F.: The treatment of childhood schizophrenia by metrazol shock modified by B-Erythroidin. Am. J. Psychiat. *98*:397, 1941.
Cotton, H. A., Draper, J. W., and Lynch, J. M.: Internal pathology in the functional psychoses. M. Rec. *97*:719, 1920.
Courvoisier, S., Ducrot, R., Fournel, J., and Julou, L.: Proprietes pharmacodynamiques generales de la Prochlorpemazine (6140 R.P.). Canad. Roy. Soc. Biol. *151*:1144, 1957.
——, ——, ——, and ——: Propriétés pharmacologiques générales de la diméthylsulfamido-3-(méthyl-4″-pipérazinyl-3′-propyl) -10-phénothiazine (7843 R.P.). Ann. méd.-psychol. *116/II*:600, 1958.
——, ——, and Julou, L.: Psychotropic Drugs, Elsevier Publishing Co., 1957.
——, Foumel, J., Ducrot, R., Kolsky, M., and Koetschet, P.: Propriétés Pharmacodynamiques du chlorhydrate de chlor-2 (diméthylemino-3 propyl)-10 phénothiazine. Arch. Internationales de Pharmacodynamie et de Thérapie. *92*:305, 1953.
Craddock, W. L., and Gilbert, H. P.: Transient auricular fibrillation complicating electric shock therapy. Am. J. Psychiat. *104*:744, 1948.
Crane, G. E.: Psychiatric side effects of iproniazid. Am. J. Psychiat. *112*:494, 1956.
Cranswick, E. H., Cooper, T. B., and Simpson, G. M.: Two-year follow-up study of protein-bound iodine elevation in patients receiving perphenazine. Amer. J. Psychiat. *122*:300, 1965.
——, and Hall, T. C.: Deoxycortone with ascorbic acid in mental disorder. Lancet *1*:540, 1950.
——, and Simpson, G. M.: Perphenazine and thyroid function. Amer. J. Psychiat. *120*:1133, 1964.
——, ——, and Nies, A.: An abnormal thyroid finding produced by a phenothiazine. J.A.M.A. *181*:554, 1962.
Crawford, J. S., and Rudofsky, S.: Placental transmission and neonatal metabolism of promazine. Brit. J. Anaesth. *37*:303, 1965.
——, and ——: The mode of administration or promazine as a factor in determining the extent of placental transmission. Brit. J.

Anaesth. *37*:310, 1965.
Cremerius, J., and Jung, R.: Über die Veränderungen des Elektroencephalograms nach Elektroschockbehandlung. Nervenarzt *18*: 193, 1947.
Creutzfeldt, H. G.: Psychochirurgie. Med. Klin. *44*:520, 1949.
Crisp, A. H., and Roberts, E. J.: The response of an adrenalectomized patient to ECT. Amer. J. Psychiat. *119*:784, 1963.
Crocket, R., Sandison, A., and Walk, A.: Hallucinogenic Drugs in Psychotherapeutic Use. London, H. K. Lewis, 1963.
Cronholm, B., and Molander, L.: Memory disturbances after electroconvulsive therapy. Acta Psychiat. Scan. *40*:212, 1964.
——, and Ottosson, J. O.: The experience of memory function after electroconvulsive therapy. Brit. J. Psychiat. *109*:251, 1963.
Cronick, C. H., Scherb, R. F., and Karnosh, L. J.: Modification of the Manic-Depressive Cycle by Metrazol. Dis. Nerv. Syst. *1*:10, 1940.
Cropper, C. F. J., and Hughes, M.: Cardiac arrest (with apnoea) after E.C.T. Brit. J. Psychiat. *110*:222, 1964.
Crossland, J. Elliot, K. A. C., and Pappius, H. M.: Acetylcholine content of the brain during insulin hypoglycemia. Am. J. Physiol. *183*:32, 1955.
Crow, H. J., Cooper, T., and Phillips, A. G.: Progressive leucotomy. *In* J. Masserman (Ed.): Current Psychiatric Therapies, Vol. III, New York, Grune & Stratton, 1963.
Cummins, J. F., and Friend, D. G.: Use of chlorpromazine in chronic alcoholics. Am. J. Ment. Sc. *227*:561, 1954.
Cunningham, M. A., Pillai, V., and Blachford Rogers, W. J.: Haloperidol in the treatment of children with severe behaviour disorders. Brit. J. Psychiat. *114*:845, 1968.
Cunningham, M. L.: Acute hepatic necrosis following treatment with amitriptyline and diazepam. Brit. J. Psychiat. *111*:1107, 1965.
Czerwenka-Wenkstetten, H., Hofmann, G., and Kryspin-Exner, K.: Ein Fall von Valium-Entzugsdelir. Wien. med. Wschr. *115*:994, 1965.
Dally, P. J., and Sargant, W.: A new treatment of anorexia nervosa. Brit. Med. J. *1*:1770, 1960.
Dameshek, W., and Myerson, A.: Insulin hypoglycemia; mechanism of neurologic symptoms. Arch. Neurol. & Psychiat. *33*:11, 1935.
Daneman, E. A.: Treatment of depressed patients with Iprindole. Psychosomatics *8*:216, 1967.
Danik, J. J., and Goverdham, M.: Haloperidol in the treatment of 120 psychotic patients. Amer. J. Psychiat. *120*:389, 1963.
Danziger, L.: Some theoretical considerations of dementia precox. Dis. Nerv. Syst. *7*:357, 1946.
——, and Kindwall, J. A.: Prediction of the immediate outcome of shock therapy in dementia precox. Dis. Nerv. Syst. *7*:299, 1946.
——, and ——: Thyroid therapy in some mental disorders. Dis. Nerv. Syst. *14*:3, 1953.
——, ——, and Lewis, H. R.: Periodic relapsing catatonia: Simplified diagnosis and treatment. Dis. Nerv. Syst. *9*:330, 1949.
Darling, H. F.: Shock treatment in psychopathic personality. J. Nerv. & Ment. Dis. *101*:247, 1945.
——: Fluphenazine: a preliminary study. Dis. Nerv. Syst. *20*:167, 1959.
Darvill, F. T., Jr.: Double-blind evaluation of methylphenidate (Ritalin) hydrochloride. J.A.M.A. *169*:1739, 1959.
Dattner, B.: The management of neurosyphilis. New York: Grune & Stratton, 1944.
David, H. P.: A critique of psychiatric and psychological research on insulin treatment in schizophrenia. Am. J. Psychiat. *110*:773, 1954.
Davidoff, E., and Raffaele, A.: Electric shock therapy in involutional psychoses. J. Nerv. & Ment. Dis. *99*:397, 1944.
Davidson, G. M.: Insulin therapy in schizophrenia and the reticulo-endothelial system. J. Nerv. & Ment. Dis. *92*:193, 1940.
Davies, B. M.: Oral Sernyl in obsessive states. J. Ment. Sci. *107*:109, 1961.
Davies, D. M., and Allaye, R.: Amitriptyline poisoning. Lancet *2*:543, 1963.
Davies, T. S.: A clinical evaluation of nialamide, a monoamine oxidase inhibitor, in psychiatry. J. Soc. Ciencias Med. de Lisboa, Nov. 274, 1959.
Davis, J. M., Bartlett, E., and Termini, B. A.: Overdosage of psychotropic drugs: A review. Part I: Major and minor tranquilizers. Part II: Antidepressant and other psychotropic agents. Dis. Nerv. Syst. *29*:157, and 246, 1968.
Davis, P. A.: Electroencephalographic studies on three cases of frontal lobotomy. Psychosom. Med. *3*:38, 1941.
——, and Sulzbach, W.: Changes in the electro-encephalogram during metrazol therapy, Arch. Neurol. & Psychiat. *43*: 341, 1940.
Davidson, K.: Episodic depersonalization. Brit. J. Psychiat. *110*:505, 1964.
——: EEG activation after intravenous amitriptyline. Electroenceph. clin. Neurophysiol. *19*:298, 1965.
——, Leyburn, P., and McClelland, H. A.: Thiothixene in schizophrenia. Brit. Med. J. *2*:489, 1967.
Dax, E. C., and Smith, E. J. R.: The operation of prefrontal leucotomy. Brit. J. Surg. *36*:74, 1948.
Daxelmüller, L.: Zur Therapie schwererer Schmerzzustände mit Tofranil. Med. Welt *N.F.17*:2339, 1966.
De Boor, W.: Pharmakopsychologie und Psychopathologie. Berlin, Springer, 1956.
De Bougard and Fournial, P.: États Parkinsoniens Apparus au Cours de Traitements à la Chlorpromazine. Presse Méd. *62*: 1358, 1954.
Dedichen, H. A.: Comparison of 1495 shock-treated and 969 non-shock-treated psychoses in Norwegian hospitals. Acta psychiat. & neurol., Supp. 37, 1946.
Degkwitz, R.: Experimentelle Untersuchungen zur photodynamischen Wirkung von

Psycholeptika. *In* H. Kranz and K. Heinrich (Eds.): Begleitwirkungen und Misserfolge der psychiatrischen Pharmakotherapie, pp. 115. Stuttgart: G. Thieme Verlag 1964.
——, and Luxenburger, O.: Das terminale extrapyramidale Insuffizienz- bzw. Defektsyndrom infolge chronischer Anwendung von Neurolepticis. Nervenarzt *36*: 173, 1965.
——, and Wenzel, W.: Persistent extrapyramidal side effects after long-term application of neuroleptics. *In* H. Brill, J. O. Cole, P. Deniker, H. Hippius, and P. B. Bradley (Eds.): Neuro-Psychopharmacology, *V*: 608 (CINP Congr., Washington 1966). Amsterdam, Excerpta Med. Found., Internat. Congr. Ser. No. 129, 1967.
DeJong, R. N.: Phenurone in the treatment of psychomotor attacks. Am. J. Psychiat. *107*:825, 1951.
Delay, J.: L'électro-choc. Paris: Masson et Cie., 1946.
——: Méthodes biologiques en clinique psychiatrique. Paris: Masson et Cie., 1950.
——: Introduction. Encéphale *45*:303, 1956.
——, and Deniker, P.: Le traitement des psychoses par une méthode neurolytique dérivèe de l'hibernothérapie. Congrés des médecins alienistes et neurologistes. Luxembourg. Juillet, 1952.
——, and ——: 38 cas de psychoses traités par la cure prolongée et continué de 4568 R.P. Ann. Méd.-Psychol. *110*:364, 1952.
——, ——, Busson, J. F., and Haim, A.: Le traitement des états dépressifs par les dérivés de l'acide iso-nicotinique: isoniazide et iproniazide. Ann. Méd-Psychol. *1*:125, 1959.
——, ——, Fourment, J., Green, A., and Ropert, M.: Nouveaux types d'accidents nerveux dus à un médicament neuroleptiques, la prochlorpérazine. Ann. méd.-psychol. *115/I*:510, 1957.
——, ——, Ginestet, D., Perier, M., Peron-Magnan, P., and Dalle, B.: Evaluation clinique précoce d'une nouvelle formule neuroleptique le thiothixène. Ann. méd.-psychol. *124/II*:196, 1966.
——, ——, Greene, A., and Mordret, M.: Le syndrome excito-moteur provoqué par les médicaments neuroleptiques. Presse méd. *65*:1771, 1957.
——, ——, and Harl, J. M.: Traitement des états d'excitation et d'agitation par une méthode médicamenteuse dérivèe de l'hibernothérapie. Ann. Méd.-psychol. *110*: 267, 1952.
——, ——, and Lemperiere, T.: Etude de l'efficacité de l'imipramine (G.22.355) dans le traitement des états dépressifs. Ann. Méd.-psychol. *117*:521, 1959.
——, ——, and ——: Le traitement des états dépressifs et mélancoliques en fonction des nouveaux médicaments antidépresseurs. Presse. méd. *67*:1586, 1959.
——, ——, and Ropert R.: Four years experience with chlorpromazine in treatment of psychoses. Presse méd. *64*:493, 1956.
——, ——, ——, Barande, R., and Eurieult, M.: Effects psychiques de la nouvelle phénothiazine sulfonidée (7843R.P.) Ann. méd.-psychol. *116*:601, 1958.
——, ——, ——, Beck, H., Barande, R., and Eurieult, M.: Syndromes neurologiques expérimentaux et thérapeutique psychotique. Presse mèd., 4 & 6, 123 & 201, 1959.
——, ——, and Thuillier, J.: Similitude des accidents nerveux de la prochlorpérazine avec certains troubles post-encéphalitiques. Ann. méd.-psychol. *115/I*: 506,1957.
——, ——, ——, Pauwels, R., and Haim, A.: A new neuroleptic phenothiazine: methopromazine (4632.RP). 54th Congress of Psychiatrists and Neurologists of France. Bordeaux, 1956.
——, ——, and Wiart, C.: Complèments à notre expérience de la réserpine. Encèphale *45*:1042, 1956.
——, Pichot, P., and Collet e Silva: Le choc amphétaminique dans la psychose maniaco-depressive et dans les catatonies. Ann. med.-psychol. *105*:415, 1947.
——, ——, and Lemperiere, T.: La psilocybene, historique, pharmacophysiologie, clinique. Presse med. p. 1731 and 1811, 1959.
——, ——, ——, and Elissalde, B.: Essais cliniques d'un nouveau neuroleptique, la thioridazine. Ann. méd.-psychol. *117*:724, 1959.
——, ——, ——, and ——: L'action du halopéridol dans les psychoses. Symposium International sur le Halopéridol. Acta Medica Belgica. 21, 1960.
——, ——, ——, and ——: Halopéridol et chimiothérapie des psychoses. Presse méd. *68*:1353, 1960.
——, ——, ——, ——, and Peigne, F.: Un neuroleptique majeur non phénothiazinique et non réserpinique, l'halopéridol, dans le traitement des psychoses. Ann. méd.-psychol. *118/I*:145, 1960.
——, ——, and Ropert, R.: New neuroleptic drug in psychiatry: ethylene-3-dimethylamino-3-propyl-10-phenothiazine acid maleate (1522.CB). Presse Méd. *65*:491 1957.
—, Puech, P., Desclaux, P., and Morice, J.: Cerebral pneumotherapy. Lisbon: Psycho-surgery, 1949.
——, Seggiaro, J. A., and Deniker, P.: Réactions biologiques au cours des traitements par le coma hypoglycémique prolongé. Ann. Méd. Psychol. *110*:427, 1952.
——, Sizaret, P., Deniker, and Lainé, B.: Essais de traitement par le dinitrile succinique. Ann. méd.-psychol. *2*:566, 1949.
——, Thuillier, J., Pichot, P., Lemperiere, T., and Brion, M. S.: Premiers résultats en clinique psychiatrique du para-chlorophénoxy-acétate de diméthylaminoéthyle (A.N.P. 235). Ann. méd.-psychol. *118/I*: 133, 1960.
Dell, P. Bonvallet, M., and Hugelin, A.: Démonstration d'un mécanisme adrènergique au niveau des formations réticulées du tronc cérèbral. Conséquences pharmacologiques et psychopathologiques. Encé-

phale. *45*:1119, 1956.
Delmas-Marsalet, P.: Electro-choc et thérapeutiques nouvelles en neuropsychiatrie. Paris: J. B. Bailliere et fils, 1946.
Delmond, J.: Electrochoc. *In* Encyclopédie Médico-Chirurgicale. Paris, 1955.
Delong, S. L.: Chlorpromazine-induced eye changes. *In* H. Brill, J. O. Cole, P. Deniker, H. Hippius, and P. B. Bradley (Eds.): Neuro-Psychopharmacology, *V*:656 (CINP Congr. Washington 1966). Amsterdam, Excerpta Med. Found., Internat. Congr. Ser. No. 129, 1967.
De Natale, L., and Paolozzi, C.: Su di un caso di catatonia posttraumatica. Rass. Neuropsichiat. *15*:265, 1961.
Denber, H. C. B.: *In* Chlorpromazine and Mental Health. Philadelphia: Lea and Febiger, 1955.
——: Some preliminary results with a new phenothiazine derivative: proclorperazine. Psychiat. Research Rep., A.P.A. 9, 1958.
——, and Bird, E. G.: Chlorpromazine in the treatment of mental illness, Am. J. Psychiat. *112*:465, 1955; *112*:1021, 1956; *113*:972, 1957.
——, and Collard, J.: Différences de bioréactivité au halopéridol entre deux groupes de psychotiques, américain et européen. Acta neurol. psychiat. belg. *62*:577, 1962.
——, Florio, D., and Rajotte, P.: Third evaluation of Haloperidol. Amer. J. Psychiat. *119*:172, 1972.
——, and Merlis, S.: Studies on mescaline. VI. Therapeutic aspects of the mescaline-chlorpromazine combination. J. Nerv. & Ment. Dis. *122*:463, 1955.
——, Rajotte, P., and Kauffman, D.: Clinical experience with a new phenothiazine. Am. J. Psychiat. *115*:1116, 1959.
——, ——, and ——: Problems in evaluation of R-1625. Amer. J. Psychiat. *116*:356, 1959.
——, ——, and Ross, E.: Some observations on the chemotherapy of depression: results with "Taractan." Comprehensive Psychiat. *1*:308, 1960.
——, Ross, E., and Rajotte, P.: Study of butyrylperazine (Bayer 1362). Amer. J. Psychiat. *117*:1119, 1961.
Denham, J.: The use of prochlorperazine (Stemetil) in chronic psychotic disorders. J. Ment. Sc. *104*:1190, 1958.
——, and Carrick, D. J. E. L.: Therapeutic value of thioproperazine and the importance of the associated neurological disturbances. J. Ment. Sci. *107*:326, 1961.
Deniker, P.: Hibernothérapies et Médicaments Neuroleptiques en Thérapeutique Psychiatrique. Encéphale *46*:1, 1957.
Denmark, J. C.: The treatment of depressive states with imipramine hydrochloride (Tofranil). J. Ment. Sc. *105*:1123, 1959.
Dent, J. Y.: Anxiety and its treatment. Brit. J. Addiction *50*:43, 1953.
Denys, W. J.: La thioridazine et son utilisation concomitante à la thérapeutique occupationelle. Acta neurol. psychiat. belg. *66*:803, 1966.
Denzel, H. A.: High-dose fluphenazine without apparent toxicity. Amer. J. Psychiat. *123*:10, 1967.
Deschamps, A.: Hibernation artificielle en psychiatrie. Presse mèd. *60*:944, 1952.
——, and Madre, J.: Résultats d'un nouveau Neuroleptique (Lévomépromazine: 7044. RP) dans des Cas de Démence Précoce Grave. Presse mèd. *66*:196, 1958.
Deshaies, G.: Les effets cliniques du 8909 R.P. Encéphale *51*:602, 1962.
——, Benda, P., Tardy, C., and Carrot, P.: The method of administration of 7843.RP. Ann. Méd.-psychol. *117*:901, 1959.
——, and Le Pourbiet: L'Encéphalo-pneumotherapie. Ann. Méd.-psychol. *2*:280, 1951.
——, and Renard, E.: La tension céphalorachidienne dans l'électro-choc. Ann. méd.-psychol. *106*:18, 1948.
——, and Renault, M.: La tension artérielle des électrochoques. Ann. méd.-psychol. *106*:137, 1948.
Desrulles, M., and Fellion, G.: A propos des traitements actuels de l'alcoolisme. Ann. Méd.-Psychol. *109*:638, 1957.
Destounis, N.: Thioridazine and amenorrhea. Amer. J. Psychiat. *120*:188, 1963.
Diethelm, O.: An historical view of somatic treatment in psychiatry. Am. J. Psychiat. *95*:1165, 1939.
Ditman, K.S.: Inhibition of ejaculation by chlorprothixene. Amer. J. Psychiat. *120*: 1004, 1964.
Divry, P., Bobon, J., and Collard, J.: Le "R 1625": nouvelle thérapeutique de l'agitation psychomotrice. Acta neurol. psychiat. belg. *58*:878, 1958.
——, ——, and ——: Rapport sur l'Activité Neuro-Psychopharmacologique du Halopéridol (R.1625). Acta Neurol. Belg. *60*:7, 1960.
——, ——, ——, and Demaret, A.: Psychopharmacologie d'un troisième neuroleptique de la série des butyrophénones: le R 2498 ou tripéridol. Acta neurol. psychiat. belg. *60*:465, 1960.
Dobkin, A. B., Gilbert, E. G. B., and Lamoureaux, L.: Physiological effects of chlorpromazine. Anaesthesia *9*:157, 1954.
Dobrina, D., and Antonini, M.: L'imipramina nelle sindromi parkinsoniane. Rivista Neurol. *32*:586, 1962.
Doepfmer, R.: Der Thioridazin-Aspermatismus. (Beitrag zur Behandlung der Ejaculation praecox). Zschr. Haut-Geschl. Krkh. *36*:265, 1964.
Dohan, F. C., Winick, W. Purcell, M., Bennett, I. F., and Hecker, A. O.: Response of blood eosinophiles and plasma 17-hydroxycorticoids to insulin shock therapy. A.M.A. Arch. Neurol. & Psychiat. *73*:47, 1955.
Dole, V. P., and Nyswander, M.: A medical treatment for diacethylmorphine (heroin) addiction. J.A.M.A. *193*:646, 1965.
Dolenz, B. J.: Unilateral ECT. Amer. J. Psychiat. *120*:1133, 1964.
——: Flurothyl (Indoklon) side-effects. Amer. J. Psychiat. *123*:1453, 1967.
Domaszewicz, A., and Erb, A.: Über die kombinierte Schizophreniebehandlung mittels Kardiazol und Insulin. Roczu. psychiat. *31*:108, 1938.

Domino, E. F.: Neurobiology of phencyclidine (Sernyl), a drug with an unusual spectrum of pharmacological activity. *In* C. C. Pfeiffer and J. R. Smythies (Eds.): Internat. Rev. Neurobiol. Vol. 6:303. New York, Academic Press, 1964.

Domm, S., and Gellhorn, E.: Influence of insulin and of stimulation of the sympathetic nervous system on the blood, study of sugar content, carbon dioxide tension and pH. Arch. neurol. & Psychiat. *43*:726, 1940.

Donaggio, A.: In materia di discussione sulla neuropsicochirurgia. Gior. di psichiat. e di neuropat. *67*:288, 1939.

Dongaji, D. R., and Saraf, K. R.: Electroplexy in schizophrenia after fronto-temporal lobectomy. Indian J. Psychiat. *8*:127, 1966.

Donnadieu and Hauser: Trouble végétatifs persistants après électro-choc. Ann. méd.-psychol. *106*:73, 1948.

Donnelly, J.: Psychiatric therapy in the geriatric patient. Geriatrics *2*:655, 1954.

——: Discussion on physiochemical research in insulin therapy. *In* M. Rinkel and H. E. Himwich, eds.: Insulin Treatment in Psychiatry. New York: Philosophical Library, 1959.

——, Lpool, D. P. M., and Radley-Smith, E. J.: Thrombotic "hydrocephalus" in insulin therapy. Lancet *2*:904, 1950.

Donovan, J. F., Galbraith, A. J., and Jackson, H.: Some observations on leucotomy and investigations by pneumoencephalography. J. Ment. Sc. *95*:655, 1949.

Dorfman, W.: Clinical experience with amitriptyline (Elavil). (A preliminary report). Psychosomatics *1*:153, 1960.

——: A new parenteral antidepressant (Elavil). Dis. Nerv. Syst. *22*:145, 1961.

Doughty, R. B.: The incidence of jaundice associated with chlorpromazine therapy. *In* Chlorpromazine and Mental Health. Philadelphia: Lea and Febiger, 1955.

Doussinet P., d'Alteroche, R., and Soucachet, P.: Twelve cases of epileptic reactions with temporal electrical localisation in mental patients treated with chlorpromazine. Sem Hôp., Paris *32*:3334, 1956.

Drake, F. R., and Ebaugh, F. G.: Pheochromocytoma and electroconvulsive therapy. Am. J. Psychiat. *113*:301, 1956.

Dransfield, G. A.: A clinical trial comparing prochlorperazine (Stemetil) with chlorpromazine (Largactil) in the treatment of chronic psychotic patients. J. Ment. Sc. *104*:1183, 1955.

Dubost, P., and Pascal, S.: Dosage du Largactil dans les Liquides Biologiques. Ann. Pharm. Franc. *11*:615, 1953.

Ducrot, R., and Koetschet, P.: Anti-emetic properties of a new phenothiazine derivative 3-chloro-10-(3-N-methyl-piperazinyl-propyl)-phenothiazine (6140.RP). Int. Physiol. Cong. Brussels, 1956.

Dukor, B.: Die Prognose der Geisteskrankheiten. Schweiz. med. Wchnschr. *1*:25, 1939.

Duncan, C. P.: The effect of electroshock convulsions on the maze habit in the white rat. J. Exper. Psychol. *35*:267, 1945.

——: Habit reversal induced by electroshock in rats. J. Comp. & Physiol. Psychol. *41*:11, 1948.

Dunlop, E.: Electroshock and Monoamine Oxidase Inhibitors in the Treatment of Depressed Reactions. Dis. Nerv. Syst. (suppl.) *21*:130, 1960.

——: Combination of antidepressants with electroshock therapy. Dis. Nerv. Syst. *21*: 513, 1960.

——: Intravenous use of nialamide in depression. Psychosomatics *2*:438, 1961.

Durell, J., and Pollin, W.: A trial on chronic schizophrenic patients of oxypertine, a psychotropic drug with an indole ring. Brit. J. Psychiat. *109*:687, 1963.

Dussik, K., Greaney, J. F., Grunberg, E., and Schneller, P.: Serial Glucagon tolerance tests in schizophrenics. *In* M. Rinkel (Ed).: Biological Treatment of Mental Illness. New York, L.C. Page & Co., 1966.

Dussik, K. T.: Über Veränderungen des Zuckergehaltes des Liquor cerebrospinalis während der Insulinschockbehandlung der Schizophrenie. Klin. Wchnschr. *17*:769, 1938.

——: Three and a half years of hypoglycemic therapy of schizophrenia; results and problems. Am. J. Psychiat. *94*:269, 1938.

——: The place of Sakel's insulin coma therapy in an active treatment unit of today. *In* M. Rinkel: Insulin Treatment in Psychiatry. New York: Philosophical Library, 1959.

——, and Sakel, M.: Ergebnisse der Hypoglykämieschockbehandlung der Schizophrenie. Ztschr. f. d. ges. Neurol. u. Psychiat. 155, 1936.

Dynes, J. B.: Affective sequelae of convulsant drug therapy. J. Ment. Sc. *85*: 489, 1939.

Easton, N. L., and Sommers, J.: The significance of vertebral fractures as a complication of metrazol therapy. Am. J. Psychiat. *98*:538, 1942.

Ebaugh, F. G., Barnacle, C. H., and Neuburger, K. T.: Fatalities following electric convulsive therapy. Arch. Neurol. & Psychiat. *49*:107, 1943.

Ebtinger, R.: Aspects psychopathologiques du post-électrochoc. Imprimerie Alsatia: Colmar, 1958.

——: Psychopathologie des Post-Elektroschocks. Nervenarzt *31*:193, 1960.

Edelstein, E. L., and Assael, M.: Ataractic effect of prothipendyl on hospitalized patients. Dis. Nerv. Syst. *23*:163, 1962.

Edisen, C. B., and Samuels, A. S.: A clinical evaluation of dartal chemotherapy for emotional disorders. A.M.A. Arch Neurol. & Psychiat. *80*:481, 1958.

Editorial, Brit. Med. J. *2*:35, 1957.

Editorial Board: Lobotomy: surgery for the insane, Stanford Law Review *1*:463, 1949.

Edwards, G.: Comparison of the effect of imipramine and desipramine on some symptoms of depressive illness. Brit. J. Psychiat. *111*:889, 1965.

——: Electro-convulsive therapy in the treatment of bizarre psychogenic movements.

Brit. J. Psychiat.: In press.
Egan, G.: Results of isolation of the orbital lobes in leucotomy. J. Ment. Sc. *95*:115, 1949.
Egsgaard, J., Martensen-Larsen, O., and Osterfeld, J.: Emotional disorders affectable by convulsion therapy. Acta psychiat. et neurol., Suppl. *47*:443, 1947.
Ehrhardt, H.: Der intraoculare, Druck im Elektroschock. Ztschr. f. Nervenheilk. *159*: 75, 1948.
——: Ergebnisse bei det Elektroschockbehandlung. Nervenarzt *19*:513, 1948.
Eilenberg, D.: Nialamide in the intravenous treatment of depression. Proc. Staff Meet. Mayo Clin. *37*:367, 1962.
Eisen, S. B., Sabshin, M., and Heath, H.: A comparison of the effects of investigators' and therapists' attitudes in the evaluation of tranquillisers prescribed to hospital patients. J. Nerv. & Ment. Dis. *128*:256, 1959.
Eisenberg, L., Ascher, E., and Kanner, L.: A clinical study of Gilles de la Tourette's disease (maladie des tics) in children. Amer. J. Psychiat. *115*:715, 1959.
Ekinci, M., Hsu, J. J., Bruck, M., and Braun, R. A.: Diazepam as an anti-convulsant agent in ECT. Am. J. Psychiat. *120*:903, 1964.
Elam, C. B., Wortz, E. C., and Brown, W. L.: A study of the interaction of electro convulsive shock with chlorpromazine and reserpine in rats. Psychopharmacologia *1*:102, 1959.
El-Deiry, N. K., Forrest, A. D., and Littmann, S. K.: Clinical trial of a new antidepressant (WY. 3263). With assessment of doctor-patient interaction. Brit. J. Psychiat. *113*:999, 1967.
Elithorn, A.: Prefrontal leucotomy and depression. Proceed. Roy. Soc. Med. *52*:203, 1959.
——, and Slater, E.: Prefrontal Leucotomy. Views of patients and their relatives. Brit. Med. J. *2*:739, 1956.
Elkes, J., and Elkes, C.: Effect of chlorpromazine on behaviour of chronically overactive psychotic patients. Brit. Med. J. *2*:560, 1954.
Elliot, R. N., Schrut, A. H., and Marra, J.: Fatal acute aspetic necrosis of the liver associated with chlorpromazine. Am. J. Psychiat. *112*:940, 1956.
Elmadjian, F., Hope, J. M., and Pincus, G.: The action of mono-ammonium glycyrhizinate on adrenalectomized subjects and its synergisen with hydrocortisone. J. Clin. Endocrin. & Metabol. *16*:338, 1956.
Elpern, S., and Chodosh, H. L.: Peroneal nerve paralysis as a complication of electroshock therapy. Confinia neurol. *18*:46, 1958.
Ende, M., Klauber, B., and Gendel, B. R.: Electric shock therapy of acute psychosis associated with pernicious anemia: Arch. Neurol. & Psychiat. *63*:110, 1950.
Engelhardt, D. M.: Drug treatment of chronic ambulatory patients. Am. J. Psychiat. *123*:1329, 1967.
Engelmeier, M. P.: Lytische Therapie in der Nervenklinik. Monatsschrift f. Psychiatrie. *131*:89, 1956.
Engler, M.: Prefrontal leucotomy in mental defectives. J. Ment. Sc. *94*:844, 1948.
Enss, H., Hartmann, K., Hippius, H., and Richter, H.-E.: Klinische Erfahrungen mit einem neuen Piperazin-Derivat des Phenothiazins in der Neuro-Psychiatrie. Arch. Psychiat. Nervenkr. *197*:534 1958.
Epstein, J.: Complications and unusual phenomena arising in the course of metrazol treatment of the psychoses—Their classification and management. J. Nerv. & Ment. Dis. *94*:562, 1941.
——: Electric shock therapy in the psychoses. J. Nerv. & Ment. Dis. *98*:115, 1943.
——: Unipolar electrocerebral stimulation. Dis. Nerv. System *15*:146, 1954.
Epstein, S. J., and de Quevedo, A.: The control of enuresis with imipramine in the presence of organic bladder disease. Amer. J. Psychiat. *120*:908, 1964.
Erb, A.: Zur Psychopathologie der hypoglykämischen Zustände bei Schizophrenen (auf Grund von Beobachtungen während der Insulintherapie). Ztschr. f. Neurol. 162, 1938.
——, and Pozniak, J.: Versuch einer Cardiazolbehandlung der Epilepsie. Ztschr. f. d. ges. Neurol. u. Psychiat. *166*:581, 1939.
Esquibel, A. J., Krantz, J. C., Jr., Truitt, E. B., Jr., Ling. A. S. C., and Kurland, A. A.: Hexafluorodiethyl ether (Indoklon): Its use as a convulsant in psychiatric treatment. J. Nerv. & Ment. Dis. *126*:530, 1958.
——, Kurland, A. A., and Mendelsohn, D.: The use of glucagon in terminating insulin coma. Dis. Nerv. Syst. *19*:485, 1958.
Evans, V. L.: Convulsive shock therapy in elderly patients— Risks and results. Am. J. Psychiat. *99*:537, 1943.
Evreux, J.-C.: Effets cardiaques de l'imipramine et de ses dérivés. Contribution expérimentale à l'étude de leur toxicité. Collection de Médecine Légale et de Toxicologie Médicale. Paris, Masson et Cie, 1967.
Ewald, G.: Zur Theorie der Schizophrenie und der Insulinschockbehandlung. Allg. Ztschr. f. Psychiat. 110, 1939.
——, and Haddenbrock, S.: Die Electrokrampftherapie. Ihre Grundlagen und ihre Erfolge. Ztschr. f. d. ges. Neurol. u. Psychiat. *174*:635, 1942.
Ewing, J. A., and Haizlip. T. M.: A controlled study of the habit forming propensities of meprobamate. Am. J. Psychiat. *114*:835, 1958.
Ey, H. and Bérard, E.: Les nouvelles techniques de cure de sommeil dans la pratique psychiatrique. Évolution Psychiatrique *4*:661, 1952.
——, and Faure, H.: Les diverses méthodes d'emploi de la chlorpromazine en thérapeutique psychiatrique et leurs indications. Encéphale *45*:361, 1956.
——, and ——: Sleep therapy and the use of chlorpromazine. Internat. Rec. Med. *170*:1, 1957.
Eyman, E. V., and Morris, H. H., Jr.: Deaths

associated with electric shock therapy. Arch. Neurol. & Psychiat. *64*:263, 1950.
Eyres, A. E.: A resumé of 6 fatalities in electric shock therapy treatment. Confin. Neurol. *16*:149, 1956.
——, Knight, J., and Reiter, R.: High frequency (sedac) testing and treatment. J. Neuropsychiat. *1*:311, 1960.
Fabbri, W.: Sulla terapia acetilcolinica di Fiamberti. Rass. studi psichiat. *46*:251, 1957.
Fabing, H. D.: Combined coramine-electroshock therapy in the treatment of psychotic excitement. Am. J. Psychiat. *105*: 435, 1948.
——: Clinical experience with Meratran. Dis. Nerv. Syst. *16*:10, 1955.
——: Frenquel, blocking agent against experimental LSD-25 and mescaline psychosis. Neurology *5*:319, 1955.
——, and Hawkins, J. R.: A year's experience with Frenquel in clinical and experimental schizophrenic psychoses. Dis. Nerv. Syst. *16*:329, 1955.
——, ——, and Moulton, J. A. L.: Clinical studies on α(2-piperidyl) benzylhydrol hydrochloride, a new anti-depressant drug. Am. J. Psychiat. *111*:832, 1955.
Fabisch, W.: The effect of chlorpromazine on the electroencephalogram of epileptic patients. J. Neurol. Neurosurg. & Psychiat. *20*:185, 1957.
Fairman, D., Livingston, K., and Popper, J. L.: Skin temperature changes after unilateral and bilateral prefrontal lobotomy. In Greenblatt et al.: Studies in lobotomy. New York: Grune & Stratton, 1950.
Falconer, M. A., and Schurr, P. H.: Surgical treatment of mental illness. Recent Progress in Psychiatry, London: *3*:352, 1959.
Farber, I. J.: Drug Fatalities. Am. J. Psychiat. *114*:371, 1958.
Fariello, V.: Contributo alla conoscenza sulla terapia insulinica nelle malattie mentali. Cervello *17*:150, 1938.
Farrell, M. J., and Vassat, E.: Effect of insulin shock on the heart and blood pressure in treatment of schizophrenia. Arch. Neurol. & Psychiat. *43*:784, 1950.
Fartuyn, J. D.: Hypoglycemia and the autonomic nervous system. J. Nerv. & Ment. Dis. *93*:1, 1941.
Fasanaro, G.: La prognosi nella schizofrenia con le moderne terapie. Acta neurol. *2*:813, 1947.
Fattovich, G.: Alcune considerazioni sugli stati terminali nei dementi precoci trattati con l'insulina. Note e riv. psychiat. *75*:39, 1939.
Faure, H. Faure, M. L., Fournier, M., and Eppe, J. P.: Sur quelques Essais d' Application du 7044.RP dans un Pavillon d'Enfants Déficients. Ann. méd.-psychol. *115(2)*:500, 1957.
——, Stoppa, L., Martin, D., Igert, C., Boutillier, H., and Rappard, P.: Réponse de la cortico-surrénale a l'électro-choc sous curare chez des malades maniaco-depressifs. Ann. Biol. clin. 1:43, 1956.
Favre, A.: Traitement ambulatoire de la schizophrénie, Monatschr. f. Psychiat. u. Neurol. *105*:305, 1942.
Favre-Tissot, M., Broussolle, P., Robert, J.-M., and Dumont Vinatier-Bron, L.: Psychopharmakologie und Teratogenese. Ergebnis einer klinischen Umfrage. *In* H. Kranz and K. Heinrich (Eds.): Begleitwirkungen und Misserfolge der psychiatrischen Pharmakotherapie, pp. 40. Stuttgart, Thieme, 1964.
Fazekas, J. F., Shea, J. G., and Sullivan, P. D.: Ataractics in medical practice. GP *14*:75, 1956.
——, Sullivan, P. D., and Schultz, J. D.: Use of dimethylamino-N-propyl phenothiazine in the management of patients with acute mental disturbance. M. Ann. Dist. Columbia. *25*:67, 1956.
Fazio, C., Giberti, F., and Loebe, C.: Un nuovo trattamento farmacologico (derivato iminotibenzilico G.22355) nella cura degli stati depressivi. Minerva med. *49*:65 & 3143, 1958.
——, ——, Rossi, R., and De Carolis, V.: Imipramine et Electrochoc dans le traitement des depressions. Ann. Médico-psychol. Paris *2*:731, 1964.
Fedotov, D. D., Stanichevskaya, N. N., and Borinevitch, V. V.: Preliminary report on the use of Meratran in some mental diseases. Zh. Neuropat. Psikhiat. *58*:592, 1958.
Feer, H., Fuchs, M., and Strässle, M.: Klinische Untersuchungen mit chlorprothixen (Taractan). Schweiz. med. Wschr. *90*:600, 1960.
Feinberg, I.: Current status of the Funkenstein test. A.M.A. Arch Neurol. Psychiat. *80*:488, 1958.
Feinblatt, T. M., Feinblatt, H. M., and Ferguson, E. A., Jr.: A new antiphobic agent: benactyzine. Dis. Nerv. Syst. *19*: 394, 1958.
Feldman, F., Susselman, S., and Barrera, S. E.: Socio-economic aspects of the shock therapies in schizophrenia. Am. J. Psychiat. *104*:402, 1947.
Feldman, P. E.: A comparative study of various ataractic drugs. Am. J. Psychiat. *113*:589, 1957.
——: Clinical evaluation of Pacatal. Am. J. Psychiat. *114*:143, 1957.
——: Two-year fate study of thorazine-treated patients. Am. J. Psychiat. *114*:237, 1957.
——: Safety and toxicity of trifluoperazine. *In:* Trifluoperazine: Clinical and pharmacological Aspects. Philadelphia: Lea and Febiger, 1958.
——: Clinical evaluation of cyclohexalamine. Am. J. Psychiat. *116*:454, 1959.
——: The treatment of anergic schizophrenia with imipramine. J. Clin. & Exper. Psychopath. *20*:235, 1959.
——: Treatment of anergic schizophrenia with nialamide. Dis. Nerv. Syst. *20*:41, 1959.
——: Comparison of effect of 2-methyl-3-piperidino-pyrazine on target symptoms of anergic schizophrenics. Ann. N.Y. Acad. Sci. *107*:1117, 1963.
Felger, H. L.: Thioridazine (Mellaril) in the geriatric patient. Dis. Nerv. Syst. *27*:537, 1966.

Felici, M.: Hematic modifications in electric shock therapy. Riv. sper. di freniat. *64*:513, 1940.

Ferguson, J. K. W.: A new drug for the treatment of alcoholism. Canad. M.A.J. *74*:793, 1956.

Ferguson, J. T.: Successful therapeutic regimen for the management of behavior problems in the elderly. J. Am. Geriat. Soc. *4*:1080, 1956.

——: A preliminary evaluation of acepromazine (Plegicil). Am. J. Psychiat. *115*:548, 1958.

Ferguson, R. S.: A clinical trial of reserpine in the treatment of anxiety. J. Ment. Sc. *102*:30, 1956.

Fernandes, B.: Anatomo-physiologie cérébrale et fonctions psychiques dans la leucotomie pré-frontale. Internat. Congr. Psychiat. Paris, 1950.

——, and Leitao, G.: Incidents and accidents in chlorpromazine therapy. J. Clin. & Exper. Psychopathol. *17*:70, 1956.

——, and Polonio, P.: Indications for the treatment of mental diseases by physical methods. J. Ment. Sc. *92*:794, 1946.

Ferraro, A.: Pathologic considerations on insulin treatment of schizophrenia. Am. J. Psychiat. *96*:103, 1939.

——: Neuropathologic findings in the brain of three additional cases of schizophrenia treated with insulin. J. Neuropath. & Exper. Neurol. *1*:188, 1942.

——: A new method of treatment of affective psychoses and psychoses with depressive features. Am. J. Psychiat. *107*:136, 1950.

——, and Roizin, L.: Cerebral morphologic changes in monkeys subjected to a large number of electrically induced convulsions. Am. J. Psychiat. *106*:278, 1949.

Ferrier, D.: The functions of the brain. London: Smith, Elder & Co., 1886.

Fetter, D.: Gastric secretion during electric shock therapy. Am. J. Digest. Dis. & Nutrition *11*:405, 1944.

——, and De Jongh, H.: Effect of electric shock therapy on muscle movements. Am. J. Digest. Dis. & Nutrition *11*:406, 1944.

Fetterman, J. L.: Electro-coma therapy of psychoses. Ann. Int. Med. *17*:775, 1942.

——, Victoroff, V. M., and Bregman, E.: Electrocoma therapy: Six-year follow-up of series of private psychotic patients treated with electrocoma therapy. Ohio State M. J. *45*:229, 1949.

Feuerlein, W.: Die Erfolgaussichten bei der Insulinbehandlung der Schizophrenie. Nervenarzt *29*:255, 1958.

Feuerlein, W., and Heczko, W.: Zur Technik der Insulinkur nach Sakel. Nervenarzt *31*:559, 1960.

Fiamberti, A. M.: Proposta di una tecnica operatoria modificata e semplificata per gli interventi alla Moniz sui lobi prefrontali in malati de mente. Rassegna di studi psichiat. *26*:797, 1947.

——: Accessi a carattere epilettico provocati con l'introduzione sottoccipitale di sostanze vasodilatatrici. Riv. sper. di freniat. 61, 1939.

——: Considerazioni sulla leucotomia prefrontale con il metodo transorbitario Gior. di psichiat. e di neuropat. *67*:291, 1939.

——: Sull'mechanismo d'azione terapeutica della "burrasca vascolare" provocata con derivati della colina. Gior. di psichiat. e di neuropat. *67*:270, 1939.

——: Indicazioni e tecnica della leucotomia prefrontale transorbitaria. Rassegna di neuropsichiat. *1*:181, 1947.

——: L'acetylcholine dans la physio-pathogénése et dans la thérapie de la schizophrénie. Congrés Internat. Paris, 1950.

Fieve, R. R., Platman, S. R., and Plutchik, R. R.: The use of lithium in affective disorders. I. and II. Amer. J. Psychiat. *125*: 487 and 492, 1968.

Fincle, L. P., and Johnson, C. C.: Psychiatric and behavioral effects of chlorprothixene concentrate suspension in chronic hospitalized schizophrenics. Dis. Nerv. Syst. *26*:225, 1965.

Finiefs, L. A.: The results of treatment of 1000 cases of schizophrenia. J. Ment. Sc. *94*:575, 1948.

Fink, L., and Vlavianos, G.: Clinical impressions of the response to promazine therapy Am. J. Psychiat. *114*:1031, 1958.

Fink, M.: Electroencephalographic and behavioral effects of Tofranil. Canad. M.A.J. (suppl.) *4*:166, 1959.

Fink, M.: Effect of anticholinergic compounds on post-convulsive electroencephalogram and behavior of psychiatric patients. Electroenceph. Clin. Neurophysiol. *12*:359, 1960.

——: Qualitative electroencephalography and human psychopharmacology; frequency spectra and drug action. Med. Exper. *5*:364, 1961.

——: The mode of action of convulsive therapy. J. Neuropsych. *3*:231, 1962.

——: Cholinergic aspects of convulsive therapy. J. Nerv. Ment. Dis. *142*:475, 1966.

——, and Kahn, R. L.: Relation of E.E.G. delta activity to behavioral response in electroshock: quantitative serial studies. Arch. Neurol. & Psychiat. *78*:516, 1957.

——, and ——: Behavioral patterns in convulsive therapy. A.M.A. Arch. Gen. Psychiat. *5*:30, 1961.

——, ——, and Green. M. A.: Experimental studies of the electroshock process. Dis. Nerv. Syst. *19*:1, 1958.

——, Zaks, A., Sharoff, R., Mora, A., Bruner, A., Levit, S., and Freedman, A. M.: Behavioral and EEG studies of naloxone in heroin dependence. In press: Clin. Pharmacol. and Therapeut.

Finkelstein, B. A.: Ditran, a psychotherapeutic advance. J. Neuropsychiat. *2*:144, 1961.

Finley, K. H., and Brenner, C.: Histologic evidence of damage to the brain in monkeys treated with metrazol and insulin. Arch. Neurol. & Psychiat. *45*:403, 1941.

Fischer, A., and Gottreich, N. S.: Anemia as a complication of prochlorperazine therapy. Am. J. Psychiat. *116*:932, 1960.

Fischer, M.: Das Verhalten des Liquorzuckers und sein Verhalten zum Blutzucker im Verlauf des Insulinkomas bei

Schizophrenen. Monatschr. f. Psychiat. 100, 1938.

Fish, B.: Drug Therapy in child psychiatry. Compreh. Psychiat. *1*:55, 1960.

Fisher, K. J., and Greiner, A.: Acute lethal catatonia treated by hypothermia. Canad. M.A.J. *82*:630, 1960.

Fisher, R. A., and Teller, E.: Clinical experience with ataractic therapy in tuberculous psychiatric patients. Dis. Chest. *35*:134, 1959.

Flach, F. F.: Clinical effectiveness of Reserpine. Ann. New York Acad. Sc. *61*:161, 1955.

——: Calcium metabolism in states of depression. Brit. J. Psychiat. *110*:588, 1964.

Flament, J., Lofft, J. G., and von Mendelssohn, F.: Clinical investigation of the psychopharmacological effects of Winthrop 18, 501-2. *In* P. B. Bradley, F. Flügel, and P. H. Hoch (Eds.): Neuro-Psychopharmacology, Vol. 3: 275, (CINP, München 1962). Amsterdam, Elsevier, 1964.

Fleck, U.: Bedeutet ambulante Elektroschockbehandlung einen Kunstfehler? Nervenarzt *21*:412, 1950.

Flegel, H.: Haloperidol in Erhaltungsdosen. Med. Klin. *55*:2250, 1960.

——, Harling, H. O., and Wödl, H.: Truxal in psychiatrischem Krankenhaus und ambulanter Nachbehandlung. Psychiat. Neurol. (Basal) *142*:176, 1961.

——, and Neller, K.: Zur Dipiperon. Behandlung chronisch Schizophrener mit Kontrollvergleich zwischen prä- und permedikativen Individualverläufen. Nervenarzt *34*:85, 1963.

Fleischhacker, H. H.: Some neurological and neurovegetative phenomena occurring during and after electroshock. J. Nerv. & Ment. Dis. *102*:185, 1945.

Fleischl, H.: Effects of thioridazine on chronically regressed patients. J. Amer. Geriat. Soc. *15*:29, 1967.

Fleming, B. G., Spencer, A. M., and Whitelaw, E. M.: A controlled comparative investigation of the effects of promazine, chlorpromazine and a placebo in chronic psychosis. J. Ment. Sc. *105*:349, 1959.

Flegel, H.: Klinische Erfahrungen mit Nitoman, einem neuartigen Psychopharmakon. Nervenarzt *31*:556, 1960.

Fleming, G. W. T. H.: Prefrontal leucotomy. J. Ment. Sc. *90*:486, 1944.

——, Golla, F., and Grey, Walter W.: Electric convulsion therapy of schizophrenia. Lancet, Dec. 1939, p. 1353.

——, and Phillips, D. G.: Transorbital leucotomy. J. Ment. Sc. *95*:197, 1949.

Flescher, J.: Die "Entladungsfunktion" des Krampfanfalles. Schweiz. Arch. f. Neurol. u. Psychiat. *50*:60, 1942.

——: Further contribution to the psychodynamics of convulsive treatment. J. Nerv. & Ment. Dis. *109*:550, 1949.

Floody, R. J., Dixon, R. E., and Mattia, V. D., Jr.: Marsilid toxicity. Dis. Nerv. Syst. *19*:541, 1958.

Flordh, P.: Curareprophylaxe bei Elektroschockbehandlung. Nord. psykiat. medlemsbl. *3*:227, 1949.

——: Einige Bemerkungen über die Wirbelfrakturen bei Elektroschock. Nord. psychiat. medlemsbl. *3*:169, 1949.

Flügel. F.: Neue klinische Beobachtungen zur Wirkung des Phenothiazinkörpers Megaphen auf psychische Krankheitsbilder. Med. Klin. *48*:1027, 1953.

——: Thérapeutique par médication neuroleptique obtenue en réalisant systèmatiquement des ètats Parkinsoniformes. Encèphale. *45*:1090, 1956.

——: Die medikamentöse Therapie der endogenen Psychosen. Nervenarzt *30*:241, 1959.

——, and Bente, D.: Das akinetisch-psychiatrische Syndrom und seine Bedeutung für die pharmakologisch-psychiatrische Forschung. Dt. Med. Wchschr. *51*:2071, 1956.

——, ——, Itil, T., and Molitoris, B.: Klinische und elektroencephalographische Untersuchungen in der Reihe der acylierten Piperazino-Phenothiazin-Derivate. *In* E. Rothlin (Ed.): Neuro-Psychopharmacology, vol. 2:236, (CINP, Basel 1960). Amsterdam, Elsevier, 1961.

——, ——, and Molitoris, B.: Zur Stellung des Thioridazins in der Pharmakotherapie depressiver Erkrankungen. Med. exp. *2*: 153, 1960.

Flügel, K. A., and Pfeiffer, W. M.: Klinische Erfahrungen mit dem Butyrophenon Benperidol. Arzneim.-Forsch. *17*:483, 1967.

Fodor, A.: Centrophenoxinbehandlung halluzinatorischer und deliriöser Zustände. Therap. Umschau *23*:102, 1966.

Ford, H.: Comparative results of drug therapy and electroshock therapy. Dis. Nerv. Syst. *23*:650, 1962.

Forrer, G. R.: Atropine toxicity in the treatment of mental disease. Am. J. Psychiat. *108*:107, 1951.

——, Miller, J. J., Grisell, J. L., Bynum, H. J., Goldner, R. D., and Schwarz, H.: Symposium on atropine toxicity therapy. J. Nerv. & Ment. Dis. *124*:256, 1956.

Forrest, F. M., and Forrest, I. S.: A simple test for the detection of chlorpromazine in urine. Am. J. Psychiat. *113*:931, 1957.

Forrest, I. S., and Forrest, F. M.: A rapid urine color test for imipramine (Tofranil, Geigy). Am. J. Psychiat. *116*:840, 1960.

Forrest, F. M., Forrest, I. S., and Mason, A. S.: Review of rapid urine tests for phenothiazine and related drugs. Amer. J. Psychiat. *118*:300, 1961.

Forssman, H.: Follow-up study of 16 children whose mothers were given electric convulsive therapy during gestation. Acta psychiat. et neurol. scandinav. *30*:437, 1955.

Forstmeyer, W. M.: Untersuchungen über die Permeabilität der Blut-Liquorschranke bei der Schizophrenie und deren Beeinflussung durch die Insulinschocktherapie. Schweiz. Arch. f. Neurol. u. Psychiat. *39* (Erg. 4):95, 1937.

Foster, A. R., and Lancaster, N. P.: Disturbance of motor function during treatment with imipramine. Brit. Med. J. *53*: 1452, 1959.

Foster, C. A., O'Mullane, E. J., Gaskell, P., and Churchill-Davidson, H. C.: Chlorpromazine: a study of its action on the circulation of man. Lancet *2*:614, 1954.

Foster, N. W., and Gayle, R. F., Jr.: Dangers in combining reserpine (Serpasil) with electroconvulsive therapy. J.A.M.A. *159*:1520, 1955.

——, and ——: Chlorpromazine and reserpine as adjuncts in electroshock treatment. South. Med. J. *49*:731, 1956.

Fournier, N.: Pharmaco-radiographic Gastro-intestinale Effets de la Chlorpromazine (4560.RP). Languedoc med. *36*:153, 1953.

Fox, R.: Treatment of chronic alcoholism. Med. Clin. North Amer., Philadelphia, Saunders, May 1958.

——: Multidisciplinary alcoholism treatment. Bull. N.Y. State Distr. Br. *11*:1, 1968.

Fox, V.: Treatment of withdrawal symptoms in the management of alcoholism. J.M.A. Georgia. *45*:139, 1956.

Fox, W., Gobble, I. F., and Clos, M.: A clinical comparison of trifluperidol, haloperidol, and chlorpromazine. Curr. Ther. Res. *6*:409, 1964.

Frandsen, E.: Toxic amblyopia during anti-depressant treatment with pheniprazine (Catron®). Acta Psychiat. Scand. *38*:1, 1962.

Frank, J.: Clinical survey and results of 200 cases of prefrontal leucotomy. J. Ment. Sc. *92*:497, 1946.

——: Some aspects of lobotomy (prefrontal leucotomy) under psychoanalytic scrutiny. Psychiatry *13*:35, 1950.

Franke, H., and Fuchs, J.: Ein neues anti-diabetisches Prinzip. Dt. Med. Wchhschr. *80*: 1449, 1955.

Frankl, L., and Mayer-Gross, W.: Personality change after prefrontal leucotomy. Lancet *2*:820, 1947.

Franks, C. M.: Alcohol, alcoholism and conditioning. J. Ment. Sc. *104*:15, 1958.

Fraser, H. F., and Grider, J. A.: Treatment of drug addiction. Am. J. Med. *14*:571, 1953.

——, and Isbell, H.: Chlorpromazine and reserpine: failure of each in treatment of abstinence from morphine. Arch. Neurol. & Psychiat. *76*:257, 1956.

——, and Rosenberg, D. E.: Observations on the human pharmacology and addictiveness of methotrimeprazine. Clin. Pharmacol. Ther. *4*:596, 1963.

Frederking, W.: Über die Verwendung von Rauschdrogen (Meskalin und Lysergsäurediäthylamid) in der Psychotherapie. Psyche *7*:342, 1953.

Freed, H.: The use of Ritalin intravenously as a diagnostic adjuvant in psychiatry. Am. J. Psychiat. *114*:944, 1958.

——, and Woffard, C. W.: Subarachnoid hemorrhage during shock therapy for schizophrenia. Arch. Neurol. & Psychiat. *39*:813, 1938.

Freedman, A. M., Effron, A., and Bender, L.: Pharmacotherapy in children with psychiatric illness. J. Nerv. Ment. Dis. *122*:479, 1955.

——, Fink, M., Sharoff, R., and Zaks, A.: Cyclazocine and Methadone in narcotic addiction. J.A.M.A. *202*:191, 1967.

——, ——, ——, and ——: Clinical studies of cyclazocine in the treatment of narcotic addiction. Amer. J. Psychiat. *124*:1499, 1968.

Freedman, D. A.: An evaluation of the efficacy of Harmonyl in psychiatric treatment. Am. J. Psychiat. *115*:248, 1958.

Freedman, D. X., and Benton, A. J.: Persisting effects of reserpine in man. N. Engl. J. Med. *264*:529, 1961.

Freeman, H.: Resistance to insulin in mentally disturbed soldiers. Arch. Neurol. & Psychiat. *56*:74, 1946.

——: Critique of tranquilizing drugs, chlorpromazine and reserpine, in neuropsy,-chiatry. New England J. Med. *255*:877, 1956.

Freeman, R. K., Jones, T. E., and Palmer, J. J.: Three year follow-up of patients developing eosinophilia during insulin coma therapy. A.M.A. Arch. Neurol. & Psychiat. *71*:501, 1954.

Freeman, W.: Transorbital lobotomy. Am. J. Psychiat. *105*:734, 1949.

——: Mass action versus mosaic function of the frontal lobe. J. Nerv. & Ment. Dis. *110*:413, 1949.

——: Psychosurgery. Am. J. Psychiat. *106*: 534, 1950.

——: Frontal Lobotomy 1936-1956. A follow-up study of 3000 patients from one to twenty years. Am. J. Psychiat. *113*:877, 1957.

——: Multiple lobotomies. Amer. J. Psychiat. *123*:11, 1967.

——, and Watts, J. W.: Psychosurgery. Springfield: C. C Thomas, 1942 and 1950.

——, and ——: Psychosurgery: An evaluation of 200 cases over seven years. J. Ment. Sc. *379*:532, 1944.

——, and ——: Schizophrenia in childhood; its modification by prefrontal lobotomy. Dig. Neurol. & Psychiat. *15*:202, 1947.

——, and Williams, J. M.: Human sonar: The amygdaloid nucleus in relation to auditory hallucinations. J. Nerv. & Ment. Dis. *116*:456, 1952.

Freudenberg, R.: The use of Vitamin B and preparations of the suprarenal cortex in insulin shock therapy. Am. J. Psychiat. *94* (Supp.): 317, 1938.

——: On the curability of mental diseases by "shock" treatment. J. Ment. Sc. *87*:529, 1941.

——: Ten years' experience of insulin therapy in schizophrenia. J. Ment. Sc. *93*:9, 1947.

——: Observations on the relation between insulin coma dosage and prognosis in schizophrenia. J. Ment. Sc. *98*:441, 1952.

Freyhan, F. A.: Effectiveness of diphenyl hydantoin in management of nonepileptic psychomotor excitement states. Arch. Neurol. & Psychiat. *53*:370, 1945.

——: Prefrontal lobotomy and transorbital leucotomy: a comparative study of 175 patients. Am. J. Psychiat. *111*:22, 1954.

——: Course and outcome of schizophrenia. Amer. J. Psychiat. *112*:161, 1955.

——: Comments on the biological and psychopathological basis of individual variation in chlorpromazine therapy. Encéphale *45*:913, 1956.
——: Psychomotilität, extra-pyramidale Syndrome und Wirkungsweisen neuroleptischer Therapien (Chlorpromazine, Reserpine, Prochlorperazine). Nervenarzt *28*: 504, 1957.
——: The neuroleptic action and effectiveness of prochlorperazine in psychiatric disorders. Psychiat. Research Rep., A.P.A. 9, 1958.
——: The pharmacological modification of mental depressions with imipramine. Proceed. 1st Internat. Congr. Neuro-Pharmac. Rome, 1958.
——: The clinical effectiveness of Tofranil in the treatment of depressive psychoses. Canad. Psychiat. A. J. *4*:86, 1959.
——: Therapeutic implications of differential effects of new phenothiazine compounds. Am. J. Psychiat. *115*:577, 1959.
——: The modern treatment of depressive disorders. Am. J. Psychiat. *116*:1057, 1960.
——: Loss of ejaculation during mellaril treatment. Amer. J. Psychiat. *118*:171, 1961.
——, Catalano, F., and Mayo, J. A.: Summary report of clinical investigation of the effects of magnesium pemoline (Abbott "Cylert") on memory impairment of geriatric patients. Compr. Psychiat. 1969, in press.
Freymuth, H. W., Waller, H., Baumecker, P., and Stein, H.: Effects of iproniazid on chronic and regressed schizophrenics. Dis. Nerv. Syst. *20*:123, 1959.
Friedgold, C. E., and Ripstein, C. B.: Use of chlorpromazine in the withdrawal of addicting drugs. Preliminary report. New Eng. J. Med. *252*:230, 1955.
Friedhoff, A. J., and Zitrin, A.: Comparison of effects of paraldehyde and chlorpromazine in delirium tremens. New York State J. Med. *59*:1060, 1959.
Friedlaender, J. W., and Bonay, R. S.: Psychosis following lobotomy in a case of sexual psychopathy. Arch. Neurol. & Psychiat. *59*:302, 1948.
Friedman, Ch., De Mowbray, M.-S., and Hamilton, V.: Imipramine (Tofranil) in depressive states. A controlled trial with inpatients. J. Ment. Sci. *107*:948, 1961.
Friedman, E.: Irritative therapy of schizophrenia. New York State J. Med. *37*:1813, 1937.
——: Unidirectional electro-stimulated convulsive therapy. J. Nerv. & Ment. Dis. *109*:540, 1949.
——: Multipolar electrocoma therapy. Confinia neurol. *14*-264, 1954.
——: Ambulatory maintenance by electrocoma therapy Dis. Nerv. Syst. *23*:50, 1962.
——, and Barry, H.: Pneumographic patterns during convulsive therapy of schizophrenia. J. Nerv. & Ment. Dis. *94*:688, 1941.
——, and Wilcox, P. H.: Electrostimulated convulsive doses in intact humans by means of unidirectional currents. J. Nerv. & Ment. Dis. *96*:56, 1942.
Friedman, H. T., and Marmelzat, W. L.: Adverse reactions to meprobamate. J.A.M.A. *162*:628, 1956.
Friedman, S., Moore, B. E., Ranger, C. O., and Russman, C.: A progress study of lobotomized and control patients. Am. J. Psychiat. *108*:10, 1951.
Fritsch, G., and Hitzig, F.: Über die elektrische Erregbarkeit des Grosshirns. Arch. f. Anat. u. wissensch. physiol. Med., p. 300, 1870.
Frosch, J., and Impastato, D.: The effects of shock treatment on the ego. Psychoanalytic Quart. *17*:226, 1948.
Frost, I.: Carbutamide in treatment of schizophrenia. Brit. Med. J. *1*:381, 1958.
Frostig, J. P.: Experiences with insulin therapy in schizophrenia with special reference to clinical problems. Am. J. Psychiat. *94*(Supp.):220, 1938.
——: Clinical observations in insulin treatment of schizophrenia. Am. J. Psychiat. *96*:1167, 1940.
——, Harreveld, A. van, Reznik, S., Tyler, D. B., and Wiersma, C. A. G.: Electronarcosis in animals and in man. Arch. Neurol. & Psychiat. *51*:232, 1944.
——, Persyko, J., and Persyko, H.: The quotient of blood sugar fall. A contribution to the question of insulin sensitization. Am. J. Psychiat. *94*:226, 1938.
Frühmann, E., and Gross, H.: Perphenazine for psychoses. J.A.M.A. *171*:450, 1959.
Frumusan, P., Cattan, R., and Bucaille, M.: Première tentative chirurgicale sur le cerveau pour le traitement des ulcères gastriques et duodénaux rebelles. Sem. hôp. Par. *33*:521, 1957.
Fry. W. J.: Ultrasound in neurology. Neurology *6*:693, 1956.
Fryer, D. G., and Timberlake, W. H.: A trial of imipramine (Tofranil) in depressed patients with chronic physical disease. J. Chron. Dis. *16*:173, 1963.
Fuhry, H.: Über psychische Insulinresistenz. Nervenarzt *10*:527, 1937.
Fullerton, A. G.: Psychiatric uses of Meratran. J. Ment. Sc. *102*:801, 1956.
Fulton, J. F.: Functional localization in the frontal lobes and cerebellum. Oxford: Oxford University Press, 1949.
Funkenstein, D., Greenblatt, M., Rost, S., and Solomon, H. C.: Psychophysiological study of mentally ill patients. Am. J. Psychiat. *106*:116, 1949.
——, ——, and ——: Autonomic nervous system changes following electric shock treatment. J. Nerv. & Ment. Dis. *108*:409, 1948.
——, ——, and ——: A test which predicts the clinical effects of electroshock treatment on schizophrenic patients. Am. J. Psychiat. *106*:889, 1950.
——, ——, and ——: An autonomic nervous system test of prognostic significance in relation to electroshock treatment. Psychosom. Med. *14*:347, 1952.
Furst, W.: The force required to crush vertebrae. Psychiatric Quart. *14*:397, 1940.
——: Therapeutic re-orientation in some

depressive states: Clinical evaluation of a new mono-amine oxidase inhibitor (W-1544-A) [phenelzine (Nardil)]. Am. J. Psychiat. *116*:429, 1959.

Furtado, D.: Results of leucotomy. A twelve years follow-up. Lisbon: Psychosurgery, 1949.

——: Chlorpromazine dans les dépressions des hypertendus. Encéphale *45*:572, 1956.

Fuster, J.: Pyreto-electric shock therapy in schizophrenia. Lancet *1*:757, 1944.

Gade, E. B., and Heinrich, K.: Neuroleptic therapy contrasted with earlier methods. *In* N. S. Kline, ed.: Psychopharmacology Frontiers. Boston: Little, Brown & Co., 1959.

Gaitz, C. M., Pokorny, A. D., and Mills, M.: Death following electroconvulsive therapy, A.M.A. Arch. Neurol. & Psychiat. *75*:493, 1956.

Galbraith, A. J., Hewat, J. K., and MacNamara: Stemetil in the treatment of chronic psychotics. J. Ment. Sc. *105*:256, 1959.

Gallagher, W. J., Schroeppel, A. E., and Pfeiffer, C. C.: Effects of reserpine, iproniazid (Marsilid) and triiodothyronine (Trionine), and of reserpine alone. A.M.A. Arch. Gen. Psychiat. *1*:215, 1959.

Gallant, D. M., Bishop, M. P., Nesselhof, W., Jr., and Sprehe, D. J.: Further observations on trifluperidol: A butyrophenone derivative. Psychopharmacologia *7*:37, 1965.

——, ——, and Steele, C. A.: DPN (NAD-oxidized form): a preliminary evaluation in chronic schizophrenic patients. Curr. Ther. Res. *8*:542, 1966.

——, ——, Timmons, E., and Gould, A. R.: Thiothixene (P-4657 B): a controlled evaluation in chronic schizophrenic patients. Curr. Ther. Res. *8*:153, 1966.

——, ——, ——, and Steele, C. A.: Trifluperidol: A butyrophenone derivative. Amer. J. Psychiat. *120*:485, 1964.

Gallinek, A.: Electric convulsive therapy in geriatrics. New York State J. Med. *47*: 1233, 1947.

——: Controversial indications for electric convulsive therapy. Am. J. Psychiat. *109*: 361, 1952.

——: Organic sequelae of electric convulsive therapy including facial and body dysgnosias. J. Nerv. & Ment. Dis. *115*:377, 1952.

——: Management of fear in electroshock therapy. Dis. Nerv. System (Suppl.) *18*:26, 1957.

——: Marsilid (iproniazid) and electroshock. Am. J. Psychiat. *115*:1011, 1959.

Galperin, E. A.: On pulmonary complications in electroconvulsive therapy. Nevropat. i psikhiat. *2*:52, 1949.

Gann, G.: Zur Differentialdiagnose und Therapie der Depressionen.—Der parenterale Niamidstoss. Wien. med. Wschr. *114*:588, and 609, 1964.

Garattini, S., and Ghetti, V.: Psychotropic drugs. Amsterdam: Elsevier, 1957.

——, Kato, R., Lamesta, L., and Valzelli, L.: Electroshock, brain serotin and barbiturate narcosis. Experentia *16*:156, 1960.

Gardes, A., and Schnetzler, J. P.: Reveil électrique du coma insulinique. Ann. méd. psychol. *113*:2, 1955.

Gardner, A.: Meprobamate. Am. J. Psychiat. *114*:524, Dec. 1957.

Garmany, G.: Personality change and prognosis after leucotomy. J. Ment. Sc. *94*:428, 1948.

——, and Early, D. F.: Electronarcosis. Lancet *1*:444, 1948.

——, May, A. R., and Folkson, A.: Use and action of chlorpromazine in psychoneuroses. British Med. J. *2*:439, 1954.

Garry, J. W., and Leonard, T. J.: Trial of amitriptyline in chronic depression. Brit. J. Psychiat. *109*:54, 1963.

Gassel, M. M.: Deterioration after electroconvulsive therapy in patients with intracranial meningioma. A.M.A. Arch. Gen. Psychiat. *3*:504, 1960.

Le Gassicke, L., Ashcroft, G. W., Eccleston, D., Evans, J. I., Oswald, I., and Ritson, E. B.: The clinical state, sleep and amine metabolism of a tranylcypromine ('Parnate') addict. Brit. J. Psychiat. *111*: 357, 1965.

Gastager, H., Haas, I., and Weinkamer, E.: Erfahrungsbericht über die Anwendung von Distraneurin in der Psychiatrie. Wien. klin. Wchnschr. *76*:639, 1964.

Gastaut, H.: Combined photic and metrazol activation of the brain. EEG & Clin. Neurophysiol. *2*:249, 1950.

——, Naquet, R., Poire, R., and Tassinari, C. A.: Treatment of status epilepticus with Diazepam (Valium). Epilepsia *6*:167, 1965.

Gault, J. E.: Agranulocytosis due to amitriptyline. Lancet *2*:44, 1963.

Gayle, R. F., and Campbell, R. E.: Electroconvulsive therapy. Dis. Nerv. Syst. *12*:3, 1951.

Gayral, L., and Lambert, P.: Le dichlorhydrate de fluphenazine. (Etude des doses élevées et des traitements de longue durée). *In* H. Brill, J. O. Cole, P. Deniker, H. Hippius, and P. B. Bradley (Eds.): Neuro-Psychopharmacology, *V*:1128 (CINP, Washington 1966). Amsterdam, Excerpta Med. Found. Internat. Congr. Ser. No. 129, 1967.

Gearren, J. B.: Trifluoperazine in emotionally disturbed office patients. Dis. Nerv. Syst. *20*:66, 1959.

Geiger, A.: Chemical changes accompanying activity in the brain. *In* D. Richter, ed.: Metabolism of the Nervous System. New York: Pergamon Press, 1957.

Geissmann, P., and Kammerer, Th.: L'imipramine dans la névrose obsessionnelle étude de 30 cas. Encéphale *53*:369, 1964.

Geller, W.: Therapeutische Ergebnisse mit dem Neuroleptikum Truxal. Med. Klin. *55*:554, 1960.

Gellhorn, E.: The physiological basis of shock therapy. Proc. Roy. Soc. Med. *42*:Supp., 1949.

——: Autonomic imbalance and the hypothalamus. Implications for physiology, medicine, psychology and neuropsychiatry. Minneapolis: University of Minnesota Press, 1957.

——, and Lambert, E. H.: The vasomotor system in anoxia and asphyxia. Urbana, Ill.: University of Illinois Press, 1939.

Geocaris, K. H., and Kooiker, J. D.: Blood pressure response of chronic schizophrenic patients to epinephrine and mecholyl. Am. J. Psychiat. *112*:808, 1956.

Geoghegan, J. J., and Stevenson, G. H.: Prophylactic electroshock. Am. J. Psychiat. *105*:494, 1949.

Georgi, F.: The problem of convulsions and insulin therapy. Am. J. Psychiat. *94* (Supp.):67 and 76, 1938.

——: Rôle du chimisme sanguin. J. suisse de med. 539, 1944.

Gerard, R. W.: Mechanism of action of "shock therapies." Arch. Neurol. & Psychiat. *42*:564, 1939.

Gerle, B.: Clinical observations of the side-effects of haloperidol. Acta Psychiat. Scand. *40*:65, 1964.

Gershberg, H., and Long, C. N. H.: The activation of the adrenal cortex by insulin hypoglycemia. J. Clin. Endocrinol. *8*:587, 1948.

Gershon, S., and Yuwiler, A.: Lithium ion: A specific psychopharmacological approach to the treatment of mania. J. Neuropsychiat. *1*:229, 1960.

Gerstacker, W.: Die schizophrene Denkstörung in der Elektrokrampfbehandlung. Arch. f. Psychiat. u. Ztschr. f. d. ges. Neurol. u. Psychiat. *183*:423, 1950.

Gerstenbrand, F., Hoff, H. and Prosenz, P.: Therapeutische Erfahrungen mit Lucidril bei neuro-psychiatrischen Krankheitsbildern. Wien. med. Wschr. *113*:539, 1963.

Gerstmann, I.: Die Malaria-Behandlung der Progressiven Paralyse. Vienna: Julius Springer, 1928.

Gerz, H. O.: The use of a phenothiazine compound in the rehabilitation of schizophrenic patients. Amer. J. Psychiat. *119*: 167, 1962.

——: A preliminary report on the management of geriatric patients with oxazepam. Amer. J. Psychiat. *120*:1110, 1964.

——: Evaluation of a new phenothiazine derivative in the treatment of schizophrenia. Amer. J. Psychiat. *121*:174, 1964.

Giacobini, A. E., and Osterman, E.: Neurological disturbances in connection with hibernial treatment. Nord. med. *52*:1547, 1954.

——, and Salenn, I.: Treatment of delirium tremens. Acta Psychiat. Scand. *37*:198, 1961.

Giannelli, V., and Sani, C.: Sur la thérapeutique convulsante de la schizophrénie et d'autres maladies mentales par le cardiazol. Schweiz. Arch. f. Neurol. u. Psychiat. *49*:92, 1942.

Gibbs, F. A., and Anderson, E. M.: Treatment of hypsarrhythmia and infantile spasms with a Librium ® analogue. Neurology *15*:1173, 1965.

——, Everett, G. M., and Richards, R. K.: Phenurone in epilepsy. Dis. Nerv. Syst. *10*:47, 1949.

——, and Murray, E. L.: Hypoglycemic convulsions; three case reports. E.E.G. and Clin. Neurophysiol. *6*:674, 1954.

Giberti, F., Gregoretti, L., and Boeri, G.: L'impiego della dietilamide dell'acido lisergico nelle psiconervosi. Sistema nervoso, *8*:191, 1956.

Giljarowski, W. A., Liwenzew, N. M., Segal, J. J., and Kirillowa, S. A.: Elektroschlaf. Berlin: VEB Verlag Volk u. Gesundheit, 1956.

Gillespie, L.: Discussion of Greenblatt I. J. and Kahn A.: Clinical toxicity studies of a monoamine oxidase inhibitor. Ann. New York Acad. Sc. *80*:954, 1959.

Gillhespy, R. O., and Mustard, D. M.: The evaluation of imipramine in the treatment of Parkinson's disease. Brit. J. Clin. Pract. *17*:205, 1963.

Gilmore, T. H., and Shatin, L.: Quantitative comparison of clinical effectiveness of chlorpromazine and promazine. J. Ment. Sc. *105*:508, 1959.

Gilmour, S. J. G.: Clinical trial of mebanazine.—A new monoamine oxidase inhibitor. Brit. J. Psychiat. *111*:899, 1965.

Gjessing. R.: Disturbances of somatic function in catatonia with a periodic course and their compensation. J. Ment. Sc. *84*:608, 1938.

Glaser, G. H., and Hoch, P. H.: Observations on effect of corticotropin in schizophrenia A.M.A. Arch. Neurol. & Psychiat. *66*:697, 1951.

——, Randt, C. T., Hoefer, P. F. A., Merritt, H. H., and Traeger, C. H.: The influence of adrenocorticotropic hormone (ACTH) on central nervous system and Neuromuscular function. Tr. Am. Neurol. A., 1950.

Glatzel, J.: Klinische Erfahrungen mit einem neuen Thymoleptikum. Schweiz. Arch. Neurol. Neurochir. Psychiat. *100*:167, 1967.

Glesinger, B.: Evaluation of lithium in treatment. Med. J. Australia *1*:277, 1954.

Gliedman, L. H., and Gantt, W. H.: Effects of reserpine and chlorpromazine on orientating behavior and retention of conditioned reflexes. South. M. J. *49*:880, 1956.

Globus, J. H., Harreveld, A. van, and Wiersma, C. A. G.: The influence of electric current application on the structure of the brain of dogs. J. Neuropath. & Exper. Neurol. *2*:263, 1943.

Glueck, B. C.: The effect of the hypoglycemic therapy on the psychotic process. Am. J. Psychiat. *94*:171, 1937.

Glueck, B. C., Jr.: Psychopathologic reactions and electric shock therapy. New York State J. Med. *42*:1553, 1942.

——, Reiss, H., and Bernard, L. E.: Regressive electric shock therapy. Psychiat. Quart. *31*:117, 1957.

Goar, E. L., and Fletcher, M. C.: Toxic chorioretinopathy following the use of NP 207. Amer. J. Opthal. *44*:603, 1957.

Goddard, E. S.: Trifluoperazine in psychoneurotic outpatients. Canad. M.A.J. *81*: 467, 1959.

Goethe, H.: Zur antemetischen Wirkung einer Fluor-Phenothiazin-Verbindung. Arzneim.-Forsch. *14*:962, 1964.

Gold, L.: Autonomic balance in patients

treated with insulin shock as measured by mecholyl chloride. A.M.A. Arch. Neurol. & Psychiat. *50*:311, 1943.
Goldberg, S. C., Klerman, G. L., and Cole, J. O.: Changes in schizophrenic psychopathology and ward behaviour as a function of phenothiazine treatment. Brit. J. Psychiat. *111*:120, 1965.
Golden, L. A.: Neurologic manifestations in hypoglycemic shock. Ann. Int. Med. *11*: 819, 1937.
Goldfarb, W.: The Vitamin B_1 requirement during therapeutic insulin shock therapy. Am. J. Psychiat. *99*:698, 1943.
Goldman, D.: Effects of large doses of protamine zinc insulin in nondiabetic individuals. Endocrinology *26*:612, 1940.
——: Brief stimulus electric shock therapy. J. Nerv. & Ment. Dis. *110*:36, 1949.
——: Electro-narcosis: Results in 125 cases with psychosis or psychoneurosis. Am. J. M. Sc. *217*:405, 1949.
——: Treatment of psychotic states with chlorpromazine. J.A.M.A. *157*:1274, 1955.
——: Comparison of clinical effects of chlorpromazine and reserpine in psychiatric patients. Am. J. Med. Sc. *233*:137, 1957.
——: Clinical experience with trifluoperazine: treatment of psychotic states. *In:* Trifluoperazine. Philadelphia: Lea and Febiger, 1958.
——: Effect of prochlorperazine (Compazine) on psychotic states. Psychiat. Research Rep., A.P.A. 9, 1958.
——: Physiologic-anatomic hypothesis. *In* N. S. Kline, ed.: Psychopharmacology Frontiers. Boston: Little, Brown & Co., 1959.
——: Pharmacologic treatment of depression. Dis. Nerv. Syst. Supp. *21*:74, 1960.
——: Evaluation of protriptyline: Practical problems and some theoretical implications. Compr. Psychiat. *8*:27, 1967.
——, and Baber, E. A.: Electric convulsion therapy in psychoses. Am. J. M. Sc. *203*: 354, 1942.
Goldner, M. G., and Rickets, H. T.: Significance of insulin inhibition by blood of schizophrenic patients. Arch. Neurol. & Psychiat. *48*:552, 1942.
Goldner, R. D.: Scopolamine sleep treatment in private practice. Internat. J. Neuropsychiat. *3*:234, 1967.
Goldstein, K.: Frontal lobotomy and impairment of abstract attitude. J. Nerv. & Ment. Dis. *110*:93, 1949.
Golla, F. L.: The range and technique of prefrontal leucotomy. J. Ment. Sc. *89*:189, 1943.
——, Grey, Walter W., and Fleming, G. W. T. H.: Electrically induced convulsions. Proc. Roy. Soc. Med. *33*:251, 1940.
Gonda, T. A.: Prediction of short-term outcome of electroconvulsive therapy. J. Nerv. Ment. Dis. *138*:586, 1964.
Gonda, V. E.: Treatment of mental disorders with electrically induced convulsions. Dis. Nerv. Syst. *2*:84, 1941.
Gonzales, J. R., and Imahara, J. K.: Electroshock therapy with the phenothiazines and reserpine. Amer. J. Psychiat. *121*:253, 1964.
Good, W. W., Sterling, M., and Holtzman, W. H.: Termination of chlorpromazine with schizophrenic patients. Am. J. Psychiat. *115*:443, 1958.
Goodwin, D. W.: Metronidazole in the treatment of alcoholism. Am. J. Psychiat. *123*: 1276, 1967.
Gordon, H. L.: Fifty shock therapy theories. Mil. Surg. *103*:397, 1948.
Gordon, M., Zeller, W., and Donnelly, J.: A biochemical evaluation of the activity of certain tranquilizers and their relationship to hormonal function. Am. J. Psychiat. *114*:201, 1957.
Gore, C. P., Egan, G. P., and Walton, D.: The place of reserpine in the treatment of the chronic psychotic patient. Am. J. Psychiat. *114*:333, 1957.
Gosline, E., Walters, C. J., and Saunders, J. C.: Clinical Report on methoxypromazine: a new phenothiazine. Am. J. Psychiat. *115*:939, 1959.
Gottfarb, G., Lehnert, E., and Wohlfahrt, S.: Acroagonin-behandling vid depressioner. Nord. med. *43*:462, 1950.
Gottfried, S. P., and Willner, H. H.: Blood chemistry of schizophrenic patients before, during and after insulin shock therapy. A.M.A. Arch. Neurol. & Psychiat. *62*:808, 1949.
Gottfries, C. G.: Clinical trial with monoamino oxidase inhibitor tryanylcypromine on a psychiatric clientele. Acta psychiat. scand. *39*:463, 1963.
Gottlieb, G., and Wilson, J.: Cerebral dominance: Temporary disruption of verbal memory by unilateral electroconvulsive shock treatment. J. Comp. & Physiol. Psychol. *60*:368, 1965.
Gottlieb, J. S.: The use of sodium amytal and benzedrine sulfate in the symptomatic treatment of depressions. Dis. Nerv. Syst. *10*:50, 1949.
——, and Hope, J. M.: Prognostic value of intravenous administration of sodium amytal in cases of schizophrenia. Arch. Neurol. & Psychiat. *46*:86, 1941.
——, and Huston, P. E.: Treatment of schizophrenia. A comparison of 3 methods: brief psychotherapy, insulin coma and electric shock. J. Nerv. & Ment. Dis. *113*: 221, 1951.
Gouldman, C., Henderson, H., Christian, D., and Smith, J. A.: The use of oral hypoglycemic agents in the treatment of schizophrenia. Am. J. Psychiat. *114*:1116, 1958.
Gour, K. N., and Chaudhry, H. M.: Study of calcium metabolism in electric convulsive therapy (ECT) in certain mental diseases. J. Ment. Sc. *103*:275, 1957.
Gradwell, B. G.: Psychotic reactions in phenelzine. Brit. Med. J. *2*:1018, 1960.
Graff, T. D., Phillips, O. C., and Gentry, W. D., Jr.: Clonic convulsions after the oral use of perphenazine (Trilafon). J.A.M.A. *169*:834, 1959.
Graham, G. S.: Chlorpromazine jaundice in a general hospital. Brit. Med. J. *2*:1080, 1957.
Grahmann, H., and Peters, U. H.: Durch

Psychopharmaka induzierte und provozierte Psychosen, ihre Psychopathologie und ihre therapeutische Bedeutung. Nervenarzt *33*:398, 1962.

Gralnick, A.: Fatalities associated with electric shock treatment of psychoses. Arch. Neurol. & Psychiat. *51*:397, 1944.

——: a seven year survey of insulin treatment in schizophrenia. Am. J. Psychiat. *101*:449, 1945.

——: Shock therapy in psychoses complicated by pregnancy. Am. J. Psychiat. *102*:780, 1946.

Grantham, E. C.: Prefrontal lobotomy for the relief of pain with a report of a new operative technique. J. Neurosurg. *8*:405, 1951.

Grassi, J. R.: Impairment of abstract behavior following bilateral prefrontal lobotomy. Psychiatric Quart. *24*:74, 1950.

Gratton, L.: Neuroleptiques, Parkinsonnisme et Schizophrènie. Union Mèd. *89*:679, 1960.

Greaves, D. C., Regan, P. F., and West, L. J.: An evaluation of subcoma insulin therapy. Am. J. Psychiat. *112*:135, 1955.

Green, I.: Experiences in the management of geriatric patients with chronic brain syndrome. Amer. J. Psychiat. *122*:586, 1965.

Green, J. P., Paasonen, M. K., and Giarman, N. J.: Blood 5-hydroxytryptamine (serotonin) levels after reserpine and electroshock therapy: Proc. Soc. Exper. Biol. & Med. *94*:428, 1957.

Green, M.: Inhibition of ejaculation as a side-effect of mellaril. Amer. J. Psychiat. Amer. J. Psychiat. *118*:172, 1961.

Greenberg, H. R.: Erectile impotence during the course of Tofranil therapy. Amer. J. Psychiat. *121*:1021, 1965.

——, and Carrillo, C.: Thioridazine-induced inhibition of masturbatory ejaculation in an adolescent. Amer. J. Psychiat. *124*:991, 1968.

Greenblatt, M., Arnot, R. E., Poppen, J. L., and Chapman, W. P.: Report on lobotomy studies at the Boston Psychopathic Hospital. Am. J. Psychiat. *104*:361, 1947.

——, ——, and Solomon, H. C.: Studies in lobotomy. New York: Grune & Stratton, 1950.

——, Grosser, G. H., and Wechsler, H.: Differential response of hospitalized depressed patients to somatic therapy. Amer. J. Psychiat. *120*:935, 1964.

——, and Solomon, H. C.: Frontal lobes and schizophrenia. New York, Springer, 1953.

Greene, R., and Dalton, K.: The premenstrual syndrome. Brit. Med. J. *1*:1007, 1953.

Greenhouse, H. R.: Treatment of the post-intoxication state in alcoholics with mephenesin. Quart. J. Stud. Alc. *14*:596, 1953.

Greiner, A. C., and Berry, K.: Skin pigmentation and corneal and lens opacities with prolonged chlorpromazine therapy. Canad. Med. Ass. J. *90*:663, 1964.

Greville, G. D., and Last, S. L.: Leucotomy as an instrument of research. Proc. Roy. Soc. Med. *40*:145, 1947.

Grinker, R. R., and McLean, H. V.: The course of a depression treated by psychotherapy and metrazol. Psychosomatic Med. *2*:119, 1940.

——, and Spiegel, J. P.: Men under stress. Philadelphia: Blakiston, 1945.

Gross, H., and Kaltenbaeck, E.: Taractan (Chlorprothixene) as a neuroleptic drug in clinical psychiatry. Dis. Nerv. Syst. *22*:502, 1961.

Gross, H., and Kaltenbäck, E.: Erfahrungen mit dem Thioxanthenderivat Chlorprothixen (Taractan) in der klinischen Psychiatrie. Wien. klin. Wschr. *73*:64, 1961.

——, and ——: Sordinal®, ein neues Neuroleptikum der Thiaxanthenreihe. Wien. klin. Wschr. *74*:549, 1962.

——, and ——: Flupenthixol (Fluanxol®), ein neues Neuroleptikum aus der Thiaxanthenreihe. (Klinische Erfahrunger bei einem psychiatrischen Krankengut). Acta psychiat. scand. *41*:42, 1965.

——, and ——: Klinische Beurteilung eines Neuroleptikums aus der Butyrophenonreihe: Triperidol. Wien, med. Wschr. *116*: 998, 1966.

——, and Langner, E.: Klinische und ambulante Behandlung endogener Psychosen mit Dipiperon. Wien med. Wschr. *114*:686, 1964.

——, and ——: Trifluoperazin (Jatroneural) bei der Behandlung schizophrener Psychosen. Wien. med. Wschr. *115*:397, 1965.

Gross, M., and Finn, M. H. P.: Oral metrazol therapy in psychotic senile and arteriosclerotic patients. J. Am. Ger. Soc. *2*:514, 1954.

——, Hitchman, I. L., Reeves, W. P., Lawrence, J., and Newell, P. C.: Discontinuation of treatment with atractic drugs. Am. J. Psychiat. *116*:931, 1960.

Gross-May, G.: Über epileptiforme Anfälle bei der Insulintherapie der Schizophrenie. Nervenarzt *11*:400, 1938.

Grosser, H. H., and Ryan, E.: Drug treatment of anxiety: A controlled study of opipramol and chlordiazepoxide. Brit. J. Psychiat. *111*:134, 1965.

Grotjahn, M.: Psychiatric observations in a case of involutional melancholia treated with metrazol. Bull. Menninger Clin. *3*:122, 1939.

Grünewald, G., Grünewald-Zuberbier, E., and Rode, I.: Beeinflussung der Handlungskontrolle durch Chlorprothixen bei unruhigen verhaltensschwierigen Kindern. Arch. Psychiat. Nervenkr. *211*:23, 1968.

Grünthal, E.: Untersuchungen über die besondere psychologische Wirkung des Thymoleptikum Tofranil. Psychiat. et Neurol. *136*:402, 1958.

Guerra, L. A.: Psychopathological observations in patients treated with insulin. Rev. de neuro-psyquiat. *5*:75, 1942.

Guiraud, P., and Mallet, J.: A propos d'un état stuporeux prolongé survenu chez une epileptique et de sa disparition par électrochoc. Ann. med.-psychol. *106*:202, 1948.

Gunn, D. R.: Functional psychoses: the role of trifluoperazine in the treatment of refractory mental patients. *In:* Trifluoperazine. Philadelphia: Lea and Febiger, 1958.

Gupta, J. C., Deb, A. K., and Kahali, B. S.:

Preliminary observations on use of rauwolfia serpentina benth. in treatment of mental disorders. Ind. med. Gaz. *78*:547, 1943.

Gurevitz, S., and Helme, W. H.: Effects of electroconvulsive therapy on personality and intellectual functioning of the schizophrenic child. J. Nerv. & Ment. Dis. *120*: 213, 1954.

Guth, E., and Hoffmann, G.: Erfahrungen bei der Anwendung von SD 709 beim depressiven Syndrom. Wien. klin. Wschr. *78*:14, 1966.

Guttmann, E., Mayer-Gross, W., and Slater, E. T. O.: Short-distance prognosis of schizophrenia. J. Neurol. & Psychiat. *2*:25, 1939.

——, and Reitmann, F.: Blood pressure in cardiazol epilepsy. J. Ment. Sc. *85*:787, 1939.

Gysin, W. M., and Wilson, J. L.: Hyaluronidase in insulin coma therapy. Dis. Nerv. Syst. *15*:138, 1954.

Haase, H.-J.: Über Vorkommen und Deutung des psychomotorischen Parkinsonsyndroms bei Megaphen bezw. Largactil-Dauerbehandlung. Nervenarzt *25*:486, 1954.

——: Vorteile und Nachteile der extrapyramidalen Symptomatik bei der Behandlung mit Chlorpromazin und Reserpin. Arch. f. Psychiat. u. Ztschr. f. d. ges. Neurol. *197*:367, 1958.

——: Das therapeutische Achsensyndrom neuroleptischer Medikamente und seine Beziehungen zu extrapyramidaler Symptomatik. Fortschr. Neurol. Psychiat. *29*:245, 1961.

——, Bergener, M., and Sauerland, L.: Klinisch-neuroleptische Prüfung von Tiotixen, einem Thiaxanthen-Derivat, unter besonderer Berücksichtigung der neuroleptischen Schwelle. Arzneim.-Forsch. *17*: 1043, 1967.

——, Frank, Th., Knaack, M., Lehnhardt, Ch., and Richter-Peill, H.: Klinische Prüfung eines neuen Langzeitneuroleptikums (Fluspirilene) unter besonderer Berücksichtigung der neuroleptischen Schwelle. Nervenarzt *39*:275, 1968.

——, Mattke, D., and Schönbeck, M.: Klinisch-neuroleptische Prüfungen am Beispiel der Butyrophenonderivate Benzperidol und Spiroperidol. Psychopharmacologia *6*:435, 1964.

Habel, L.: Kritische Bemerkungen zur Reserpinbehandlung in der Psychiatrie. Nervenarzt *31*:27, 1960.

Haddenbrock, S.: Über die soziale Bedeutung der modernen psychiatrischen Schock- und Krampftherapie. Med. Rundschau *1*:80, 1947.

——: Radikaltherapie durch Defrontalisation? Theoretisches und Kritisches zur präfrontalen Leukotomie (Moniz). Med. Klin. *44*:69, 1949.

——, and Kemmann, W.: Über die Wirkung der Elektrokrampfbehandlung auf das pathologische Elektrokardiogramm. Nervenarzt *21*:442, 1950.

Hader, M., and Madonick, J. J.: Experience with amitriptyline in elderly patients. Amer. J. Psychiat. *122*:1289, 1966.

——, Schulman, P. M., and Madonick, M. J.: Paranoid conditions of late life treated with trifluoperazine. Dis. Nerv. Syst. *27*:460, 1966.

Hadorn, W.: Untersuchungen des Herzens im hypoglykämischen Schock. Anhang: Das EKG bei der Cardiazolschockbehandlung der Schizophrenie. Arch. f. Kreislaufforsch. *2*:1, 1937.

——: Insulin and the circulation. Am. J. Psychiat. *94* (Supp.):89, 1938.

Häfliger, F., and Burckhardt, V.: Iminodibenzyl and related compounds. *In* M. Gordon Ed.): Psychopharmacological Agents, Vol. I: 35, Medicinal Chemistry; A Series of Monographs, Vol. 4. New York, Academic Press, 1964.

Häfner, H., and Brehm, I.: Thromboembolic complications in neuroleptic treatment. Compr. Psychiat. *6*:25, 1965.

Hagopian, P. B., and Crossfield, R. M.: Experience with chlorprothixene in a state hospital. Amer. J. Psychiat. *119*:466, 1962.

Hagopian, V., Stratton, D. B., and Busiek, R. D.: Five cases of pigmentary retinopathy associated with thioridazine administration. Amer. J. Psychiat. *123*:97, 1966.

Haider, I.: Thioridazine and sexual dysfunctions. Internat. J. Neuropsychiat. *2*:255, 1966.

——: A controlled trial of fluphenazine enanthate in hospitalized chronic schizophrenics. Brit. J. Psychiat. *114*:837, 1968.

Haines, H. H.: An unusual complication of convulsive therapy. Psychiatric Quart. *18*:273, 1944.

Hakim, R. A.: Indigenous drugs in the treatment of mental diseases. Read at the 6.Gujarat and Sanrashtra Provincial Medical Conference, Baroda, India, 1953.

Hald, J., Jacobsen, E., and Larsen, V.: Sensitizing effect of tetraethylthiuramdisulphide (Antabuse) to ethyl alcohol. Acta pharmacol. et toxicol. *4*:285, 1948.

Hales, W. M., and Simon, W.: Minnesota multiphasic personality inventory patterns before and after insulin shock therapy. Am. J. Psychiat. *105*:254. 1948.

Haley, T. J., Komesu, N., and Williams, P.: Pharmacological effects of Melleril. Fed. Proc. *18*:399, 1959.

Halliday, A. M., Davison, K., Browne, M. W., and Kreeger, L. C.: A comparison of the effects on depression and memory of bilateral E.C.T. and unilateral E.C.T. to the dominant and non-dominant hemispheres. Brit. J. Psychiat. *114*:997, 1968.

Halpern, F.: Rorschach interpretations of the personality structure of schizophrenics who benefit from insulin therapy. Psychiatric Quart. *14*:826, 1940.

Halpern, L.: Electroshock as a diagnostic aid in schizophrenia. Monatschr. f. Psychiat. u. Neurol. *118*:61. 1949.

——, Rozanski, J., and Liban, E.: Lésion vasculaire unilatérale du cerveau survenue á la suite du traitement par l'électrochoc. Rev. neurol. *87*:294, 1952.

Halstead, W. C.: Brain and intelligence. Chicago: University of Chicago Press, 1947.
——, Carmichael, H. T., and Bucy, P. C.: Prefrontal lobotomy. A preliminary appraisal of the behavioral results. Am. J. Psychiat. *103*:217, 1946.
Hamilton, D. M.: The use of electric shock therapy in psychoneurosis. Am. J. Psychiat. *103*:665, 1947.
Hamilton, M.: Quantitative assessments of the Mecholyl (Funkenstein) test. Acta Psychiat. Scan. *35*:156, 1960.
——, Smith, A. L. G., Lapidus, H. E., and Cadogan, E. P.: A controlled trial of thiopropazate dihydrochloride (Dartalan), chlorpromazine and occupational therapy in chronic schizophrenics. J. Ment. Sc. *106*:40, 1960.
——, and White, J. M.: Factors related to the outcome of depressions treated with ECT. J. Ment. Sci. *106*:1031, 1960.
Hamon, J., Paraire, J., and Velluz, J.: Remarques sur l'action du 4560. RP sur l'agitation maniaque. Ann. méd. psychol. *110*:331, 1952.
Hamsa, W. R., and Bennett, A. E.: Traumatic complications of convulsive shock therapy. J.A.M.A. *112*:2224, 1939.
Hanlon, Th. E., Kurland, A. A., Esquibel, A. J., and Ota, K. Y.: A comparative study of chlorpromazine and triflupromazine in the management of the chronic hospitalized psychotic patient. J. Nerv. Ment. Dis. *127*:17, 1958.
——, Michaux, M. H., Ota, K. Y., Shaffer, J. W., and Kurland, A. A.: The comparative effectiveness of eight phenothiazines. Psychopharmacologia *7*:89, 1965.
——, Schoenrich, C., Freinek, W., Turek, I., and Kurland, A. A.: Perphenazine-benztropin mesylate treatment of newly admitted psychiatric patients. Psychopharmacologia *9*:328, 1966.
Hård, G.: Nytt tandmelianlägg för electrochockbehandlung. Sven. läk tidn. *51*:1422, 1954.
Hardi, I.: Psychologische Beobachtungen der Schrift und Zeichnung nach vorangegangener Elektroschock-Therapie. Arch. Psychiat. Nervenkr. *203*:610, 1962.
Hardon, J.: Komplikationen bei der Insulinschockbehandlung. Psych. Bl. (UD) *42*: 131, 1938.
Hare, E. H., Seager, C. P., and Leitch, A.: Reserpine in anxiety states. Lancet *1*:545, 1956.
Hargreaves, G. R., Hamilton, M., and Roberts, J. M.: Benactyzine as an aid in treatment of anxiety states. Preliminary report. Brit. Med. J. *1*:306, 1957.
Hargreaves, M. A.: An investigation into the effects of azacyclonal in the hallucinations of chronic schizophrenic patients. J. Ment. Sc. *105*:201, 1959.
Hargrove, E. A., Bennet, A. E., and Ford, F. R.: The value of subconvulsive electrostimulation in the treatment of some emotional disorders. Am. J. Psychiat. *109*: 612, 1953.
——, ——, and Steele, M.: Investigation of CO_2 as adjunct to psychotherapy in some neuroses. Am. J. Psychiat. *110*:844, 1954.
Harman, Ch., and Winn, D. A.: Clinical experience with chlorprothixene in disturbed children. A comparative study. Internat. J. Neuropsychiat. *2*:72, 1966.
Harms, E.: The origin and early history of electrotherapy and electroshock. Am. J. Psychiat. *111*:933, 1955.
Harrer, G.: Zur Inkompatibilität zwischen Monoaminooxydase-Hemmern und Imipramin. Wien. med. Wschr. *111*:551, 1961.
—— (Ed.): Neuleptil-Therapie. Österr. Mhft. f. Ärztl. Fortb. 1966. Sonderschrift. Wien, Facultas—Buch- und Zeitschriftenverlag für Medizin und Pharmazie.
——: Zur Therapie von Schmerzzuständen mittels Psychopharmaka. *In* G. Harrer (Ed.): Neuleptil-Therapie. Österr. Mhft. f. Ärztl. Fortb. *1966*:33. Wien, Facultas—Buch- und Zeitschriftenverlag für Medizin und Pharmazie.
——: Inkompatibilitätserscheinunger bei Psychopharmaka. *In* H. Brill, J. O. Cole, P. Deniker, H. Hippius, and P. B. Bradley (Eds.): Neuro-Psychopharmacology, *V*:588, (CINP, Washington 1966). Amsterdam, Excerpta Med. Found. Internat. Congr. Ser. No. 129, 1967.
——, Harrer, H., and Fischbach, R.: Die Beeinflussung pharmakodynamischer Kreislauf-belastungen durch Antidepressiva. Wien. med. Wschr. *114*:717, 1964.
——, Lenz, H., and Leuschner, I.: Zur Pharmakotherapie depressiver Zustandsbilder mit dem Iminodibenzylderivat Tofranil. Wien. med. Wschr. *109*:542, 1959.
Harrington, J. A., and Mayer-Gross, W.: Benactyzine in anxiety states. Lancet *2*:183, 1959.
Harris, A.: Cardizaol treatment of schizophrenia. J. Ment. Sc. *84*:735, 1938.
Harris, M. M.: Insulin sensitivity of patients with mental disease. Arch. Neurol. & Psychiat. *48*:761, 1942.
——, and Harris, R. S.: Effect of insulin hypoglycemia and glucose on various amino acids in blood of mental patients. Proc. Soc. Exper. Biol. & Med. *64*:471, 1947.
——, Horwitz, W. A., and Milch, E. A.: Regarding sodium amytal as a prognostic aid in insulin and metrazol shock therapy of mental patients (dementia praecox). Am. J. Psychiat. *96*:327, 1939.
Harris, R. E., Bowman, K. M., and Simon, A.: Studies in electronarcosis therapy. J. Nerv. & Ment. Dis. *107*:371, 1948.
Hartelius, H.: Further experiences of the use of malononitrile in the treatment of mental illnesses. Am. J. Psychiat. *107*:95, 1950.
——: Cerebral changes following electrically induced convulsions. Acta Psychiatr., Suppl. 77, 1952.
Hartert, D., and Browne-Mayers, A. N.: The Use of methylphenidate (Ritalin) hydrochloride in alcoholism J.A.M.A. *166*:1982. 1958.
Hartmann, E.: Reserpine: Its effect on the sleep-dream cycle in man. Psychopharmacologia *9*:242, 1966.
Hartnett, B. S.: Liver damage and eosino-

philia following chlorpromazine therapy: report of a case. Brit. Med. J. *1*:1458, 1955.
Hassin, G. B.: Cerebral changes in fatal cases following treatment with barbital, soluble barb. U.S.P. insulin and metrazol. Arch. Neurol. & Psychiat. *42*:679, 1939.
Hassler, R.: Über die anatomischen Grundlagen der Leukotomie. Fortschr. d. Neurol. u. Psychiat. *18*:351, 1950.
Hastings, D. W.: Circular manic-depressive reaction modified by "prophylactic electroshock." Amer. J. Psychiat. *118*:258, 1961.
——, and Rivers, T. D.: A technique for the modification of metrazol therapy procedure. Am. J. Psychiat. *97*:904, 1941.
Haug, J. O.: Kontrollerte kliniske forsok med thioridazin (Mellaril) -et nett phenothiazinderivat. Tschr. Norske. Laegeforg. *79*: 317, 1959.
Hawkins, J. R., and Tibbetts, R. W.: CO_2 inhalation therapy in neuroses-controlled clinical trial. J. Ment. Sc. *102*:52, 1956.
——, and ——: Intravenous acetylcholine therapy in neurosis. J. Ment. Sc. *102*:45, 1956.
Haydu, G. G., Brinitzer, W., Gibbon, J., and Goldschmidt, L.: A clinical trial of chlorprothixine. Amer. J. Psychiat. *118*:460, 1961.
Hayes, K. J.: Current path in electric convulsion shock. Arch. Neurol. & Psychiat. *63*:102, 1950.
Hayman, M., and Wilkins, P. A.: Polyneuropathy as a complication of disulfiram therapy of alcoholism. Quart. J. Stud. Alc. *17*:601, 1956.
Heath, E. S., Adams, A., and Wakeling, P. L. G.: Short courses of E.C.T. and simulated E.C.T. in chronic schizophrenia. Brit. J. Psychiat. *110*:800, 1964.
Heath, R. G., and Norman, E. C.: Electroshock therapy by stimulation of discrete cortical sites with small electrodes. Proc. Soc. Exper. Biol. & Med. *63*:496, 1946.
——, and Pool, J. L.: Treatment of psychoses with bilateral ablation of a focal area of the frontal cortex. Psychosom. Med. *10*:254, 1948.
Hebb, D. O.: Man's frontal lobes. Arch. Neurol. & Psychiat. *54*:10, 1945.
Heberden, P., and Cooper, W.: Attempted suicide with meprobamate treated with Leptazol. Brit. Med. J. *1*:1513, 1957.
Hedegaard, P., and Hjerrild, N.: Some cerebral complications in shock therapy. Acta psychiat. et neurol. *20*:167, 1945.
Hegarty, J. G.: ME.4703—a new phenothiazine derivative. J. Ment. Sc. *104*:870, 1958.
——, and Dabbs, A. R.: A controlled study of the effectiveness of trifluopromazine hydrochloride. J. Ment. Sc. *105*:811, 1959.
Heggtveit, H. A.: Coronary occlusion during EST. Amer. J. Psychiat. *120*:78, 1963.
Heilbrunn, G., and Feldman, P.: Electric shock treatment in general paresis. Am. J. Psychiat. *99*:702, 1943.
——, and Hletko, P.: Disappointing results with bilateral prefrontal lobotomy in chronic schizophrenia. Am. J. Psychiat. *99*:569, 1943.
——, and Liebert, E.: Biopsies on the brain following artificially produced convulsions. Arch. Neurol. & Psychiat. *46*:548, 1941.
——, and Weil, A.: Pathologic changes in the central nervous system in experimental electric shock. Arch. Neurol. & Psychiat. *47*:918, 1942.
Heimann, H.: Erfahrungen mit det frontalen Lobotomie bei Schizophrenen. Monatschr. f. Psychiat. u. Neurol. *121*:163, 1951.
——: Psychochirurgie. *In* Psychiatrie der Gegenwart I/2. Springer, Berlin, 1963.
Heinrich, K.: Die gezielte Symptomprovokation mit monoaminooxydasehemmenden Substanzen in Diagnostik und Therapie schizophrener Psychosen. Nervenarzt *31*: 507, 1960.
——: Zur Symptomprovokation in der Therapie der Schizophrenie. *In* Proc. Third World Congr. of Psychiatry, Montreal, Canada 4.-10. June 1961, Vol. II:1105. Canada, Univ. of Toronto Press; McGill Univ. Press, 1961.
——: Probleme und Ergebnisse der Therapie endogener Psychosen mit neueren psychotropen Substanzen. Med. Welt 335, 1961.
——, Wegener, I., and Bender, H.-J.: Späte extrapyramidale Hyperkinesen bei neuroleptischer Langzeittherapie. Pharmakopsychiatrie *1*:169, 1968.
Hekimian, L. J., Gershon, S., and Floyd, Jr., A.: Some clinical and physiologic effects of a thioxanthene derivative, thiothixene (P-4657 B), in 20 newly hospitalized male schizophrenics. J. Clin. Pharmacol. *7*:52, 1967.
Heldt, T. J.: Therapeutic use of prolonged sodium amytal narcosis. Am. J. Psychiat. *104*:27, 1947.
Heller, G. C., Walton, D., and Black, D. A.: Meprobamate in the treatment of tension states. J. Ment Sc. *103*:581, 1957.
Heller, J.: Another case of inhibition of ejaculation as a side effect of mellaril. Amer. J. Psychiat. *118*:173, 1961.
Helmchen, H., and Hippius, H.: Unerwartete neurologische Begleiterscheinungen der Pharmakotherapie von Psychosen. *In* H. Kranz and K. Heinrich (Eds.): Neurolepsie und Schizophrenie, pp 77. Stuttgart, Thieme 1962.
——, and ——: Bemerkungen zur psychiatrischen Nosologie an Hand unerwarteter psychischer Wirkungen bei antidepressiver Pharmakotherapie. Arzneim.-Forsch. *14*: 520, 1964.
——, and ——: Die unerwünschten psychischen Wirkungen der Psychopharmaka. Internist *8*:336, 1967.
——, and ——: Depressive Syndrome im Verlauf neuroleptischer Therapie. Nervenarzt *38*:455, 1967.
——, and Künkel, H.: Pneumoencephalographische und electroencephalographische Untersuchungen bei Phenothiazin-Behandelten. I. Herdbefunde. II. Paroxysmale Dysrhythmie. Med. Exp. *5*:406, and 412, 1961.
——, and ——: Zur Analyse elektroencephalographischer Veränderungen unter psychiatrischer Pharmakotherapie. *In* D.

Bente and P. B. Bradley (Eds.): Neuro-Psychopharmacology, Vol. 4:377, (CINP Congr. Birmingham 1964). Amsterdam, Elsevier, 1965.
Hemphill, R. E.: Studies in certain pathophysiological and psychological phenomena in convulsive therapy. J. Ment. Sc. *86*:799, 1940.
——: Electric convulsion therapy. Lancet, Aug. 8, 1942, p. 152.
——: Prefrontal leucotomy. M. Press *217*: 480, 1947.
——, and Stuart, J. R.: Simulated amnesia for identity treated by electrically induced epilepsy. Brit. M. J. *1*:938, 1949.
——, and Walter, W. G.: Epanutin and electric convulsive therapy. Lancet 240, 1941.
——, and ——: The treatment of mental disorders by electrically induced convulsions. J. Ment. Sc. *87*:256, 1941.
Henne, M., Martel, J., Le Renard, C., and Bouju, B.: Bilan clinique de l'action de la thioridazine à doses moyennes et fortes pendant quatre ans chez 150 malades mentaux. Ann. méd.-psychol. *124/I*:239, 1966.
Henscher, J., and Kielholz, P.: Praktische Erfahrungen und experimentelle Untersuchungen bei modifizierten Elektroschockbehandlungen. Schweiz. Med. Wchnschr. *79*:853, 1949.
Herman, E., and Pleasure, H.: Clinical evaluation of thioridazine and chlorpromazine in chronic schizophrenics. Dis. Nerv. Syst. *24*:54, 1963.
Herman, M., and Nagler, S. H.: Psychoses due to amphetamine. J. Nerv. & Ment. Dis. *120*:268, 1954.
Hernández-Peón, R., and Naranjo, R.: Depressant action of Insidon on limbic mechanisms regulating automatic and endocrine functions. Med. Pharmacol. Exp. *14*:45, 1966.
Herz, A.: Drugs and the conditioned avoidance response. *In* C. C. Pfeiffer and J. R. Smythies (Eds.): International Review of Neurobiology, Vol. 2:229. New York, Academic Press, 1960.
Heuyer, G., Dauphin, and Lebovici, S.: La pratique de l'électrochoc chez l'enfant. Ztschr. f. Kinderpsychiat. *14*:60, 1947.
——, Dell C., and Pringuet, G.: Emploi de la chlorpromazine en neuro-psychiatrie infantile. Encéphale *45*:576, 1956.
——, Lebovici, S., and Amado, G.: Les électrochocs en sommation. Ann. méd.-psychol. *106*:205, 1948.
Hewat, J. K., Leach, P. W. W., and Simpson, R. W.: Chlorpromazine, reserpine and isoniazid treatment in mental disorder. Brit. Med. J. *2*:1119, 1955.
Heyck, H.: Über einen Hirnbefund ohne Ganglienzellausfälle nach 355 Elektro-Krampfbehandlungen. Monatsschr. Psychiat. u. Neurol. *129*:128, 1955.
Hibbard, R. W.: Humane techniques in electroconvulsive therapy. W. Virginia Med. J. *56*:438, 1960.
Hickman, J. W., Atkinson, R. P., Flint, L. D., and Hurxthal, L. M.: Transient schizophrenic reaction as a major symptom of Cushing's syndrome. N. Engl. J. Med. *264*:797, 1961.
Hicks, W. R., and Barnes, E. H.: A double-blind study of the effect of imipramine on enuresis in 100 naval recruits. Amer. J. Psychiat. *120*:812, 1964.
Hierons, R.: Electrical convulsive therapy. Lancet *1*:158, 1947.
Hift, St., and Kryspin-Exner, K.: Prothipendyl-hydrochlorid, ein neues Neuroleptikum. Wien. med. Wschr. *108*:664, 1958.
——, ——, and Solms, W.: Meprobamate in der Psychiatrie. Wien. med Wschr. *107*: 485, 1957.
Hilbert, G. H.: False-positive pregnancy tests caused by Sparine and Thorazine. Am. J. Clin. Path. *31*:466, 1959.
Hill, D., Pond, D. A., Mitchell, W., and Falconer, M. A.: J. Ment. Sci. *103*:18, 1957.
Hill, H.: The histamine and insulin treatment of schizophrenia and other mental diseases. London: Bailliere, Tindall & Cox, 1940.
Hill, R. M., Desmond, M. M., and Kay, J. L.: Extrapyramidal dysfunction in an infant of a schizophrenic mother. J. Pediat. *69*:589, 1966.
Himwich, H. E.: Effect of shock therapies on the brain. *In*: Biology of Mental Disease. New York: Paul B. Haabe, 1952.
——: Stimulants Res. Publ. Assoc. Res. Nerv. Ment. Dis. *37*:356, 1959.
——: Loci of actions of psychotropic drugs in the brain. Fol. psychiat. neurol. japon. *19*:217, 1965.
——, Alexander, F. A. D., and Lipetz, B.: Effects of acute anoxia produced by breathing nitrogen on the course of schizophrenia. Proc. Soc. Exper. Biol. & Med. *39*:367, 1938.
——, Bowman, K. M., Daly, C., Fazekas, J. F., Wortis, J., and Goldfarb, W.: Changes in cerebral blood flow and arterio-venous oxygen difference during insulin hypoglycemia. Proc. Soc. Exper. Biol. & Med. *45*:468, 1940.
——, and Himwich, W. A. (Eds.): Progress in Brain Research, Vol. *8*:250, "Biogenic Amines". Amsterdam, Elsevier, 1964.
——, Rinaldi, F., and Willis, D.: An examination of phenothiazine derivatives with comparisons of their effects on the alerting reaction, chemical structure, and therapeutic efficacy. J. Nerv. & Ment. Dis. *124*:53, 1956.
Himwich, W. A.: Biochemical changes in the brain occurring during insulin hypoglycemia. *In* Rinkel and Himwich: Insulin Treatment in Psychiatry. New York: Philosophical Library, 1959.
——, and Glisson, S. N.: Effect of haloperidol on caudate nucleus. Int. J. Neuropharmacol. *6*:329, 1967.
——, and Petersen, J. A. C.: Recovery from insulin coma and hematoencephalic exchange. Dis. Nerv. Syst. *19*:104, 1958.
Hinko, E. N., and Lopschutz, L. S.: Five years after shock therapy. Am. J. Psychiat. *104*:387, 1947.
Hinsie, L. E.: Malaria treatment of schizophrenia. Psychiatric Quart. *1*:120, 1927.

——, Barach, A. L., Harris, M. M., Brand, E., and McFarland, R. A.: The treatment of dementia praecox by continuous oxygen administration in chambers and oxygen and carbon dioxide inhalations. Psychiatric Quart. *8*:34, 1934.

Hinton, J. M.: A controlled trial of meprobamate in anxious out-patients. J. Neurol. Neurosurg. & Psychiat. *21*:301, 1958.

——: A comparison of perphenazine (Fentazine), sodium amylobarbitone and a placebo in anxious and depressed outpatients. J. Ment. Sc. *105*-872, 1959.

Hiob, J., and Hippius, H.: Klinische Erfahrungen mit dem Rauwolfia-Alkaloid Reserpine in der Psychiatrie. Dtsch. Med. Wchnschr. 1497, 1955.

——, and ——: Über die Behandlung von Psychosen mit dem Phenothiazinderivat "Pacatal". Med. Klin. *50*:1746, 1955.

Hippius, H.: Die Stellung des Propericiazin im System der Neuroleptika. *In* G. Harrer (Eds.): Neuleptil-Therapie. Österr. Mhft. f. Ärzt. Fortb. *1966*:7. Wien, Facultas—Buch- und Zeitschriftenverlag für Medizin und Pharmazie.

——: Psychiatric side effects of psychotropic drugs. *In* "Psychosomatic Medicine", pp 133. Proc. First Internat. Congr. of the Academy of Psychosomatic Medicine, Mallorca/Spanien 1966. Amsterdam, Excerpta Med. Found. Internat. Congr. Ser., No. 134, 1967.

——, and Jantz, H.: Die heutige Behandlung der Depressionen. Nervenarzt *30*:4, 1959.

——, and Kanig, K.: Die Agranulocytose unter neuro-psychiatrischer Phenothiazine-Therapie. Ärztl. Wchnschr. *13*:501, 1958.

——, and ——: Neue Phenothiazin-Derivate für die psychiatrische Pharmako-Therapie. Fortschr. Neurol., Psychiat. u. ihr. Grenzgeb. *26*:582, 1958.

——, ——, and Selbach, H.: Dynamic action of phenothiazines and reserpine. *In* N. S. Kline, ed.: Psychopharmacology Frontiers. Boston: Little, Brown & Co., 1959.

——, ——, and ——: Humorale "Nebenwirkungen" der psychiatrischen Pharmakotherapie. *In* H. Kranz and K. Heinrich (Eds.): Begleitwirkungen und Misserfolge der psychiatrischen Pharmakotherapie, pp 71. Stuttgart, Thieme, 1964.

——, and Selbach, H.: Zur medikamentösen Dauertherapie bei Psychosen. Med. Exp. *5*:298, 1961.

Hirose, S.: Studies on personalities of patients treated by prefrontal lobotomy. Psychiat. et Neurolog. Japon. *56*:379, 1954.

——: Orbito-ventromedial undercutting 1957-1963. Amer. J. Psychiat. *121*:1194, 1965.

——: Present trends in psychosurgery. Folia Psychiatrica et Neurologica Japonica *20*: 361, 1966.

Hirsch, J. M., and Quintero, Muro, E.: El problema de las fracturas y luxaciones en la terapeutica convulsivante y su prevencion. Rev. "Policlinica Caracas" *65*:1, 1942.

Hirschfeld, G.: Observations with non-convulsive electric-stimulation. Psychiatric Quart. Suppl., part 2, 1950.

——, and Bell, J.: Differential cerebral stimulation. Dis. Nerv. Syst. *12*:264, 1951.

——, Giffen, M. B., Kleinmann, M. V., and Harris, B.: Electric stimulation and insulin coma. Psychiat. Quart. *30*:260, 1956.

Hirschmann, J.: Über Insulinbehandlung bei Schizophrenie. Psychiat.-neurol. Wchnschr. *39*:13, 1937.

Hishikawa, Y., Ida, H., Nakai, K., and Kaneko, Z.: Treatment of narcolepsy with imipramine (Tofranil) and desmethylimipramine (Pertofrane). J. Neurol. Sci. *3*:453, 1966.

Hnatko, S. I., Stirrat, J. H., Verchomin, J.: Agranulocytosis associated with imipramine (Tofranil). Canad. Med. Ass. J. *92*:33, 1965.

Hoagland, H., Cameron, D. E., and Rubin, M. A.: Electroencephalogram of schizophrenics during insulin treatment. Am. J. Psychiat. *94*:183, 1937.

——, Malamud, W., Kaufman, C., and Pincus, G.: Changes in the electroencephalogram and the excretion of 17-ketosteroids accompanying electroshock therapy of agitated depressions. Psychosom. Med. *8*:246, 1946.

——, and Pincus, G.: Pituitary-adrenocortical function in patients with severe personality disorders. Proc. First Clin. ACTH Conference. Philadelphia: Blackiston Co., 1950.

Hoaken, P. C. S.: Jaundice during imipramine treatment. Canad. Med. Ass. J. *90*:1367, 1964.

Hobson, J. A., and Prescott, F.: Comparison of decamethonium iodide with d-tubocurarine in controlling electrically induced convulsions. Lancet *1*:819, 1949.

Hoch, P. H.: Atropinversuche bei Katatonen und anderen Geisteskranken. Allgem. Ztsch. Psychiat. *96*:388, 1932.

——: Treatment of schizophrenia with prolonged narcosis. Psychiatric Quart. *9*:386, 1935.

——: Neurological observations in hypoglycemic states. Psychiatric Quart. *12*:690, 1938.

——: Clinical and biological interrelations between schizophrenia and epilepsy. Am. J. Psychiat. *99*:507, 1943.

——: The present status of narcodiagnosis and therapy. J. Nerv. & Ment. Dis. 103: 248, 1946.

——: The effects of electric convulsive therapy on the functioning of mental patients. J. Personality *17*:48, 1948.

——: Theoretical aspects of frontal lobotomy and similar brain operations. Am. J. Psychiat. *106*:448, 1949.

——: Evaluations of the results of topectomy operations. Surg., Gynec. & Obstet. *92*:608, 1951.

——: The effect of chlorpromazine on moderate and mild mental emotional disturbance. Chlorpromazine and Mental Health. New York: Lea & Febiger, 1955.

——: Drugs and psychotherapy. Am. J. Psychiat. *116*:305, 1959.

——, Pool, J. L., Ransohoff, J., Cattell, J. P., and Pennes, H. H.: The psychosurgical treatment of pseudoneurotic schizo-

phrenia. Am. J. Psychiat. *111*:653, 1955.
——, ——, and Rouke, F. L.: Psychogalvanometric investigations in psychoses and other abnormal mental states. Psychosomatic Med. *6*:237, 1944.
——, and Polatin, P.: Pseudoneurotic forms of schizophrenia. Psychiatric Quart. *23*: 248, 1949.
Hodge, J. R.: Akathisia. Am. J. Psychiat. *116*:337, 1959.
Hodges, H. H., and Lazerte, G. D.: Jaundice and agranulocytosis with fatality following chlorpromazine therapy. J.A.M.A. *158*: 114, 1955.
Hodges, J. R., Jones, M., Elithorn, A., and Bridges, P.: Effect of electroconvulsive therapy on plasma cortisol-levels. Nature *204*:754, 1964.
Hoenig, J., and Leiberman, D. M.: The epileptic threshold in schizophrenia. J. Neurol., Neurosurg, Psychiat. *16*:30, 1953.
——, and Visram, S.: Amitriptyline versus imipramine in depressive psychoses. Brit. J. Psychiat. *110*:840, 1964.
Hoff, H., and Hofmann, G.: Die Anwendung der Neuroleptika in der psychiatrischen und allgemeinen Praxis. Wien. Med. Wschr. *113*:269, 1963.
——, Tschabitscher, H., and Kryspin-Exner (Eds.): Muskel und Psyche. Symp. an der Psychiatrischen und Neurologischen Klinik der Universität Wien, 18./19. Oktober 1963. Basel and New York. S. Karger, 1964.
Hoffer, A.: The effects of nicotinic acid on the frequency and duration of re-hospitalization of schizophrenic patients; a controlled comparison study. Intern. J. Neuropsychiat. *2*:234, 1966.
——, and Osmond, H.: Treatment of schizophrenia with nicotinic acid. A ten year follow-up. Acta psychiat. scand. *40*:171, 1964.
——, and ——: Nicotinamide adenine dinucleotide in the treatment of chronic schizophrenic patients. Brit. J. Psychiat. *114*:915, 1968.
——, and Parsons. S.: Histamine therapy for schizophrenics. Canad. M.A.J. *72*:325, 1955.
Hoffet, H., and Cornu, F.: Klinische Effahrungen mit dem Thioxanthenderivat Ro 4-0403 (Taractan). Schweiz. med. Wschr. *90*:602, 1960.
Hoffman, F. H., and Wunsch, C. A.: Nonconvulsive electro-stimulation in insulin coma. Dis. Nerv. Syst. *11*:302, 1950.
Hoffmann, M. H., Sandler, N., and Hecht, H.: Paroxysmal auricular fibrillation complicating metrazol shock therapy. Am. J. Psychiat. *97*:372, 1940.
Hofman, E.: Über Beziehungen zwischen Blutzuckerbewegung und klinischen Symptomen so wie dem Heilungsverlaufe bei der Insulinbehandlung Schizophrener. Ztschr. f. d. ges. Neurol. u. Psychiat. *164*:537, 1939.
Hofstatter, L., Smolik, E. A., and Busch, A. K.: Prefrontal lobotomy in treatment of chronic psychoses. Arch. Neurol. & Psychiat. *53*:125, 1945.
Hökfelt, B.: Selective depletion of the adrenaline content of the suprarenal gland by the injection of insulin in the cat. Endocrinol. *53*:536, 1953.
Holland, H. C., Newman, E. G., and Hohman, L. B.: Effects of lobotomy in childhood. Dis. Nerv. Syst. *19*:201, 1958.
Hollister, L. E.: Complications from the use of tranquilizing drugs. New England. J. Med. *257*:170, 1957.
——: Hematemesis and melena complicating treatment with rauwolfia alkaloids. Arch. Int. Med. *99*:218, 1957.
——: Letter. J.A.M.A. *169*:1235, 1959.
——: Complications from psychotherapeutic drugs—1964. Clin. Pharmacol. *5*:322, 1964.
——: Toxicity of psychotherapeutic drugs. Practitioner *194*:72, 1965.
——, and Bennett, J. L.: Thyroid function and psychotherapeutic drugs. J.A.M.A. *185*:890, 1963.
——, ——, Kimbell, Jr., J., Savage, Ch., and Overall, J. E.: Diazepam in newly admitted schizophrenics. Dis Nerv. Syst. *24*:746, 1963.
——, Erickson, G. V., and Motzenbecker, F. P.: Trifluoperazine in chronic psychiatric patients. J. Clin. Exp. Psychopath. *21*:15, 1960.
——, and Kosek, J. C.: Sudden death during treatment with phenothiazine derivatives. J.A.M.A. *192*:1035, 1965.
——, Kreiger, G. E., Kringel, A., and Roberts, R. H.: Treatment of chronic schizophrenic reactions with reserpine. Annals New York Acad. Sc. *61*:92, 1955.
——, Motzenbecker, R. F., and Degan, R. O.: Withdrawal reactions from chlordiazepoxide ("Librium"). Psychopharmacologia *2*: 63, 1961.
——, Overall, J. E., Bennett, J. L., Kimbell, I., Jr., and Shelton, J.: Triperidol in newly admitted schizophrenics. Amer. J. Psychiat. *122*:96, 1965.
——, ——, Johnson, M., Katz, G., Kimbell, Jr. I. H., and Honigfeld, G.: Evaluation of desipramine in depressive states. J. New Drugs, *3*:161, 1963.
——, ——, ——, Pennington, V., Katz, G., and Shelton, J.: Controlled comparison of amitriptyline, imipramine, and placebo in hospitalized depressed patients. J. Nerv. Ment. Dis. *139*:370, 1964.
——, ——, Kimbell, I., Jr., Bennett, J. L., Meyer, F., and Caffey, E., Jr.: Oxypertine in newly admitted schizophrenics. J. New Drugs *3*:26, 1963.
——, Traub, L., and Prusmack, J. J.: Use of thioridazine for intensive treatment of schizophrenics refractory to other tranquilizing drugs. J. Neuropsychiat. *1*:200, 1960.
Holmberg, G.: The factor of hypoxemia in electroshock therapy. *110*:115, 1963.
——, and Thesleff, S.: Succinylcholine-iodide as a muscular relaxant in electroshock therapy. Am. J. Psychiat. *108*:842, 1952.
Holoubek, J. E., Thomas, O. C., and Segura, J.: Toxic reaction to 2-Methyl-2-n-propyl-1, 3, propanediol dicarbamate

(Miltown and Equanil). Ann. Int. Med. *46*:1002, 1957.
Holsbrook, C. S.: Twelve years' experience with electrosleep (shock) therapy J. Louisiana M. Soc. *106*:7, 1954.
Holson, J.: Curare-controlled electrical convulsive therapy. J. belge de neurol. et de psychiat. *47*:618, 1947.
Holstein, A. P., and Chen, C. H.: Haloperidol —A preliminary clinical study. Amer. J. Psychiat. *122*:462, 1965.
Holt, J. P., and Wright, E.: Preliminary results with fluphenazine (Prolixin) in chronic psychotic patients. Am. J. Psychiat. *117*:157, 1960.
Holt. W. L., Jr., McCandless, F. D., Yacoubian, J., and Mebed, A. A. M.: A comparison of "Anectine" (succinylcholine) and "Flaxidil" effects on blood pressure, pulse, and respiration in 30 cardiac and 49 other patients given electroconvulsive therapy. Conf. neurol. *13*:313, 1953.
Holt, W. L., Rinkel, M., Nicholson, M., and Solomon, H. C.: Decamethonium bromide (C-10) in electric convulsive therapy. Am. J. Psychiat. *107*:821, 1951.
Holzbauer, M., and Vogt, M.: The concentration of adrenaline in the peripheral blood during insulin hypoglycemia. Brit. J. Pharmacol. & Chemother. *9*:249, 1954.
Holzer, W.: Über eine Entwicklungsreihe von Elecktroschockgeräten. Allg. Ztschr. f. Psychiat. *121*:124, 1942.
——, and Polzer, K.: Elektroschock und Elektrokardiogramm. Arch. f. Kreislaufforsch. *8*:382, 1941.
Horányi, B.: On prefrontal leucotomy, Monatschr. f. Psychiat. u. Neurol. *118*: 105, 1949.
Hordern, A.: Treatment of depressive states. J. Chron. Dis. *18*:315, 1965.
——, Burt, C. G., Gordon, W. F., and Holt, N. F.: Amitriptyline in depressive states: Six-month treatment results. Brit. J. Psychiat. *110*:641, 1964.
——, Holt, N. F., Burt, C. G., and Gordon, W. F.: Amitriptyline in depressive states. Phenomenology and prognostic considerations. Brit. J. Psychiat. *109*:815, 1963.
——, King, A., Holt, N. F., Collins, J., and Toussaint, J.: Thioproperazine in chronic schizophrenia. Brit. J. Psychiat. *110*:531, 1964.
Horsley, J. P.: Narco-analysis. London & New York: Oxford University Press, 1943.
Hormia, A.: Observations on combined treatment with chlorpromazine, reserpine and insulin coma. Duodecim. *72*:948, 1956.
Horwitz, W. A.: Physiologic responses as prognostic guides in the use of antidepressant drugs. Amer. J. Psychiat. *125*:60, 1968.
——, Blalock, J. R., and Harris, M. M.: Occurrence of relapses in patients treated with insulin hypoglycemic shock. Psychiatric Quart. *12*:716, 1938.
——, and Kalinowsky, L. B.: Combined insulin coma and electric convulsive therapy in schizophrenia. Am. J. Psychiat. *104*:682, 1948.
Houillon, Salles, and Selin: Considérations sur l'emploi de la centrophénoxine en cure hospitalière et ambulatoire. Ann. méd.-psychol. *121/II*:63, 1963.
Houston, F.: Group behaviour in chronic schizophrenics treated with Meratran. Brit. Med. J. *1*:949, 1956.
Hsu, J. J., Nol, E., Martinez, M. L., Lessien, B., Paragas, P. G., Puhac, M., and Braun, R. A.: One-year study of fluphenazine enanthate. Dis. Nerv. Syst. *28*:807, 1967.
Hubble, D.: Toxicity of phenothiazine. Lancet *2*:600, 1941.
Huggins, P. K., Sandifer, M.G., and Pearson, W. S.: Electroschock with and without barbiturate anesthesia. J. Nerv. Ment. Dis. *138*:141, 1964.
Hughes, F. W., and Forney, R. B.: Delayed audiofeedback (DAF) for induction of anxiety. Effect of nortriptyline, ethanol, or nortriptyline-ethanol combinations on performance with DAF. J.A.M.A. *185*:556, 1963.
Hughes, J., Wigton, R., and Jardon, F.: Electroencephalographic studies on patients receiving electric shock treatment. Arch. Neurol. & Psychiat. *46*:748, 1941.
Hugues, A., Chauvergne, J., Lissilour, J., and Lagarde, C.: L'imipramine utilisée comme antalgique majeur en carcinologie. Presse méd. *71*:1073, 1963.
Hunt, P. V.: A comparison of the effects of oxypertine and trifluoperazine in withdrawn schizophrenics. Brit. J. Psychiat. *113*:1419, 1967.
Hunt, R. C.: *In* Freeman, W., and Watts, J. W.: Psychosurgery, p. 164, Springfield, Ill., Charles C Thomas, 1942.
Hunter, R., Earl, C. J., and Janz, D.: A syndrome of abnormal movements and dementia in leucotomized patients treated with phenothiazines. J. Neurol. Neurosurg. Psychiat. *27*:219, 1964.
——, ——, and Thornicroft, S.: An apparently irreversible syndrome of abnormal movements following phenothiazine medication. Proc. Roy. Soc. Med. *57*:758, 1964.
Hussar, A. E., and Pachter, M.: Myocardial infarction and fatal coronary insufficiency during electroconvulsive therapy. J.A.M.A. *204*:146, 1968.
Huston, J. R., and Bell, G. E.: The effect of thioridazine hydrochloride and chlorpromazine on the electrocardiogram. J.A.M.A. *198*:16. 1966.
Huston, P. E., and Locher, L. M.: Involutional psychosis. Arch. Neurol. & Psychiat. *59*:385, 1948.
——, and Strother, C. R.: The effect of electric shock on mental efficiency. Am. J. Psychiat. *104*:707, 1948.
Hutchinson, J. T., and Smedberg, D.: Phenelzine (Nardil) in the treatment of endogenous depression. J. Ment. Sc. *106*: 704, 1960.
Hutton, E. L.: Contra-indications for leucotomy, J. Ment. Sc. *93*:333, 1947.
——, and Bassett, M.: The effect of leucotomy on creative personality. J. Ment. Sc. *94*:332, 1948.
Hyden, H., and Hartelius, H.: Stimulation of the nuclein-production in the nerve cells on malononitrile and its effect on

psychic functions in mental disorders. Acta Psychiat. et Neurol., Suppl. 58, 1948.
Hyvert, M.: La chlorpromazine, traitement des psychoses chroniques. Encéphale *45*: 617, 1956.
Ilem, P. G., and Sainz, A.: The psychiatric application of Vesprin. Psychiat. Quart. *33*:9, 1959.
Illberg, P.: The use of perphenazine in the treatment of drug resistant schizophrenics. Amer. J. Psychiat. *120*:810, 1964.
Imlah, N. W.: Preliminary report on phenoxypropazine. Amer. J. Psychiat. *119*:1091, 1963.
Immich, H., Eckmann, F., Schäpperle, O., Schwarz, H., und Tempel, H.: Psychopharmakologis che Gemeinschaftsuntersuchung mit einem Antidepressivum (BAY 1521). Arzneim.-Forsch. (in press).
Impastato, D. J.: Study of over 2000 cases of electrofit-treated patients. New York State J. Med. *43*:2057, 1943.
——: The safer administration of succinylcholine without barbiturates—A new technic. Am. J. Psychiat. *113*:461, 1956.
——: Reports on use of sedac high frequency stimulator. Dis. Nerv. Syst. *18*:314, 1957.
——: Electric and chemical convulsive therapy in psychiatry. Dis. Nerv. Syst. *22*:91, 1961.
——: Indications and complications of EST and pharmacotherapy. Dis. Nerv. Syst. *23*:653, 1962.
——: Tendon reflexes and safe EST. Dis. Nerv. Syst. *24*:618, 1963.
——, and Almansi, R.: The electrofit in the treatment of mental disease. J. Nerv. & Ment. Dis. *95*:395, 1942.
——, and Berg, S.: Methods of administration of succinylcholine dichloride in electroshock therapy with a description of a simple and modified technique and a succinylcholine dichloride test. Am. J. Psychiat. *112*:893, 1956.
——, Frosch, J., Almansi, R. J., and Wortis, S. B.: The electrofit in depression—Comparison of hospital and privately treated patients. New York State J. Med. Jan. 15, 1945, p. 179.
——, and Karliner, W.: Control of memory impairment in EST by unilateral stimulation of the non-dominant hemisphere. Dis. Nerv. Syst. *27*:182, 1966.
Isaacs, B., MacArthur, J. G., and Taylor, R. M.: Jaundice in relation to chlorpromazine therapy. Brit. Med. J. *2*:1122, 1955.
Isbell, H.: Comparison of the reactions induced by psilocybin and LSD-25 in man. Psychopharmacologia *1*:29, 1959.
——, and White, W. M.: Clinical characteristics of addictions. Am. J. Med. *14*:558, 1953.
Ison, M. G.: The effect of Thorazine on Wechsler scores. Am. J. Ment. Def. *62*:543, 1957.
Ito, K., Yoshimura, Y., Yamashita, I., Moroji, T., and Endo, M.: Effect of electric convulsive therapy and insulin shock therapy on the pituitary gonadotropin production of psychotic patients. Fol. Psychiat. Neuro. Japon. *18*:287, 1964.
Ivanov-Smolenskii, A.: Observations on insulin and prolonged narcosis therapy in schizophrenia. Sovet. psikhonevrol. *15*:16, 1939.
Jackman, A. L.: Neurotic index evaluation of the effect of CO_2 therapy of 500 patients. *In* Meduna: Carbon Dioxide Therapy. Springfield: Charles C Thomas, 1958.
Jacobs, J. S. L., and Gilson, W. E.: Treatment of schizophrenia with intensive electric convulsive therapy. Wisconsin M. J. *45*:395, 1946.
Jacobs, M. A., and Pillard, R.: Approach to studying drug effects in ambulatory patients. Arch. Gen. Psychiat. *13*:163, 1965.
Jacobsen, C. F.: Functions of frontal association area in primates. Arch. Neurol. & Psychiat. *33*:558, 1935.
Jacobsen, E.: Benactyzine. Antibiot. Med. *5*:89, 1958.
——: Benactyzine. *In* M. Gordon (Ed.): Psychopharmacological Agents, Vol. I: 287, Medicinal Chemistry; A Series of Monographs, Vol. 4. New York, Academic Press, 1964.
——, Kehlet, H., Larsen, V., Munkva, D., and Skinhoj, K.: The autonomic reaction of psychoneurotics to a new sedative: benactyzine NFN, Suavitil (R) (benzilic acid diethylaminoethylester hydrochloride). Acta psychiat. et neurol. scandinav. *30*:627, 1955.
——, and Martensen-Larsen, O.: Treatment of alcoholism with tetraethylthiuram disulfide (Antabuse). J.A.M.A. *139*:918, 1949.
Jacquel, M. and G., Amoussou and Racadot: L'association coramine-électrochoc dans le traitement des états d'excitation. Presse méd. *57*:521, 1949.
Jahn, D.: Köperliche Umstellungen durch die Insulin- und Kardiazolbehandlung in ihrer Bedeutung für die Prognose der Schizophrenie. Allg. Ztschr. f. Psychiat. *107*:114, 1938.
Janis, I. L.: Memory loss following electric convulsive treatments. J. Personality, *17*: 29, 1948.
——: Psychologic effects of electric convulsive treatments. J. Nerv. & Ment. Dis. *111*:359, 1950; *111*:383, 1950 and *111*: 469, 1950.
Janjigian, E. R.: Report of three cases of trigeminal neuralgia apparently cured by electroshock therapy. Am. J. Psychiat. *106*:143, 1949.
Jansen, J., and Waaler, B.: Pathologisch-anatomische Veränderungen bei Todesfällen nach Insulin- und Cardiazol-Behandlong. Arch. f. Psychiat. *111*:62, 1940.
Janssen, P. A. J.: Vergleichende pharmakologische Daten über sechs neue basische 4'Fluorobutyrophenon-Derivate. Haloperidol, Haloanison, Triperidol, Methylperidid, Haloperidid und Dipiperon. 1. und 2. Mitteilung. Arzneim.-Forsch. *11*:819, and 932, 1961.
——: Haloperidol and related butyrophenones. *In* M. Gordon (Ed.): Psychopharmacological Agents, Vol. II: pp 199, Medical Chemistry, A Series of Mono-

graphs, Vol. 4. New York, Academic Press, 1967.

Janzarik, W.: Die Bedeutung der neuroplegischen Therapie für die Psychopathologie des schizophrenen Wahns. Encéphale *45*:635, 1956.

Jaquith, W. L., Nail, H. R., Smith, B. S., and Taylor, M. R.: Perphenazine therapy among outpatients. Amer. J. Psychiat. *123*:1023, 1967.

Jasinski, D. R., Martin, W. R., and Haertzen, C. A.: The human pharmacology and abuse potential of N-Allylnoroxymorphone (Naloxone). J. Pharm. Exper. Therap. *157*:420, 1967.

Jelliffe, S. E.: Discussion on insulin and hypoglycemic shock therapy. Arch. Neurol. & Psychiat. *38*:200, 1937.

Jenner, F. A., Kerry, R. J., and Parkin, D.: A controlled trial of methaminodiazepoxide (chlordiazepoxide, "Librium") in the treatment of anxiety in neurotic patients. J. Ment. Sci. *107*:575, 1961.

Jens, R.: Desoxycorticosterone in certain psychotic cases. Northwest. Med. *48*:609, 1949.

Jentoft, B.: Convulsive treatment in 56 tuberculous mental patients. J. Ment. Sc. *95*:651, 1949.

Jessel, H. J.: Erfahrungen mit Prothipendyl in der Psychiatrie. Dtsch. med. Wschr. *85*:192, 1960.

Jessner, L., and Ryan, V. G.: Shock treatment in psychiatry. New York: Grune & Stratton, 1941.

Jetter, Walter W.: Fatal circulatory failure caused by electric shock therapy. Arch. Neurol. & Psychiat. *51*:551, 1944.

Joel, S. W.: Twenty month study of iproniazid therapy. Dis. Nerv. Syst. *20*:521, 1959.

Johnson, M. H., and Boucher, J. V.: A fatality associated with antidepressant therapy. Amer. J. Psychiat. *120*:1125, 1964.

Jones, C. H., and Shanklin, T. G.: Transorbital lobotomy. Northwest Med. *47*:421, 1948.

——, and ——: Theoretical considerations in the therapeutic use of peripheral electrical stimulation in psychiatry. Dis. Nerv. System *18*:342, 1957.

Jones, G. L.: Symposium: Complications of and contraindications to electric shock therapy. Arch. Neurol. & Psychiat. *49*:788, 1943.

Jones, G. N., and McCowan, P. K.: Leucotomy in the periodic psychoses. J. Ment. Sc. *95*:101, 1949.

Jones, M.: Intravenous insulin in the treatment of schizophrenia. Lancet *2*:361, 1940.

Jorstad, J., and Retterstol, N.: Intra-arterial blood pressure measurements during electroshock convulsive treatment with and without a muscle relaxant (succinylcholine iodide). Scandinav. J. Clin. & Lab. Invest. *8*:95, 1956.

Joshi, V. G.: Controlled clinical trial of isocarboxazid ("Marplan") in hospital psychiatry. J. Ment. Sci. *107*:567, 1961.

Joynt, R. J., and Clancy, J.: Extreme eosinophilia during imipramine therapy. Amer. J. Psychiat. *118*:170, 1961.

Juba, A.: Über nach Elektroschock auftretende kortikale Funktionsstörungen (Gerstmannsches Syndrom, Gesichts- und Raumagnosien). Schweiz. Arch. f. Neurol. u. Psychiat. *61*:217, 1948.

Judah, L. Murphree, O., and Seager, L.: Psychiatric response of geriatric-psychiatric patients to Melleril (TP-21 SANDOZ), Amer. J. Psychiat. *115*:1118, 1959.

Jude, J.-P., Gatineaux, J.-M., and Maupome, J.-J.: Le dominal chez les enfants débiles caractériels. Ann. méd.-psychol. *121/II*: 588, 1963.

Jung, R.: Gedanken zur psychiatrischen Schockbehandlung. Sonderdr. Festschr. f. Kurt Schneider. Scherer, 1947.

——: Hirnelektrische Untersuchungen über den Electrokrampf. Arch. f. Psychiat. u. Ztschr. Neurol. *183*:206, 1949.

Junkenitz, K. W., and Schäffer, S.: Ein "kleines Thymolepticum" aus der Sicht des praktischen Arztes: Ergebnisse einer Gemeinschaftsarbeit von 21 praktischen Ärzten. Med. Welt 2638:*1964*.

Kähler, H. J.: Störwirkungen von Psychopharmaka und Analgetika. Stuttgart, Wissenschaftl. Verlagsges. m. b. H., 1967.

Kahn, R. L., and Fink, M.: Changes in language during electroshock therapy. *In* Hoch, P., and Zubin, J. (Eds.). Psychopathology of Communication. New York, Grune & Stratton, 1958.

——, ——, and Weinstein, E. A.: Relation of Amobarbital test to clinical improvement in electroshock. A.M.A. Arch. Neurol. & Psychiat. *76*:23, 1956.

Kaldeck, R., et al.: Physical risks of electroconvulsive therapy. New England J. Med. *239*:778, 1948.

Kalinowsky. L. B.: Electric convulsion therapy in schizophrenia. Lancet *2*:1232, 1939.

——: Convulsions in nonepileptic patients on withdrawal of bartiturates, alcohol, and other drugs. Arch. Neurol. & Psychiat. *48*:946, 1942.

——: Organic psychotic syndromes occurring during electric convulsive therapy. Arch. Neurol. & Psychiat. *53*:269, 1945.

——: Failures with electric shock therapy. *In* Hoch, P. (ed.): Failures in Psychiatric Treatment. New York: Grune & Stratton, 1948.

——: The function of the occupational therapies as an adjunct to shock therapies and prefrontal lobotomy. Am. J. Occup. Ther. *2*:261, 1948.

——: Variations of body weight and menstruation in mental illness and their relations to shock treatments. J. Nerv. & Ment. Dis. *108*:423, 1948.

——: Die Elektrokrampfbehandlung in ihrer Beziehung zur Neurologie. Monatschr. f. Psychiat. u. Neurol. *117*:268, 1949.

——: Relation of lobotomies to the shock therapies. Proc. Roy. Soc. Med. *42* Suppl.: 43, 1949.

——: Das Problem der Hirnschädigung bei Schockbehandlungen. Nervenarzt *22*:201, 1951.

——: Problems of psychotherapy and transference in shock treatments and psychosurgery. Psychosomat. Med. *18*:399, 1956.

——: The danger of various types of medication during electric convulsive therapy. Am. J. Psychiat. *112*:745, 1956.

——: Appraisal of the "tranquilizers" and their influence on other somatic treatments in psychiatry. Am. J. Psychiat. *115*: 294, 1958.

——: Organic (non-drug) therapy of depression. Canad. Psychiat. A. J. *4*:138, 1959.

——: Electric convulsive therapy after ten years of pharmacotherapy. Amer. J. Psychiat. *120*:944, 1964.

——: Die Problematik der chronischen endogenen Psychosen mit besonderer Berücksichtigung der Verhältnisse in den USA. Forum d. Psychiat. *19*:10, 1967.

——: Pharmacotherapy and other somatic treatments. Int. Pharmacopsychiatry. *1*:73, 1968.

——, Barrera, S. E., and Horwitz, W. A.: The "petit mal" response in electric shock therapy. Am. J. Psychiat. *98*:708, 1942.

——, ——, and ——: Electric convulsive therapy of the psychoneuroses. Arch Neurol. & Psychiat. *52*:498, 1944.

——, Horwitz, W. A., Krantz, J. C., Jr., and Kurland, A. A.: A new inhalant convulsive therapy with hexafluorodiethyl ether (Indoklon). Proceed. 1st Internat. Congr. Neuro-Pharmac. Rome, 1958.

——, and Kennedy, F.: Observations in electric shock therapy applied to problems of epilepsy. J. Nerv. & Ment. Dis. *98*:56, 1943.

——, and Putnam, T. J.: Attempts at treatment of schizophrenia and other non-epileptic psychoses with dilantin. Arch. Neurol. & Psychiat. *49*:414, 1943.

——, and Scarff, J. E.: The selection of psychiatric cases for prefrontal lobotomy. Am. J. Psychiat. *105*:81, 1948.

——, and Worthing, H. J.: Results with electric convulsive treatment in 200 cases of schizophrenia. Psychiatric Quart. 17: 144, 1943.

Kalk, H.: Hepatitis und posthepatitische Leberkrankheiten. Verhandl. deutsch. Gesellsch. inn. Med. *63*:177, 1957.

Kalpa, I.: The influence of shock treatment on the activity in hospitals for mental diseases. Acta psychiat. et neurol. Suppl. *47*:416, 1947.

Kalus, F.: Erfahrungen mit den neuzeitlichen Psychosebehandlungen. Psychiat., Neurol. et Med.-Psychol. *1*:65, 1948.

Kamin, I., and Shaskan, D. A.: Death due to massive overdose of meprobamate. Am. J. Psychiat. *115*:1123, 1959.

Kamm, I., and Mandel, A.: Thioridazine in the treatment of behavior disorders in epileptics. Dis. Nerv. Syst. *28*:46, 1967.

Kammerer, Th. and Ebtinger, R.: Treatment of delirium tremens with chlorpromazine. Press méd. *62*:1210, 1954.

Kane, F. J., Jr.: Transient neurological symptoms accompanying ECT. Amer. J. Psychiat. *119*:786, 1963.

——, and Taylor, T. W.: An unusual reaction to combined imipramine-thorazine therapy. Amer. J. Psychiat. *120*:186, 1963.

Kant, F.: Protracted shocks occurring during insulin shock therapy and their treatment. J. Nerv. & Ment. Dis. *91*:712, 1940.

——, Phillips, P. L., and Stolzheise, R. M.: Problems of shock treatment in schizophrenics. J. Nerv. & Ment. Dis. *91*:329, 1940.

Kaplan, N. M.: Hypotension as a complication of promazine therapy. Arch Intern. Med. *103*:219, 1959.

Kaplan, S. M., Mass, J. W., Pixley, J. M., and Ross, W. D.: Use of imipramine in diabetics. Effects on glycosuria and blood sugar levels. J.A.M.A. *174*:511, 1960.

Karagulla, S.: Evaluation of electric convulsion therapy as compared with conservative methods of treatment in depressive states. J. Ment. Sc. *97*:1060, 1950.

Karliner, W.: Present status of Indoklon convulsive treatments. Dis. Nerv. Syst. *27*:470, 1966.

——, and Padula, L. J.: Improved technique for Indoklon convulsive therapy. Am. J. Psychiat. *116*:358, 1959.

——, and ——: Further clinical studies of hexafluorodiethyl ether convulsive treatments. J. Neuropsychiat. *3*:159, 1962.

Karnosh, L. J., and Gardner, W. J.: The effects of bilateral stellate ganglion block on mental depression. Cleveland Clin. Quart. *14*:133, 1947.

Kastein, G. W.: Die Insulin- und Kardiazol-(Corvis-) behandlung bei Schizophrenie (Experimente bei Kaninchen). Nederl. tijdschr. v. geneesk. 6016, 1937.

——: Insulinvergiftung. Ztschr. f. d. ges. Neurol. u. Psychiat. *163*:322, 1938.

Katz, H.: Examination of insulin-treated schizophrenics by the Rorschach method. Monatschr. f. Psychiat. u. Neurol. *104*:15, 1941.

Katzenelbogen, S.: Critical appraisal of "shock therapies" in major psychoses. Psychiatry *2*:493, 1939; *3*:211, 1940.

——, Baur, A. K., and Coyne, A. R. M.: Electric shock therapy. Arch. Neurol. & Psychiat. *52*:323, 1944.

Kautzky, R.: Spontanhypoglykämische Anfälle im Gefolge einer Insulinschockbehandlung. Ztschr. f. d. ges. Neurol. u. Psychiat. *106*:141, 1949.

Kay, W. W.: The endocrinology of deep insulin coma therapy. *In* M. Reiss, ed.: Psychoendocrinology. New York: Grune & Stratton, 1958.

——, and Thurley, A. S.: Some biochemical aspects of hypoglycemic coma. Proceed. Royal Soc. Med. *44*:969 and *44*:973, 1951.

Keddie, K. M. G., and Cooper, A. J.: A controlled in-patient pilot study with the antidepressant mebanazine, a mono amine oxidase inhibitor of the hydrazine group—Part I. Internat. J. Neuropsychiat. *2*:346, 1966.

Keehn, J. D.: An investigation into the value of "objective test psychoticism" in predicting response to insulin coma therapy. J. Ment. Sc. *101*:871, 1955.

Kellner, E.: Preludinsucht und Preludinpsychose. Ther. Gegenw. *99*:524, 1960.

Kelly, D. H. W., and Sargant, W.: Present treatment of schizophrenia—a controlled follow-up study. Brit. Med. J. *1*:147, 1965.
——, Walter, C. J. S., and Sargant, W.: Modified leucotomy assessed by forearm blood flow and other measurements. Brit. J. Psychiat. *112*:871, 1966.
Kelly, H. G., Fay, J. E., and Laverty, S. G.: Thioridazine hydrochloride (Mellaril): Its effect on the electrocardiogram and a report of two fatalities with electrocardiographic abnormalities. Canad. Med. Ass. J. *89*:546, 1963.
Kelsey, J. R., Jr. Moyer, J. H., Brown, W. G., and Bennett, H. D.: Chlorpromazine jaundice. Gastroenterology *29*:865, 1955.
Kennard, M. A., and Willner, M. D.: Significance of changes in electroencephalogram which result from shock therapy. Am. J. Psychiat. *105*:40, 1948.
Kennedy, A.: The treatment of mental disorders by induced convulsions. J. Neurol., Neurosurg. & Psychiat. *3*:49, 1940.
Kennedy, C. J. C., and Anchel, D.: Regressive electric-shock in schizophrenics refractory to other shock therapies. Psychiatric Quart. *22*:317, 1948.
Kennedy, F.: The Neuroses. Med. Clin. N. America *28*:452, 1944.
——, and Wiesel, B.: A report on the results of the electric shock treatment on mental and emotional symptoms. New York State J. Med. *42*:1665, 1942.
Kent, E. A., and Gitman, L.: Chemopsychiatric institutional care of the aged: A three- and one-half-year study of promazine treatment. Geriatrics *15*:480, 1960.
Kenyon, V. B., Lozoff, M., and Rapaport, D.: Metrazol convulsions in the treatment of the psychosis of dementia paralytica. Arch. Neurol. & Psychiat. *46*:884, 1941.
Kepler, E. J., and Moersch, F. P.: Psychiatric manifestations of hypoglycemia. Am. J. Psychiat. *94*:89, 1937.
Kessler, M., and Gellhorn, E.: The effect of electrically and chemically induced convulsions on conditioned reflexes. Am. J. Psychiat. *99*:687, 1943.
Kety, S. S., Javoy, F., Thierry, A.-M., Julou, L., and Glowinski, J.: A sustained effect of electroconvulsive shock on the turnover of norepinephrine in the central nervous system of the rat. Proc. Nat. Acad. of Sciences *58*:1249, 1967.
Keup, W.: Liver function and blood proteins during chlorpromazine therapy in schizophrenia. Monatsschr. Psychiat. Neurol. *129*:476, 1955.
——: Amorphes Insulin und Hyaluronidase in der Insulinbehandlung der Psychosen. Schweiz. Med. Wchnschr. *35*:1957, 1957.
——: Effect of phenothiazine derivatives on liver function. Dis. Nerv. Syst. *20*:161, 1959.
——: Cross Index of Psychotropic Compounds and Chemical relatives. Plenum Press, New York, in press.
Khazan, N., Primo, C., Danon, A., Assael, M., Sulman, F. G., and Winnik, H. Z.: The mammotropic effect of tranquillizing drugs. Arch. Internat. Pharmacodyn. *136*:291, 1962.
Kielholz, P.: Über Ergebnisse der Behandlung akuter Katatonien mit der Durchblutungsmethode. Schweiz. Arch. f. Neurol. u. Psychiat. *63*:230, 1949.
——, and Battegay, R.: Behandlung depressiver Zustandsbilder unter spezieller Berücksichtigung von Trofranil, einem neuen Antidepressivum. Schweiz. Med. Wschr. *31*:763, 1958.
Kierland, R. R., and O'leary, P. A.: Oral treatment of neurosyphilis with aureomycin. Am. J. Syph. *35*:544, 1951.
Killam, E. K.: Drug action on the brain-stem reticular formation. Pharmacol. Rev. *14*: 175, 1962.
Kiloh, L. G., and Ball, J. R. B.: Depression treated with imipramine: A follow-up study. Brit. Med. J. *1*:168, 1961.
——, ——, and Garside, R. F.: Prognostic factors in treatment of depressive states with imipramine. Brit. Med. J. *1*:1225, 1962.
——, Davison, K., and Osselton, J. W.: An electroencephalographic study of the analeptic effects of imipramine. Electroenceph. Clin. Neurophysiol. *13*:216, 1961.
——, and Garside, R. F.: The independence of neurotic depression and endogenous depression. Brit. J. Psychiat. *109*:451, 1963.
——, Roy, J. R., and Carney, M. W. P.: A pilot trial of G. 33040 in the treatment of depressive illness. J. Neuropsychiat. *5*:18, 1963.
Kimbell, I., Jr., and Pokorny, A. D.: The use of Marplan in chronically depressed patients. Dis. Nerv. Syst. (suppl.) *21*:70, 1960.
Kindwall, J. A.: Carbon-dioxide narcosis therapy. Am. J. Psychiat. *105*:682, 1949.
King, P. D.: Phenelzine and ECT in the treatment of depressions. Amer. J. Psychiat. *116*:64, 1959.
——: A comparison of REST and ECT in the treatment of schizophrenias. Amer. J. Psychiat. *116*:358, 1959.
Kingsley, G. R., and Freed, H.: Effects of insulin and metrazol therapy on cerebrospinal fluid proteins. Arch. Neurol. & Psychiat. *45*:289, 1941.
Kingstone, E.: The use of fluphenazine enanthate in an out-patient clinic. Int. J. Clin. Pharmacol. *1*:413, 1968.
Kino, F. F.: Reflex studies in electrical shock procedure. Brain *66*:152, 1943.
——: Eye movements in electrical shock procedure. J. Ment. Sc. *379*:592, 1944.
——: The nasopalpebral reflex: its application to neuropsychiatry, particularly to insulin shock treatment. J. Ment. Sc. *95*: 143, 1949.
——, and Thorpe, F. T.: The occurrence of the grasping reflex in the postconvulsive stage of electrically induced seizures and its behavior in various mental diseases. J. Ment. Sc. *88*:541, 1942.
Kinross-Wright, V., Vogt, A. H., and Charalampous, K. D.: A new method of drug therapy. Amer. J. Psychiat. *119*:779, 1963.
——: Chlorpromazine treatment of mental

disorders. Am. J. Psychiat. *111*:907, 1955.
——: Chlorpromazine in psychiatric disorders. Med. Clin. N. Amer. *41*:295, 1957.
——: Newer phenothiazine drugs in treatment of nervous disorders. J.A.M.A. *170*: 1283, 1959.
——, Cohen, I. M., and Knight, J. A.: The management of neurotic and psychotic states with RO.5-0690 (Librium). Dis. Nerv. Syst. (Suppl.), *21*:23, 1960.
——, and Moyer, J. H.: Observations upon the therapeutic uses of benactyzine (suavitil). Am. J. Psychiat. *114*:74, 1957.
——: Clinical trial of a new phenothiazine compound: Np-207. Psychiat. Res. Rep. Amer. Psychiat. Ass. *4*:89, 1956.
Kinsey, L. J.: Incidence and cause of death in shock therapy. Arch. Neurol. & Psychiat. *46*:55, 1941.
Kisker, G. W.: Psychoneurological problems related to surgical transsection of prefrontal association areas in man. J. Nerv. & Ment. Dis. *99*:343, 1945.
Klaesi, J.: Über die therapeutische Anwendtung der "Dauernarkose" mittels Somnifen bei Schizophrenen. Ztschr. f. d. ges. Psychiat. u. Neurol. *74*:557, 1922.
Klein, D. F.: Delineation of two drug-responsive anxiety syndromes. Psychopharmacologia *5*:397, 1964.
——: Visual hallucinations with imipramine. Amer. J. Psychiat. *121*:911, 1965.
Klein, J. J., Segal, R. L., and Pichel Warner, R. R.: Galactorrhea due to imipramine. N. Engl. J. Med. *271*:510, 1964.
Klein, M. R., and Tardieu, G.: La leucotomie chez l'enfant et ses indications. Semaine d. hôp. Paris *25*:113, 1949.
Klein, R., and Early, D. F.: Observations on the electrically-produced epileptic convulsion. J. Ment. Sc. *94*:805, 1948 and *95*:638, 1949.
Kleinschmidt, H. J., Miller, J. S. A., Orens, M. H., and Cohen, L.: Electric and metrazol shock treatment despite physical contraindications. Psychiatric Quart. *23*: 145, 1949.
Kleist, K.: Bericht über die Gehirnpathologie in ihrer Bedeutung für Neurologie und Psychiatrie. Ztschr. f. d. ges. Neurol. u. Psychiat. *158*:159, 1937.
Klemperer, E.: Versuch einer Behandlung des Delirium tremens mit Insulin. Psychiat.-Neurol. Wchnschr. *50*:549, 1926.
Klerman, G. L., and Cole, J. O.: Clinical pharmacology of imipramine and related antidepressant compounds. Pharmacol. Rev. *17*:101, 1965.
Klett, C. J., and Moseley, E. C.: The right drug for the right patient. J. Consult. Psychol. *29*:546, 1965.
Kline, N. S.: Use of rauwolfia serpentina benth. in neuropsychiatric conditions. Ann. New York Acad. Sc. *59*:107, 1954.
—— (Ed.): Psychopharmacology. Am. A. Advance. Sc. Washington, 1956.
—— (Ed.): Psychopharmacology Frontiers. Boston, Little, Brown and Co., 1959.
——, Barclay, G. L., Cole, J. O., Esser, A. H., Lehmann, H., and Wittenborn, J. R.: Controlled evaluation of nicotinamide adenine dinucleotide in the treatment of chronic schizophrenic patients. Brit. J. Psychiat. *113*:731, 1957.
——, Barsa, J. A., Bruckman, N. S., and Saunders, J. C.: The use of prochlorperazine (Compazine) in a variety of psychiatric conditions. Psychiat. Research Rep., A.P.A. 9, 1958.
——, and Jacobs, M. J.: Use of Pacatal (N-methylpiperidyl-(3)-Methylphenothiazine) in psychiatric patients. Am. J. Psychiat. *112*:63, 1955.
——, and Simpson, G. M.: A long-acting phenothiazine in office practice. Amer. J. Psychiat. *120*:1012, 1964.
——, and Stanley, A. M.: Applications of psychic energizers such as iproniazid (Marsilid). *In* Bradley, Deniker, and Raduco-Thomas, eds.: Neuropharmacology. Amsterdam: Elsevier, 1959.
Klotz, M.: Serial electroencepalographic changes due to electrotherapy. Dis. Nerv. System *16*:120, 1955.
Klüver, H., and Bucy, P. C.: Preliminary analysis of functions of the temporal lobes in monkeys. Arch. Neurol. & Psychiat. *42*:979, 1939.
Knight, G.: 330 cases of restricted orbital cortex undercutting. Proc. Roy. Soc. Med. *53*:727, 1960.
——: Stereotactic tactotomy in the surgical treatment of mental illness. Neurol., Neurosurg., Psychiat. *28*:304, 1965.
——: Intractable psychoneurosis in the elderly and infirm: Treatment by stereotactic tractotomy. Brit. Geriat. Pract. *3*:7, 1966.
——: Observations on surgical technique. J. Ment. Sc. *89*:174, 1943.
Kobler, F.: Histologischer Gehirnbefund nach Insulinkoma. Arch. f. Psychiat. *107*:688, 1938.
Kohlmann, Th., and Rett, A.: Über den Einfluss sogenannter Psychoenergizer auf die klinische und psychische Situation gehirngeschädigter Kinder. Wien. med. Wschr. *113*:356, 1963.
——, and ——: Klinische und pharmakopsychologische Untersuchungen mit Truxal bei gehirngeschädigten Kindern. Wien. klin. Wschr. *76*:789, 1964.
Kolb, L. C.: An evaluation of lobotomy and its potentialities for future research in psychiatry and the basic sciences. J. Nerv. & Ment. Dis. *110*:112, 1949.
——, and Vogel, V. H.: The use of shock therapy in 305 mental hospitals, Am. J. Psychiat. *99*:90, 1942.
Kolle, K., and Ruckdeschel. K. T.: Erfolge der Insulinkur bei Schizophrenie. Dt. med. Wchnschr. *81*:89, 1956.
Komora, E. J., and Padula, L. J.: Combined use of metrazol and succinylcholine in the therapy of mental disorders. *18*:21, 1957.
Kopeloff, N., and Kirby, G. H.: Focal infection and mental disease. Am. J. Psychiat. *3*:149, 1923.
Kopmann, E., and Hughes, F. W.: Potentiating effects of alcohol on tranquilizers and other central depressants. A.M.A. Arch. Gen. Psychiat. *1*:7, 1959.

Koranyi, E. K., Smith, R. L., and Sarwer-Foner, G. J.: Clinical assessment of D-206. A new pyridyl-amine. Med. Serv. J. *14*:130, 1958.
Kordas, S. K., Kazamias, N. G., Georgas, J. G., and Papadokostakis, J. G.: Clopenthixol: A controlled trial in chronic hospitalized schizophrenic patients. Brit J. Psychiat. *114*:833, 1968.
Korenyi, C., and Whittier, J. R.: Drug treatment in 117 cases of Huntington's disease with special reference to fluphenazine (Prolixin). Psychiat. Quart. *41*:203, 1967.
Kornmuller, A. E.: Ansatz zu einer spezifischen Therapie von Psychosen. Dt. med. Wchnschr. *75*:994, 1950.
Koupernik, C.: La psycho-pharmacologie: Stratégie et tactique médicales Evol. psychiat. *31*:661, 1966.
Kovits, B., Carter, J. T., and Addison, W. P.: Comparison of chlorpromazine and reserpine in chronic psychosis. A.M.A. Arch. Neurol. Psychiat. *74*:467, 1955.
Kraines, S. H.: Mental Depressions and Their Treatment. New York, Macmillan, 1957.
——: The continuing importance of Shock Therapy in the treatment of depressive states. Dis. Nerv. Syst. *23*:649, 1962.
Krakowski, A. J.: Protriptyline in treatment of severe depressions. A long-range pilot study. Amer. J. Psychiat. *121*:807, 1965.
Kral, V. A., and Durost, H. B.: A comparative study of the amnestic syndrome in various organic conditions. Amer. J. Psychiat. *110*:41, 1953.
——, and Elvidge, A. R.: Four years experience with pre-frontal leucotomy. Amer. J. Psychiat. *112*:375, 1955.
Kramer, M., Whitman, R. M., Baldridge, B., and Ornstein, P. H.: Drugs and dreams III: The effects of imipramine on the dreams of depressed patients. Amer. J. Psychiat. *124*: 1385, 1968.
Krantz, J. C., Jr., Manchey, L., Truitt, E. B., Ling, A. S. C., and Kurland, A. A.: The availability of hexafluorodiethyl ether by intravenous injection as a convulsant in psychiatric treatment. J. Nerv. & Ment. Dis. *129*:92, 1959.
——, Truitt, E. B., Jr., Speers, L., and Ling, A. S. O.: New pharmacoconvulsive agent. Science *126*:353, 1957.
Kranz, H.: Die Narkoanalyse als diagnostisches und kriminalistisches Verfahren. Tübingen: Recht u. Staat, J. C. B. Mohr, 1950.
Kraulis, W.: Protracted shock in the treatment of schizophrenia and results of the therapy in Riga, Latvia. Am. J. Psychiat. *94* (Supp.):324, 1938.
Kraus, J.: Komplikationen bei der Cardiazolbehandlung nach von Meduna. Psychiat. en neurol. bl. *42*:81, 1938.
Krauss, P.: Wann Kardiazol-, wann Elektrokrampf? Nervenarzt *18*:163, 1947.
——: Zur Krampfbehandlung der Verstimmungszustände und psychogenen Reaktionen. Nervenarzt *18*:127, 1947.
Krayenbühl, H., and Stoll, W. A.: Psychochirurgie bei unerträglichen Schmerzen. Acta Neurochirg. *1*:1, 1950.
Kreienberg, W., and Ehrhardt, H.: Die Gehirndurchblutung im Elektroschock. Nervenarzt *18*:154, 1947.
——, and ——: Diuresehemmung durch Elektroschock. Klin. Wchnschr. *26*:239, 1948.
Kris, E. B.: Simplifying chlorpromazine maintenance therapy. Am. J. Psychiat. *114*:836, 1958.
——, and Carmichael, D. M.: Follow-up study on Thorazine treated patients. Am. J. Psychiat. *114*:449, 1957.
Kristjansen, P.: Experimentation clinique du R.1625 (Halopéridol) Symposium International sur le Halopéridol, Acta Medica Belgica. p. 82, 1960.
Kristof, F. E., MacPherson, A. S., and Brown, M.: Clinical evaluation of a new antidepressant: G-33040. Amer. J. Psychiat. *118*:1134, 1962.
Kronfeld, A.: Psychopathologie der Heilungsvorgänge bei Insulintherapie der Schizophrenie—Arbeiten aus dem Forschungsinstitut Gannuschkin. Moscow: 1938.
——, and Sternberg, E.: Erfahrungen mit der Insulinschocktherapie bei der Schizophrenie. Schweiz. Arch. f. Neurol. *39* (Erg.-H.):187, 1937.
Kruse, W.: "Paradoxical" effect of chlorpromazine in a case of periodic catatonia. Am. J. Psychiat. *114*:463, 1957.
——: Experience with trifluoperazine in 110 female schizophrenics. Am. J. Psychiat. *115*:1031, 1959.
——: Preliminary report on a new psychotropic compound (RO 4-0403/4). Amer. J. Psychiat. *116*:849, 1960.
——: Die Wirkung des Trifluoperazins auf die Gehörstäuschungen Schizophrener. Nervenarzt *31*:180, 1960.
——: Persistent muscular restlessness after phenothiazine treatment: report of 3 cases. Am. J. Psychiat. *117*:152, 1960.
——: Development of Parkinsonism after gradual reduction of fluphenazine dosage. Amer. J. Psychiat. *119*:995, 1963.
——, and Hoermann, M. G.: Clinical evaluation of four anti-depressant drugs. Current Therapeutic Research, *2*:111, 1960.
Küchle, H. J., and Rohrschneider, W.: Elektroschock und Augenbinnendruck. v. Graefes Arch. f. Ophthalmol *159*:88, 433, 1957; *106*:96, 186, 1958.
Kuhn, R.: Über die Behandlung depressiver Zustände mit einem Iminodibenzyl-derivat G.22355). Schweiz. med. Wschr. *87*:1135, 1957.
——: The treatment of depressive states with G.22355 (imipramine hydrochloride). Am. J. Psychiat. *115*:549, 1958.
Kulcsar, S., Polishuk, W., and Rubin, L.: Aspects endocriniens du traitement à la chlorpromazine. Presse méd. *65*:1288, 1957.
Küppers, E.: Die Insulin- und Cardiazolbehandlung der Schizophrenie. Allg. Ztschr. f. Psychiat. *107*:76, 1938.
——: Die Schockbehandlung des manisch-depressiven Irreseins. Allg. Ztschr. f. Psychiat. *112*:436, 1939.
Kurland, A. A., Destounis, N., Shaffer, J. W.,

and Pinto, A.: A critical study of isocarboxazid (Marplan) in the treatment of depressed patients. J. Nerv. Ment. Dis. *145*:292, 1967.
——, Hanlon, T. E., Esquibel, A. J., Krantz, J. C., Jr., and Sheets, C. S.: Comparative study of hexafluorodiethyl ether (Indoklon) and electroconvulsive therapy. J. Nerv. & Ment. Dis. *129*:95, 1959.
——, Pinto, A., Dim, B. H., and Johnson, C. A.: Pilot study of Navane (thiothixene) in chronic schizophrenics and acute psychotic patients. Curr. Ther. Res. *9*:298, 1967.
——, and Richardson, J. H.: A comparative study of two long acting phenothiazine preparations, fluphenazine-enanthate and fluphenazine-decanoate. Psychopharmacologia *9*:320, 1966.
——, and Vasconcellos, J.: Clinical experience with α-phenothiazine sulfonamide dimethanesulfonate in chronic psychotic patients. J. Nerv. & Ment. Dis. *127*:378, 1958.
Kurtis, L. B.: Clinical study of the response to nortriptyline of autistic children. Internat. J. Neuropsychiat. *2*:298, 1966.
Kwalwasser, S.: Report on 441 cases treated with metrazol. Psychiat. Quart. *14*:527, 1940.
——, Monroe, R. R., and Neander, J. F.: Lung abscess as a complication of electroshock therapy. Am. J. Psychiat. *106*:750, 1950.
——, and Robinson, L. C.: General survey of insulin treated patients after five years. Psychiatric Quart. *23*:672, 1949.
Labhardt, F.: Technik, Nebenerscheinungen und Komplikationen der Largactiltherapie. Schw. Arch. Neurol. und Psychiat. *73*:338, 1954.
——: Chlorpromazine in psychic diseases *In* N. S. Kline, ed.: Psychopharmacology Frontiers. Boston: Little, Brown & Co., 1959.
Laborit, H.: L'hibernation artificielle. Acta Anaesthesiologica Belgica *2*:710, 1951.
——, and Huguenard, P.: L'Hibernation artificielle par Moyens Pharmacodynamics et Physiques. Presse méd. *59*:1329, 1951.
Laffan, R. J., High, J. P., and Burke, J. C.: The prolonged action of fluphenazine enanthate in oil after depot injection. Internat. J. Neuropsychiat. *1*:300, 1965.
Lambert, P. A., Beaujard, M., Achaintre, A., Broussolle, P., Perrin, J., Berthier, C., Balvet, P., Revol, L., and Requet, A.: Essais thérapeutiques d'un nouveau dérivé de la Phénothiazine: la lévomépromazine ou 7044.RP. Ann. méd-psychol. *115*:291, 1957.
——, and Guyotat, J.: Un nouvel antidépresseur sédatif dérivé de l'iminodibenzyle: Le 7162 R.P. Essais thérapeutiques. Presse méd. *69*:1425, 1961.
——, ——, and Charriot, G.: La triméproprimine (7162 R.P.), un nouvel antidépresseur à propriétés sédatives et tranquillisantes. Ann. méd.-psychol. *119*:713, 1961.
Lambo, T. A., Chlorpromazine jaundice. Letter, Brit. Med. J. *2*:1048, 1957.
Lambros, V. S.: The use of reserpine in certain neurological disorders: organic convulsive states, enuresis and head injuries. Ann. New York Acad. Sc. *6*:211, 1955.
Lancaster, N. P., and Foster, A. R.: Suicidal attempt by imipramine overdosage. Brit. Med. J. *2*:1458, 1959.
Lancaster, N. P., Steinert, R. R., and Frost, I.: Unilateral electro-convulsive therapy. J. Ment. Sci. *104*:221, 1958.
Landis, C.: Psychological observations on psychosurgery patients. Psychiatric Quart. *25*:409, 1951.
——, Zubin, J., and Mettler, F. A.: The functions of the human frontal lobe. J. Psychol. *30*:123, 1950.
Lang, H. B.: Clinical report on parenteral nortriptyline. Dis. Nerv. Syst. *26*:435, 1965.
Langfeldt, E.: The prognosis in schizophrenia, and the factors influencing the course of the disease. Acta psychiat. et neurol., Supp., *13*, 1937.
Langley, G. E., and Robin, A. A.: A pilot trial of orphenadrine (Disipal) in patients treated with reserpine. J. Ment. Sc. *106*: 682, 1960.
Langsley, D. G., Enterline, J. D., and Hickerson, G. X.: Comparison of chlorpromazine and EST in treatment of acute schizophrenia and manic reactions. A.M.A. Arch. Neurol. & Psychiat. *81*:384, 1959.
Lanzkron, J.: A case of hip-fracture occurring during electric shock treatment with an amputation stump. Am. J. Psychiat. *111*:702, 1955.
Lapipe, M., and Rondepierre, J.: Contribution a l'étude physique, physiologique et clinique de l'électro-choc. Paris: Librairie Maloine, 1943.
Laqueur, H. P., Dussik, K. T., LaBurt, H. A., and McLaughlin, W. F.: Tactical and strategical considerations in the use of insulin therapy. *In* M. Rinkel (Ed.): Biological Treatment of Mental Illness. New York, L. C. Page & Co., 1966.
——, and LaBurt, H. A.: Coma therapy with multiple insulin doses. J. Neuropsych. *1*:135, 1960.
——, and ——: Experiences with low-zinc insulin, with semi-lente insulin, with glucagon and adrenalin-thiamine in insulin coma treatment. J. Neuropsychiat. *2*:86, 1960.
Larragoiti, R. J.: Medicacion previa para la electroshock terapia. Rev. de med. y cir. de la Habana *50*:115, 1945.
——: La terapeutica convulsivante par estimulo breve. Arch. Soc. estud. clin. Habana *41*:239, 1948.
——: Lobotomia transorbitaria. Medicina Latina, 1950.
Larsen, E. F., and Vraa-Jensen, G.: Ischaemic changes in the brain following electroshock therapy. Acta psychiat. et neurol. scandinav. *28*:75, 1953.
Larson, A. N., Hamlon, J. S., and Sines, L. K.: A note on the clinical effects of perphenazine at very high dosages. Am. J. Psychiat. *116*:456, 1959.
Lasagna, L., and DeKornfeld, Th. J.: Metho-

trimeprazine. A new phenothiazine derivatives with analgesic properties. J.A.M.A. *178*:887, 1961.
Lascelles, C. F., and Levene, L. J.: A study of the use of azacyclonal hydrochloride (Frenquel) in chronic schizophrenia. J. Ment. Sc. *105*:247, 1959.
Lasky, J. J., Klett, C. J., Caffey, Jr., E. M., Bennett, J. L., Rosenblum, M. P., and Hollister, L. E.: Drug treatment of schizophrenic patients. A comparative evaluation of chlorpromazine, chlorprothixene, fluphenazine, reserpine, thioridazine and triflupromazine. Dis. Nerv. Syst. *23*:698, 1962.
Lathrop, D. D.: Evaluation of Deprol in psychiatric out-patients. Comments on a double-blind technique. Dis. Nerv. Syst. *20*:216, 1959.
Laties, V. G., and Weiss, B.: A critical review of the efficacy of meprobamate (Miltown, Equanil) in the treatment of anxiety. J. Chron. Dis. *7*:500, 1958.
Lauter, H.: Die psychiatrische Pharmakotherapie und ihre Stellung im Behandlungsplan endogener Psychosen. Münch. med. Wschr. *104*:2236, 1962.
LaValette, R. De: Dynamics of the effect of electroshock in schizophrenia. Rev. Cubana di Neurol. e Psiquiat, *23*, 1946.
La Verne, A. A.: Rapid coma technic of carbon dioxide therapy. *In* Meduna: Carbon Dioxide Therapy. Springfield: Charles C Thomas, 1958.
——: Narco-Stimulation. Amer. J. Psychiat. *115*:738, 1959.
——, and Herman, M.: An evaluation of carbon dioxide therapy. Am. J. Psychiat. *112*:107, 1955.
Lawrence, R. D., Meyer, A., and Nevin, S.: The neuropathology of hypoglycemia. Quart. J. Med. *35*:181, 1942.
Leahy, M. R., and Martin, I. C. A.: Double-blind comparison of nortriptyline and amitriptyline in depressive illness. Brit. J. Psychiat. *113*:1433, 1967.
——, Rose, J. T., and Plowman, R.: A preliminary study of phenoxypropazine in the treatment of depression. Amer. J. Psychiat. *119*:986, 1963.
Le Beau, J.: Psycho-chirurgie et fonctions mentales. Techniques, résultats, applications physiologiques. Paris: Masson, 1954.
Lecomte, G., Certhaux, A., and Garrabè, J.: Chlorpromazine en perfusion continuée dans quelques états psychopatiques. Encéphale *45*:382, 1956.
Leduc, S.: Production du sommeil et de l'anesthésie générale et locale par le courant électrique. Compt. rend. Acad. de sc. *199*:135, 1902; *878*:135, 1902.
Leestma, J. E., and Koenig, K. L.: Sudden death and phenothiazines. A current controversy. Arch. Gen. Psychiat. *18*:137, 1968.
Leger, Y.: A four-year appraisal of thioridazine. Amer. J. Psychiat. *123*:728, 1966.
Leggeri, G.: Electrochoc-thérapie intensive (méthode d'annihilation) dans le traitement de sujets criminels particuliers. Ann. med.-psychol. *114*:1, 1956.
Lehmann, H. E.: A dynamic concept of the action of chlorpromazine at physiological and psychological levels. Encéphale *45*: 1113, 1956.
——, and Ban, T. A. (Eds.): Toxicity and adverse reaction studies with neuroleptics and antidepressants. Quebec, Psychopharmac. Res. Ass. Publ. No. 3, 1968.
——, ——, and Naltchayan, E.: Metronidazole in the treatment of the alcoholic. Psychiat. & Neurol. *152*:395, 1966.
——, and Bos, C.: The advantages of nitrous oxide inhalation in psychiatric treatment. Am. J. Psychiat. *104*:164, 1947.
——, Cahn, C. H., and de Verteuil, R. L.: The treatment of depressive conditions with imipramine (G.22355). Canad. Psychiat. Ass. J. *3*:155, 1958.
——, and Hanrahan, G. E.: Chlorpromazine. New inhibiting agent for psychomotor excitement and manic states. Arch. Neurol. & Psychiat. *71*:227, 1954.
——, and Knight, D. A.: Psychophysiologic testing with a new phrenotropic drug. *In:* Trifluoperazine. Philadelphia: Lea and Febiger, 1958.
Leibbrand, W.: Gerichtspsychiatrische Folgen der ambulaten Behandlung mit Elektroschock. Nervenarzt *20*:63, 1949.
Leiberman, D. M.: Tranquillising drugs in psychiatry. Brit. Med. J. *1*:512, 1956.
——, Hoenig, J., and Auerbach, I.: Insulin coma and ECT in schizophrenia. J. Neurol. Neurosurg. and Psychiat. *20*:108, 1957.
Leinefelder, P. J., and Burian, H. M.: Mellaril intoxication of retina with full restitution of function. Invest. Ophthal. *3*:466, 1964.
Lemere, F.: Effects on electroencephalogram of various agents used in treating schizophrenia. J. Neurophysiol. *1*:590, 1938.
——: Isoniazid treatment in psychiatric patients. A.M.A. Arch. Neurol. & Psychiat. *71*:624, 1954.
——: The treatment of psychotic complications of porphyria with electroshock. Am. J. Psychiat. *111*:41, 1954.
——: Habit forming properties of meprobamate. Arch. Neurol. & Psychiat. *76*:205, 1956.
——: JB-516 and iproniazid. Am. J. Psychiat. *115*:554, 1958.
——: Negative results in the treatment of depression with imipramine hydrochloride (Tofranil). Am. J. Psychiat. *116*:258, 1959.
——: Tranylcypromine (Parnate) a new monoamine oxidase inhibitor. Am. J. Psychiat. *117*:249, 1960.
Lenke, D., Brock, N., and Neteler, B.: Zur Pharmakologie und Toxikologie des Neurolepticums 3-Chlor-10-(γ-[N′-β′-(1″-methyl-2″-oxo-imidazolidyl-3″),-aethyl-N-piperazinyl]-propyl)-phenothiazin-dihydrochlorid. I. Mitteilung: Pharmakologie. Arzneim.-Forsch. *17*:317, 1967.
Leon, C. A.: A non-reported side effect of imipramine. Amer. J. Psychiat. *118*:455, 1961.
Leonard, R.: Thioridazine in the plateaued patient. Dis. Nerv. Syst. *29*:462, 1968.
Lerman, J.: Insulin resistance. The role of

immunity in its production. Am. J. Ment. Sc. *207*:354, 1954.
Lesse, S.: An evaluation of promazine hydrochloride in psychiatric practice. Am. J. Psychiat. *113*:984, 1957.
——: Electroshock therapy and the tranquilizing drugs. J.A.M.A. *170*:1791, 1959.
Lester, D.: Study of prolonged coma following insulin shock. Am. J. Psychiat. *95*:1083, 1939.
Letailleur, N., Le Borgney, and Lebrun, C.: Essai de la Lévomèpromazine (7044.RP) dan les états dépressifs. Sem. des Hôp.-Sem. Méd. *34*:758, 1958.
——, Morin, J., Demay, J., and Monnerie, R.: La chlorpromazine dans le traitement des délires aigus et subaigus alcooliques. Encéphale *45*:738, 1956.
Leuner, H.: Die Experimentelle Psychose. Berlin-Göttingen-Heidelberg, Springer, 1962.
——: Über den Missbrauch von LSD-25. Pharmakopsychiatrie *1*:275, 1968.
——: Ist die Verwendung von LSD-25 für die experimentelle Psychiatrie und in der Psychotherapie heute noch vertretbar? Nervenarzt *39*:356, 1968.
Levin, S., Greenblatt, M., Healey, M. M., and Solomon, H. C.: Electroencephalographic effects of bilateral prefrontal lobotomy. Am. J. Psychiat. *106*:174, 1949.
Levine, J., and Ludwig, A. M.: The LSD controversy. Compr. Psychiat. *5*:314, 1964.
——, Rinkel, M., and Greenblatt, M.: Psychological and physiological effects of intravenous pervitin. Am. J. Psychiat. *105*:429, 1948.
Levinson, F., and Meyer, V.: Personality changes in relation to psychiatric status following orbital cortex undercutting. Brit. J. Psychiat. *111*:207, 1965.
Levy, L., Cameron, D. E., and Aitken, R. C. B.: Observation on two psychotomimetic drugs of piperidine derivation—CI.395 (Sernyl) and CI.400. Am. J. Psychiat. *116*: 843, 1960.
Levy, N. A., and Grinker, R. R.: Psychological observations in affective psychoses treated with combined convulsive shock and psychotherapy. J. Nerv. & Ment. Dis. *97*:623, 1943.
——, Serota, H. M., and Grinker, R. R.: Disturbances in brain function following convulsive shock therapy. Arch. Neurol. & Psychiat. *47*:1009, 1942.
Levy, S.: Fatal massive gastric hemorrhage as an immediate complication of *metrazol* shock therapy. Am. J. Psychiat. *107*:468, 1950.
——, and Perry, H. A.: Narco-synthesis immediately following insulin shock. J. Nerv. & Ment. Dis. *106*:137, 1947.
——, and Perry, H. A.: Psychosis with hematoporphyuria. Clinical report of a case. Arch. Neurol. & Psychiat. *61*:699, 1949.
Lewin, W.: Observations on selective leucotomy. J. Neurol., Neurosurg., & Psychiat. *24*:37, 1961.
Lewis, A.: *In*: P. B. Bradley, P. Deniker, and C. Radouc-Thomas: Neuropsychopharmacology. Amsterdam: Elsevier, 1959.
Lewis, N. D. C.: The present status of shock therapy of mental disorders. Bull. New York Acad. Med. *19*:227, 1943.
Leyrie, J.: Les indications d'une hydrazine I.M.A.O. (nialamide) dans le traitement des névroses asthéniques et hypochondriaques. (A propos de 70 cures ambulatoires). Ann. méd.-psychol. *123/1*:745, 1965.
Liberson, W. T.: Brief stimulus therapy. Am. J. Psychiat. *105*:28, 1948.
——, and Wilcox, P. H.: Electric convulsive therapy: comparison of "brief stimuli technique" with Friedman Wilcox-Reiter technique. Dig. Neurol. & Psychiat. *8*:292, 1945.
Lidbeck, W. L.: Pathologic changes in the brain after electric shock. J. Neuropath. & Exper. Neurol. *3*:81, 1944.
Liebaldt, G.: Reserpintodesfälle. Nervenarzt *29*:110, 1958.
——: Permeabilitätsverhalten bei Resperpin- und Orphenadrin-Anwendung. Tierexperimentelle Untersuchungen. Med. Welt 1876:1960.
Liebert, E.: Spontaneous convulsions following metrazol treatment. J.A.M.A. *118*: 119, 1942.
Liepmann. W.: Über das Koma and Reflexanomalien bei der Insulinschocktherapie. Schweiz. Arch. f. Neurol. u. Psychiat. *40*:133, 1947.
Lieser, H.: Heilkrämpfe als lebensrettende Therapie. Med. Wchnschr. *6*:350, 1957.
Lindemann, E.: Psychological changes in normal and abnormal individuals under the influence of sodium amytal. Am. J. Psychiat. *11*:6, 1932.
Lindner, M.: Das "organische Schocksyndrom" im Rorschachtest. Arch. f. Psychiat. *181*:577, 1949.
Lindstrom, P.: Prefrontal ultrasonic irradiation—a substitute for lobotomy. A.M.A. Arch. Neurol. & Psychiat. *72*:399, 1954.
——, Moench, L. G., and Rovnanek, A.: Prefrontal sonic treatment. Amer. J. Psychiat. *120*:487, 1963.
Ling, T. M., and Buckman, J.: The treatment of anxiety with lysergic acid and methyl Phenidate. Practitioner *191*:201, 1963.
Lingjaerde, O.: Tetrabenazine: a new atarache with reserpire-like action. Nord. med. *62*:1576, 1959.
——: Tetrabenazine (Nitomane) in the treatment of psychoses. With a discussion on the central mode of action of tetrabenazine and reserpine. Acta Psychiat. Scand. *39*: sppl. 170, 1963.
——, and Schiøth, A.: Perphenazine: a new ataractic. Tidaakr. norske laegefor. *78*:278, 1958.
Lingley, J. R., and Robbins, L. L.: Fractures following electroshock therapy. Radiology *48*:124, 1947.
Linn, L., and Ottenheimer, J. G.: Cardiac complications in electroshock therapy. Dis. Nerv. Syst. *10*:8, 1949.
——, and Rosen, S. R.: Brief shock therapy—adjuvant to psychotherapy. Psychiatric Quart. *24*:506, 1950.
Lipton, M. B., Tamarin, S., and Lotesta, P.:

Test evidence of personality change and prognosis by means of the Rorschach Wechsler Bellevue test on 17 insulin treated paranoid schizophrenics. Psychiat. Quart. *25*:434, 1951.
Livingston, K. E.: Cingulate cortex isolation for treatment of psychoses and psychoneuroses. Res. Publ. Ass. Nerv. Ment. Dis. *31*:374, 1953.
Ljungberg, E.: Some observations on the behavior of the blood glutathione, particularly during insulin shock therapy. Acta psychiat. et neur., Suppl. *47*:172, 1947.
Loevenhart, A. S., Lorenz, W. F., and Waters, R. W.: Cerebral stimulation. J.A.M.A. *92*:880, 1929.
Loewenbach, H.: and Lyman, R. S.: The electroencephalogram in electrically induced convulsions on rabbits. J. Neurol., Neurosurg. & Psychiat. *3*:336, 1940.
——, and Stainbrook, E. J.: Observations on mental patients after electro-shock. Am. J. Psychiat. *98*:828, 1942.
Loftus, T. A., Clark, D. L., Crouse, F. R., Dillon, T. E., Jones, D. J., and LeFever, H. E., Jr.: Negative results with chlorpromazine and benactyzine in a group of chronic psychotics. Paper read at the A.P.A. Philadelphia, April 1959.
Logothetis, J.: Spontaneous epileptic seizures and electroencephalographic changes in the course of phenothiazine therapy. Neurology *17*:869, 1967.
Lomas, J.: Treatment of schizophrenia: Pacatal and chlorpromazine compared. Brit. Med. J. *2*:78, 1957.
Longmire, Jr., W. T., and Davis, H. K.: Acute imipramine intoxication. Amer. J. Psychiat. *120*:400, 1963.
Loo, P., Menier, J., and Fanous, O.: Un cas d'intoxication par le Tofranil. Ann. méd. psychol. *122/II*: 69, 1964.
Loomer, H. P., Saunders, J. C., and Kline, N. S.: A clinical and pharmacodynamic evaluation of iproniazid as a psychic energizer. A.P.A. Psychiatric Research Reports. *8*:129, 1957.
Loomis, T. A., and West, T. C.: Comparative sedative effects of a barbiturate and some tranquilliser drugs on normal subjects. J. Pharmacol. & Exp. Therap. *122*: 525, 1958.
López-Ibor, J.: Limited indications for the use of leucotomy. Lisbon: Psychosurgery, 1949.
——: Indications respectives des méthodes de choc. Congrès Internat. de Psychiat. *4*:85, 1950.
Lorentzen, K. A.: The central nervous system during insulin shock. Acta psychiat. et neurol., Suppl. *64*, 1950.
Lotsof, E. J., and Yobst, J.: Electric shock therapy and the mecholyl test. Psychosom. med. *19*:374, 1957.
Lovett Doust, J. W., and Schneider, R. A.: Rhythmic sensory bombardment therapy. Am. J. Psychiat. *110*:854, 1954.
Lowinger, L., and Huddleson, J. H.: Complications in electric shock therapy. Am. J. Psychiat. *102*:594, 1946.
Luby, E. D., Cohen, B. D., Rosenbaum, G. Gottlieb, J. S., and Kelley, R.: Study of a new schizophrenomimetic drug—Sernyl. A.M.A. Arch. Neurol. & Psychiat. *81*:363, 1959.
Lucas, A. R.: Gilles de la Tourette's disease in children: Treatment with haloperidol. Amer. J. Psychiat. *124*:243, 1967.
Luhan, J. A., and Tuteur, W.: Insulin coma therapy in advanced pregnancy without harm to mother or child. J.A.M.A. *159*: 112, 1955.
Lundbaek, K., and Magnussen, G.: Carbohydrate metabolism in insulin shock therapy. Acta med. Scandinav. *105*:447, 1940.
Lund-Johansen, P.: Shock after administration of phenothiazines in patients with pheochromocytoma. Acta med. Scand. *172*: 525, 1962.
Lunn, V.: Experimental studies on electroshock treatment. II. Variations in the skin temperature following E.C.T. Acta psychiat. et neurol. *26*:7, 1951.
——: and Trolle, E.: On the initial impairment of consciousness following electric convulsive therapy. Acta psychiat. et neurol. *24*:33, 1949.
Lustig, B.: Über therapeutische Methoden in der neueren sowietischen Psychiatrie. Fortschr. Neurol. u. Psychiat. *26*:209, 1958.
Luttges, M. W., and McGaugh, J. L.: Permanence of retrograde amnesia produced by electro-convulsive shock. Science *156*:408, 1967.
Lüttke, S., and Koch, R. D.: Psychiatrische Schockbehandlung mit Bemegrid. Dtsch. Gesundheitswesen *17*:1027, 1962.
Lyerly, J. G.: Transsection of the deep association fibers of the prefrontal lobes in certain mental disorders. South. Surgeon *8*:426, 1939.
Lyon, R. L. L.: Drug treatment of Huntington's chorea. A trial with thiopropazate. Brit. Med. J. *1*:1308, 1962.
Lytton, G. J., and Knobel, M.: Diagnosis and treatment of behaviour disorders in children. Dis. Nerv. Syst. *20*:334, 1959.
Mackay, G. W.: Leucotomy in the treatment of psychopathic feebleminded patients in a state mental deficiency institution. J. Ment. Sc. *94*:834, 1948.
MacKinnon, I. H., Hoch, P. H., Cammer, L., and Waelsch, H. B.: The use of malononitrile in the treatment of mental illnesses: Preliminary report. Am. J. Psychiat. *105*: 686, 1949.
Maclay, W. S.: Death due to treatment. Proc. Royal Soc. Med. *46*:13, 1953.
Madgwick, J. R. A., McNeill, D. L. M., Driver, M., and Preston, G. C.: Stelazine (trifluoperazine): a preliminary report on a clinical trial. J. Ment. Sc. *104*:1195, 1958.
Maggs, R.: Treatment of manic illness with lithium carbonate. Brit. J. Psychiat. *109*: 56, 1963.
——, and Ellison, R. M.: Five year follow-up of results of reserpine therapy in mental hospital practice. J. Ment. Sc. *106*:590, 1960.
Maholick, L. T., and Warkentin. J.: Hypnosis in electric shock treatment. Am. J. Psychiat. *105*:623, 1949.

Mahoney, V. P., and Herskovitz, H. H.: Hypoglycemic shock therapy produced by insulin administered intravenously. J. Nerv. & Ment. Dis. *95*:265, 1942.

Maier, H. W.: Discussion. Encéphale *31*: 294, 1936.

Malamud, N.: Fatalities resulting from treatment with subshock doses of insulin. Am. J. Psychiat. *105*:373, 1948.

Malamud, W., Barton, W. E., Fleming, A. M., Middleton, P. McK., Friedman, T. T., and Schleifer, M. J.: The evaluation of the effects of derivatives of Rauwolfia in the treatment of schizophrenia. Am. J. Psychiat. *114*:193, 1957.

——, and Zheutlin, A.: Fatal cardiac complications during electroshock treatment. J. Nerv. & Ment. Dis. *117*:458, 1953.

Malitz, S., Esecover, H., Wilkens, B., and Hoch, P. H.: Some observations on psilocybin, a new hallucinogen in volunteer subjects. Compr. Psychiat. *1*:8, 1960.

——, and Hoch, P. H.: Preliminary evaluation of new phenothiazine derivative NP. 207. Psychiat. Quart. 30:633, 1956.

——, ——, and Lesse, S.: A two-year evaluation of chlorpromazine in clinical research and practice. Am. J. Psychiat. *113*:540, 1956.

——, and Wilkens, B.: Preliminary evaluation of Tofranil in a combined in-patient and out-patient setting. Canad. Psychiat. Ass. J. *4*:152, 1959.

Malzberg, B.: Outcome of insulin treatment of 1000 patients with dementia praecox. Psychiatric Quart. *12*:528, 1938.

——: The outcome of electric shock therapy in the New York Civil State Hospitals. Psychiatric Quart. *17*:154, 1943.

Mandel, W., and Evans, Ph.: Comparison of butyrylperazine and trifluoperazine in chronic schizophrenic subjects. Amer. J. Psychiat. *119*:70, 1962.

Mandell, A. J., Markham, C., and Fowler, W.: Parkinson's syndrome, depression, and imipramine. A preliminary report. California Med. *95*:12, 1961.

Mann, A. M., Catterson, A. G., and MacPherson, A. S.: Toxicity of imipramine: report on serious side effects and massive overdosage. Canad. M.A.J. *81*:23, 1959.

——, and Lehmann, H.: The eosinophile level in psychiatric conditions. Canad. M.A.J. *66*:52, 1952.

Mann, S. H., Depasquale, N., and Paterson, R.: Cerebrospinal fluid-glutamic oxalacetic acid transaminase in patients receiving electroconvulsive therapy and in neurologic diseases. Neurology *10*:381, 1960.

Manning, E. L., and Hollander, W. M.: Glaucoma and electroshock therapy. Am. J. Ophth. *37*: 857, 1954.

Maragoni, B. A.: Use of perphenazine in 60 patients with anxiety and tension. Amer. Pract. & Digest of Treatment. 8:1959, 1957.

Marchand, L., and Guirand, P.: Neurinome malin du quatriéme ventricule avec propagation intrabulbaire chez un schizophréne. Mort au cours d'un électrochoc. Ann. Méd.-psychol. *115*:108, 1957.

Margolis, L. H., and Goble, J. L.: Lenticular opacities with prolonged phenothiazine therapy. A potential hazard with all phenothiazine derivatives. J.A.M.A. *193*: 7, 1965.

Maria, B., Böhm, T., and Andorjani, F.: La terapia acetilcolinica negli ammalati di mente con speciale riguardo al meccanismo d'azione. Riv. Sper. Freniat. *84*:746, 1960.

Mariotti, E., and Sciuti, M.: La terapia intracerebrale nelle malattie mentali. Contributo alla neurchirurgia delle psicosi. Riv. sper. di fren. *61*:870, 1937.

Markham, J. D., and Hoff, E. C.: Toxic manifestations in the antabuse-alcohol reaction. Study of electrocardiographic changes. J.A.M.A. *152*:1597, 1953.

Marks, L. J., Weiss, D. M., Leftin, J. H., and Rossmeisl, E. C.: The adrenocortical response to insulin coma. J. Clin. Endocrinol & Metabol. *18*:235, 1958.

Marley, E.: Modification of insulin resistance. J. Ment. Sc. *102*:576, 1956.

——, and Bartholomew, A. A.: Clinical aspects of susceptibility to methylpentynol. J. Neur. Neurosurg. & Psychiat. *21*:129, 1958.

——, and Chambers, J. S. W.: Toxic effects and side effects of methylpentynol. Brit. Med. J. *2*:1467, 1956.

Marquis, D. G., Kelly, E. L., Miller, J. G., Gerard, R. W., and Rapoport, A.: Experimental studies of behavioral effects of meprobamate on normal subjects. Ann. New York Acad. Sc. *67*:701, 1957.

Marshall, W., and Tarwater, J. S.: Use of histamine phosphate and peptone solution in the treatment of neuroses and psychoses. J. Nerv. & Ment. Dis. *88*:36, 1938.

Martin, K. E., Overley, H. O., and Krone, R. E.: Pipradol combined therapy for geriatric and agitated patients. Int. Rec. Med. Gen. Practice Clin. *170*:33, 1957.

Martin, W. L., Ford, H. F., McDanald, E. C., Jr., and Towler, M. L.: Clinical evaluation of unilateral EST. Amer. J. Psychiat. *121*: 1087, 1965.

Martin, W. R., Gorodetsky, C. M., and McClane, T. K.: An experimental study in the treatment of narcotic addicts with cyclazocine. Clin. Pharmacol. Ther. *7*:455, 1966.

Marx, H.: Über die neuroleptische Behandlung der Psychosen und die Bedeutung der Dauermedikation. Weiterer Bericht über die Prüfung des Thiaxanthenderivates Ciatyl. Med. Welt *17 N.F.*:446, 1966.

Marzynsky, M.: Results of the insulin shock therapy in schizophrenia. Am. J. Psychiat. *94*:240, 1938.

Mason, E.: Peroneal nerve palsy seen in patients treated with electroconvulsive therapy. Am. J. Psychiat. *112*:299, 1955.

Mason, T. H., and Hamby, W. B.: Relief of morphine addiction by prefrontal lobotomy. J.A.M.A. *136*:1039, 1948.

Mason-Browne, H. L.: Perphenazine in Practice. Canad. M. A. J. *79*:985, 1958.

Massazza, A.: Il sistema neuromusculare durante l'insulinoterapia. Atti del convegno sulla terapia moderna della schizophrenia. Milano: 1937.

Masserman, J. H., Arieff, A., Pechtel, C., and Klehr, H.: The effects of direct interrupted electroshock on experimental neuroses. J. Nerv. & Ment. Dis. *112*:384, 1950.

——, and Jacques, M. G.: Effects of cerebral electroshock on experimental neuroses in cats. Am. J. Psychiat. *104*:92, 1947.

Mathews, F. P.: Dartal: a clinical appraisal. Amer. J. Psychiat. *114*:1034, 1958.

Matthew, J. R., and Constan, E.: Complications following ECT over a three-year period in a state institution. Amer. J. Psychiat. *120*:1119, 1964.

Matthew, J. R., and Constan, E.: Pharmacogenetics in pre-ECT-medication. Amer. J. Psychiat. *121*:490, 1964.

Matthews, A. E. B.: Double-blind trials of promazine in labour. Brit. Med. J. *2*:423, 1963.

Maurice, H.: Des complications phlebitiques au cours des traitements par les neuroleptiques. Encéphale *45*:797, 1956.

May, A. R., Whiteley, J. S., and Gradwell, B. G.: Trifluoperazine (Stelazine) in psychoneuroses: a clinical assessment. J. Ment. Sc. *105*:1059, 1959.

May, P. R., and Tuma, A. H.: Treatment of schizophrenia. An experimental study of 5 treatment methods. Brit. J. Psychiat. *111*:503, 1965.

May, R. H., Selymes, P., Weekley, R. D., and Potts, A. M.: Thioridazine therapy: results and complications. J. Nerv. & Ment. Dis. *130*:230, 1960.

Mayer, E. E.: Prefrontal lobotomy and the courts. J. Crim. Law and Criminol. *38*:576, 1948.

Mayer-Gross, W.: Convulsive therapy in outpatient department. Brit. M. J. *1*:62, 1941.

——: Retrograde amnesia. Lancet *2*:603, 1943.

——: Electric convulsion treatment in patients over 60. J. Ment. Sc. *91*:101, 1945.

——: A propos de la théorie de l'effet de la leucotomie sur les symptomes psychotiques. Encéphale *38*:317, 1949.

——: Insulin coma therapy of schizophrenia: Some critical remarks on Dr. Sakel's report. J. Ment. Sc. *97*:132, 1951.

McAndrew, J., Berkey, B., and Matthews, C.: The effects of dominant and nondominant unilateral ECT as compared to bilateral ECT. Amer. J. Psychiat. *124*:69, 1967.

McCable, E. S., and Wilson, W.: Dangerous cardiac effects of tetraethylthiuram disulfide (Antabuse) therapy in alcoholism. Arch. Int. Med. *94*:259, 1954.

McClure, C. W., Papas, P. N., Speare, G. S., Palmer, E., Slattery, J. J., Konefal, S. N., Henken, B. S., Wood, C. A., and Ceresia, G. B.: Treatment of depression—new technics and therapy. Am. Pract. & Digest Treat. *10*:1525, 1959.

McDonald, I. M., Perkins, M., Marjerrison, G., and Podilsky, M.: A controlled comparison of amitriptyline and electroconvulsive therapy in the treatment of depression. Amer. J. Psychiat. *122*:1427, 1966.

McFoos, L. G.: Prochlorperazine (Compazine) in emotional disturbances. Dis. Nerv. Syst. *18*:430, 1957.

McGrath, D.: Spontaneous hypoglycaemia and diabetes mellitus associated with the insulin coma therapy of schizophrenia. J. Ment. Sc. *96*:285, 1950.

McIntyre, H. D., Mayfield, F. H., and McIntyre, A. P.: Ventromedial quadrant coagulation in the treatment of psychoses and neuroses. Am. J. Psychiat. *111*:112, 1954.

McKegney, F. P., and Panzetta, A. F.: An unusual fatal outcome of electro-convulsive therapy. Amer. J. Psychiat. *120*:398, 1963.

McKenzie, M. E., and Roswell-Harris, D.: A contolled trial of prothipendyl (Tolnate) in mentally subnormal patients. Brit. J. Psychiat. *112*:95, 1966.

McKissock, W.: Technique of pre-frontal leucotomy. J. Ment. Sc. *89*:194, 1943.

——: Rostral leucotomy. Lancet *2*:91, 1951.

——: Discussion on psychosurgery. Proceed. Roy. Soc. Med. *53*:206, 1959.

McLardy, T.: Thalamic projections to frontal cortex in man. IVe Congrès Neurol. Internat., Paris *11*:24, 1949.

——: Uremic and trophic deaths following leucotomy. J. Neurol., Neurosurg. & Psychiat. *13*:106, 1950.

——, and Davies, T. L: Clinical and pathological observations on relapse after successful leucotomy. J. Neurol., Neurosurg. & Psychiat. *12*:231, 1949.

——, and Meyer, A.: Anatomical correlates of improvement after leucotomy. J. Ment. Soc. *95*:182, 1949.

McLean, R. E. G.: Imipramine hydrochloride ('Tofranil') and enuresis. Amer. J. Psychiat. *117*:551, 1960.

McNair, D. M., Goldstein, A. P., Lorr, M., Cibelli, L. A., and Roth, I.: Some effects of chlordiazepoxide and meprobamate with psychiatric outpatients. Psychopharmacologia *7*:256, 1965.

McNair, F. E.: Intravenous chlorpromazine. Canad. M. A. J. *79*:291, 1958.

McNeil, B. H., Dewan, J. G., Meyers, C. R., Procter, L. D., and Goodwin, J. E.: Parallel psychological, psychiatric and physiological findings in schizophrenic patients under insulin shock treatment. Am. J. Psychiat. *98*:393, 1941.

McNichol, R.: Delayed complications of E.C.T.—"Crush Syndrome". Amer. J. Psychiat. *115*:346, 1958.

McPherson, F. M., and LeGassicke, J.: A single-patient, self-controlled and self-recorded trial of Wy 3498. Brit. J. Psychiat. *111*: 149, 1965.

Medlicott, R. W.: Electronarcosis treatment of schizophrenia. New Zealand M. J. *46*:280, 1947.

——: Brief stimuli electroconvulsive therapy. New Zealand M. J. *47*:29, 1948.

——: The place of electronarcosis in psychiatric treatment. New Zealand M. J. *53*:128, 1954.

Meduna, L. J.: Die Konvulsionstherapie der Schizophrenie. Halle: Carl Marhold, 1937.

——: General discussion of the cardiazol

therapy. Am. J. Psychiat. *94* (Supp.):40, 1938.
——: Pharmaco-dynamic treatment of psychoneurosis. Dis. Nerv. Syst. *8*:2 1947.
——: Carbon dioxide therapy. Springfield, Ill.: Charles C Thomas, 1950.
——: Clinical and biochemical indications of the convulsive and of the carbon dioxide treatments. Congrès Internat. de Psychiat. *4*:135, 1950.
——: Physiologic background to CO_2 treatment of neuroses. Am. J. Psychiat. *110*: 664, 1954.
——, ed.: Carbon Dioxide Therapy. Springfield: Charles C Thomas, 1958.
——, and Abood, L. G.: Studies of a new drug (Ditran) in depressive states. J. Neuropsychiat. *1*:20, 1959.
——, and Friedmann, E.: The convulsive-irritative therapy of the psychoses. J.A.M.A. *112*:6, 1939.
Meggendorfer, F.: Zur Klinik des Elektrokrampfes. Nervenarzt *15*:49, 1942.
Meier-Ruge, W.: Medikamentöse Retinopathie. Zwanglose Abhandlungen aus dem Gebiet der normalen und pathologischen Anatomie, Heft 18. Stuttgart, Thieme, 1967.
Mellinger, Th. J.: Serum concentrations of thioridazine after different oral medication forms. Amer. J. Psychiat. *121*:1119, 1965.
——, Mellinger, E. M., and Smith, W. T.: Urine tests for chlorprothixene. Amer. J. Psychiat. *120*:1111, 1964.
Melrose, A. G., and Roy, J. R.: Late prognosis of chlorpromazine jaundice. Brit. Med. J. *1*:818, 1959.
Mendel, W. M.: Observations on the comparative effects of tranquilizers on patients previously treated with prochlorperazine. Am. J. Psychiat. *115*:406, 1958.
Mendels, J.: Thioproperazine-induced lactation. Amer. J. Psychiat. *121*:190, 1964.
——: Electroconvulsive therapy and depression. Brit. J. Psychiat. *111*:675, 1965.
Mendes, J. M., Fragoso, and Rosario, J. A.: Psychopathologic study of certain depressions treated with Nialamide. J. da Soc. das Ciencias Med. de Lisboa (supp.), Nov. 1959.
Meneghini, P., and Fasce, M.: Influenze della shock terapia elettrica, insulinica e cardiazolica sull'emopoiesi midollare. Arch. "E. Maragliano" pat. *3*:731, 1948.
Menguy, R. B., Bollman, J. L., Grindlay, H. H., and Cain, J. B.: Biliary stasis produced by chlorpromazine. Proc. Staff Meet. Mayo Clinic. *30*:601, 1955.
Menninger, W. C.: Arterial hypertension following metrazol shock therapy. Arch. Neurol. & Psychiat. *49*:120, 1943.
Menzies, E. C.: Treatment of schizophrenia by hypoglycemia. Canad. M.A.J. *42*:320, 1940.
Merli, S.: Todesfall nach Elektroschock. Wien, Klin. Wschr. 797, 1961.
Merrem, G.: Die frontopolare Lobotomie. Psychiat., Neurol. u. med. Psychol, *2*:257, 1950.
Mercier, J., and Dessaigne, S.: Sur le mécanisme de l'action neurodépressive centrale du dicarbamate de méthyl-N-propyl propanediol (meprobamate). Arch. Int. Pharmacodyn. *121*:38, 1959.
Messmer, E.: Die Anwendung von Prothipendyl zur Behandlung unruhiger, schlafgestörter Zerebralsklerotiker. Med. Welt 2571:1960.
Mettler, F. A. (Ed.): Selective partial ablation of the frontal cortex. New York: Paul B. Hoeber, 1949.
——, and Rowland, L. P.: Relation of the trephine opening (Freeman-Watts lobotomy point) to the underlying cerebrum. Tr. Am. Neurol. A. p. 156, 1949.
Meulenbeld, G. J.: The treatment of presenile and senile depressions with orphenadrine. Disipal Symposium. Amersfoort, Holland: Brocades, 1957.
Meyer, A.: Anatomical lessons from prefrontal leucotomy. Congrès Internat. de Psychiat. Paris: Hermann & Cie., 1950.
——, and Beck E.: Prefrontal leucotomy and related operations. Anatomical aspects of success and failure. London: Oliver and Boyd, 1954.
——, ——, and McLardy, T.: Prefrontal leucotomy: A neuro-anatomical report. Brain *70*:18, 1947.
——, and McLardy, T.: Posterior cuts in prefrontal leucotomy: A clinicopathological study. J. Ment. Sc. *94*:555, 1948.
——, and ——: Clinico-anatomical studies of frontal lobe function based on leucotomy material. J. Ment. Sc. *95*:403, 1949.
——, and ——: Neuropathology in relation to mental disease. Recent Progr. Psychiat. *2*:284, 1950.
——, and Teare, D.: Cerebral fat embolism after electrical convulsion therapy. Brit. M.J. July, 14, 1945, p. 42.
Meyer, H. H.: Die Winterschlafbehandlung in der Psychiatrie und Neurologie. Dt. Med. Wchnschr. *78*:1097, 1953.
——: Die Behandlung exogener Psychosen mit Phenothiazinderivaten. Encéphale *45*: 524, 1956.
——: Die Insulin- und Heilkrampftherapie und ihre Stellung zur Pharmakotherapie. Arch. f. Psychiat. u. Ztsch. f. d. ges. Neurol. *210*:126, 1967.
Meyer, J. E.: Über Schockamnesien und ihre Beziehung zum Heilverlauf der Psychosen. Arch. Psychiat. *186*:254, 1951.
——, Simon, G., and Stille, D.: Die Therapie der Schizophrenie und der endogenen Depression zwischen 1930 und 1960. Vergleichend-statistische Untersuchungen an einer Universitätsnervenklinik und einem Nervenkrankenhaus. Arch. Psychiat. Nervenkr. *206*:165, 1964.
Meyer, L. M., Heeve, W. L., and Bertscher, R. W., Aplastic anemia after meprobamate therapy. New England J. Med. *256*:1232, 1957.
Meyer-Mickeleit, R. W.: Das Elektroencephalogramm beim Elektrokrampf des Menschen. Arch. Psychiat. *183*:12, 1949.
Michael, S. T.: Impotence during electric shock therapy. Psychiatric Quart. *25*:24, 1951.

——: The menstrual cycle and recovery during shock treatment. Dis. Nerv. Syst. *15*:342, 1954.
Michel, H.: Erfahrungen über die Wirksamkeit der präfrontalen Leukotomie bei chronischen Schizophrenien. Schweiz. Arch. f. Neurol. u. Psychiat. *61*:256, 1948.
Middlefell, R.: The treatment of endogenous depression with phenelzine and its side effects. Proceed. Roy. Coll. of Surg., May 27, 1960.
——, and Edwards, K. C. S.: Hydroxyzine (Atarax) in the relief of tension associated with anxiety neurosis and mild depressive states. J. Ment. Sc. *105*:792, 1959.
Mielke, F. A.: Über das Rauwolfia-Alkaloid Reserpin (Serpasil) in der Psychiatrie. Arch. f. Psychiat. u. Z. Neurol. *194*:263, 1956.
Milch, E. C.: Changes in retinal arteries before convulsions induced by electric shock. Arch. Neurol. & Psychiat. *45*:848, 1941.
Miles, J. E.: Psychosis with phantom limb pain treated by chlorpromazine. Am. J. Psychiat. *112*:1027, 1956.
Miletto, G., and Sacco, J.-J.: Le benzpéridol dans les états d'agitation en neurologie, psychiatrie et gérontologie. Ann. méd.-psychol. *121/II*:228, 1963.
Millar, J.: Trial of fluphenazine in schizophrenia. Brit. J. Psychiat. *109*:428, 1963.
Millar, R. A.: The fluormetric estimation of epinephrine in peripheral venous plasma during insulin hypoglycemia. J. Pharmacol. & Exper. Therap. *118*:435, 1956.
Miller, E. C., and Mathas, J. L.: The use of effectiveness of electrosleep in the treatment of some common psychiatric problems. Amer. J. Psychiat. *122*:460, 1965.
Millet, J. A. B., and Mosse, E. P.: On certain psychological aspects of electroshock therapy. Psychosomatic Med. *6*:226, 1944.
Milligan, W. L.: Psychoneuroses treated with electrical convulsions. Lancet *2*:516, 1946.
——: Treatment of psychoneurosis. Modified CO_2 abreactive technique. Brit. M. J., June *23*:1426, 1951.
Milne, H. B., and Berliner, F.: A clinical trial of Stemetil (prochlorperazine). J. Ment. Sc. *104*:873, 1958.
Misès, R., and Borenstein, S.: Cures prolongées et doses fortes de thioridazine en neuro-psychiatrie infantile. Ann. méd.-psychol. *123/I*:147, 1965.
——, Peron, P., and Perit, J.-M.: Le traitement de l'automutilation chez l'enfant par la lévomépromazine. Ann. méd.-psychol. *119/II*:968, 1961.
Moehlig, R. C.: The anxiety state: its similarity with that produced by rauwolfia drugs. Med. Times. *85*:495, 1957.
Moersch, F. P., and Kernohan, J. W.: Hypoglycemia, neurologic and neuropathologic studies. Arch. Neurol. & Psychiat. *39*:242, 1938.
Moffat, J., and MacLeod, E. C.: "Discontinuous" thioproperazine: A controlled trial in chronic schizophrenia. Brit. J. Psychiat. *110*:851, 1964.
Mølholm Hansen, J., and Siersbaek-Nielsen, K.: Serum protein-bound iodine and serum thyroxine during perphenazine therapy. Acta endocrinol. *55*:136, 1967.
Møller-Madsen. A.: Disulfiram and anaesthesia. Quart. J. Stud. Alc. *18*:349, 1957.
Moniz, E.: Tentatives opératoires dans le traitement de certaines psychoses. Paris: Masson et Cie., 1936.
——: Präfrontale Leukotomie. Arch. f. Psychiat. *181*:591, 1949.
Monnier, M., and Krupp, P.: Elektrophysiologische Analyse zur Wirkung verschiedener Neuroleptika (Chlorpromazin, Reserpin, Tofranil, Meprobamate). Schweiz. med. Wchnschr. *89*:430, 1959.
Monro, A. B.: Electronarcosis in the treatment of schizophrenia. J. Ment. Sc. *96*:254, 1950.
Monroy, M., Teboul, R., Calfayan, J., Ave, M., and Pottier, N.: Bilan de l'utilisation prolongée du Benpéridol dans un service de psychiatrie. Ann. méd.-psychol. *125/I*: 562, 1967.
Montagu, J. D.: Electrical termination of hypoglycemic coma. J. Ment. Sc. *99*:112, 1953.
Montilla, E., Frederik, W. S., and Cass, L. J.: Analgesic effect of methotrimeprazine and morphine. A clinical comparison. Arch. Intern. Med. *111*:725, 1963.
Monza, C.: In tema di leucotomia transorbitaria. Minerva med. *2*:637, 1949.
Moore, C. D., and Friedman, S.: A note on the occurrence of ruptured duodenal ulcer in two patients previously treated with metrazol. Psychiatric Quart. *15*:380, 1941.
Moore, J. N. P., and Martin, E. A.: Trial of reserpine in treatment of schizophrenia. Brit. Med. J. *1*:8, 1957.
Moore, L. E.: Fluphenazine in the treatment of hospitalized mental patients. Amer. J. Psychiat. *119*:987, 1963.
Moore, M. T.: Discussion: Alpers and Hughes—Changes in the brain after electrically induced convulsions in cats. Arch. Neurol & Psychiat. *47*:384, 1942.
——: Electrocerebral shock therapy. A reconsideration of former contraindications. Arch. Neurol. & Psychiat. *57*:693, 1947.
——: A new instrument for performing transorbital leucotomy. Am. J. Psychiat. *105*:741, 1949.
——, Hill, R. L., and Lutz, W. M.: Transorbital leucotomy in a State Hospital program. J.A.M.A. *146*:324, 1951.
Moore, N. P.: Maintenance treatment of chronic psychotics by electrically induced convulsions. J. Ment. Sc. *89*:257, 1943.
Moorehead, C. N., and Knox, S. J.: Imipramine-induced auricular fibrillation. Amer. J. Psychiat. *122*:216, 1965.
Morel. F.: A propos du traitement chirurgical de la démence précoce. Schweiz. Arch. f. Neurol. u. Psychiat. *39*:208, 1937.
Moriarty, J. D.: Evaluation of CO_2 inhalation therapy. Am. J. Psychiat. *110*:765, 1954.
——, and Mebane, J. C.: Clinical uses of deanol (Deaner). Am. J. Psychiat. *115*:941, 1959.
——, and Siemens, J. C.: Electroencephalographic study of electric shock therapy. Arch. Neurol. & Psychiat. *57*:712, 1947.

——, and Weil, A. A.: Combined convulsive therapy and psychotherapy of the neuroses. Arch. Neurol. & Psychiat. *49*:685, 1943.

Morrow, L. E.: Fluphenazine in the long-term treatment of non-hospitalized psychiatric patients. Amer. J. Psychiat. *120*:1008, 1964.

de Morsier, G., and Bersot, H.: Cerebral disorders in provoked hyperinsulinemia. Am. J. Psychiat. *94* (Supp.):143, 1938.

Mosketi, K. V., Belskaya, G. M., and Mouravieva, I. D.: L'expérience de l'application de lithium iodatum pour le traitement de certains états psychotiques. Zh. Nevro-pat. Psikhiat. *63*:92, 1963.

Mosovich, A., and Katzenelbogen, S.: Electroshock therapy, clinical and electroencephalographic studies. J. Nerv. & Ment. Dis. *107*:517, 1948.

Mosse, E. P.: Electroshock and personality structure. J. Nerv. & Ment. Dis. *104*:296, 1946.

Moyer, J. H., Kent, B., Knight, R., Morris, G., Huggins, R., and Handley, C. A.: Laboratory and clinical observations on chlorpromazine (SKF-2061-A), hemodynamic and toxicological studies. Am. J. Ment. Sc. *227*:283, 1954.

——, Kinross-Wright, V., and Finney, R. M.: Chlorpromazine as a therapeutic agent in clinical medicine. A.M.A. Arch. Int. Med. *95*:202, 1955.

——, Pevey, K., and Kinross-Wright, V.: Tranquilizing (ataractic) agents: current evaluation of their clinical use in patients who are not hospitalized. G. P. *15*:97, 1957.

Muir, A.: Acute choreo-athetosis during reserpine therapy. Lancet *2*:507, 1955.

Müller, H.: Die Frage der Dosierung der Insulinbehandlung der Schizophrenie. Allg. Ztschr. f. Psychiat. 108:296, 1938.

——, Müller, J. M., Schlitter, E., and Bein, H. J.: Reserpin, der sedative Wirkstoff aus Rauwolfia Serpentina Benth. Experimentia *8*:338, 1952.

Müller, M.: Insulin- und Cardiazolschockbehandlung der Schizophrenie. Fortschr. d. Neurol., Psychiat. u. Ihrer Grenzgeb. *9*:131, 1937.

——: The insulin therapy of schizophrenia. Am. J. Psychiat. *94* (Supp.): 15, 1938.

——: Die Insulin- und Cardiazolbehandlung in der Psychiatrie. Fortschr. d. Neurol., Psychiat. u. ihrer Grenzgeb. *11*:361, 1939.

——: Die Indikationen der Elektroschockbehandlung bei Depressionen. Schweiz. Arch. f. Neurol. u. Psychiat. *58*:286, 1947.

——: Über die präfrontale Leukotomie. Nervenarzt *19*:97, 1948.

——: Prognose und Therapie der Geisteskrankheiten. Stuttgart: Georg Thieme, 1949.

——: Die Körperlichen Behandlungsverfahren in der Psychiatrie I: Die Insulinbehandlung. Stuttgart: Georg Thieme, 1952.

——: Insulinbehandlung. *In* Psychiatrie der Genewart. I/2 Berlin, Springer, 1963.

Mulvaney, R. B. J.: Treatment of narcotic withdrawal symptoms with thioridazine. Dis. Nerv. Syst. *27*:329, 1966.

Munkvad, Ib.: Treatment of psychoses and psychoneuroses with a new sedative (Suavitil). Acta psychiat. et neurol. scandinav. *30*:729, 1955.

Muratorio, A.: Preliminary report on the use of hydroxyzine hydrochloride in psychiatric therapy. Bull. de la Soc. Medico-Chir. de Pise. *24*: No. 2, 1956.

Murlin, J. R., Clough, H. D., Gibbs, C. B. F., and Stokes, A. M.: Aqueous extracts of pancreas. I. Influence on the carbohydrate metabolism of depancreatized animals. J. Biol. Chem. *56*:253, 1923.

Murphy, J. A., Beardwood, J. T., and Miller M. M.: Report on insulin sensitivity with attempt at passive transfer. J. Allergy *5*:606, 1934.

Murphy, J. P.: Electroencephalograph in lobotomy. Dig. Neurol. & Psychiat. *17*: 419, 949.

Myers, J. D., Olson, R. E., Lewis, J. H., and Moran, T. J.: Xanthomatous biliary cirrhosis following chlorpromazine, with observations indicating overproduction of cholesterol, hyperprothrombinemia, and the development of portal hypertension. Transactions of the Association of American Physicians. *70*:243, 1957.

Myerson, A.: Effect of benzedrine sulphate on mood and fatigue in normal and neurotic persons. Arch. Neurol. & Psychiat. *36*:816, 1936.

——: Experiences with electric shock therapy in mental diseases. New England J. Med. *224*:1081, 1941.

——: Borderline cases treated by electric shock. Am. J. Psychiat. *100*:355, 1943.

——: Prolonged cases of grief reaction treated by electric shock. New England J. Med. *230*:253, 1944.

——, and Myerson, P. G.: Prefrontal lobotomy in the chronic depressive states of old age. New England J. Med. *237*:511, 1947.

Nadeau, G., and Rouleau, Y.: Insulin tolerance in schizophrenia. J. Clin. & Exper. Psychopathol. *14*:69, 1953.

Nahunek, K.: Pentazol-ataraktische Behandlung der Psychosen. Psychiat. Neurol. *137*: 33, 1959.

Nandy, K., and Bourne, G. H.: Effect of centrophenoxine on the lipofuscin pigments in the neurones of senile guinea-pigs. Nature *210*:313, 1966.

Napier, F. J.: Death from electrical convulsion therapy. J. Ment. Sc. *90*:875, 1944.

Nash, H.: The design and conduct of experiments on the psychological effects of drugs. J. Nerv. & Ment. Dis. *128*:129, 1959.

Natenshon, A. L.: Clinical evaluation of Ritalin. Dis. Nerv. Syst. *17*:392, 1956.

The National Institute of Mental Health, Psychopharmacology Service Center, Collaborative Study Group: Phenothiazine treatment in acute schizophrenia. Effectiveness. Arch. Gen. Psychiat. *10*:246, 1964.

Nayrac, P., and Graux, P.: Indications et contra-indications de la Chlorpromazine en psychiatrie. Encéphale *45*:518, 1956.

——, Lorrain, A., and Arnott, G.: Résultats cliniques obtenus chez 82 malades as cours de traitements par le melléril. Considéra-

tions E.E.G. Ann. méd.-psychol. *120/I*: 342, 1962.
Negrin, J.: Studies on shock therapy. J. Nerv. & Ment. Dis. *101*:14, 1945.
——: Selected intracranial cerebral electroshock therapy. A.M.A. Arch. Neurol. & Psychiat. *70*:538, 1953.
Neki, J. S., and Kishore, B.: Narcostimulation in depressive states. Amer. J. Psychiat. *124*:1196, 1968.
Neri, A.: Primi risultati ottenuti con l'impiego del largactil in malati mentali. Encéphale *45*:682, 1956.
Neuburger, K. T., Whithead, R. W., Rutledge, E. K., and Ebaugh, F. G.: Electric shock: pathologic changes in brains of dogs given repeated shocks. Am. J. Ment. Sc. *204*:381, 1942.
Neumann, H.: Klinische und pathophysiologische Aspekte der Therapie schizophrener Kernpsychosen mit Nicotinsäureamid. Nervenarzt *38*:511, 1967.
——, and Peters, U. H.: Neuere Gesichtspunkte bei der Benandlung des Delirium tremens. Med. Welt 1559:1961.
Neveu. P.: Insulinothérapie. *In:* Encyclopédie Médico-Chirurgicale. Paris, 1955.
Newman, R. A., and Fisher, W. R.: Imipramine as a psychoto-mimetic drug in borderline schizophrenics. Amer. J. Psychiat. *121*:77, 1964.
Neymann, C. A.: Artificial fever. Baltimore: Charles C Thomas, 1938.
——, Urse, V. G., Madden, J. J., and Countryman, M. A.: Electric shock therapy in the treatment of schizophrenia, manic depressive psychoses and chronic alcoholism. J. Nerv. & Ment. Dis. *98*:618, 1943.
Nickel, J., Breyer, U., Claver, B., and Quadbeck, G.: Zur Wirkung von Aminoaethanol-Derivaten auf das Zentralnervensystem. Arzneim.-Forsch. *13*:881, 1963.
Nicolajev, V.: Zur Erfolgsprognose der Insulinschockbehandlung und zur Deutung des Heilungsvorganges (Untersuchungen über Schrankenpermeabilität und Liquoreiweiss). Schweiz. Arch. f. Neurol. *39* (Erg.-H): 206, 1937.
——: A special glial alteration after repeated insulin shock in animals. Am. J. Psychiat. *96* (Supp.):302, 1938.
Nielsen, J. M., and Ingham, S. D.: Death from complications of metrazol treatment; autopsy. Bull. Los Angeles Neurol. Soc. *5*:130, 1940.
Nieschulz, O.: Weitere Beiträge zum Wirkungsspektrum des 10-[1-Methylpiperidyl-(3)-methyl]-phenothiazins. Arzneim.-Forsch. *15*:271, 1965.
Nieschulz, O., Hoffmann, I., and Popendiker, K.: Pharmakologische Untersuchungen einiger N-Alkyl-piperidyl-carbazol-Derivate. Arzneimittel Forsch. *9*:219, 1959.
——, Popendiker, K., and Sack, K. H.: Pharmakoloische Untersuchungen über N-alkyl-piperidyl-Phenothiazin Derivate. Arzneimitt. Forsch. *4*:232, 1954.
Nistri, M., and Sgambati, M.: Clinical evaluation of nialamide in psychiatry. J. da Soc. das Ciências Med. de Lisboa (suppl.) Nov.:157, 1959.
——, and de Luca, P.-L.: A propos de l'inhibition de l'éjaculation pendant le traitement thioridazinique: Son éventuelle valeur thérapeutique. Encéphale *53*:203, 1964.
Niswander, G. D., and Karacan, I.: Clinical experience with fluphenazine. Dis. Nerv. Syst. *20*:1, 1959.
Noack, C. H., and Trautner, E. M.: The lithium treatment of maniacal psychoses. Med. J. Austral. *2*:2;9, 1951.
Noce, R. H., Williams, D. B., and Rapaport, W.: Reserpine (Serpasil), in management of the mentally ill and mentally retarded. J.A.M.A. *156*:821, 1954; *158*:11, 1955.
Norman, J., and Worthington, R. V., Electric shock treatment in 100 cases. Dis. Nerv. Syst. *5*:236, 1944.
Notkin, J., Watts, L. E., Shannon, G. W., Niles, C. E., and De Natale, F. J.: A comparative study of the combined metrazolhypoglycemic shock treatment and spontaneous improvements in schizophrenia. J. Nerv. & Ment. Dis. *97*:62, 1943.
Nussbaum, K., and Kurland, A. A.: Intravenous administration of Indoklon 10% solution. Amer. J. Psychiat. *120*:69, 1963.
——, Wittig, B. A., Hanlon, Th. E., and Kurland, A. A.: Intravenous nialamide in the treatment of depressed female patients. Compr. Psychiat. *4*:105, 1963.
Nuyts, A.: The treatment of chronic psychoses with Dipiperon-R 3345. Acta neurol. psychiat. belg. *63*:326, 1963.
Nyiro, J.: Beitrag zur Wirkung der Krampftherapie der Schizophrenie. Schweiz. Arch. f. Neurol. u. Psychiat. *40*:180, 1937.
Nyman, E., and Silfversköld, B. P.: Kreislaufstörungen bei Krampfanfällen epileptischen Typs. Acta med. scandinav. *114*:223, 1943.
Nyström, S.: On relation between clinical factors and efficacy of ECT in depression. Acta Psychiat. Scand. *40* (Suppl. 181):11, 1964.
Oberholzer, W.: Arbeiten zur Insulinschocktherapie der Schizophrenia. Allg. Ztg. Psychiat. 114, 1940.
In Obersteg, J., and Bäumler, J.: Über Suizide mit Psychopharmaka. Münch. med. Wschr. *106*:969, 1964.
Obrador, S.: Temporal lobotomy. J. Neuropath. & Exper. Neurol. *6*:185, 1947.
Ødegaard, O.: Leucotomy in Norway from a psychiatrist's point of view. Lisbon: Psychosurgery, 1949.
——: Psychochirurgie. I. Indikationen, psychologische Untersuchungen und Ergebnisse. Nord. psykiatr. Medlemsbl. *3*:65, 1949.
——: Results of treatment in mental hospitals in Norway before and after the introduction of shock treatment. Mental Hygiene *38*:447, 1954.
——: A statistical study of factors influencing discharge from psychiatric hospitals. J. Ment. Sci. *106*:1124, 1960.
Ody, F.: Le traitement de la démence précoce par résection du lobe préfrontal. Arch. ital. di chir. *53*:321, 1938.

Offner, F.: Stimulation with minimum power. J. Neurophysiol. *9*:387, 1946.

Ohno, Y.: A therapeutic approach to anergic, chronic schizophrenics with trifluoperazine. Fol. psychiat. neurol. japon. *18*:112, 1964.

Oles, M.: Klinische Erfahrungen mit dem Neuroleptiuum Haloperidol (R.1625). *In:* Symposium International sur le Halopéridol. Acta Medica Belgica, 1960.

Oliver, W.: Account of the effects of camphor in a case of insanity. London M. J. *6*:120, 1785.

Ollendorf, R. H. V.: High dosage chlorpromazine therapy in acute and chronic schizophrenia. Am. J. Psychiat. *116*:720, 1960.

Olsen, C. W.: Insulin shock therapy; prevention of secondary hypoglycemic shock. Bull. Los Angeles Neurol. Soc. *7*:99, 1942.

——: An unusual reaction to electroshock treatment. Unilateral convulsion and transient hemiplegia. Bull. Los Angeles Neurol. Soc. *9*:171, 1944.

Olsen, N. S., and Klein, J. R.: Effect of insulin hypoglycemia on brain glucose, glycogen, lactate and phosphates. Arch. Biochem. *13*:343, 1947.

Oltman, J. E. Brody, B. S., Friedman, S., and Green, W. F.: Frontal lobotomy. Am. J. Psychiat. *105*:742, 1949.

——, and Friedman, S.: Analysis of temporal factors in manic-depressive psychosis, with particular reference to the effect of shock therapy. Am. J. Psychiat. *107*:57, 1950.

——, and Friedman, S.: Use of Marplan in depressive states (a preliminary report). Dis. Nerv. Syst. *21*:81, 1960.

——, and ——: Pargyline in the treatment of depressive illnesses. Amer. J. Psychiat. *120*:493, 1963.

——, and ——: Protein-bound iodine in patients receiving perphenazine. J.A.M.A. *185*:726, 1963.

——, and ——: Further report on protein-bound iodine in patients receiving perphenazine. Amer. J. Psychiat. *121*:176, 1964.

O'Neill, F. J.: Serious complications of insulin shock therapy. Psychiatric Quart. *12*:455, 1938.

Opinsky, M., Serbin, A. F., and Rosenfeld, J. E.: Arterial thrombosis with gangrene after use of promazine (Sparine) hydrochloride. J.A.M.A. *168*:1224, 1958.

Opitz, K., and Loeser, A.: Abschwächung der blutzuckersenkenden Wirkung antidiabetischer Substanzen durch Neuroleptica. Dtsch. med. Wschr. *87*:105, 1962.

O'Reilly, P. O., Michaud, M., Wojcicki, H. M., and Keogh, R. P.: Acetylpromazine (Acepromazine) in the treatment of chronic mental illness. Canad. Med. Ass. J. *79*:381, 1958.

——, Wojcick, H. M., Hrychuk, W., and Keogh, R. P.: Perphenazine treatment of psychoses. Canad. M. A. J. *77*: 952, 1957.

Orenstein, L. L., and Schilder, P.: Psychological considerations of the insulin treatment in schizophrenia. J. Nerv. & Ment. Dis. *88*:397, 1939.

Osgood, C. W.: An analysis of disappointing results with metrazol in the treatment of certain depressions. J. Nerv. & Ment. Dis. *95*:192, 1942.

——: Unusual reactions to electroshock. J. Nerv. & Ment. Dis. *100*:343, 1944.

Ostergaard, Jansen O.: The treatment of neurotic manifestations with benactyzine. Dt. Med. Wchnschr. *82*:1269, 1957.

Osterman, E., Bollander Löfvenberg, S., and Lassenius, B.: Therapeutical trials with SCTZ—a new hypnotic—in psychotic illness. Nord. Med. *62*:1191, 1959.

Ostertag, B.: Pathologie der Schockbehandlung. Zentralbl. f. ges. Neurol. u. Psychiat. Oct.:5, 1949.

Ostow, M.: The effects of the newer neuroleptic and stimulating drugs on psychic function. *In* G. J. Sarwer-Foner, ed.: The Dynamics of Psychiatric Drug Therpay. Springfield, Ill.: Charles C Thomas, 1960.

——: Drugs in Psychoanalysis and Psychotherapy. New York, Basic Books, 1962.

——, and Kline, N.: The psychic action of reserpine and chlorpromazine. *In* N. S. Kline, ed.: Psychopharmacology Frontiers. Boston, Little, Brown & Co., 1959.

Ott, T.: Contribution à l'étude de la physiopathologie due liquide céphalo-rachidien au cours du traitement insulinique de la schizophrénie. Dissertation. Lausanne: 1938.

Ottosson, J. O.: Experimental studies of the mode of action of electroconvulsive therapy. Acta Psychiat. et Neurol. scandinav. Suppl. 145, Vol. 35, 1960.

——: Electroconvulsive therapy of endogenous depression. J. Ment. Sci. *108*:694, 1962.

——: Electroconvulsive therapy—electrostimulatory or convulsive therapy? J. Neuropsychiat. *3*:216, 1962.

Overall, J. E., Hollister, L. E., Meyer, F., Kimbell, Jr., I., and Shelton, J.: Imipramine and thioridazine in depressed and schizophrenic patients. J.A.M.A. *189*:605, 1964.

——, ——, Shelton, J., Johnson, M., and Kimbell, I.: Tranylcypromine compared with dextroamphetamine in hospitalized depressed patients. Dis. Nerv. Syst. *27*:653, 1966.

Overholser, W.: Administrative and forensic psychiatry. Am. J. Psychiat. *106*:541, 1950.

Owen, T. V., and Stemmerman, M. G.: Electric convulsive therapy in stammering. Am. J. Psychiat. *104*:410, 1947.

Owensby, N. M.: Homosexuality and lesbianism treated with metrazol. J. Nerv. & Ment. Dis. 92:65, 1940.

Pacella, B. L.: Sequelae and complications of convulsive shock therapy. Bull. New York Acad. Med. *20*:575, 1944.

——: Follow-up study of a series of patients treated by electrically induced convulsions and by metrazol convulsions. Am. J. Psychiat. *99*:513, 1943.

——: Spontaneous convulsions following convulsive shock therapy. Am. J. Psychiat. *101*:783, 1945.

——: "Nonshock" therapies in clinical prac-

tice. Am. J. Psychiat. *111*:845, 1955.
——, and Barrera, S. E.: Some considerations of the electroencephalogram in the convulsive state (electrically induced seizures). J. Nerv. & Ment. Dis. *95*:125, 1942.
——, Piotrowski, Z., and Lewis, N. D. C.: The effects of electric convulsive therapy on certain personality traits in psychiatric patients. Am. J. Psychiat. *104*:83, 1947.
Pacheco e Silva, A. C.: Indications of insulin therapy. *In* M. Rinkel: Insulin Treatment in Psychiatry. New York: Philosophical Library, 1959.
Paganini, A. E., and Zlotlow, M.: Two-year follow-up study of the relationship of chlorpromazine and the incidence of convulsions in 50 post-lobotomy patients. Am. J. Psychiat. *114*:839, 1958.
Page, L. G. M., and Russell, R. J.: Intensified electrical convulsion therapy in the treatment of mental disorders. Lancet *254*:597, 1948.
Pakesch, E. F.: Köpertemperatur bei Schockbehandlung. Wien. Ztschr. f. Nervenheilk. *2*:314, 1949.
Paley, H. M., Hankoff, L. D., Kawi, A. A., and Mendelsohn, F. S.: The therapeutic profile of Haloperidol. A preliminary study of a butyrophenone derivative in inpatients and out-patients. J. Neuropsychiat. *4*:39, 1962.
Palisa, Ch.: The awakening from the hypoglycemic shock. Am. J. Psychiat. *94* (Supp.):96, 1938.
Palmer, D. M., Riepenhoff, J. P., and Hanahan, P. W.: Insulin shock therapy. A statistical survey of 393 cases. Am. J. Psychiat. *106*:918, 1950.
Palmer, H. D., Hastings, D. W., and Sherman, S. H.: Therapy in involutional melancholia. Am. J. Psychiat. *97*:1086, 1941.
Papez, J. W.: A proposed mechanism of emotion. Arch. Neurol. & Psychiat. *38*:725, 1937.
Pappalardo, P.: Stato funzionale del s.r.i. nelle malattie mentali e meccanismo terapeutico delle terapie da shock. Acta neurol. *2*:908, 1947.
Pare, C. M. B.: Acetylcholine as therapeutic agent in mild psychiatric disorder. J. Ment. Sc. *102*:847, 1956.
——, and Jenner, G. C.: Intramuscular nialamide in depressed patients. (A biochemical study). Dis Nerv. Syst. *27*:193, 1966.
Parfitt, E. H.: The neurological and psychological effects of hypoglycaemia. Proc. Roy. Soc. Med. 31, 1937.
Pargiter, R. A.: Parenteral methylphenidate hydrochloride (Ritalin) in chronic underactive schizophrenics. Dis. Nerv. Syst. *20*:69, 1959.
Parker, C. S.: Observations on autonomic functions during hypoglycemic treatment of schizophrenics. J. Ment. Sc. *86*:645, 1940.
Parland, O.: Shock therapy for soldiers suffering from psychosomatic disturbances during the war. Acta psichiat. et neurol., Suppl. *47*:511, 1947.
Parsons, E. H.: Clinical report on the use of the dimethyl ether of D-tubocurarine iodide in electroshock therapy. Am. J. Psychiat. *107*:184, 1950.
——, Gildea, E. F', Ronzoni, E., and Hulbert. S. Z.: Comparative lymphocytic and biochemical responses of patients with schizophrenia and affective disorders to electro-shock insulin shock, and epinephrine. Am. J. Psychiat. *105*:573, 1949.
Partridge, M.: Prefrontal leucotomy. Oxford: Blackwell, 1950.
Pasquarelli, B. Campbell, R. J., Polatin, P., and Horwitz, W. H.: Further appraisal of the cardiac output. A-V oxygen difference, arterial pressure and peripheral resistance. J. Clin. Invest. *27*:290, 1948.
Patel, N., Mock, Jr., D. C., and Hagans, J. A.: Comparison of benzphetamine, phenmetrazine, D-amphetamine, and placebo. Clin. Pharmacol. *4*:330, 1963.
Paterson, A. Spencer: Electronarcosis. Lancet *2*:198, 1947.
——: Electro-shock and electronarcosis in the treatment of mental disorders. Edinburgh M. J. *55*:38, 1948.
——: Electrical and Drug Treatments in Psychiatry. Amsterdam, Elsevier, 1963.
Patton, G. O., and Garneau, J.: Resocialization project replaces insulin coma therapy in a mental hospital. III. Statistical comparisons. Canad. Serv. M. J. *13*:319, 1957.
Pauleikhoff, B.: "Ist die elektrische Behandlung bei endogenen Psychosen heute entbehrlich?" Nervenarzt *32*:329, 1961.
Paulson, G.: Treatment of post-traumatic headache with imipramine. Amer. J. Psychiat. *119*:368, 1962.
Pauly, R.: Nouvelle note sur les dangers de la thérapeutique par le largactil (à propos d'un infarctus du myocarde survenu au cours d'une cure ambulatoire). J. Méd. Bordeaux *131*:587, 1954.
——: Remarques à propos d'une statistique personnelle sur les avantages, les limites et les accidents de l'hibernothérapie á la chlorpromazine. J. Méd. Bordeaux *131*: 235. 1954.
Payne, P.: Trifluoperazine in treatment of the acutely ill psychotic: a preliminary report. Canad. M. A. J. *81*:42, 1959.
Pearce, J. D. W., and Thornton, H. L.: Chlorpromazine in ECT. Brit. Med. J. *1*:1218, 1955.
Pearl, D. Vanderkamp, H., Olsen, A. L., Greenberg, P. D., and Armitage, S. G.: The effects of reserpine on schizophrenic patients. A.M.A. Arch. Neurol. & Psychiat. *76*:198, 1956.
Peck, R. E.: Carbon dioxide therapy: a cooperative statistical study. *In* Meduna: Carbon Dioxide Therapy. Springfield, Ill.: Charles C Thomas, 1958.
Penfield, W., Cameron, D. E., Prados, M. D., and Malmo, R. B.: Symposium on gyrectomy. A. Research, Nerv. & Ment. Dis. Proc. *27*:519, 1948.
——, and Flanigan, H.: Surgical therapy of temporal lobe seizures. Arch. Neurol. & Psychiat. *64*:491, 1950.
Penick, S. B., and Hinkle, Jr., L. E.: The effect of expectation on response to phenmetrazine. Psychosom. Med. *26*:369, 1964.

Pennington, V. M.: Clinical results of triflupromazine (Vesprin) in 132 psychotic patients. Am. J. Psychiat. *115*:740, 1959.
——: Meprobamate-benactyzine (Deprol) in the treatment of chronic brain syndrome, schizophrenia and senility. J. Am. Geratrics Soc. *7*:656, 1959.
——: Prochlorperazine in the treatment of the schizophrenias. Am. J. Psychiat. *115*: 820, 1959.
Penrose, L. S.: Survey of patients treated with shock therapy in the Ontario hospitals, 1938-1941. Ontario: Department of Health, 1942.
——, and Marr, W. B.: Results of shock therapy evaluated by estimating chances of patients remaining in hospital without such treatment. J. Ment. Sc. *89*:374, 1943.
Pepeu, G., Friedman, D. X., and Giarman, N. J.: Biochemical and pharmacological studies of dimethylaminoethanol (Deanol). J. Pharmac. Exp. Ther. *129*:291, 1960.
Perk, D.: Mepacrine psychosis. J. Ment. Sc. *93*:756, 1947.
Perlson, J.: Case of schizophrenia treated with 248 electric shock treatments. Arch. Neurol. & Psychiat. *54*:409, 1945.
Perlstein, M. A.: Use of meprobamate (Miltown) in convulsive disorders. J.A.M.A. *161*:1040, 1956.
Perrin, G. M.: Cardiovascular aspects of electric shock therapy. Acta Psychiat. Scan. *36* (Suppl. 152):7, 1961.
Perry, H. A., and Levy, S.: Intravenous alcohol and early convulsive shock in the treatment of exhaustion due to mental disorder. J. Nerv. & Ment. Dis. *110*:497, 1949.
Pessin, J., and Reese, H. H.: Fatal complication following metrazol treatment for schizophrenia. Am. J. Psychiat. *96*:393, 1939.
Petersen, M. C., and Buchstein, H. H.: Prefrontal lobotomy in chronic psychoses. Am. J. Psychiat. *99*:426, 1942.
——, Dodge, H. W., Jr., Sem-Jacobsen, C. W., Lazarte, J. A., and Holman, C. B.: Clinical results of selective leucotomy based on intracerebral electrography. J.A.M.A. *159*:774, 1955.
——, and Love, J. G.: Graded lobotomy. Am. J. Psychiat. *106*:65, 1949.
——, and Lutz, E. H.: Intravenous injection of insulin in the treatment of schizophrenia. J. Nerv. & Ment. Dis. *97*:141, 1943.
Petersen, M. C., and McBrayer, J. W.: Treatment of affective depression with trans-dl-phenylcyclopropylamine hydrochloride: a preliminary report. Am. J. Psychiat. *116*:67, 1959.
Petersen, P. V., and Møller Nielsen, I.: Sordinol, a new neuroleptic drug in the thioxanthene series. Ugesk. Laeger *123*: 1669, 1961.
——, and ——: Thioxanthene derivatives. *In* M. Gordon (Ed.): Psychopharmacological Agents, Vol. I: pp 301, Medical Chemistry, A Series of Monographs, Vol. 4. New York, Academic Press, 1964.
Petri-Canella and Levi, M. G.: Sulla terapia convulsivante con cardiazol nelle malattie mentali. Rassegna di studi psichiat. 27, 1938.
Petrie, A.: Preliminary report of changes after prefrontal leucotomy. J. Ment. Sc. *95*:449, 1949.
——, and Le Beau, J.: The effects on personality of chlorpromazine as compared with various brain operations. Encéphale *45*:987, 1956.
Petrilowitsch, N.: Zur Indikationsbreite antriebsintensiver Thymoleptika bei der Therapie depressiver Verstimmungen. Dargestellt am Wirkungsspektrum des Nortriptylin. Med. Welt *N.F. 18*:286, 1967.
Peyton, W. T., Noran, H. H., and Miller, E. W.: Prefrontal lobectomy (excision of the anterior areas of the cerebrum). Am. J. Psychiat. *104*:513, 1948.
Pfeiffer, C. C., and Jenney, E. H.: The inhibition of the conditioned response and the counteraction of schizophrenia by muscarinic stimulation of the brain. Ann. New York Acad. Sc. *66*:573, 1957.
Pfister, H. O.: Die neuro-vegetativen Störungen der Schizophrenien und ihre Beziehungen zur Insulin-Kardiazol- und Schlafkurbehandlung. Schweiz. Arch. f. Neurol. *39* (Erg.-H):77, 1937.
——: Über die Verwendung von Amytal in der Psychiatrie. Monatschr. f. Psychiat. u. Neurol. *106*:40, 1942.
Phillips, R. M., Judy, F. R., and Judy, M. E.: Meprobamate addiction. Northwest Med. *56*:453, 1957.
Piaget, R. M.: Zur Frage einer Leberstütztherapie bei Schizophrenie. Confinia neurol. *10*:33, 1950.
Piehler, R.: Über das Traumerleben Leukotomierter. Nervenarzt *21*:517, 1950.
Pilkington, T. L.: Prochlorperazine (Stemetil) in mental deficiency. J. Ment. Sc. *105*:215, 1959.
Pilling, L. F. M., Barry, M. J., Jr., and Parkin, T. W.: Electroshock therapy of a depressed patient with complete heart block. Amer. J. Psychiat. *119*:788, 1963.
Piotrowski, Z.: The prognostic possibilities of the Rorschach method in insulin treatment. Psychiatric Quart. *12*:679, 1938.
——: Rorschach method as prognostic aid in insulin shock treatment of schizophrenics. Psychiatric Quart. *15*:807, 1941.
Pippard, J.: Second leucotomies. J. Ment. Sci. *101*:788, 1955.
——: Leucotomy in Britain today. J. Ment. Sci. *108*:249, 1962.
Piret, J., Delay, J., Pichot, P., and Lemperiere, Th.: Étude clinique des effets thérapeutiques du chlorhydrate de 3-chloro-5(γ-diméthylaminopropyl)-10,11-dihydro-5H-dibenzo-[b,f]-azépine. (G. 34. 586). *In* J. J. Lopez Ibor (Ed.): Psychiatry, part *3*: 2041, Proc. 4th World Congr. Psychiat., Madrid 1966. Amsterdam, Excerpta Med. Found. Internat. Congr. Ser. No. 150, 1968.
Pisetsky, J. E.: Disappearance of painful phantom limbs after electric shock treatment. Am. J. Psychiat. *102*:599, 1946.
Pisk, G.: Über ein "Zeitraffer" Phänomen nach Insulinkoma. Ztschr. f. d. ges. Neurol.

u. Psychiat. *156*:777, 1936.
Plattner, P.: Amnestisches Syndrom nach Insulin- und Kardiazolbehandlung. Ztschr. f. d. ges. Neurol. u. Psychiat. *162*:727, 1938.
——, and Fröhlicher, E.: Zur Insulinschockbehandlung der Schizophrenie. Ztschr. f. d. ges. Neurol. u. Psychiat. *160*:735, 1938.
Pleasure, H.: 233 patients with mental illness treated with electroconvulsive therapy in the presence of tuberculosis. Am. J. Psychiat. *111*:177, 1954.
——: *In:* Chlorpromazine and Mental Health. Philadelphia: Lea and Febiger, 1955.
Pletscher, A.: Beeinflussung des 5-hydroxytryptamin-Stoffwechsels im Gehirn durch Isonikotinsäurehydrazid. Experientia *12*: 479, 1956.
——, Brossi, A., and Gey, K. F.: Benzoquinolizine derivatives: A new class of monoamine decreasing drugs with psychotropic action. *In* C. C. Pfeiffer and J. R. Smythies (Eds.): Internat. Rev. of Neurobiology, Vo.l 4: pp 275. New York, Academic Press, 1962.
——, Gey, K. F., and Zeller, P.: Monoaminoxydase-Hemmer. Chemie, Biochemie, Pharmakologie, Klinik. *In* E. Jucker (Ed.): Fortschr. Arzneimittelforsch. Vol. *2*:417 (Progress in Drug Res.). Basel-Stuttgart, Birkhäuser Verlag, 1960.
Plice, S. G., and Pfister, C. W.: Electrocardiographic absormalities in the mentally ill: is "myocardial damage" sometimes of psychogenic origin? Illinois M. J. *99*:212, 1951.
Plichet, A.: Un nouveau traitement des psychonéuroses: le chlorhydrate de l'acide benzilique dièthylaminoethylester. Presse mèd. *63*:1748, 1955.
Ploog, D., and Selbach, H.: Über den Funktionswandel des vegetativen Systems im Sympatol-Versuch während der Elektroschockbehandlung. Dt. Ztschr. Nervenh. *167*:302, 1952.
Plummer, A. J., Maxwell, R. A., and Earl, A. E.: Some pharmacological interrelationships between methylphenidate (Ritalin) and reserpine. Am. J. Med. Sc. *233*: 179, 1957.
Polatin, P., Friedman, M. M., Harris, M. M., and Horwitz, W. A.: Vertebral fractures produced by metrazol-induced convulsions in treatment of psychiatric disorders. J.A.M.A. *112*:1684, 1939.
——, and Hoch, P.: Electroshock therapy in pregnant mental patients. New York State. J. Med. *45*:1562, 1945.
——, and Linn, L.: An orthopedic and neurological follow-up study of vertebral fractures in shock therapy. Am. J. Psychiat. *105*:824, 1949.
——, and Spotnitz, H.: Effects of combined ambulatory insulin and electroshock therapy in the treatment of schizophrenia. New York State J. Med. *46*:2648, 1946.
——, ——, and Wiesel, B.: Ambulatory insulin treatment of mental disorders. New York State J. Med. *40*:843, 1940.
——, ——, and ——: Effects of intravenous injection of insulin in treatment of mental disease. Arch. Neurol. & Psychiat. *43*:925, 1940.
——, Strauss, H., and Altman, L. L.: Transient organic mental reactions during shock therapy of the psychoses: Psychiatric Quart. *14*:457, 1940.
Pöldinger, W.: Ein Neurolepticum mit antidepressiver Wirkung "Taractan" (Ro 4-0403). Praxis *49*:468, 1960.
——: Klinische Erfahrungen mit dem Iminostilbenderivat G 33040. Therap. Umschau *19*:34, 1962.
——: Akute Intoxikationen mit Psychopharmaka. Ther. Umschau *22*:155, 1965.
——: Vergleichende klinisch-psychiatrische Erfahrungen mit Thioxanthen-Derivaten unter besonderer Berücksichtigung von Flupenthixol. Arzneim.-Forsch. *17*:1133, 1967.
Pollack, B.: Preliminary report on 500 patients treated with Thorazine at Rochester State Hospital. Psychiat. Quart. *29*:439, 1955.
——: Recurrent thorazine-induced agranulocytosis. Am. J. Psychiat. *113*:557, 1956.
——: The effect of chlorpromazine in reducing the relapse rate in 716 released patients. Am. J. Psychiat. *114*:749, 1958.
——: Clinical findings in the use of Tofranil in depressive and other psychiatric states. Am. J. Psychiat. *116*-312, 1959.
Polonio, P., and Slater, A.: A prognostic study of insulin treatment in schizophrenia. J. Ment. Sc. *100*:442, 1954.
Polzer, K.: Elektrokardiographische Veränderungen unter Elektroschocktherapie depressiver Zustände. Wien. Ztschr. f. Nerv. *1*:256, 1948.
Pool, J. L.: Topectomy. Proc. Roy. Soc. Med. *42* Suppl.:1, 1949.
——, Heath, R. G., and Weber, J. J.: Topectomy: surgical indications and results. Bull. New York Acad. Med. *25*:335, 1949.
Poppen, J. L.: Technic of prefrontal lobotomy. J. Neurosurg. *5*:514, 1948.
Popper, H.: Hepatic injury in patients who have received iproniazid. Ann. N.Y. Acad. Sci. *80*:928, 1959.
Porot, M.: Traitement des accidents graves du coma insulinique. Ann. méd.-psychol. *106*:596, 1948.
Porteus, S. D., and Peters, H. N.: Maze test validation and psychosurgery. Genet. Psychol. Monogr. *36*:3, 1947.
Portnow, S. L., Ardis, M. B., and Lubach, J. E.: The effect of deanol on the activity of chronic schizophrenia patients. Am. J. Psychiat. *116*:748, 1960.
Posnyakova: *In* B. Lustig: New Research in Soviet Psychiatry. Report of Ost-Europa Institut, Berlin, 1957.
Post, F., Rees, W. L., and Schurr, P. H.: An evaluation of bimedial leucotomy. Brit. J. Psychiat. *114*:1223, 1968.
Pötzl, O.: Über die Erfolge der Schock-Therapie bei Geisteskrankheiten. Wien. med. Wchnschr. *94*:11, 1944.
Poussaint, A. F., and Ditman, K. S.: A controlled study of imipramine (Tofranil) in the treatment of childhood enuresis. J. Pediat. *67*:283, 1965.

——, ——, and Greenfield, R.: Amitriptyline in childhood enuresis. Clin. Pharmacol. *7*:21, 1966.

Powell, L. W., Mann, G. T., and Kays, S.: Acute meprobamate poisoning. New England Med. J. *259*:716, 1958.

Power, T. D.: Reversal of evolution in insulin coma. J. Nerv. & Ment. Dis. *121*:535, 1955.

Pozniak, J., and Erb, A.:Versuch einer Cardiazolbehandlung der Epilepsie. Ztschr. f. d. ges. Neurol. u. Psychiat. *166*:581, 1939.

Pratt, J. T., Bishop, M. P., and Gallant, D. M.: Trifluperidol and Haloperidol in the treatment of acute schizophrenia. Amer. J. Psychiat. *121*:592, 1964.

Prensky, A. L., Raff, M. C., Moore, M. J., and Schwab, R. S.: Intravenous diazepam in the treatment of prolonged seizure activity. N. Engl. J. Med. *276*:779, 1967.

Pressman, M. D., and Weiss, L. B.: Experience with Elavil: Treatment of fifty-one cases of depression. Amer. J. Psychiat. *118*:74, 1961.

Price, H. G., and Knouss, R.: Selection of music to accompany electro-shock therapy. Occup. Therap. *29*:220, 1950.

Proctor, L. D., Dewan, J. G., and McNeel, B. H.: Variations in glucose tolerance observations in schizophrenics before and after shock treatment. Am. J. Psychiat. *100*:652, 1944.

——, and Goodwin, J. S.: Comparative electroencephalic observations following electro-shock therapy using raw 60 cycle alternating and unidirectional fluctuating currents. Am. J. Psychiat. *99*:525, 1943.

Proctor, R. C.: A new therapeutic approach to certain cases of alcoholism. South. med. J. *49*:73, 1956.

——, and Odland, T.: Frenquel. Dis. Nerv. Syst. *17*:25, 1956.

Pscheidt, G. R.: Monoamine oxidase inhibitors. *In* C. C. Pfeiffer and J. R. Smythies (Eds.): Internat. Review of Neurobiology, Vol. 7:191. New York, Academic Press, 1964.

Puech, P., Guilly, P., Desclaux, P., and Morice, J.: La psychochirurgie. Monde méd. Paris Bo. 12, 1947.

——, Morice, J., Thuillier, J., and Sizaret, P.: Accidents de l'insulinothérapie ou de l'électro-choc et troubles de l'hydrodynamique cérébro-méningée. Ann. méd. psychol. *107*:273, 1949.

Pulver, S. E., and Jacobs, E. G.: Effect of nonconvulsive electric stimulation upon some side-effects of ECT. Dis. Nerv. Syst. *22*:382, 1961.

Putnam, T. J.: Procain base in iodized oil introduced transorbitally as a test for the effects of lobotomy. Tr. Am. Neurol. A., p. 125, June 1950.

Quandt, J., and Sommer, H.: Zur Frage der Hirngewebsschädigungen nach electrischer Krampfbehandlung. Ztschr. Neurol. u. Psychiat. *34*:513, 1966.

——, von Horn, L., and Schliep, H.: Bemerkungen zur Behandlung mit Phenothiazin-Verbindungen innerhalb der Psychiatrie unter besonderer Berücksichtigung eines neuartigen Thiophenylpyridylamin-Derivates. Psychiat. Neurol. (Basel) *135*:197, 1958.

Quarrington, B.: CO_2 therapy with stutterers. Dis. Nerv. Syst. *15*:123, 1954.

Quinn, G. P., Shore, P. A., and Brodie, B. B.: Biochemical and pharmacological studies of Ro 1-9569 (Tetrabenazine) nonindole tranquilizing agent with reserpine-like effects. J. Pharmacol. Exp. Ther. *127*: 103, 1959.

Quinn, P. J. G., Johnston, J., Latner, G., and Kiloh, L. G.: A comparative controlled trial of methotrimeprazine (Veractil) in chronic schizophrenia. J. Ment. Sc. *106*: 160, 1960.

Rabin, A. I.: Patients who received more than 100 electric shock treatments. J. Personal. *17*:42, 1948.

Radinger, N., Rochlin, D., and Kline, N. S.: Treatment of depressed and regressed patients with iproniazid and reserpine. Dis. Nerv. Syst. *20*:31, 1959.

Radomski, J. L., Fuyat, H. N., Nelson, A. A., and Smith, P. K.: The toxic effects, excretion and distribution of lithium chloride. J. Pharmacol. *100*:429, 1950.

Rajotte, P., Giard, N., and Tetreault, L.: Etude comparative double aveugle de la propériciazine et de la chlorpromazine dans les troubles caractériels. Acta neurol. psychiat. belg. *65*:1006, 1965.

Ramapuram, G. M., Metcalfe, E. V., Stevenson, J. A. F., and Hobbs, G. E.: A clinical trial of the epinephrine-mecholyl test in a mixed group of psychiatric patients. Canad. Psychiat. Ass. J. *3*:94, 1958.

——: Pharmacology of Methaminodiazepozide. Dis. Nerv. Syst. (Suppl.) *21*:7, 1960.

Ramirez, E., Mariategui, J., and Bachmann, C.: Glucagon in terminating insulin coma. *In* Rinkel, M. (Ed.): Biological Treatment of Mental Illness. New York, L. C. Page, 1966.

Randall, L. O., Cameron, D. E., and Looney, J. M.: Changes in blood lipids during insulin treatment of schizophrenia. Am. J. M. Sc. *195*:802, 1938.

——, Heise, G. A., Schallek, W., Bagdon, R. E., Banziger, R., Boris, A., Moe, R. A., and Abrams, W. B.: Pharmacological and clinical studies on ValiumT.M.. A new psychotherapeutic agent of the benzodiazepine class. Curr. Ther. Res. *3*:405, 1961.

——, Schallek, W., Heise, G. A., Keith, E. F., Bagdon, R. E.: The psychosedative properties of methaminodiazepoxide. J. Pharmacol. Exp. Ther. *129*:163, 1960.

——, ——, Scheckel, C., Banziger, R., Boris, A., Moe, R. A., Bagdon, R. E., Schwartz, M. A., und Zbinden, G.: Zur Pharmakologie von Valium, einem neuen Psychopharmakon der Benzodiazepinreihe. Schweiz. med. Wschr. *93*:794, 1963.

Randell, J. B.: Euphoriant effects of "Preludin". Brit. Med. J. *2*:508, 1957.

Rathod, N., and Rees, L.: A controlled study of the prognostic significance of autonomic responses in the chlorpromazine treatment of disturbed psychotic patients. J. Ment. Sc. *104*:705, 1958.

Rauch, H. J.: Hirnschädigungen bei Schockbehandlung der Psychosen. Arztl. Wchnschr. *3*:65, 1948.

Ravaris, C. L., Weaver, L. A., and Brooks, G. W.: A controlled study of fluphenazine enanthate in chronic schizophrenic patients. Dis. Nerv. Syst. *26*:33, 1965.

——, ——, and ——: Further studies with fluphenazine enanthate: II. Relapse rate in patients deprived of medication. Amer. J. Psychiat. *124*: 248, 1967.

Ravn, J.: Truxal, ein neuartiges Psychopharmakon. Wien. klin. Wschr. *72*:192, 1960.

——: Chlorprothixene: A new psychotropic entity. Amer. J. Psychiat. *118*:227, 1961.

——, and Rud, Ch.: Sordinol, a new psychopharmacologic drug. Ugesk. Laeg. *123*: 1663, 1961.

Ray, P. C.: The hypnotic action of rauwolfia serpentina (Dhan Marua). Patna J. Med. *6*:193, 1931.

Rea, E. L., and Fazekas, J. F.: Effects of parenterally administered reserpine. A.M.A. Arch. Int. Med. *95*:538, 1955.

Reed, G. E., and Dancey, T. E.: Compression fractures of the vertebral bodies following induced and "idiopathic" convulsions. Canad. M. A. J. *42*:38, 1940.

Rees, L.: Electronarcosis in the treatment of schizophrenia. J. Ment. Sc. *95*:625, 1949.

——: Physiological concomitants of electronarcosis. J. Ment. Sc. *95*:162, 1949.

——, Annear, M. W., and Crosse, G.: Trichlorethylene narcosis as a therapeutic aid in psychiatry. J. Ment. Sc. *94*:502, 1950.

——: The premenstrual tension syndrome and its treatment. Brit. Med. J. *1*:1014, 1953.

——, A controlled trial of chlorpromazine in the management of patients suffering from asthma associated with anxiety and tension symptoms. Encéphale *45*:555, 1956.

——: Chlorpromazine and allied phenothiazine derivatives. Brit. Med. J. *2*:522, 1960.

——, and Davies, B.: A controlled trial of phenelzine ("Nardil") in the treatment of severe depressive illness. J. Ment. Sci. *107*:560, 1961.

——, and ——: A controlled study of amitriptyline in severe depressive states. Internat. J. Neuropsychiat. *1*:158, 1965.

——, and Lambert, C.: A controlled study of the value of chlorpromazine in the treatment of anxiety-tension states. Encéphale *45*:547, 1956.

——, and Rathod, N.: Autonomic responses as a prognostic aid in chlorpromazine therapy of psychoses. Encéphale *45*:968, 1956.

Rees, T. P.: Symposium on pre-frontal leucotomy. The indications for pre-frontal leucotomy. J. Ment. Sc. *89*:161, 1943.

Reese, H. H.: Hypoglycemia and convulsive therapy in schizophrenia. J.A.M.A. *112*: 493, 1939.

Reeves, J. E.: Thioridazine (Mellaril) in general office practice. Arizona Medicine. *17*:2:90, 1960.

Reichlin, S., and O'Neal, L.: Thyroid hormone levels of the blood after electroshock induced convulsions in man. J. Clin. Endocrin. *22*:385, 1962.

Reinert, R. E.: EEG changes with promazine. Am. J. Psychiat. *115*:742, 1959.

Reiss, M.: Application of endocrinological research methods in psychiatry. J. Endocr. (Oxford) *7*:235, 1951.

——: Endocrine concomitants of certain physical psychiatric treatments. J. Clin. Exp. Psychopath. *17*:254, 1956.

——, Hemphill, R. E., Maggs, R., Haigh, C. P., and Reiss, J. M.: Comparative action of E.C.T. and of pituitary anterior lobe hormones on thyroid function. Brit. M. J. *2*:634, 1951.

Reitan, R. M.: The comparative effects of placebo, ultran, and meprobamate on psychologic test performances. Antibiotic Med. Clin. Therapy *4*:158, 1957.

Reitmann, F.: Zur Frage der Insulinschockwirkung. Psychiat.-neurol. Wchnschr. *40*: 51, 1938.

——: Cardiazol therapy in schizophrenia. Lancet *1*:439, 1939.

——: Orbital cortex syndrome following leucotomy. Am. J.Psychiat. *103*:238, 1946.

——: Leucotomy as an instrument of research: Physiological research. Proc. Roy. Soc. Med. *40*:147, 1947.

——: The "creative spell" of schizophrenics after leucotomy. J. Ment. Sc. *93*:55, 1947.

——: Evaluation of leucotomy results. Am. J. Psychiat. *105*:86, 1948.

——, and Richards, B. W.: Observations on the mechanism of electrically induced convulsions. J. Nerv. & Ment. Dis. *102*: 421, 1945.

Remmen, E., Cohen, S., Ditman, K. S., and Franty, J. R.: Psychochemotherapy—The Physicians' Manual. Los Angeles, Western Medical Publications, 1962.

Remvig, J., and Sonne, L. M.: Chlorprothixene ("Truxal") compared to chlorpromazine. Psychopharmacologia *2*:203, 1961.

Rémy, M.: Essai d'un nouveau dérivé de la phénothiazine, le Melleril, en clinique psychiatrique. Schweiz. med. Wschnschr. *88*:1221, 1958.

Rennie, T. A. C.: Prognosis in manic-depressive and schizophrenic conditions following shock treatment. Psychiatric Quart. *17*:642, 1943.

Rett, A.: Nialamide in the treatment of cerebrally-defective children. J. da Soc. das Ciências Méd. de Lisboa, Nov.: 265, 1959.

Reuse, J. J.: Aspects de la pharmacodynamie des dérivés phénothiaziniques. Encéphale *45*:320, 1956.

Reznikoff, L.: Comparison of metrazol convulsive therapy with electric shock in treatment of schizophrenia. Arch. Neurol. & Psychiat. *49*:587, 1943.

——: Experience with trifluoperazine in the treatment of 100 chronic anergic schizophrenic patients. Am. J. Psychiat. *116*: 1024, 1960.

Riboli, B.: Terapia elettrica transcerebrale con corrente alternata a bassa intensitá. Rass. neuropsychia. *5*:404, 1951.

Rice, D.: The use of lithium salts in the

treatment of manic states. J. Ment. Sc. *1*:604. 1956.
Richter, H. R., and Müller, H. R.: Zur Beeinflussung extrapyramidaler Bewegungsstörungen durch ein neues Neuroplegicum der Thiophenylpyridylamin-Reihe (Prothipendyl, "Dominal forte" Homburg). Ein klinisch-experimenteller Bericht. Schweiz. med. Wschr. *89*:794, 1959.
Rickels, E., Ewing, J. H., Clark, T., and Smock, C. D.: Evaluation of tranquilizing drugs in medical out-patients. J.A.M.A. *171*:1649, 1959.
Rickels, K., Raab, E. DeSilverio, R., and Etemad, B.: Drug treatment in depression. Antidepressant or tranquilizer? J.A.M.A. *201*:675, 1967.
Rickles, N. K., and Polan, C. G.: Causes of failure in treatment with electric shock. Arch. Neurol. & Psychiat. *59*:337, 1948.
Ridenour, R. H.: Brief psychotherapy with Thorazine. M. Ann. Dist. Columbia. *26*: 234, 1957.
Rieger, J. A.: A resume of insulin shock treatment at Central Oklahoma State Hospital. J. Oklahoma M. A. *42*:196, 1949.
Riese, W.: Report of two new cases of sudden deaths after electric shock treatment with histopathological findings in the central nervous system. J. Neuropath. & Exper. Neurol. *7*:98, 1948.
——, and Fultz, G. S.: Electric shock treatment succeeded by complete flaccid paralysis, hallucinations and sudden death. Am. J. Psychiat. *106*:206, 1949.
Riggs, B. C., and Schlomer, G. M.: Hazards of curarization before electroschock. Dis. Nerv. Syst. *8*:382, 1947.
Rinaldi, F., and Himwich, H. E.: A comparison of effects of reserpine and some barbiturates on the electrical activity of the cortical and subcortical structures of the brain of rabbits. Ann. New York Acad. Sc. *61*:27, 1955.
——, Rudy, L. H., and Himwich, H. E.: The use of Frenquel in the treatment of disturbed patients with psychoses of long duration. Am. J. Psychiat. *112*:343, 1955.
Rinkel, M.: Symposium on chemical concepts of psychosis, Zürich, 1957. New York: McDowell, Obolensky, 1958.
——: Biological Treatment of Mental Illness. New York, L. C. Page & Co., 1966.
——, Greenblatt, M., Coon, G. P., and Solomon, H. C.: Relation of the frontal lobe to the aunonomic nervous system in man. Arch. Neurol. & Psychiat. *58*:570, 1947.
——, and Himwich, H. E.: Insulin treatment in Psychiatry. New York: Philosophical Library, 1959.
Rinsley, D. B.: Extended experience with thioridazine in the treatment of hospitalized adolescents. Dis. Nerv. Syst. *29*:36, 1968.
Rivers, T. D.: Effect of Vitamin B, sucrose and sorbitol on certain complications of insulin hypoglycemia. Arch. Neurol. & Psychiat. *44*:910, 1940.
Rizzatti, E.: L'operazione frontale bilaterale di Egas Moniz nelle psicosi postencefalitiche. Schizofrenie *6*:203, 1937.
——: Chirurgia delle psicosi. Gior. di psichiat. e di neuropat. *67*:125, 1939.
——, and Borgarello, G.: Duecento malati dimente operati di leucotomia prefrontale alla Moniz: data statistici e clinici. Nevrasse *1*:11, 1940.
Robb, R. W., Kovitz, B., and Rapaport, D.: Histamine in the treatment of psychosis. Am. J. Psychiat. *97*:601, 1940.
Roberts, A. H.: The value of ECT in delirium. Brit. J. Psychiat. *109*:653, 1963.
Roberts, E. L.: A case of chronic mania treated with lithium citrate and terminating fatally. Med. J. Australia *2*:261, 1950.
Roberts, J. M.: Prognostic factors in the electro-shock treatment of depressive states. J. Ment. Sci. *105*:703, 1959.
Robie, T. R.: Is shock therapy on trial? Am. J. Psychiat. *106*:902, 1950.
——: Treatment of acute barbiturate poisoning by nonconvulsive electrostimulation. Postgrad. Med. *9*:253, 1951.
——: Pseudo-tabes syndrome as complication of tranquilizer drug therapy. Am. J. Psychiat. *113*:463, 1956.
——: Chemotherapy in melancholia. Dis. Nerv. Syst. *21*:124, 1960.
Robin, A. A., and Langley, G. E.: A controlled trial of imipramine. Brit. J. Psychiat. *110*:419, 1964.
——, and Wiseberg, S.: A controlled trial of methyl phenidate (Ritalin) in the treatment of depressive states. J. Neurol. Neurosurg. & Psychiat. *21*:55, 1958.
Robinson, G. W., Jr.: Treatment of delirium tremens with insulin in subshock doses. Am. J. Psychiat. *97*:136, 1940.
——, and De Mott, J. D.: How important is liver damage in the use of anectine controlled electroshock? Confinia neurol. *14*:275, 1954.
Robinson, M. F.: What price lobotomy? J. Abnorm. & Soc. Psychol. *41*:421, 1946.
Robinson, R. C. V.: Adjunctive therapy of dermatoses with Librium. Dis. Nerv. Syst. (suppl.) *21*:43, 1960.
Robitscher, J. B., ahd Pulver, S. E.: Orphenadrine in the treatment of depression. Am. J. Psychiat. *114*:1113, 1958.
Rockwell, F. W.: Dibenamine therapy in certain psychopathologic syndromes. Psychosom. Med. *10*:230, 1948.
Rodnick, E. H.: The effect of metrazol shock upon habit systems. J. Abnorm. & Soc. Psychol. *37*:560, 1942.
Roebuck, B. E., Chambers, J. L., and Williams, E.: An evaluation of the therapeutic use of triflupromazine in mental disease. J. Nerv. & Ment. Dis. *129*:184, 1959.
Roizin, L., True, C., and Knight, M.: Structural effects of tranquilizers. *In* The Effect of Pharmacologic Agents on the Nervous System. Chapter XVIII ,Proc. Assoc. Res. Nerv. Ment. Dis. Baltimore, Williams & Wilkins, 1959.
Römer, R.: Zum Thema "Psychochirurgie." Med. Klin. *42*:561, 1947.
Ropert, P.: Drug addiction, psychotic illness

and brain self-stimulation. Canad. Med. Ass. J. *95*:1030, 1966.
Ropert, R., and Berges, J.: Place de la Nortriptyline dans le groupe des anti-dépresseurs, considérations cliniques et électro-encéphalographiques. Ann. méd.-psychol. *125/1*:750, 1967.
Rose, J. T., and Westhead, T. T.: Treatment of depression. A comparative trial of imipramine and desipramine. Brit. J. Psychiat. *113*:659, 1967.
Rose, L., and Watson, A.: Flurothyl-induced convulsions. Clin. Trials J. p. 749, 1967.
Rosie, J. M.: The results of prefrontal leucotomy in 68 patients not discharged from hospital. J. Ment. Sc. *95*:431, 1949.
Rosner, B. S., Fierman, L. B., and Kramer, J. F.: Clinical evaluation of Meratran and Frenquel on a chronic psychotic population. Am. J. Psychiat. *113*:993, 1957.
Ross, J. R.: The pharmacological shock treatment of schizophrenia. Am. J. Psychiat. *95*:769, 1939.
——, and Malzberg, B.: A review of the results of the pharmacological shock therapy and the metrazol convulsive therapy in New York State. Am. J. Psychiat. *96*: 297, 1939.
Rossmann, J. M., and Chine, W. B.: The pharmacological "shock" treatment of chronic schizophrenia. Am. J. Psychiat. *94*:1323, 1938.
Roth, G.: The treatment of psychiatric conditions with Nozinan. Wien. med. Wchnschr. *109*:1021, 1959.
Roth, M.: Changes in EEG under barbiturate anaesthesia produced by electro-convulsive treatment and their significance for the theory of ECT action. EEG Clin. Neurophysiol. *3*:261, 1951.
——: A theory of ECT action and its bearing on the biological significance of epilepsy. J. Ment. Sci. *98*:44, 1952.
——: Affective disorders arising in the senium. J. Ment. Sc. *102*:141, 1956.
——, Kay, D. W. K., Shaw, J., and Green, J.: Prognosis and pentothal induced electroencephalographic changes in electroconvulsive treatment. EEG and Clin. Neurophys. *9*:225, 1957.
Rothenberg, P. A., and Hall. Ch.: Agranulocytosis following use of imipramine hydrochloride (Tofranil). Amer. J. Psychiat. *116*: 847, 1960.
Rothman, T.: Nine years experience with the treatment of refractory psychoneuroses and personality disorders with sodium pentothal, methamphetamine and methylphenidate (Ritalin). *In* P. B. Bradley, P. Deniker and C. Radouco-Thomas (Eds.): Neuro-Psychopharmacology, Vol. 1: 668 (CINP Congr., Rom 1958). Amsterdam, Elsevier, 1959.
——: Preliminary study of the effectiveness of isocarboxazid in depressive syndromes. J. Neuropsychiat. *1*:148, 1960.
——, Grayson, H., and Ferguson, J.: An evaluation of the effectiveness of isocarboxazid (Marplan) in the depressive syndromes. Compr. Psychiat. *2*:27, 1961.
——, and Sward, K.: Studies in pharmacological psychotherapy. Arch. Neurol. and Psychiat. *75*:95, 1956.
Rothschild, D., and Kaye, A.: The effects of prefrontal lobotomy on the symptomatology of schizophrenic patients. Am. J. Psychiat. *105*:752, 1949.
Rothstein, C., and Lacerva, S. P.: Prochlorperazine in a psychotic geriatric group. J. Maine Med. Assoc. *50*:4, 1959.
Roubîĉek, J.: Pharmacologically activated psychotherapy. Proc. IV World Congr. of Psychiat. Ed.: Lopez-Ibor, Excerpta Medica Translation, Amsterdam: *4*:2841, 1966.
Roulet, N., Alvarez, R. R., Duffy, J. P., Lenkoski, L. D., and Bidder, T. G.: Imipramine in depression: A controlled study. Amer. J. Psychiat. *119*:427, 1962.
Rowe, R. P., Bloom, B. M., P'An, S. Y., and Finger, K. F.: Pharmacological studies with nialamide, a new antidepressant agent. Proc. Soc. Exper. Biol. & Med. *101*:832, 1959.
Rubenovitch, P.: Étude de quelques réactions psychologiques, provoquées par le choc insulinique chez les schizophrènes. Évolution psychiatrique 2, 1938.
Rubin, M., and Slonicki, A.: A proposed mechanism for the skin-eye syndrome. *In* H. Brill, J. O. Cole, P. Deniker, H. Hippius, and P. B. Bradley (Eds.): Neuro-Psychopharmacology, *V*: 661 (CINP. Congr. Washington 1966). Amsterdam, Excerpta Med. Found., Internat. Congr. Scr. No. 129, 1967.
Ruchwarger, A.: Use of Deprol (meprobamate combined with benactyzine hydrochloride) in the office treatment of depression. Med. Ann. District of Columbia *28*:438, 1959.
Rudberg-Lindqvist, B. E., and Lindqvist, G.: The antidepressive effect of amitriptyline in an adrenalectomized patient. Amer. J. Psychiat. *120*:912, 1964.
Rudolf, G. de M.: The treatment of mental defectives with aneurin for one year. J. Ment. Sc. *96*:265, 1950.
Rudy, L. H., Himwich, H. E., and Tasher, D. C.: Clinical evaluation of two phenothiazine compounds, promazine and mepazine. Am. J. Psychiat. *113*:979, 1957.
——, Rinaldi, F., Costa, E., Himwich, H. E., Tuteur, W., and Glotzer, J.: The use of trifluoperazine in the treatment of acute and chronic psychotics. *In:* Trifluoperazine. Philadelphia: Lea and Febiger, 1958.
Ruffin, A.: Erfahrungen mit Insulinschockbehandlung bei Schizophrenie. Allg. Ztschr. f. Psychiat. *107*:110, 1937.
Runge, H.: Zur Prognose der Schizophrenie (Nachuntersuchung schockbehandelter Psychosen). Nervenarzt 151, 1942.
Rüsken, W.: Über die Beeinflussung schizophrener Krankheitszustände durch die Leukotomie. Nervenarzt *21*:508, 1950.
Rylander, G.: Personality changes after operations on the frontal lobes. Acta Psychiat. & Neurol. Suppl. 15, London, 1939.
——: Mental changes after excision of cerebral tissue. Acta Psychiat. & Neurol. Suppl. 25, Copenhagen, 1943.

——: Personality analyses before and after frontal lobotomy. A. Research Nerv. & Ment. Dis., Proc. 26, 1947.

Sackler, A. M., Sackler, M. D., Sackler, R. R., and Van Ophuijsen, J. H. W.: Nonconvulsive biochemotherapy with histamine and electric convulsive therapy. J. Nerv. & Ment. Dis. *110*; 149 and 195, 1949.

Sagebiel, J. L.: Regressive convulsive therapy and lobotomy in the treatment of mental disorders. Dis. Nerv. Syst. *22*:193, 1961.

St. Jean, A., Sterlin, C., Noe, W., and Ban, T. A.: Clinical studies with propericiazine (R.P.8909). Dis. Nerv. Syst. *28*:526, 1967.

St. Laurent, J., Cahn, C.-H., and Ban, T. A.: Treatment of psychiatric patients with a phenothiazine derivative (prochlorperazine) with special reference to after care. Amer. J. Psychiat. *118*:938, 1962.

Sainz, A.: Benzquinamide: A preliminary report. Amer. J. Psychiat. *119*:777, 1963.

Sainz, A. A.: Clinical applications of chlorpromazine in psychiatry. Psychopharmacology *42*:39, 1956.

——: Diagnosis and treatment of endogenous depressions with mono-amino-oxidase inhibitors. Dis. Nerv. Syst. *20*:537, 1959.

——: Speculation on the mode of action. *In:* Psychopharmacology Frontiers (ed. by N. S. Kline) Boston: Little, Brown & Co., 1959.

——: The phrenopraxic activity of a nonnoxious anti-depressant. Ann. New York Acad. Sc. *80*:780, 1959.

Sakel, M.: Neue Behandlung der Morphinsucht. Ztschr. f. d. ges. Neurol. u. Psychiat. *143*:506, 1933.

——: Zur Methodik der Hypoglykämiebehandlung von Psychosen. Wien. klin. Wchnschr. *49*:1278, 1936.

——: Zur Bedeutung des epileptischen Anfalls als therapeutischer Faktor in der medikamentösen Schocktherapie der Schizophrenie. Klin. Wchnschr, *2*:1277, 1937.

——: Neue Behandlungsmethode der Schizophrenie. Mortiz Perles, Wien and Leipzig: 1935.

——: The nature and origin of the hypoglycemic treatment of psychoses. Am. J. Psychiat. *94* (Supp.):24, 1938.

——: The pharmacological shock treatment of schizophrenia. Nervous and Mental Disseases Monograph Series, No. 62. New York: Nervous Mental Diseases Publishing Company, 1938.

——: Insulinotherapy and shock therapies. Congrès Internat. de Psychiat. *4*:163, 1950.

——: Schizophrenia. New York, Philosophical Library, 1958.

——, and Dussik, K. T.: Ergebnisse der Hypoglykämieschockbehandlung der Schizophrenie. Ztschr. f. d. ges. Neurol. u. Psychiat. *155*:351, 1936.

Sal y Rosas, F.: El cardiazol en la epilepsia. Rev. di psiquiat. y criminol. *4*:709, 1939.

——: Notes on the application of the Sakel Method in mental patients in Peru. *In* M. Rinkel: Insulin Treatment in Psychiatry. New York: Philosophical Library, 1959.

Salm, H.: Die Elektrokrampfbehandlung im Erleben der Behandelten. Psychiat., Neurol. u. med. Psychol. *2*:245, 1950.

Salzman, L.: Evaluation of shock therapy. Am. J. Psychiat. *103*:669, 1947.

Salzmann, M. M.: A controlled trial with trimipramine, a new antidepressant drug. Brit. J. Psychiat. *111*:1105, 1965.

Samuels, A. S.: Acute chlorpromazine poisoning. Am. J. Psychiat. *113*:746, 1957.

Sandifer, M. G., Jr., Albert, R. F., and Wilson, I. C.: Patient preference: Indoklon vs. electroshock therapy. J. Nerv. Ment. Dis. *134*:184, 1962.

Sandifer, M. G., Wilson, I. C., and Gambill, J. M.: The influence of case selection and dosage in an antidepressant drug trial. Brit. J. Psychiat. *111*:142, 1965.

Sandison, R. A.: The psychology of electric convulsion treatment. J. Ment. Sc. *96*:734, 1950.

——, and McGregor, J. S.: A year's experience of intravenous insulin in the hypoglycemic shock treatment of schizophrenia. J. Ment. Sc. *88*:26, 1942.

——,Spencer, A. M., and Whitelaw, J. D. A.: The therapeutic value of lysergic acid diethylamide in mental illness. J. Ment. Sci. *100*:491, 1954.

Sands, S. L., and Malamud, W.: A rating scale analysis of the clinical effects of lobotomy. Am. J. Psychiat. *105*:760, 1949.

Sano, I., Kakimoto, Y., Okamoto, T., Najajimo, H., and Kudo, Y.: Excretion of 5 oxyindol acetic acid in the urine of schizophrenics with consideration of the influence of chlorpromazine and reserpine on the metabolism of serotonin. Schweiz. med. Wchnschr. *87*:214, 1957.

Sargant, W.: Seven years of experience with modified insulin treatment in neuroses and early psychoses. Am. J. Psychiat. *105*:821, 1949.

——: Discussions on indications for shock therapy. J. Ment. Sc. *97*:135, 1951.

——: Leucotomy in psychosomatic disorders. Lancet *2*:87, 1951.

——: Sedatives and tranquillisers. Brit. Med. J. *2*:1031, 1095, 1958,

——: The present indications for leucotomy. Lancet *1*:1197, 1962.

——, and Craske, N.: Modified insulin therapy in war neuroses. Lancet *2*:212, 1941.

——, and Slater, E.: An introduction to somatic methods of treatment in psychiatry. Baltimore: Williams and Wilkins Co., 1944.

——, and ——: An introduction to physical methods of treatment in psychiatry. Edinburgh: E. & S. Livingstone, Ltd., 1963.

——, and Stewart, C. M.: Chronic battle neurosis treated with prefrontal leucotomy. Brit. M. J. *2*:866, 1947.

——, Walter, C. J. S., and Wright, N.: New treatment of some chronic tension states. Brit. Med. J. *1*:322, 1966.

Sarro, R., and De La Cruz, M.: Clinical experience with a new orthothymic drug: Covatin (N. 68). Medicamenta, *14*:295, 1956.

Sarwer-Foner, G. J.: The dynamics of psy-

chiatric drug therapy. Springfield: Charles C Thomas, 1960.
——, Grauer, H., Mackay, J., and Korcanyi, E. K.: Depressive states and drugs. Med. Serv. J. Canada *15*:539, 1959.
——, Hajnsek, F., Groszman, M., Grauer, H., and Koranyi, E. K.: Clinical investigation of levomepromazine (Nozinan) in open psychiatric settings. Med. Serv. J. *17*:798, 1961.
——, and Korcanyi, E. K.: Clinical investigation of azacyclonal hydrochloride. Canad. P. A. J. *1*:92, 1956.
——, and Ogle, W.: Psychosis and Enhanced Anxiety produced by reserpine and chlorpromazine. Canad. M. A. J. *74*:526-532, 1956.
Sattes, H.: Die Behandlung der Chorea maior mit dem Monoamin-Freisetzer "Nitoman". Psychiat. Neurol. *140*:13, 1960.
Saul, G. D., and Feld, M.: The limbic system and EST seizures. Compr. Psychiat. *1*:281, 1960.
Saunders, J. C.: Etiology of psychosis theorized from drug actions. *In* N. S. Kline, ed. Psychopharmacology Frontiers. Boston: Little, Brown & Co., 1959.
Savitzky, N., and Karliner, W.: Reflex studies in electroshock treatments. Arch. Neurol. & Psychiat. *59*:481, 1948.
——, and Tarachow, S.: The question of shorter courses of electroshock therapy in the depressions. J. Nerv. & Ment. Dis. *101*:115, 1945.
Scarff, J. E.: Unilateral prefrontal lobotomy for the relief of intractable pain and termination of narcotic addiction. Surg., Gynec. & Obst. *89*:385, 1949.
——, and Kalinowsky, L. B.: Prefrontal lobotomy under direct vision. New York State J. Med. *47*:2669, 1947.
Scartozzi, C.: Anestesia chirurgica con l'elettro-shock alla Cerletti. Minerva chir. *4*:371, 1949.
Schaaf, M., and Payne, Ch. A.: Dystonic reactions to prochlorperazine in hypoparathyroidism. N. Engl. J. Med. *275*:991, 1966.
Schallek, W., Kuehn, A., and Jew, N.: Effects of chlordiazepoxide (Librium) and other psychotropic agents on the limbic system of the brain. Ann. N.Y. Acad. Sci. *96*:303, 1962.
——, Zabransky, F., and Kuehn, A.: Effects of benzodiazepines on central nervous system of cat. Arch. Int. Pharmacodyn. *149*: 467, 1964.
Schalterbrand, G.: Bemerkungen zur Schockbehandlung. Ztschr. f. d. ges. Neurol. u. Psychiat. *107*:5, 1949.
Schäpperle, O., and Schwarz, H.: Klinische Untersuchung mit dem Phenothiazinderivit Ponsital. Med. Welt *18 N.F.*:821, 1967.
Scharfetter, Ch.: Vergiftung mit einem Antidepressivum. Status epilepticus bei suicidaler Amitriptylin-intoxikation. Bemerkungen zur Neurologie schwerer Vergiftungen. Arch. Psychiat. Nervenkr. *207*:79, 1965.
Schatner, M., and O'Neill, F. J.: Some observations in treatment of dementia praecox with hypoglycemia. Psychiatric Quart. *12*:5, 1938.
Scheflen, A. E., and Reiner, E. R.: Sensitivity in insulin coma therapy. J. Clin. Exper. Psychopath. *13*:225, 1952.
Schelkunov, E. L.: Adrenergic effect of chronic administration of neuroleptics. Nature *214*: 1210, 1967.
Scherbel, A. L.: Clinical experience in treatment of over 2,000 cases with amine oxidase inhibitors. Dis. Nerv. Syst. (Suppl.) *21*:67, 1960.
Scherer, I. W.: The psychological scores of mental patients in an individual and group testing situation. J. Clin. Psychol. *5*:405, 1949.
——, and Winne, J. F.: Intracerebral procaine as prognostic test for prefrontal lobotomy. A.M.A. Arch. Neurol. & Psychiat. *76*:220, 1956.
Scherr, A.: Le Largactil en psychiatrie extrahospitalière. Encéphale. *45*:388, 1956.
Scheurle, G.: Have the side effects of reserpine a therapeutic significance? Dt. med. Woch. *82*:2227, 1957.
——: The treatment of chronic schizophrenia with reserpine. Dt. med. Woch. *82*:2226, 1957.
Schiele, B. C.: The unique therapeutic properties of tranylcypromine and trifluoperazine (Parstelin). A. J. Psychiat. *117*:245, 1960.
——, Vestre, N. D., and MacNaughton, D. V.: Treatment of hospitalized schizophrenics with trifluoperazine plus tranylcypromine: A double-blind controlled study. Compr. Psychiat. *4*:66, 1963.
Schilder, P.: Notes on psychology of metrazol treatment of schizophrenia. J. Nerv. & Ment. Dis. *89*:133, 1939.
Schildge, E.: Zur Erlebnisseite der Elektrokrampfbehandlung. Tuebingen: Bericht u. d. Kongress f. Neurol., Psychiat., 1947.
——: Die Aura bei abortiven Elektroschock. Nervenarzt *29*:52, 1949.
Schildkraut, J. J., Schanberg, S. M., Breese, G. R., and Kopin, I. J.: Norepinephrine metabolism and drugs used in the affective disorders: A possible mechanism of action. Amer. J. Psychiat. *124*:600, 1957.
Schindler, W., and Häflinger, F.: Über Derivative des Iminodibenzyls. Helv. chim. Acta *37*:472, 1954.
Schlagenhauf, G., Tupin, J., and White, R. B.: The use of lithium carbonate in the treatment of manic psychoses. Amer. J. Psychiat. *123*:201, 1966.
Schläpfer, U., and Mumenthaler, M.: Klinische Prüfung der muskelrelaxierenden Wirkung von Valium "Roche" bei Spastikern. Schweiz. med. Wschr. *94*:1425, 1964.
Schlichter. W., Bristoe, M. E., Schultz, S., and Henderson, A. L.: Seizures occurring during intensive chlorpromazine therapy. Canad. M. A. J. *74*:364, 1956.
Schmid, H. E.: Contributions to the histophysiology of insulin. Am. J. Psychiat. *94* (Supp.):154, 1938.
Schmidt, M., and Daudet, G.: Action du benzpéridol (8089 CB soluté buvable dosé à 0,2 mg/ml) sur les troubles du com-

portement d'un groupe d'enfants suivis dans un service de débiles profonds. Ann. méd.-psychol. *126/I*:113, 1968.
Schmidt, R.: Insulinschock und Auge. Nervenarzt 11, 1938.
Schmidt, W. R., and Jarcho, L. W.: Persistent dyskinesias following phenothiazine therapy. Arch. Neurol. *14*:369, 1966.
Schmied, J., and Ziegler, A.: Tofranil in der Geriatrie. Praxis. 49:472, 1960.
Schmieder, F.: Zur Häufigkeit und Bedeutung der Wirbelsäulenschädigungen bei den Krampf und Schockverfahren. Allg. Ztschr. f. Psychiat. *121*:141, 1942.
Schmitt, D.: Elektrokardiographische Untersuchungen bei der Schock- und Krampfbehandlung der Schizophrenie. Ztschr. f. d. ges. Neurol. u. Psychiat. *166*: 108, 1939.
Schmitt, W.: Die Pharmakotherapie depressiver Psychosen mit einem Imino-dibenzylderivat. Nervenarzt. *30*:5, 1959.
——, Meyer, H.-H., Quadbeck, G., and Vogt, J.: Die Pharmakotherapie depressiver Psychosen mit einem neuen Iminostilben-Derivat. Med. Klin. *57*:49, 1962.
Schneider, C.: Behandlung und Verhütung der Geisteskrankheiten. Berlin: Springer, 1939.
Schneider, E.: Die Amenorrhoe bei Geisteskrankheiten und ihr Verhalten bei der Elektroschockbehandlung Zentralbl. f. *71*:964, 1949.
Schneider, J. A., Plummer, A. J., Earl, A. E., and Gaunt, R.: Neuropharmacological aspects of reserpine. Ann. New York Acad. Sc. *61*:17, 1955.
Schneider, P. B., and Crot, M.: Le résultat du traitement ambulatoire de la dépression par un dérivè de l'iminodibenzyle. Praxis. *48*:313, 1959.
Schneider, R. A.: The acute effects of reserpine and of amytal on central sympathetic reactivity. Ann. New York Acad. Sc. *61*: 150, 1955.
Schnetzler, J. P., and Lamand, J. C.: La thioridazine dans le traitement des états dépressifs. Ann. méd.-psychol. *120/I*:609, 1962.
——, ——, Cassassuce, J., and Carrel, M.: Effets des neuroleptiques en général et de la thioridazine en particulier sur la sexualité. Encéphale *53*:207, 1964.
Schönke, A.: Juristische Fragen der psychiatrischen Praxis. Nervenarzt *22*:161, 1951.
Schorer, C. E.: Report of hypomanic excitement with imipramine treatment of depression. Am. J. Psychiat. *116*:844, 1960.
Schou, M.: Meratran. Brit. Med. J. *1*:1236, 1956.
——: Lithium in psychiatric therapy. Psychopharmacol. *1*:65, 1960.
——, Juel-Nielson, N., Strömgren, E., and Voldby, H.: Treatment of manic psychoses by administration of lithium salts. J. Neurol., Neurosurg. & Psychiat. *17*:250, 1954.
——: Lithium in Psychiatry. In press.
Schrader, P. J., and Robinson, M. F.: Evaluation of prefrontal lobotomy through ward behavior. J. Abnorm. & Soc. Psychol. *40*:61, 1945.
Schroeder, K.: Über Sulfosinbehandlung der Schizophrenie (Dementia praecox). Ugesk. f. laeger. I, 1929.
Schube, P. G., McManamy, M. C., Trapp, C. E., and Myerson, A.: The effect of benzedrine sulphate on certain abnormal mental states. Am. J. Psychiat. *94*:27, 1937.
Schulman, J. L., and Greben, S. E.: The effect of glucagon on the blood glucose level and the clinical state in the presence of marked insulin hypoglycemia. J. Clin. Investig. *36*:74, 1957.
Schulte, W.: Die Elektroschockbehandlung. Psychiat., Neurol. u. med. Psychol. *1*:167, 1949.
——, and Dreyer, R.: Eine cerebrale tödliche Komplikation nach Elektroschock. Nervenarzt *21*:175, 1950.
Schulz, H., Müller, J., Roth, B., and Stein, J.: Die bioelektrisch kontrollierte Krampfbehandlung der endogenen Psychosen in Narkose und Relaxation. Arch. f. Psychiat. u. Nervenkrankh. 1968 (in press).
Schulz, H. E.: Zur Frage des epileptischen Anfalls im Insulinschock. Psychiat.-Neurol. Wchnschr. *40*:307, 1938.
Schumacher: Spontane Krampfanfälle nach Elektrokonvulsionen. Psychiat., Neurol. u. med. Psychol. *1*:94, 1949.
Schunzelaar, K.: Treatment of enuresis and encopresis with Tofranil in chronic psychiatric female inpatients. Acta neurol. psychiat. belg. *63*:333, 1963.
Schuster, J.: Zur Entdeckung der Insulinschocktherapie bei akuten Geisteskrankheiten insbesondere bei der Schizophrenie. Budapest: Selbstverlag, 1937.
Schut, J. W., and Himwich, H. E.: The effect of Meratran on 25 institutionalized mental patients. Am. J. Psychiat. *111*:837, 1955.
Schwab, H., and Riechelmann, R.: Über die Schockangst bei manisch-depressiven Psychosen. Allg. Ztschr. f. Psychiat. *125*: 115, 1949.
Schwab, O.: Über Stützreaktionen (Magnus) beim Menschen. Ztschr. f. d. ges. Neurol. u. Psychiat. *108*:585, 1927.
Schwartz, E.: Depression in Parkinsonism treated by prefrontal leucotomy. J. Ment. Sc. *91*:503, 1945.
Schwarz, B. E., Bickford, R. G., and Rome, H. P.: Reversibility of induced psychosis with chlorpromazine. Proc. Staff Mtg. Mayo Clinic. *30*:407, 1955.
Schwarz, L., Schmidt, Jr., H., and Stern, J. A.: A double-blind trial of the efficacy of promazine in the treatment of alcohol withdrawal syndrome. Dis. Nerv. Syst. *29*:173, 1968.
Scott, P. A. L., Grimshaw, L., and Molony, H. M. P.: Hypotensive episodes following treatment with meprobamate. Lancet. *2*:1158, 1956.
Scott, R. D.: The psychology of insulin coma treatment. Brit. J. M. Psychol. *23*: 15, 1950.
Scoville, W. B.: Selective cortical undercutting, Proc. Roy. Soc. Med. 42 Suppl.: 3, 1949.

——: Late results of orbital undercutting. Am. J. Psychiat. *117*:525, 1960.
——, and Wilk, E. K.: Selective cortical undercutting. Am. J. Psychiat. *107*:730, 1951.
Seager, C. P., and Leitch, A.: Benactyzine in Psychoneurosis: a controlled clinical trial in hospital patients. Brit. Med. J. *2*:1407, 1956.
Šedivec, V., and Černik, V.: Death in electroshock treatment. Českoslov. Psychiatr. *52*:25, 1956.
Segal, L. J., and Tansley, A. E.: A clinical trial with hydroxyzine (atarax) on a group of maladjusted educationally subnormal children. J. Ment. Sc. *103*:677, 1957.
Seggario, J. A.: Étude clinique et symptomatologie neurologique au cours des traitements au moyen de comas hypoglycémiques prolongués. Encéphale *42*:43, 1953.
Seid, B.: A study of the antianxiety effect of nortriptyline in urological patients. Curr. Ther. Res. *6*:156, 1964.
Seignot, M. J.-N.: Un cas de maladie des tics de Gilles de la Tourette guéri par le R.1625. Ann. méd.-psychol. *119/1*:578, 1961.
Selbach, H.: Über intravenöse PH-Messungen im experimentellen epileptischen Anfall (durch Cardiazol). Ztschr. f. d. ges. Neurol. u. Psychiat. *160*:334, 1937.
Selbach, C., and Selbach, H.: Phenothiazinwirkung und somatopsychische Dynamik. Nervenarzt *27*:145, 1959.
Selinsky, H.: The selective use of electroshock therapy as an adjuvant to psychotherapy. Bull. New York Acad. Med. *19*: 245, 1943.
Selling, L. S.: Clinical study of new tranquilizing drug: use of Miltown (2-methyl-2-N-Propyl-1, 3-Propanediol Dicarbamate). J.A.M.A. *157*:1594, 1955.
Selzer, M. L., and Inderbitzin, L. B.: Renal function after EST. Amer. J. Psychiat. *121*:266, 1964.
——, Reinhart, M. J., and Deeney, M. D.: Acute renal failure following EST. Amer. J. Psychiat. *120*:602, 1963.
Semer, J. M., Friedland, P., Vaisberg, M., and Greenberg, A.: The use of metronidazole in the treatment of alcoholism. Amer. J. Psychiat. *123*:722, 1967.
Sen, G., and Bose, K. C.: Rauwolfia serpentina: a new Indian drug for insanity and high blood pressure. Indian Med. World. *2*:194, 1930.
Seneca, H.: Hydroxyzine (Atarax) as a therapeutic agent. Antibiot. Med. *4*:25, 1957.
Sereijskii, M. I.: Results and perspectives in active therapy of psychoses. Nevropat. i Psikhiat. 17, 1948.
——, and Geschelina, L. L.: Endogene und exogene Zustandsbilder bei Insulinhypoglykämie. Arbeiten aus dem Gannuschkin Institut. Moscow: 1938.
Serova: (quoted by Lustig, B.) New research *in:* Soviet Psychiatry. Berlin: Report of Ost-Europa Institut, 1957.
Settel, E.: Clinical observations on the use of hydroxyzine (Atarax) in tension states. Amer. Practit. *8*:1584, 1957.
Severinghaus, E., and Nutley, N. J.: The present and future of Marsilid: Open discussion. J. Clin. Exper. Psychopath. *19*: 183 (Supp.), 1958.
Shagass, C., Azima, H., and Sangowicz, J.: Effect of meprobamate in sustained high dosage on the EEG and sedation threshold. Electroenceph. Clin. Neurophysiol. *11*:275, 1959.
——, and Bittle, R.: Therapeutic effects of LSD: A follow-up study. N. Jerv. & Ment. Dis. *144*:471, 1967.
——, Naiman, J., and Mihalik, J.: An objective test which differentiates between neurotic and psychotic depression. A.M.A. Neurol. & Psychiat. *75*:461, 1956.
Shanklin, J. G.: Transorbital lobotomy in institutional practice. Am. J. Psychiat. *107*:120, 1950.
Shapiro, A. K.: A contribution to a history of the placebo effect. Behavioral Science *5*:109, 1960.
——: A historic and heuristic definition of the placebo. Psychiatry *27*:52, 1964.
——, and Shapiro, E.: Treatment of Gilles de la Tourette's syndrome with haloperidol. Brit. J. Psychiat. *114*:345, 1968.
Shapiro, H. D., and Freeman, W.: Shock therapy (insulin and metrazol) in the neuroses. M. Ann. District of Columbia *8*:65, 1939.
Shapiro, M. F.: Despair, trifluoperazine, exercise, and temperature of 108° F. Amer. J. Psychiat. *124*:705, 1967.
Sharpley, P., Heistad, G., and Schiele, B. C.: Comparison of butaperazine and perphenazine: A double-blind controlled study. Psychopharmacologia *5*:209, 1964.
Shaw, E. B., Dermott, R. V., Lee, R., and Burbridge, T. N.: Phenothiazine tranquillisers as a cause of severe seizures. Pediatrics *23*:485, 1959.
Shepherd, M.: Reserpine: problems associated with the use of a so-called tranquillising agent. Proc. Roy. Soc. Med. *49*:*33*:849, 1956.
——: Clinical trial of the treatment of depressive illness. Report to the Medical Research Council by its Clinical Psychiatry. Committee. Brit. Med. J. *1*:881, 1965.
——, Goddman, N., and Watt, D. C.: The application of hospital statistics in the evaluation of pharmacotherapy in a psychiatric population. Compr. Psychiat. *2*:11, 1961.
——, Lader, M., and Rodnight, R.: Clinical Psychopharmacology. London, English Universities Press, 1968.
——, and Watt, D. C.: A controlled clinical study of chlorpromazine and reserpine in chronic schizophrenia. J. Neurol., Neurosurg. 1 *19*:232, 1956.
Shepley, W. H., and McGregor, J. S.: Electrically induced convulsions in treatment of mental disorders. Brit. M. J. *11*:1269, 1939.
Sherman, I., Mergener, J., and Levitin, D.: Effect of convulsive therapy on memory. Am. J. Psychiat. *98*:401, 1941.
Shimizu, A., Bost, K., and Himwich, H. E.: Electroencephalographic studies of halo-

peridol. Int. Pharmacopsychiat. *1*:134, 1968.

Shipley, W. C., and Kant, F.: The insulin-shock and metrazol treatments of schizophrenia with emphasis on the psychological aspects. Psychol. Bull. *37*:259, 1940.

Shoor, M., and Adams, F. H.: The intensive electric shock therapy of chronic disturbed psychotic patients. Am. J. Psychiat. *107*: 279, 1950.

Shorvon, H. J.: Prefrontal leucotomy and the depersonalization syndrome. Lancet *2*:714, 1947.

——: Psychopathologie de la dépersonanalisation. 111. Discussion in EY H. et al. Comptes rendues du Premier Congrès Mondial de Psychiat. 1. Psychopath. gén. Paris: Hermann et Cie, 1952.

Shurley, J. T., and Morris, H. M., Jr.: Autonomic function in insulin coma therapy. J. Nerv. & Ment. Dis. *14*:532, 1951.

——, and Sargant, W.: Excitatory abreaction: With special reference to its mechanism and the use of ether. J. Ment. Sc. *93*:709, 1947.

Siegmann, A.: Electro-convulsive treatment in manic depressive psychosis. Canad. Psychiat. Assoc. J. *4*:213, 1959.

Siekert, R. G., Williams, S. C., and Windle, W. F.: Histologic study of the brains of monkeys after experimental electric shock. Arch. Neurol. & Psychiat. *63*:79, 1950.

Sigg, E. B.: Pharmacological studies with Tofranil. Canad. Psychiat. Assoc. J. *4*:75, 1959.

Sigwald, J.: La cure ambulatoire par la chlorpromazine. Encéphale. *45*:392, 1956.

——, and Bouttier, D.: La phénothiazine en thérapeutique psychiatrique. Presse méd. Avril: 607, 1953.

——, ——, Raymondeaud, C., Marquez, M., and Gal J. C.: Étude de l'action sur l'akinésie parkinsonienne de deux dérivés de l'iminodibenzyl: le chlorhydrate de N-(gamma-dimethylaminopropyl)-iminodibenzyle ou Imipramine et le beta-(hydroxyethyl-4″ piperazinyl)-3′ propyl-5 iminodibenzyle, ou 8307 RP. Presse médic. *67*:1698, 1959.

——, ——, ——, and Piot, Cl.: Quatre cas de dyskinésie facio-bucco-linguomasticatrice à évolution prolongée secondaire à un traitement par les neuroleptiques. Rev. neurol. *100*:751, 1959.

——, Henne, M., Bouttier, J., Raymondeaud, C., and Quetin, A.: Action of new phenothiazine in psychiatry and neurology: therapeutic properties of maleate acid of 3-levomethyoxy (3 dimethyl-amino-2-methyl-10-propyl) phenothiazine (7044.RP). Presse Méd. *64*:2011, 1956.

——, Herbert, H., and Quetin, A.: Traitement du zona et des algies zosteriennes (ainsi que de certaines algies rebelles) par les phénothiazines. Sem. Hôp. Paris. *33*:1137, 1957.

Silberman, M., and Ransohoff, J.: Medicolegal problems in psychosurgery. Am. J. Psychiat. *110*:801, 1954.

Sillman, L. R., and Terrence, C.: An analysis of shock therapy in schizophrenia on the basis of a nitrogen inhalation control series. Psychiatric Quart. *17*:241, 1943.

Silverman, M.: The clinical response of psychoneurotics to chlorpromazine. J. Ment. Sci. *101*:640, 1955.

——: Organic stupor subsequent to a severe head injury treated with ECT. Brit. J. Psychiat. *110*:648, 1964.

Simeon, J., Keskiner, A., Ponce, D., Itil, T., and Fink, M.: Clinical trial of Navane (thiothixene) in schizophrenia. Curr. Ther. Res. *9*:10, 1967.

Simon, A., Bowman, K. M., and Halliday, N.: Studies in electronarcosis therapy. J. Nerv. & Ment. Dis. *107*:358, 1948.

Simonson, M.: Phenothiazine depressive reaction. J. Neuropsychiat. *5*:259, 1964.

Simpson, G. M.: Reactions following the intra-muscular administration of chlorprothixene. Amer. J. Psychiat. *120*:1021, 1964.

——, Amin, M., Kunz, E., and McCafferty, F. V.: Studies on a second long-acting fluphenazine. Amer. J. Psychiat. *121*:784, 1965.

——, and Kunz-Bartholini, E.: Relationship of individual tolerance, behavior and phenothiazine produced extrapyramidal system disturbance. Dis. Nerv. Syst. *29*: 269, 1968.

Simpson, R. W.: The effects of Notensil in chronic mental illness. J. Ment. Sci. *104*: 179, 1958,

Sindell, J. A.: The vasomotor factor in hypoglycemia. J. Nerv. & Ment. Dis. *105*:616, 1947.

Singh, H.: A case of inhibition of ejaculation as a side effect of Mellaril. Amer. J. Psychiat. *117*:1041, 1961.

——: Therapeutic use of thioridazine in premature ejaculation. Amer J. Psychiat. *119*:891, 1963.

Singh, K.: Clinical uses of SCTZ—a preliminary report. Am. J. Psychiat. *116*:*8*: 749, 1960.

Sjöqvist, O., af Björkesten and Fernström, U.: The diagnosis of intracerebral hematomas following frontal lobotomy. Acta chir. Scandinav. *98*:280, 1949.

Skarbek, A.: Trial of amitriptyline in chronic depression. Dis. Nerv. Syst. *24*:115, 1963.

——, and Hill, G. B.: An extended trial of oxypertine in five selected cases of chronic schizophrenia. Brit. J. Psychiat. *113*:1107, 1967.

——, and Jacobsen, M.: Oxypertine. A review of clinical experience. Brit. J. Psychiat. *111*:1173, 1965.

——, and Smedberg, D.: Amitriptyline: A controlled trial in chronic depressive states. J. Ment. Sci. *108*:859, 1962.

Skorodin, B.: Some observations on the treatment of psychotic reactions with haloperidol. Internat. J. Neuropsychiat. *3*:400, 1967.

Slater, E. T. O.: Evaluation of electric convulsion therapy as compared with conservative methods of treatment in depressive states. J. Ment. Sc. *97*:567, 1951.

Slocum, J. Bennett, C. L., and Pool, J. L.: The role of prefrontal lobe surgery as a

means of eradicating intractable anxiety. Am. J. of Psychiat. *116*:222, 1959.
Sloman, L.: Myocardial infarction during imipramine treatment of depression. Canad. M. A. J. *82*:20, 1960.
DeSmedt, R., Gambetti, P., and Claes, C.: Aspects neurologiques et neuropathologiques de l'intoxication par le nialamide. J. neurol. Sci. *2*:554, 1965.
Smigel, J. O., Lowe, K. J., and Green, M.: Emotional and pyschic problems of institutionalized geriatric patients: evaluation of hydroxyzine. J. Am. Geriat. Soc. *7*:61, 1959.
Smith, A. J., Christian, D., Rutherford, A., and Mansfield, E.: A comparison of triflupromazine (Vesprin), chlorpromazine and placebo in 85 chronic patients. Amer. J. Psychiat. *115*:253, 1958.
Smith, D. B.: Thioridazine in the treatment of anxiety in military dependents. Dis. Nerv. Syst. *28*:455, 1967.
Smith, J. A., and Barron, A. R.: The use of chlorprothixene in the disturbed geriatric patient. Amer. J. Psychiat. *122*:213, 1965.
——, Wolfard, J. A., Weber, M., and McLean, D.: Use of citrated calcium carbimide (Temposil) in treatment of chronic alcoholism. J.A.M.A. *165*:2181, 1957.
Smith, J. J.: The endocrine basis and hormonal therapy of alcoholism. New York State J. Med. *50*:1704, 1950.
Smith, K., and Biddy, R. L.: Shock treatment. *In* Spiegel, E. A. (Ed.): Progress in Neurology and Psychiatry, Vol. XIX. New York, Grune & Stratton, 1964.
Smith, L. H., Hastings, D. W., and Hughes, J.: Immediate and follow-up results of electroshock therapy. Am. J. Psychiat. *100*:351, 1943.
Smith, M. E.: Clinical Comparison of tetrabenazine (RO, 1-9569), reserpine and a placebo in chronic schizophrenics. Dis. Nerv. Syst. (suppl.) *21*:120, 1960.
——: The effects of benzquinamide. Dis. Nerv. Syst. *24*: Section two-Monogr. Suppl.: 116, 1963.
Smith, S.: The use of electroplexy (ECT) in psychiatric syndromes complicating pregnancy. J. Ment. Sc. *102*:796, 1956.
Smith, S. W.: Trifluoperazine in children and adolescents with marked behavior problems. Amer. J. Psychiat. *122*:702, 1965.
Smolik, E. A., Hofstatter, L., and Busch, A. K.: Further observations on orbital prefrontal lobotomy in treatment of chronic mental illness. Post-Grad. M. J. *3*:179, 1948.
Snow, L. H., and Rickels, K.: The controlled evaluation of imipramine and amitriptyline in hospitalized depressed psychiatric patients. A contribution to the methodology of drug evaluation. Psychopharmacologia *5*:409, 1964.
Sobel, D. E.: Fetal damage due to ECT, insulin coma, chlorpromazine or reserpine. A. M. A. Arch. Gen. Psychiat. *2*:606, 1960.
Sogliani, G.: Assoziazione armonica alle terapie da shock. Gior. di psichiat. e di neuropat. *67*:284, 1939.
——: Elettroshockterapia e cardiazol terapia. Rassegna di studi psichiat. *28*:652, 1939.
——: Il metronidazolo net trattamento dell'alcoolismo. Minerva med. *58*:1510, 1967.
Solms, H.: Die Krampfbehandlung. *In* Psychiatrie der Gegenwart I/2. Berlin, Springer, 1963.
Solomon, A. P., Darrow, C. W., and Blaurock, M.: Blood pressure and palmic sweat (galvanic) responses of psychotic patients before and after insulin and metrazol therapy. Psychosomatic Med. *1*:118, 1939.
Solomon, H. C., Rose, A. S., and Arnot, R. E.: Electric shock therapy in general paresis. J. Nerv. & Ment. Dis. *107*:377, 1948.
Somers, D. C., and Richardson, R. P.: Bilateral fracture of the femoral necks caused by metrazol convulsions. Am. J. Psychiat. *95*:1193, 1939.
Soulairac, A., Geier, S., de Mijolla, A., and Berouti, R.: Etude de l'action de la thioridazine dans certaines psychoses dépressives et dissociatives chroniques. Ann. méd.-psychol. *125/1*:258, 1967.
——, Schaub, Cl., and Morel, P.: Action d'une butyrophénone-pipérazine (2028 MD) seule ou en association, sur les états d'agitation aigue. Presse méd. *70*:805, 1962.
Spencer, A. M.: The effects of intravenous insulin in Sakel's hypoglycemic treatment. J. Ment. Sc. *93*:483, 1947.
——: Post-hypoglycaemic encephalopathy in Sakel's insulin treatment. J. Ment. Sc. *84*:513, 1948.
——: Modifications in the technique of LSD therapy. Compr. Psychiat. *5*:232, 1964.
Spernau, H.: Der Heilungsverlauf bei der Insulinbehandlung der Schizophrenie. Allg. Ztschr. f. Psychiat. *107*:283, 1938.
Spiegel, E. A., and Wycis, H. T.: Physiological and psychological results of thalamotomy. Proc. Roy. Soc. Med. (suppl.) *42*:84, 1949.
——, and ——: Stereoencephalotomy. New York: Grune & Stratton, 1952 and 1962.
——, ——, Freed, H., and Orchinik, C. W.: A follow-up study of patients treated by thalamotomy and by combined frontal and thalamic lesions. J. Nerv. and Ment. Dis. *124*:399, 1956.
Spiegel-Adolf, M., Spiegel, E. A., Oshkenez, E. W., and Lee, A. J.: Physiochemical effects of electrically induced convulsions. J. Neuropath. & Exper. Neurol. *4*:227, 1945.
——, Wilcox, P. H., and Spiegel, E. A.: Cerebrospinal fluid changes in electroshock treatment of psychoses. Am. J. Psychiat. *104*:697, 1948.
Spiegelberg, U.: Klinisch-psychiatrische Erfahrungen mit einem neuen antriebssteigernden Präparat: 2-Phenyl-3-methyltetrahydro-1,4-oxazinhydrochlorid. Nervenarzt *25*:276, 1954.
Spreng, R. W. E.: Tolserol in acute alcoholism. J. Nerv. and Ment. Dis. *118*:545, 1953.
Staehelin, B.: Mitteilungen zum Wirkungsbereich von Tofranil (Geigy) unter besonderer Berücksichtigung allergischer Probleme. Schweiz. Arch. Neurol. Psychiat. *84*:41, 1959.

Staehelin, J. E.: Insulin bei nicht schizophrenen psychischen Störungen. Schweiz. med. Wchnschr. *68*, 1938.
——, and Labhardt, F.: Les résultats atteints par les neuroplégiques dans le traitement des psychoses et des nervoses. Encéphale. *45*:511, 1956.
Stainbrook, E.: The effects of electrically induced convulsions on animal behavior. J. Personal. *17*:2, 1948.
——, and Loewenbach, H.: Writing and drawing of psychotic individuals after electrically induced convulsions. J. Nerv. & Ment. Dis. *99*:382, 1944.
Stanley, W. J., and Fleming, H.: A clinical comparison of phenelzine and electroconvulsive therapy in the treatment of depressive illness. J. Ment. Sci. *108*:708, 1962.
Staudt, V. M., and Zubin, J. A.: A biometric evaluation of the somato-therapies in schizophrenia—a critical review. Psychol. Bull. *54*:171, 1957.
Steck, H.: Die Behandlung des Delirium Tremens mit Insulin. Schweiz. Arch. f. Neurol. u. Psychiat. *29*:173, 1932.
——: Zur Insulinbehandlung akuter Psychosen. Schweiz. Arch. f. Neurol. u. Psychiat. *31*:153, 1933.
——: Le syndrome extra-pyramidal et diencephalique au cours des traitements en Largactil et en Serpasil. Ann. Méd. Psychol. *112*:737, 1954.
——: Le syndrome extra-pyramidal dans les cures de chlorpromazine et serpasil. Sa symptomatologie, clinique et son rôle thérapeutique. Encéphale. *45*:1083, 1956.
Stein, A. A., and Wright, A. W.: Hepatic pathology in jaundice due to chlorpromazine. J.A.M.A. *161*:508, 1956.
Steinfeld, J. I.: Acidosis and its therapeutic value in the treatment of psychotics. J.A.M.A. *145*:226, 1951.
Stender, A.: Über Provokation epileptiformer Anfälle durch Cardiazol. München. med. Wchnschr. *84*:1893, 1937.
——: Über die transorbitale Leukotomie und eine neur Variante. Intrafrontale Eigenblutinjektion. Nervenarzt *21*:514, 1950.
Stengel, E.: A follow-up investigation of 330 cases treated by prefrontal leucotomy. J. Ment. Sc. *96*:633, 1950.
——: Intensive E.C.T. J. Ment. Sc. *97*:139, 1951.
Stern, K. Askonas, B., and Cullen, A. M.: The influence of electroconvulsive treatment on blood sugar, total number of leucocytes and lymphocytes. Am. J. Psychiat. *105*:585, 1949.
——, Dancer, T. E., and McNaughton, F. L.: Sensory disturbances following insulin treatment of psychoses. J. Nerv. & Ment. Dis. *95*:183, 1942.
Sternbach, L. H., Randall, L. O., and Gustafson, S. R.: 1,4-Benzodiazepines (Chlordiazepoxide and related compounds). *In* M. Gordon (Ed.): Psychopharmacological Agents, Vol. I: 137, Medicinal Chemistry; A Series of Monographs, Vol. 4. New York, Academic Press, 1964.
Sterkmans, P., and Geerts, F.: Le benpéridol (R 4584) est-il le médicament spécifique des comportements hypersexuels? Acta neurol. psychiat. belg. *66*:1030, 1966.
Stevens, H., and Mosovich, A.: Clinical and EEG investigations of prefrontal lobotomy patients. Am. J. Psychiat. *104*:73, 1947.
Stevenson, G. H., and Geoghegan, J. J.: Prophylactic electroshock. Am. J. Psychiat. *107*:743, 1951.
Stief, A., and Tokay, L.: Beiträge zur Histopathologie der experimentellen Insulinvergiftung. Ztschr. f. d. ges. Neurol. u. Psychiat. *139*:434, 1932.
Stieve, R.: Weitere Beobachtungen über den Einfluss verschiedener Narkosearten auf die Ganglienzellen des autonomen Nervensystems und die Leber. Zentralbl. Chir. *80*:649, 1955.
Stockhausen, F. G.: Clinical studies with tetrabenazine (RO.1-9569). Dis. Nerv. Syst. *21*:115 (suppl.), 1960.
Stoll, W. A.: Lysergsäure-diäthylamid, ein Phantastikum aus der Mutterkorngruppe. Schweiz. Arch. f. Neurol. & Psychiat. *60*: 279, 1947.
Stone, C. P.: Losses and gains in cognitive functions as related to electroconvulsive shocks. J. Abnorm. & Soc. Psychol. *42*: 206, 1947.
Storch, A.: Communication at the Münsingen meeting. Am. J. Psychiat. *94* (Supp.): 348, 1938.
Strain, J. J., Brunschwig, L., Duffy, J. P., Agle, D. P., Rosenbaum, A. L., and Bidder, T. G.: Comparison of therapeutic effects and memory changes with bilateral and unilateral ECT. Amer. J. Psychiat. *125*: 294, 1968.
Straker, M., Davanloo, H., and Moll, A.: A double-blind comparison of a new antidepressant protriptyline with imipramine and amitriptyline. Canad. Med. Ass. J. *94*:1220, 1966.
——, and Roth, E. M.: Use of imipramine (Tofranil) in the aged chronically ill. Canad. M. A. J. *82*:362, 1960.
Stratas, N. E.: Pseudo electroconvulsive therapy using hypnosis: A controlled pilot study. Am. J. Clin. Hypnosis *5*:62, 1962.
Strauss, E. B., and Macphail, A.: Treatment of out-patients by electrical convulsant therapy with a portable apparatus. Brit M. J. *2*:779, 1940.
Strauss, H.: Office treatment of depressive states with a new drug (Imipramine). New York State J. Med. 59:2906, 1959.
——, Landis, C., and Hunt, W. A.: The metrazol seizure and its significance for the pathophysiology of epileptic attachs. J. Nerv. & Ment. Dis. *90*:439, 1939.
——, and Rahm, W. E., Jr.: The effects of metrazol injections on electroencephalograms. Psychiatric Quart. *14*:43, 1940.
Strecker, E. A., Alpers, B. J., Flaherty, J. A., and Hughes, J.: Experimental and clinical study of effects of metrazol convulsions. Arch. Neurol. & Psychiat. *41*:996, 1939.
——, Palmer, H. D., and Grant, F. C.: A

study of frontal lobotomy. Am. J. Psychiat. *98*:524, 1942.
Ström-Olen, R., Last, S. L., Broody, M. B., and Knight, G. C.: Results of prefrontal leucotomy in 30 cases of mental disorder. J. Ment. Sc. *89*:165, 1943.
——, and Tow, P. M.: Late social results of prefrontal leucotomy. Lancet *1*:87, 1949.
Stroud, G. M.: Drug eruptions due to meprobamate. New Eng. J. Med. *256*:354, 1957.
Suarez, M. V.: Prefrontal lobotomy in mental and incoercible pain. Lisbon: Psychosurgery, 1949.
Suchenwirth, R.: Thrombosen bei Neuroleptikabehandlung. *In* H. Kranz and K. Heinrich (Eds.): Begleitwirkungen und Misserfolge der psychiatrischen Pharmakotherapie, pp 109. Stuttgart, Thieme, 1964.
Sugerman, A. A.: A pilot study of floropipamide (Dipiperon). Dis. Nerv. Syst. *25*:355, 1964.
——, Stolberg, H., and Herrmann, J.: A pilot study of P-4657 B in chronic schizophrenics. Curr. Ther. Res. *7*:310, 1965.
——, Williams, B. H., and Adlerstein, A. M.: Haloperidol in the psychiatric disorders of old age. Amer. J. Psychiat. *120*:1190, 1964.
Sulser, F., Watts, J., and Brodie, B. B.: On the mechanism of antidepressant action of imipraminelike drugs. Ann. N.Y. Acad. Sci. *96*:279, 1962.
Sulzbach, W., Tillotson, K. J., Guillemin, V., and Sutherland, G. F.: A consideration of some experiences with electroshock treatment in mental diseases, with special regard to various pyschosomatic phenomena and to certain electrotechnical factors. Am. J. Psychiat. *99*:519, 1943.
Sunshine, P., and Yaffe, S. J.: Amitriptyline poisoning. Clinical and pathological findings in a fatal case. Amer. J. Dis. Childh. *106*:501, 1963.
Surat, W. S.: Über neurologische Veränderungen bei präfrontaler Lobotomie. Nevropat. i. psikhiat. *18*:17, 1949.
Sutter, J. M., and Pascalis, G.: Effects psychologiques de la chlorpromazine. Encéphale. *45*:979, 1956.
Svenneby, G., Kvamme, E., and Eitinger, L.: Levomepromazine (Nozinan) medication as a source of error in the laboratory diagnostic of phenylketonuria. Scand. J. Clin. Lab. Invest. *17*:260, 1965.
Sweet, W. H., Cotzias, G. C., Seed, J., and Yakovlev, P.: Gastro-intestinal hemorrhages, hyperglycemia, azotemia, hyperchloremia and hypernatremia following lesions of the frontal lobe in man. The Frontal Lobes. A. Research Nerv. & Ment. Dis., Proc. *27*:795, 1948.
Swinyard, E. A., Chin, L., and Fingl, E.: Withdrawal excitability following chronic administration of meprobamate to mice. Science. *125*:739, 1957.
——, Wolf, H. H., Fink, G. B., and Goodman, L. S.: Some neuropharmacological properties of thioridazine hydrochloride (Melleril). J. Pharmacol. & Exper. Therapeutics *126*:312, 1959.
Sydenstricker, V. P., and Cleckley, H. M.: The effect of nicotinic acid in stupor, lethargy and various other psychiatric disorders. Am. J. Psychiat. *98*:83, 1941.
Sykes, M. K., and Tredgold, R. F.: Restricted orbital undercutting. Brit. J. Psychiat. *110*:609, 1964.
Symes, M. H.: Monochlorimipramine: A controlled trial of a new antidepressant. Brit. J. Psychiat. *113*:671, 1967.
Szatmari, A.: Clinical and electroencephalogram investigation on Largactil in psychosis: preliminary study. Am. J. Psychiat. *112*:788, 1956.
Taen, S., and Pöldinger, W.: Dimethacrin (Istonil), ein Acridanderivat mit antidepressivem Wirkungsspektrum. Schweiz. med. Wschr. *96*:1616, 1966.
Taeschler, M., and Cerletti, A.: Differential analysis of the effects of phenothiazine-transquillisers on emotional and motor behaviour in experimental animals. Nature. *184*:823, 1959.
Talairach, J., Constans, J., and Sauguet, J.: Psychochirurgie. *In:* Encyclopédie Médico-Chirurgicale. Paris, 1955.
Talbott, J. H., and Tillotson, K. J.: Effects of cold on mental disorders (study of 10 patients with schizophrenia). Dis. Nerv. Syst. *2*:116, 1941.
Talland, G. A., Hagen, D. Q., and James, M.: Performance tests of amnesic patients with cylert. J. Nerv. & Ment. Dis. *144*:421, 1967.
Talley, J. E.: Meratran, a new cerebral stimulant: report on the results of clinical investigation. A.P.A. Psychiat. Research Reports *1*:133, 1955.
Tanck, R. H.: Psychologic changes induced by reserpine therapy on a group of severely disturbed psychotics. J. Nerv. & Ment. Dis. *126*:353, 1958.
Taubel, D. E.: Mellaril: Ejaculation disorders. Amer. J. Psychiat. *119*:87, 1962.
Taylor, I. J.: Clinical evaluation of a new phenothiazine tranquilizer, fluphenazine (Prolixin). Am. J. Psychiat. *116*:457, 1959.
Taylor, J. A. T.: Metronidazole a new agent for combined somatic and psychic therapy of alcoholism. Bull. Los Angeles Neurol. Soc. *29*:158, 1964.
Taylor, J. H.: A further report on the use of shock therapy. Dis. Nerv. Syst. *5*:56, 1944.
——: Returns of schizophrenics following shock therapy. Dis. Nerv. Syst. *6*:28, 1945.
Taylor, R. M., and Pacella, B. L.: Significance of abnormal electroencephalograms prior to electroconvulsive therapy. J. Nerv. & Ment. Dis. *107*:220, 1948.
Tedeschi, D. H., Spencer, J. N., Macko, E., Tedeschi, R. E., Leonard, C. A., McLean, R. A., Flanagan, N. A. T., Cook, L., Mattis, P. A., and Fellows, E. J.: Pharmacology of Trifluoperazine. *In:* Trifluoperazine, Philadelphia: Lea and Febiger, 1958.
Tellenbach, H.: Gezielte Behandlung von Schädigungsangst (Blaptophobie) mit Imipramin. Dtsch. med. Wschr. *91*:2032, 1966.
Temporary Commission on State Hospital Problems: Insulin shock therapy. New York: 1944.

Tennent, T.: Insulin therapy. J. Ment. Sc. *90*:465, 1944.
Terruwe, A. A. A.: Epileptische Toevallen na de Electroshocktherapie. Nederl. tijdschr. v. geneesk. *90*:608, 1946.
Teulié, M., Follin, S., and Bégoin: Étude de l'action des sels de lithium dans états d'excitation psycho-motrice. Encéphale *44*: 267, 1955.
Thal, N.: Cumulative index of anti-depressant medications. Dis. Nerv. Syst. *20*:197, 1959.
Thénon, J.: Electrochoque monolateral. Acta neuropsiqu. Argentina *2*:292, 1956.
Thiebaux, M., Boyer, R., Leborgne, F., and Rousseau, G.: L'électrochoc dans le délirium tremens et le délire éthylique subaigu. Soc. Avstr.: Ann. méd.-psychol. *114*:95, 1956.
Thiemann, H. H., Otto, L., and Fritz, H.: Tödliche Vergiftung durch Imipramin. Dtsch. Gesundh. wesen *22*:1719, 1967.
Thomas, L. J.: Preliminary observation on the use of Librium (RO.5-0690) in Internal Medicine. Dis. Nerv. Syst. *21*:40 (suppl.), 1960.
Thompson, G. N.: Electroshock and other therapeutic considerations in sexual psychopathy. J. Nerv. & Ment. Dis. *109*:531, 1949.
——, and Bielinski, B.: Improvement in psychoses following conditioned reflex treatment for alcoholism. J. Nerv. and Ment. Dis. *117*:537, 1953.
——, McGinnis, J. E., van Harreveld, A., Wiersma, C. A. G., and Tietz, E. B.: Electronarcosis: clinical comparison with electroshock. War Med. *6*:158, 1944.
Thompson, W. A.: Subconvulsive electric shock treatment of the psychoses. Am. J. Psychiat. *99*:382, 1942.
Thomsen, W., Reid, W. B., and Hebeler, J.: Effect of Tofranil on enuretic boys. Dis. Nerv. Syst. *28*:167, 1967.
Thonnard-Neumann, E.: Phenothiazines and diabetes in hospitalized women. Amer. J. Psychiat. *124*:978, 1968.
Thorpe, F. T.: Prefrontal leucotomy in treatment of post-encephalitic conduct disorder. Brit. M. J. *1*:312, 1946.
——: An evaluation of prefrontal leucotomy in the affective disorders of old age: a follow-up study. J. Ment. Sci. *104*:403, 1958.
Thorpe, J. G.: The current status of prognostic test indicators for electroconvulsive therapy. Psychom. Med. *24*:554, 1962.
Thuillier, G., and Thuillier, J.: Chimie et pharmacologie de nouveaux antidépresseurs dérivés des auxines, Arzneim.-Forsch. *14*: 556, 1964.
Ticktin, H., Epstein, J., Shea, J. G., and Fazekas, J. F.: Effect of methylphenidate hydrochloride in antagonizing barbiturate-induced depressions. Neurology. *8*:267, 1958.
——, and Schultz, J. D.: Librium, a new quieting drug for hyperactive alcoholic and psychotic patients. Dis. Nerv. Syst. *21*:49 (suppl.) 1960.
Tietz, E. B.: Further experiences with electronarcosis. J. Nerv. & Ment. Dis. *106*: 150, 1947.
——, Dornheggen, H., and Goldman, D.: Blood adrenalin levels during insulin shock treatments for schizophrenia. Endocrinology *26*:641, 1940.
Tillim, S. J., and Squires, M. T.: A clinical evaluation of hypoglycemic and convulsive therapy. Psychiatric Quart. *16*:469, 1942.
Tillotson, K. J., and Sulzbach, W.: A comparative study and evaluation of electric shock therapy in depressive states. Am. J. Psychiat. *101*:455, 1945.
Tobin, J. M., Bird, I. F., and Boyle, D. E.: Preliminary evaluation of Librium (RO.5-0690) in the treatment of anxiety reactions. Dis. Nerv. Syst. *21*:11, (suppl.) 1960.
Tolan, E. J., Olariu, J., Rees, J. M., and Peppel, H. A.: Clinical and statistical evaluation of results with Plegicil AY-57062 in chronic mental patients. Am. J. Psychiat. *116*:69, 1959.
——, and Peppel H. H.: Preliminary observations on Trifluoperazine in Schizophrenia. Am. J. Psychiat. *115*:935, 1959.
Tölle, R.: Indikationen des Perazin (Taxilan) und die Psychopathologie seiner Wirkung bei endogenen Psychosen. Nervenarzt *31*: 277, 1960.
——: Die Behandlung endogener Psychosen mit Laevomepromazin (Neurocil). Nervenarzt *33*:178, 1962.
Tomlinson, P. J.: Insulin and electric therapy in general paresis. Psychiatric Quart. *18*:413, 1943.
——: Subcoma insulin therapy: An analysis of 300 cases. Psychiatric Quart. *22*:609, 1948.
Tompkins, J. B.: A summary of 36 cases of lobotomy. Am. J. Psychiat. *105*:443, 1948.
Tooth, G. C., and Newton, M. P.: Leucotomy in England and Wales, 1942-54. Rep. Publ. Hlth. Med. Subj. 104, 1961.
Torkildsen, A.: Notes on the importance of the occipital lobes in a case of schizophrenia (Experience with a case of bilateral occipital leucotomy). Acta Psychiat. et Neurol. *24*:701, 1949.
Tow, P. M.: Personality changes following frontal leucotomy. London: Oxford, 1955.
Trabucchi, C., Zuanazzi, G. F., and Caceffo, G.: Nostre esperienze sulla cura con Tofranil. Riv. Sper. di Freniat. *83*:328, 1959.
Trelles, J. O., Saavedra, A., and Donayre, J.: First results with levomepromazine (Nozinan) in depression. Rev. de Neuro-Psiquiatria. *21*:3, 1958.
Trethowan, W. H., and Scott, P. A. L.: Chlorpromazine in obsessive-compulsive and allied disorders. Lancet *1*:781, 1955.
Treves, G.: Terapia cardiazolica nella schizofrenia e negli equivalenti epilettici. Atti del convegno sulla terapia moderna della schizofrenia. Milano: 1937.
Tsai, S. Y., Bennett, A., May, L. G., and Gregory, R. L.: Effect of insulin hypoglycemia on eosinophiles and lymphocytes of psychotics. Proceed. Soc. Exper. Biol. & Med. *74*:782, 1950.

Tuberculosis Control in Ontario Mental Hospitals: Tuberculosis Division Ontario Hospital, Woodstock, Sept. 1950.

Turner, E. A.: Prefrontal leucotomy. Brit. Med. J. *1*:1494, 1965.

Turner, W. J.: Therapeutic use of diphenylhydantoin in neuroses. Intern. J. Neuropsychiat. *3*:94, 1967.

——, Lowinger, L., and Huddleson, J. H.: The correlation of pre-electroshock electroencephalogram and therapeutic result in schizophrenia. Am. J. Psychiat. *102*:299, 1945.

——, and Merlis, S.: A clinical trial of pargyline and DOPA in psychotic subjects. Dis. Nerv. Syst. *25*:538, 1964.

Turns, D., Denber, H. C. B., and Teller, D. N.: Preliminary clinical study of propericiazine. J. New Drugs *5*:90, 1965.

Tuta, J. A., and Batko, J. M.: An acute perforated duodenal ulcer following metrazol therapy. Am. J. M. Sc. *204*:107, 1942.

Tuteur, W.: Combined reserpine-chlorpromazine therapy in highly disturbed psychotics. Am. J. Psychiat. *112*:206, 1955.

——: A case of fatal agranulocytosis due to chlorpromazine. Am. J. Psychiat. *113*:76, 1956.

——: Chlorpromazine and its derivatives. *In:* Psychopharmacology Frontiers (ed. by N. S. Kline). Boston: Little, Brown & Co., 1959.

Uhlenhuth, E. H., Canter, A., Neustadt, J. O., and Payson, H. E.: The symptomatic relief of anxiety with meprobamate, phenobarbital and a placebo. Am. J. Psychiat. *115*:905, 1959.

Uhler, C.: Carbon dioxide coma therapy. Dis. Nerv. Syst. *23*:56, 1962.

Uhrbrand, L., and Faurbye, A.: Reversible and irreversible dyskinesia after treatment with perphenazine, chlorpromazine, reserpine, and electroconvulsive therapy. Psychopharmacologia *1*:408, 1960.

Ulett, G. A.: Experience with photic stimulation in psychiatric research. Am. J. Psychiat. *114*:127, 1957.

Ulett, G. A., Smith, K., and Biddy, R.: Shock Treatment. *In* Spiegel, E. A. (Ed.): Progress in Neurology and Psychiatry, Vol. XXI. New York, Grune & Stratton, 1967.

——, Smith, K., and Gleser, G. C.: Evaluation of convulsive and subconvulsive shock therapies utilizing a control group. Am. J. Psychiat. *112*:795, 1956.

Ulrich, H.: Veränderungen des Liquorbildes und des Encephalogramms durch Cardiazolschock und Elektrokrampf. Psychiat., Neurol. u. med. Psychol. *1*:91, 1949.

Ungerleider, J. T.: Acute myocardial infarction and electroconvulsive therapy. Dis. Nerv. Syst. *21*:149, 1960.

Urquhart, R., and Forrest, A. D.: Clinical trial of promazine hydrochloride and acetylpromazine in chronic schizophrenic patients. J. Ment. Sci. *105*:260, 1959.

Uytterschaut, P., and Jacobs, R.: Etude clinique de l'activité neuropsychopharmacologique du methylpéridol (R 1658). Acta neurol. psychiat. belg. *62*:677, 1962.

Vaessen, M. L. J.: Insulin-Koma-Therapie in psychischer Hinsicht. Alkmaar: Van Putten & Oortmeijer, 1957.

Vahia, N. S.: Insulin treatment in India. *In* M. Rinkel (Ed.): Biological Treatment of Mental Illness. New York, Sakel Foundation, 1966.

Vaisberg, M.: Protriptyline in the treatment of depressive states. Dis. Nerv. Syst. *25*: 110, 1964.

Valentine, M.: Intensive electroplexy. J. Nerv. & Ment. Dis. 109:95, 1949.

——, Keddie, K. M. G., and Dunne, D.: A comparison of techniques in electroconvulsive therapy. Brit. J. Psychiat. *114*: 989, 1968.

Vallade, L., Milletto, G., Hugonenq, H., and Espinas, A.: Contribution à l'étude des effets cliniques obtenus par la prochlorpérazine (6140.RP) dans divers syndrômes psychiatriques. Presse méd. *65*:1762, 1957.

Vallat, J. N., and Lepetit: Intoxication par la chlorproazine (Largactil) au cours d'une tentative de suicide. Sem. Hôp. Paris. *30*:2307, 1954.

Van Andel, H.: Investigations into the so-called reserpine parkinsonoid in chronic schizophrenics and its treatment with orphenadrine (Disipal). Folia Psychiat. Neurol. et neurochirurg. Neerl. *62*:476, 1959.

Van de Erve, J., and Childs, D. R.: Meprobamate reactions. J. South Carolina Med. Assoc. *53*:83, 1957.

Van der Horst, L.: De hersenen na leucotomie. Nederl. tijdschr. v. geneesk, *92*: 59, 1948.

Van Meter, W. G., Owens, H. F., and Himwich, H. E.: Effects of Tofranil, an anti-depressant drug, on electrical potentials of rabbit brain. Canad. Psy. Assoc. J. *4*:133 (suppl.), 1959.

Van Reeth, P. C.: Nialamide in severe endogenous depression. J. da Soc. das Ciências Méd de Lisboa (supp.) *Nov.*:210, 1959.

Vasilyeva, Dikovitsky, and Zelyeva: Treatment of schizophrenia by combined method (insulin and cardiazol). Am. J. Psychiat. *96*:1261, 1940.

Vattuone, G.: Behavior of deep reflexes during electric shock therapy. Riv. sper. di freniat. *64*:489, 1940.

Ventriglia, C.: Su l'uso endovenoso dell'insulina per la provocazione dello shock ipoglicemico. Gior. di psichiat. e di neuropat. *67*:156, 1939.

Verrey, F.: Dégénérescence pigmentaire de la rétine d'origine médicamenteuse. Ophthalmologica (Basel) *131*:296, 1956.

Verstraeten, P.: La thérapeutique convulsivante de la psychose maniaco-depressive. Ann. méd.-psychol. *95 II*:654, 1937.

Vestre, N. D., MacNaughton, D. V., and Schiele, B. C.: A comparison of the slow-release and the regular forms of thioridazine: A double-blind controlled study in hospitalized psychiatric patients. Curr. Ther. Res. *5*:183, 1963.

Veterans Administration: Department of Medicine and Surgery. Transactions of the

Third Research Conference on Chemotherapy in Psychiatry. Washington, D.C. Veterans Administration, 1959.
de Villiers, J. C.: Intracranial haemorr age in patients treated with monoamineoxidase inhibitors. Brit. J. Psychiat. *112*:109, 1966.
Voegtlin, W. L.: The treatment of alcoholism by establishing a conditioned reflex. Am. J. Med. Sci. *199*:802, 1940.
Voelkel, A.: Zum Problem der BAL-wirkung im therapeutischen Insulinkoma. Nervenarzt *27*:369, 1956.
——: Klinische Erfahrungen mit einer Reihe von Monoamin-Freisetzern. Psychiat. Neurol. *140*:36, 1960.
——, and Dresler, J.: Clinical psychiatric experience with the benzoquinolizine derivative RO.1-9569. Nervenarzt. *30*:322, 1959.
Volmat, R., Beaudouin, J.-L., Collin, J., Allers, G., and Vittouris, N.: Essais cliniques du neuroliptique 8909 RP (propériciazine) sur une population de malades chroniques internes. Gazette Méd. France *70*:1747, 1963.
Von Euler, U. S., and Luft, R.: Effect of insulin on urinary excretion of adrenaline and noradrenaline. Metabolism *1*:528, 1952.
Waelkens, J.: Étude clinique du R.1625 (Halopéridol). Symposium international sur le Halopéridol. Acta Medica Belgica, 1960.
Wagensommer, J.: Therapeutisch unerwünschte Wirkungen der Thymoleptika. Fortschr. Neurol. Psychiat. *32*:497, 1964.
Wagner,-von., Jauregg, J.: Die Einwirkung der Malaria auf die progressive Paralyse. Psychiat.-neurol. Wchnschr. *20*:132, 1918.
Waites, L., and Keele, D. K.: Fluphenazine in management of disturbed mentally retarded children. Dis. Nerv. Syst. *24*:113, 1963.
Waldron, J., and Bates, T. J. N.: The management of depression in hospital. A comparative trial of desipramine and imipramine. Brit. J. Psychiat. *111*:511, 1965.
Waldrop, F. N., Robertson, R. H., and Vourlekis, A.: A comparison of the therapeutic and toxic effects of thioridazine and chlorpromazine in chronic schizophrenic patients. Compr. Psychiat. *2*:96, 1961.
Walker, A. E.: The primate thalamus. Chicago: University of Chicago Press, 1938.
Walker, C. F., and Kirkpatrick, B. B.: Dilantin treatment for behavior problem children with abnormal electroencephalograms. Am. J. Psychiat. *103*:484, 1947.
Wallinga, J. V.: Use of a phenothiazine derivative, thioridazine, in the treatment of childhood emotional disorders. Acta paedopsychiat. *30*:211, 1963.
Walsh, G. P., Walton, D., and Black, D. A.: The relative efficacy of Vespral and chlorpromazine in the treatment of a group of chronic schizophrenic patients. J. Ment. Sci. *105*:199, 1959.
Walsh, J.: Continuous narcosis: The advantages of oral somnifen—A comparison. J. Ment. Sc. *93*:255, 1947.
——: Transorbital leucotomy. Some results and observations. Lancet *2*:465, 1949.
Walter, W. G.: Electrically induced convulsions. Brit. J. Phys. Med. *3*:146, 1940.
Walther, R.: Elektroschock und vegetatives Nervensystem (IV and V). Psychiat., Neurol. u. med. Psychol. *1*:111, 1949; and *1*:143, 1949.
Wardell, D. W.: Untoward reactions to tranquilizing drugs. Am. J. Psychiat. *113*: 745, 1957.
Warnes, H., Lehmann, H. E., and Ban, T. A.: Adynamic ileus during psychoactive medication. Canad. Med. Ass. J. *96*:1112, 1967.
Wase, A. W., Christensen, J., and Polley, E.: The accumulation of S36 chlorpromazine in brain. A.M.A. Arch. Neurol. & Psychiat. *75*:54, 1956.
Wassing, H.: Personal communications.
Waters, M. A., and Northover, J.: Rehabilitated long-stay schizophrenics in the community. Brit. J. Psychiat. *111*:258, 1965.
Watt, D. C.: The effect of reserpine on the duration of manic attacks. J. Neurol., Neurosurg. & Psychiat. *21*:297, 1958.
Watt, M. D. B.: Reserpine and chlorpromazine in the treatment of chronic schizophrenics. Encéphale. *45*:661, 1956.
Weatherly, J., and Deabler, H. L.: Schizophrenia in identical twins, one of whom was lobotomized. J. Nerv. & Ment. Dis. *120*:262, 1954.
Webb, R. R.: Largactil in psychiatry. M. J. Australia *42*:*1*:759, 1955.
——, and Noall, M. T.: The insulin treatment of schizophrenia: A 10 year follow up. M. J. Australia *2*:130, 1949.
Weber, E.: Ein Rauwolfia Alkaloid in der Psychiatrie: seine Wirkungsähnlichkeit mit Chlorpromazin. Schweiz. Med. Wchschr. *84*:968, 1954.
Wechlser, D., Halpren, F., and Jaros, E.: Psychometric study of insulin-treated schizophrenics. Psychiatric Quart. *14*:460, 1940.
Weckowicz, T. E., and Ward, T. F.: Clinical trial of "Stelazine" on apathetic chronic schizophrenics. J. Ment. Sci. *106*:1008, 1960.
Weekley, R. D., Potts, A. M., Reboton, J., and May, R. H.: Pigmentary retinopathy in patients receiving high doses of a new phenothiazine. Arch. Ophthal. *64*:65, 1960.
Weil, A.: Die optischen Wahrnehmungsphänomene in der Hypoglykämie. Monatschr. f. Psychiat. u. Neurol. *100*:98, 1939.
——, and Brinegar, W. C.: Electroencephalographic studies following electric shock therapy. Arch. Neurol. & Psychiat. *57*:719, 1947.
——, Liebert, E., and Heilbrunn, G.: Histopathologic changes in the brain in experimental hyperinsulinism. Arch. Neurol. & Psychiat. *39*:467, 1938.
——, and Moriarty, J. D.: Insulin therapy in schizophrenic patients responding unsatisfactorily to electroshock therapy. Dis. Nerv. Syst. *5*:334, 1944.
Weil, P. L.: "Regressive" electroplexy in schizophrenia. J. Ment. Sc. *96*:514, 1950.
Weil-Malherbe, H.: The action of glutamic acid in hypoglycaemic coma. J. Ment. Sc.

95:930, 1949.
——: The concentration of adenosinetriphosphate (ATP), citrate and calcium in blood during insulin shock therapy. J. Ment. Sc. *96*:226, 1950.
——, and Bone, A. D.: The effect of insulin on the levels of adrenaline and noradrenaline in human blood. J. Endocrinol. *11*: 285, 1954.
Weinberg, A. Cammer, L., and Dell'Aria, S.: A preliminary report on hypnosis as an anesthetic agent in electroconvulsive therapy with succinylcholine. J. Neuropsychiat.: in press.
Weinberg, J., and Goldstein. H. H.: The treatment of metrazol failures with insulin. J. Nerv. & Ment. Dis. *95*:597, 1942.
Weinland, W. L., and Weinland, G.: Elektroencephalogramm und Klinik. Über electroencephalographische Beobachtungen bein Insulinschock. Arch. f. Psychiat. *183*:34, 1949.
Weinstein, E. A., Linn, L., and Kahn, R. L.: Psychosis during electroshock therapy: its relation to the theory of shock therapy. Am. J. Psychiat. *109*:22, 1952.
Weinstein. L.: Electroconvulsive and insulin comatherapy in the presence of active pulmonary tuberculosis. J. Nerv. and Ment. Dis. *118*:36, 1953.
Weinstein, M. R., and Fischer, A.: Electroconvulsive treatment of a patient with artificial mitral and aortic valves. Amer. J. Psychiat. *123*:882, 1967.
Weise, K., and Mühlbach: Zur Bedeutung der Früherkennung und Frühbehandlung schizophrener Psychosen. Duetschr. Gesundh. Wesen 891, 1967.
Weiskrantz, L., and Wilson, W. A.: The effects of reserpine on emotional behavior of normal and brain-operated monkeys. Ann. New York Acad. Sci. *61*:36, 1955.
Weiss, D. N.: Changes in the blood pressure with electroshock therapy in a patient receiving chlorpromazine hydrochloride (Thorazine). Am. J. Psychiat. *111*: 617, 1955.
Weissman, A.: Psychopharmacological effects of thiothixene and related compounds. Psychopharmacologia *12*:142, 1968.
Weisz, S., and Creel, J. N.: Maintenance treatment in schizophrenia. Dis. Nerv. Syst. *9*:10, 1948.
Weitbrecht, H. J.: Studie zur Psychopathologie krampfbehandelter Psychosen. Stuttgart: Georg Thieme, 1949.
Wender, H. B.: Experience in group psychotherapy with insulin-treated patients. Psychiatric Quart. *24*:314, 1950.
Wender, L., Balser, B. H., and Beres, D.: Extra-mural shock therapy. Am. J. Psychiat. *99*:712, 1943.
Wendkos, M. H.: The significance of electrocardiographic changes produced by thioridazine. J. New Drugs *4*:322,1964.
Werenberg, H.: Mepazine in therapy of severe mental diseases. Nord. Med. *54*: 1787, 1955.
Wespi, H.: Vorläufige Mitteilung über Beobachtungsresultate von vegetativen Funktionen bei der Insulinschockbehandlung Schizophrener. Schweiz. Arch. f. Neurol. *39* (Erg.-H.): 83, 1937.
——: Ein Fall von spontaner Wirbelfraktur im Cardiazolanfall. Schweiz. Arch. f. Neurol. u. Psychiat. *42*:404, 1938.
West, E. D., and da Fonseca, A. F.: Controlled trial of meprobamate. Brit. Med. J. *2*:1206, 1956.
——, and Dally, P. J.: Effects of iproniazid in depressive syndromes. Brit. Med. J. *1*:1491, and *2*:433, 1959.
West, F. H., Bond, E. D., Shurley, J. T., and Meyers, C. D.: Insulin coma therapy in schizophrenia. Am. J. Psychiat. *111*: 583, 1955.
Whalen, J. F., Darling, H. F., and Sanddal, J. W.: Treatment of psychopathic personality by transorbital lobotomy. Dis. Nerv. System *13*:136, 1952.
Wharton, R. N.: Electroshock treatment: Two novel problems. Amer. J. Psychiat. *125*:397, 1968.
——, and Fieve, R. R.: The use of lithium in the affective psychoses. Amer. J. Psychiat. *123*:706, 1966.
Whitehead, R. W., Neuberger, K. T., Rutledge, E. K., and Silcott, W. L.: Pharmacologic and pathologic effects of repeated convulsant doses of metrazol. Am. J. M. Sc. *199*:352, 1940.
Whitman, R. L.: Prefrontal leucotomy: Aftercare and rehabilitation. Northwest Med. *47*:419, 1948.
Whitman, R. M., Pierce, Ch. M., Maas, J. W., and Baldridge, B.: Drugs and dreams. II: Imipramine and prochlorperazine. Compr. Psychiat. *2*:219, 1961.
Whittier, J., Haydu, G., and Crawford, J.: Effect of imipramine (Tofranil) on depression and hyperkinesia in Huntington's disease. Amer. J. Psychiat. *118*:79, 1961.
Whittier, J. R., Korenyi, Ch., Haydu, G. G., and Goldschmidt, L.: Effects of long-acting injectable Prolixin in 23 psychotic patients. Dis. Nerv. Syst. *28*:459, 1967.
Whitty, C. W. M., Duffield, J. E., Tow, P. M., and Cairns, H.: Anterior cingulectomy in the treatment of mental disease. Lancet *1*:475, 1952.
Wiedeking, J.: Selbstbeobachtungen im hypoglykämischen Zustand Ztschr. f. d. ges. Neurol. u. Psychiat. *159*:417, 1937.
Wiedorn, W., and Ervin, F.: Schizophrenic-like psychotic reactions with administration of Isoniazid. A.M.A. Arch. Neurol. & Psychiat. *72*:321, 1954.
Wijsenbeek, H.: Over de praefrontale lobotomia. Utrecht: Nitgeresnij, 1949.
Wikler, A., and Frank, K.: Effects of electroshock convulsions on chronic decorticated cats. Proc. Soc. Exper. Biol. & Med. *67*:464, 1948.
Wilbur, C. B., and Fortes, A.: Convulsive shock therapy in patients over seventy years of age with affective disorders. Am. J. Psychiat. *104*:48, 1947.
Wilcox, K. W.: Intellectual functioning as related to electroconvulsive therapy. Ph.D. Thesis. Univ. of Michigan, 1953.
Wilcox, P. H.: Electroshock therapy. A review of over 23,000 treatments using uni-

directional currents. Am. J. Psychiat. *104*: 100, 1947.
——: Shock therapy. In Spiegel, E. A.: Progress in Neurology and Psychiatry, Vol. II-XIV. New York: Grune & Stratton, 1947-1960.
——: Psychopenetration. Dis. Nerv. Syst. *12*:1, 1951.
——: Coordination of electrostimulation with other techniques in the treatment of neurotic symptoms. Conf. Neurol. *14*:288, 1954.
——: Abreaction produced by low non-convulsive electrostimulation. Dis. Nerv. Syst. *19*:87, 1958.
——: Non-convulsive electro-cerebral stimulation therapy. Dis. Nerv. Syst. *19*:437, 1958.
Wilder, A.: Objective evaluation of insulin therapy of the morphine abstinence syndrome. J. Nerv. & Ment. Dis. *110*:26, 1949.
Wilder, J.: Klinik und Therapie der Zuckermangelkrankheit für den praktischen Arzt. Leipzig: 1936.
Will, O. A., and Duval, A. M.: Use of electroshock therapy in psychiatric illness complicated by pulmonary tuberculosis. J. Nerv. & Ment. Dis. *105*:637, 1947.
——, Rehfeldt, F. C., and Neumann, M. A.: A fatality in electroshock therapy. J. Nerv. & Ment. Dis. *107*:105, 1948.
Williams, L.: A review of 200 chronic alcoholics. Lancet *1*:787, 1952.
Williams, R. L., and Barrera, S. E.: Observations and opinions concerning complications and contraindications in electric convulsive therapy. Psychiatric Quart. *24*: 800, 1950.
Wilson, I. C., Gambill, J. M., and Sandifer, M. G.: Loeffler's syndrome occurring during imipramine therapy. Amer. J. Psychiat. *119*:892, 1963.
Wilson, R. E., and Shagass, C.: Comparison of two drugs with psychotomimetic effects (LSD and Ditran). J. Nerv. & Ment. Dis. *138*:277, 1964.
Wilson, S. A. K., and Walshe, F. M. R.: The phenomenon of "tonic innervation" and its relation to motor apraxia. Brain *37*: 199, 1914.
Winkelman, N. W.: Metrazol treatment in schizophrenia. Am. J. Psychiat. *95*:303, 1938.
——, and Moore, M. T.: Neurohistopathologic changes with metrazol and insulin shock therapy. Arch. Neurol. & Psychiat. *43*:1108, 1940.
——, and ——: Neurohistological findings in experimental electric shock treatment. J. Neuropath. & Exper. Neurol. *3*:199, 1944.
Winkelman, N. W., Jr.: Chlorpromazine in treatment of neuropsychiatric illness. J.A.M.A. *155*:18, 1954.
——: An appraisal of chlorpromazine. Am. J. Psychiat. *113*:961, 1957.
——: A psychoanalytic study of phenothiazine action. *In:* Psychopharmacology Frontiers. (ed. by N. S. Kline). Boston: Little, Brown & Co., 1959.
——: Evaluation of two ataractic agents: experience of one year with prochlorperazine and of seven months with benactyzine. Dis. Nerv. Syst. *20*:27, 1959.
Winkler, W.: Konstitutionstypologische Unterschiede bei der Insulinschockbehandlung. Z. menschl. Vererb.- ul Konstitu. lehre *29*:38, 1948.
——: Krampfbereitschaft und Konstitution. Arch. f. Psychiat. *184*:473, 1950.
——, and Vogel, E.: Insulinschockbehandlung und Konstitution (Insulintoleranz und Krampfbereitschaft bei 487 weiblichen Patienten). Arch. f. Psychiat. *182*:419, 1949.
Winnik, H. Z., Landau, I., Assael, M., and Tomim, B.: Micro-Vascular changes during insulin-coma treatment. *In* Rinkel, M. (Ed.): Biological Treatment of Mental Illness. New York, L. C. Page & Co., 1966.
Wintrob, R. M.: Use of a long-acting phenothiazine in acute manic states. Dis. Nerv. Syst. *28*:323, 1967.
Wirt, R. D., and Simon, W.: Differential treatment and prognosis in schizophrenia. Blackwell Scientific Publications. Springfield, 1959.
Wirth, W.: Pharmacology of new centrally active substances. Dt. Med. Wchnschr. *82*:1745, 1957.
——, Gösswald, R., Hörlein, U., Risse, K.-H., and Kreiskott, H.: Zur Pharmakologie acylierter Phenothiazin-Derivate. With summary. Arch Int. Pharmacodyn. *115*:1, 1958.
——, ——, and Vater, W.: Zur Pharmakologie acylierter Phenothiazin-Derivate. With summary. Arch. Int. Pharmacodyn. *123*:78, 1959.
Wittenborn, J. R., and Plante, M.: Patterns of response to placebo, iproniazid and electroconvulsive therapy among young depressed females. J. Nerv. Ment. Dis. *137*:155, 1963.
Wittman, M. P., and Russell, J. T.: Mental efficiency levels before and after shock therapy. Elgin Papers. *4*:70, 1941.
Wohlfahrt. S.: Psychochirurgie. Anatomische Voraussetzungen, Operationsmethoden, pathologische Befunde, u.s.w. Nord. psykiatr. medlemsbl. *3*:75, 1949.
Wohlwill, F.: Über Hirnbefunde bei Insulinüberdosierung. Klin. Wchnschr. 7:344, 1928.
Wolff, G. E.: Results of four years active therapy for chronic mental patients and the value of an individual maintenance dose of ECT. Am. J. Psychiat. *114*:453, 1957.
Wolford, J. A.: Electroshock therapy and aortic aneurysm. Am. J. Psychiat. *113*: 656, 1957.
Wolpert, A., Sheppard, Ch., and Merlis, S.: An early clinical evaluation of clopenthixol in treatment-resistant female schizophrenic patients. Amer. J. Psychiat. *124*:702, 1967.
Woods, L. W., Tyce, F. A. J., and Bickford, R. G.: Electric sleep-producing devices: an evaluation using EEG monitoring. Amer. J. Psychiat. *122*:153, 1965.
Woringer, E.: La leucotomie chimique. Rév. neurol. *80*:518, 1948.

Worthing, H. J., Bigelow, N., Binzley, R., and Brill, H.: The organization and administration of a state hospital insulin-metrazol-electric shock therapy unit. Am. J. Psychiat. *99*:692, 1943.
——, Brill, H., and Wigderson, H.: 350 cases of prefrontal lobotomy. Psychiatric Quart. *23*:617, 1949.
——, and Kalinowsky, L. B.: The question of vertebral fractures in convulsive therapy and in epilepsy. Am. J. Psychiat. *98*: 533, 1942.
Wortis, J.: Early experiences with Sakel's hypoglycemia insulin treatment of the psychoses in America. Am. J. Psychiat. *94* (suppl): 307, 1938.
——: Failures with insulin shock therapy. In Hoch, P. H.: Failures in Psychiatric Treatment. New York: Grune & Stratton, 1948.
——: The history of insulin shock treatment. *In:* M. Rinkel, Insulin Treatment in Psychiatry. New York: Philosophical Library, 1959.
——, and Goldfarb, W.: Schizophrenic brain metabolism in the course of insulin shock treatment. New York State J. Med. *42*:1053, 1942.
——, and Lambert, R. H.: Irreversible or hypoglycemic insulin coma; its cause and its response to blood transfusion. Am. J. Psychiat. *96*:335, 1939.
Wortis, S. B.: Effects of insulin, metrazol and camphor convulsions on brain metabolism. New York State J. Med. *38*:1015, 1938.
——: A list of some of the newer drugs used in psychiatric practice. Am. J. Psychiat. *115*:169, 1958.
——, Shaskan, D., Impastato, D. J., and Almansi, R.: Brain metabolism: the effects of electric shock and some newer drugs. Am. J. Psychiat. *98*:354, 1941.
Wright, R. L. D., and Kyne, W. P.: A clinical and experimental comparison of four anti-schizophrenic drugs. Psychopharmacologia *1*:437, 1960.
Wright, T., Jr.: Further statistics on electric shock therapy. Arch. Neurol. & Psychiat. *49*:790, 1943; *51*:204, 1944.
Wylie, D. W., and Archer, S.: Structure-activity relationships of 1-[(3-indolyl) alkyl]-4-arylpiperazines. A new series of tranquilizers. J. Med. Pharmaceut. Chem. *5*:932, 1962.
Wyrsch, J., Psychopathologische Bemerkungen zur körperlichen Behandlung endogener Psychosen. Nervenarzt *15*:120, 1942.
Yagdjoglou, B.: Un nouveau procédé technique dans le choc à l'insuline. Presse méd. *58*:1287, 1950.
Yahn, M. et al.: Tratamento cirurgico das moléstias mentais (leucotomia). Sao Paulo: Edigraf, 1951.
——, Pimenta, M. A., and Sette, A.: Leucotomia parietal. Arq. neuropsiquiat. *6*:225, 1948.
Yakovlev, P. I., Hamlin, H., and Sweet, W. H.: Frontal lobotomy. J. Neuropath. & Exper. Neurol. *9*:250, 1950.
Yokoi, S.: Neuropathological study of prefrontal lobotomy. J. Neuropath. & Exper. Neurol. *16*:251, 1957.
Young, D., and Scoville, W. B.: Paranoid psychosis with narcolepsy and possible danger of benzedrine treatment. M. Clin. N. Am. *22*:637, 1938.
Zador, K.: Der Lachgas (NO) Rausch in seiner Bedeutung für Psychiatrie und Neurologie, Arch. f. Psychiat. *84*:1, 1928.
Zamora, E. N., and Kaelbling, R.: Memory and electroconvulsive therapy. Amer. J. Psychiat. *122*:546, 1965.
Zeghauser, A., and Erb, A.: Untersuchungen über die Pathogenese des Insulinschocks. Klin. Wchnschr. 48, 1937.
Zeifert, M.: Etiology and prevention of "lung abscess" in metrazol therapy. Psychiatric Quart. *13*:303, 1939.
——: Metrazol remission in severe obsession-compulsion neurosis of five years' duration. J. Nerv. & Ment. Dis. *92*:290, 1940.
——: Results obtained from the administration of 12,000 doses of metrazol to mental patients. Psychiatric Quart. *15*:772, 1941.
Zeitllofer, J., Tschabitscher, H., and Wanko, T.: Zur Pathologie des protrahierten Insulinschocks. Wien. Ztschr. Nervenh. *9*:445, 1954.
Zeller, E. A., Barsky, J. Fouts, J. R., Kirchheimer, W. F., and Van Orden, L. S.: Influence of isonicotinic acid hydrazine (INH) and 1-isonicotinynl-2-isopropyl hydrazine (IIH) on bacterial and mammalian enzymes. Experientia. *8*:349, 1952.
Zeman, W.: Zur Frage der Hirngewebsschaedigung durch Heilkrampfbehandlung. Arch. f. Psychiat. & Ztschr. Neurol. *104*: 440, 1950.
Ziegler, Ch., and Lovette, J. B.: Operative complications after therapy with reserpine and reserpine compounds. J.A.M.A. *176*: 916, 1961.
Ziegler, L. H.: Discussion of physical risks in convulsive shock therapy. Arch. Neurol. & Psychiat. *48*:1019, 1942.
——: Bilateral prefrontal lobotomy. Am J. Psychiat. *100*:178, 1943.
Zigarelli, J. F.: Electroencephalography. In, Selective partial ablation of the frontal cortex. New York: Paul B. Hoeber, 1949.
Zimmerman, F. T., Burgemeister, B. B., and Putnam, T. J.: Effect of glutamic acid functioning in children and in adolescents. Arch. Neurol. & Psychiat. *56*:5, 1946.
Zimmerman, H. J., Rosenblum, L., Korn, R. J., and Feldman, P. E.: Some preliminary clinical and biochemical aspects of liver function in patients receiving iproniazid. Ann. N.Y. Acad. Sci. *80*:915, 1959.
Zimmermann, F.: Klinische und serologische Untersuchungen mit grossen Insulindosen. Monatschr. f. Psychiat. u. Neurol. 100, 1938.
Zinkin, S., and Birtchnell, J.: Unilateral electroconvulsive therapy: its effects on memory and its therapeutic efficacy. Brit. J. Psychiat. *114*:973, 1968.
Zirkle, C. L., and Kaiser, C.: Monoamine oxidase inhibitors. (Nonhydrazines). *In* M. Gordon (Ed.): Psychopharmacological Agents, Vol. I: 445, Medicinal Chemistry;

A Series of Monographs, Vol. 4. New York, Academic Press, 1964.
Ziskind, E.: Considerations in the case of EST and pharmacotherapy in depressive states. Dis. Nerv. Syst. *23*:656, 1962.
——, Somerfeld-Ziskind, E., and Ziskind, L.: Metrazol and electric convulsive therapy of the affective psychoses. Arch. Neurol. & Psychiat. *53*:212, 1945.
——, ——, and ——: Metrazol therapy in the affective psychoses. J. Nerv. & Ment. Dis. *95*:460, 1942.
Zohman, B. L., and Russek, H. I.: The influence on insulin shock therapy on the electrocardiogram. Am. Heart J. *39*:737, 1950.
Zrull, J. P., Westman, J. C., Arthur, B., and Bell, W. A.: A comparison of chlordiazepoxide, D-amphetamine and placebo in the treatment of the hyperkinetic syndrome in children. Amer. J. Psychiat. *120*: 590, 1963.
Zubiani, A.: Atarax in schizophrenia. Zürich: Int. Congress of Psychiatry, 1957.
Zubin, J.: Memory functioning in patients treated with electric shock therapy. J. Personality *17*:33, 1948.
——, and Barrera, S. E.: Effect of electric convulsive therapy on memory. Proc. Soc. Exper. Biol. & Med. *48*:596, 1941.
——, Sutton, S., Salzinger, K., Salzinger, S., Burdock, E. I., and Peretz, D.: A biometric approach to prognosis in schizophrenia. *In:* Comparative Epidemiology of the mental disorders, P. H. Hoch and Joseph Zubin, eds. New York: Grune & Stratton, 1961.
Zuckerman, F.: Amenorrhea occurring during Mellaril treatment. Amer. J. Psychiat. *118*:947, 1962.

Index